a LANGE medical book

P9-COP-383

# SYMPTOM TO DIAGNOSIS

## An Evidence-Based Guide

**Second Edition**

**Scott D. C. Stern, MD, FACP**
*Professor of Medicine*
*Co-Director, Junior Clerkship in Medicine*
*Clinical Director of Clinical Pathophysiology and Therapeutics*
*University of Chicago*
*Pritzker School of Medicine*
*Chicago, Illinois*

**Adam S. Cifu, MD, FACP**
*Associate Professor of Medicine*
*Co-Director, Junior Clerkship in Medicine*
*University of Chicago*
*Pritzker School of Medicine*
*Chicago, Illinois*

**Diane Altkorn, MD, FACP**
*Associate Professor of Medicine*
*Director, Senior Student Clerkships in Medicine*
*University of Chicago*
*Pritzker School of Medicine*
*Chicago, Illinois*

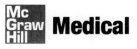

New York   Chicago   San Francisco   Lisbon   London   Madrid   Mexico City
Milan   New Delhi   San Juan   Seoul   Singapore   Sydney   Toronto

**Symptom to Diagnosis: An Evidence-Based Guide, Second Edition**

Copyright © 2010 by The McGraw-Hill Companies, Inc. All rights reserved. Printed in the United States of America. Except as permitted under the United States Copyright Act of 1976, no part of this publication may be reproduced or distributed in any form or by any means, or stored in a data base or retrieval system, without the prior written permission of the publisher.

1 2 3 4 5 6 7 8 9 0   QWD/QWD 12 11 10 9

ISBN 978-0-07-149613-1
MHID 0-07-149613-0

ISSN 1556-2719

McGraw-Hill books are available at special quantity discounts to use as premiums and sales promotions, or for use in corporate training programs. To contact a representative, please e-mail us at bulksales@mcgraw-hill.com.

This book was set in Adobe Garamond by International Typesetting and Composition.
The editors were James Shanahan and Harriet Lebowitz.
The production supervisor was Phil Galea.
Project management was provided by Madhu Bhardwaj, International Typesetting and Composition.
The text designer was Eve Siegel.
Cover art direction: Margaret Webster-Shapiro; series designer: Mary McKeon.
Quebecor World Dubuque was printer and binder.

Cover photos: Left, credit: Jose Luis Pelaez; Right, credit: Rob Melnychuk.

This book is printed on acid-free paper.

In memory of Kim Michele Stern
*Scott Stern*


In memory of my father, Dr. Robert Cifu
*Adam Cifu*


In memory of my father, Robert Seidman
*Diane Altkorn*

# Contents

Color Insert appears between pages 404 and 405

# Contributing Authors

**John Luc Benoit, MD**
Section of Infectious Diseases and Global Health
Assistant Professor of Medicine
Director, Infectious Diseases Fellowship Program
Director, Travel Clinic
*AIDS/HIV Infection* (Coauthored with Scott Stern)

**Sarah Stein, MD**
Section of Dermatology
Associate Professor of Medicine
*Rashes* (Coauthored with Adam Cifu)

# Preface

Our goal in creating *Symptom to Diagnosis* was to develop an interesting, practical, and informative approach to teaching the diagnostic process in internal medicine. Interesting, because real patient cases are integrated within each chapter, complementing what can otherwise be dry and soporific. Informative, because *Symptom to Diagnosis* articulates the most difficult process in becoming a physician: making an accurate diagnosis. Many other textbooks describe diseases, but fail to characterize the process that leads from patient presentation to diagnosis. Although students can, and often do, learn this process through intuition and experience without direct instruction, we believe that diagnostic reasoning is a difficult task that can be deciphered and made easier for students. Furthermore, in many books the description of the disease is oversimplified, and the available evidence on the predictive value of symptoms, signs, and diagnostic test results is not included. Teaching based on the classic presentation often fails to help less experienced physicians recognize the common, but atypical presentation. This oversight, combined with a lack of knowledge of test characteristics, often leads to prematurely dismissing diagnoses.

*Symptom to Diagnosis* aims to help students and residents learn internal medicine and focuses on the challenging task of diagnosis. Using the framework and terminology presented in Chapter 1, each chapter addresses one common complaint, such as chest pain. The chapter begins with a case and an explanation of a way to frame, or organize, the differential diagnosis. As the case progresses, clinical reasoning is clearly articulated. The differential diagnosis for that particular case is summarized in tables that delineate the clinical clues and important tests for the leading diagnostic hypothesis and important alternative diagnostic hypotheses. As the chapter progresses, the pertinent diseases are reviewed. Just as in real life, the case unfolds in a stepwise fashion as tests are performed and diagnoses are confirmed or refuted. Readers are continually engaged by a series of questions that direct the evaluation. Each chapter contains several cases and concludes with a diagnostic algorithm.

*Symptom to Diagnosis* can be used in three ways. First, it is designed to be read in its entirety to guide the reader through a third-year medicine clerkship. We used the Core Medicine Clerkship Curriculum Guide of the Society of General Internal Medicine/Clerkship Directors in Internal Medicine to select the symptoms and diseases we included, and we are confident that the text does an excellent job teaching the basics of internal medicine. Second, it is perfect for learning about a particular problem by studying an individual chapter. Focusing on one chapter will provide the reader with a comprehensive approach to the problem being addressed: a framework for the differential diagnosis, an opportunity to work through several interesting cases, and a review of pertinent diseases. Third, *Symptom to Diagnosis* is well suited to reviewing specific diseases through the use of the index to identify information on a particular disorder of immediate interest.

Our approach to the discussion of a particular disease is different than most other texts. Not only is the information bulleted to make it concise and readable, but the discussion of each disease is divided into 4 sections. The *Textbook Presentation*, which serves as a concise statement of the common, or classic, presentation of that particular disease, is the first part. The next section, Disease Highlights, reviews the most pertinent epidemiologic and pathophysiologic information. The third part, Evidence-Based Diagnosis, reviews the accuracy of the history, physical exam, laboratory and radiologic tests for that specific disease. Whenever possible, we have listed the sensitivities, specificities, and likelihood ratios for these findings and test results. This section allows us to point out the findings that help to "rule in" or "rule out" the various diseases. We often suggest a test of choice. It is this part of the book in particular that separates this text from many others. In the final section, Treatment, we review the basics of therapy for the disease being considered. Recognizing that treatment evolves at a rapid pace, we have chosen to limit our discussion to the fundamentals of therapy rather than details that would become quickly out of date.

The second edition differs from the previous edition in several ways. First, there are five new chapters—Hypertension, Diabetes, Rashes, HIV/AIDS, and Screening and Health Maintenance—as well as 4 pages of full-color images of rashes. Second, there is more emphasis on highlighting the pivotal points for each symptom that help to focus a broad differential diagnosis into one tailored to the individual patient. Third, history and physical exam findings so highly specific that they point directly to a particular diagnosis are indicated with the following "fingerprint" icon:

$$\triangle\!\!\!\!/\text{FP} = \text{fingerprint}$$

Fourth, the diagnostic algorithms at the end of each chapter are more uniform. Finally, all chapters have been updated to reflect new information on diagnostic testing.

For generations the approach to diagnosis has been learned through apprenticeship and intuition. Diseases have been described in detail, but the approach to diagnosis has not been formalized. In *Symptom to Diagnosis* we feel we have succeeded in articulating this science and art and, at the same time, made it interesting to read.

*Scott D. C. Stern, MD*
*Adam S. Cifu, MD*
*Diane Altkorn, MD*

# Acknowledgments

We would like to thank Sarah Stein, MD, and John Luc Benoit, MD for their co-authorship of two chapters, Rashes and AIDS, respectively. We would also like to thank the following subspecialty colleagues who helped us by reviewing chapters pertaining to their specialties and making suggestions about recent studies and subtleties of patient management. They definitely have had a positive impact on the quality of the second edition: Morton Arnsdorf, Andrew Artz, John Asplin, Jean Luc Benoit, James Brorson, Ronald Cohen, Linda Druelinger, Catherine Dubeau, Brian Gelbach, Ira Hanan, Philip Hoffman, Richard Kraig, John Lopez, Tipu Puri, Mary Strek, Helen Te, Tammy Utset, and Steven Weber. We are grateful for the support of Harriet Lebowitz and James Shanahan at McGraw-Hill, who have helped us throughout this process and believed in our vision. Thanks to Jennifer Bernstein for her meticulous copyediting. Finally, our patients deserve special praise, for sharing their lives with us, trusting us, and forgiving us when our limited faculties err, as they inevitably do. It is for them that we practice our art.

Scott Stern: I would like to thank a few of the many people who have contributed to this project either directly or indirectly. First I would like to thank my wife Laura, whose untiring support throughout the last 32 years of our lives and during this project, made this work possible. Other members of my family have also been very supportive including my children Michael, David and Elena; My parents Suzanne Black and Robert Stern and grandmother, Elsie Clamage. Two mentors deserve special mention. David Sischy shared his tremendous clinical wisdom and insights with me over 10 wonderful years that we worked together. David is the best diagnostician I have met and taught me more about clinical medicine than anyone else in my career. I remain in his debt. I would also like to note my appreciation to my late advisor, Dr. John Ultmann. Dr. Ultmann demonstrated the art of compassion in his dealings with patients on a day-to-day basis on a busy hematology-oncology service in 1983.

Adam Cifu: Excellent mentors are hard to find. I have been fortunate to have found mentors throughout my life and career guided in numerous and varied ways. My parents gave me every opportunity imaginable. Claude Wintner taught me the importance of organization, dedication, and focus and gave me a model of a gifted educator. Olaf Andersen nurtured my interest in science and guided my entry into medicine. Carol Bates showed me what it means to be a specialist in general medicine and a clinician educator. My family, Sarah, Ben, and Amelia, always remind me of what is most important. Thank you.

Diane Altkorn: I want to thank the students and house officers at the University of Chicago for helping me to continually examine and refine my thinking about clinical medicine and how to practice and teach it. I have been fortunate to have many wonderful mentors and teachers. I particularly want to mention Dr. Steven MacBride, who first taught me clinical reasoning and influenced me to become a general internist and clinician educator. As a resident and junior faculty member, I had the privilege of being part of Dr. Arthur Rubenstein's Department of Medicine at the University of Chicago. Dr. Rubenstein's commitment to excellence in all aspects of medicine is a standard to which I will always aspire. His kind encouragement and helpful advice have been invaluable in my professional development. Finally, I want to thank my family. My parents have provided lifelong support and encouragement. My husband, Bob, is eternally patient, and supportive of everything I do. And without my son, Danny, and my daughter, Emily, my life would be incomplete.

# I have a patient with a problem.
# How do I figure out the possible causes?

## THE DIAGNOSTIC PROCESS

Constructing a differential diagnosis, choosing diagnostic tests, and interpreting the results are key skills for all physicians and are some of the primary new skills medical students begin to learn during their third year. The diagnostic process, often called clinical reasoning, is complex, but it can be broken down into a series of steps, diagrammed in Figure 1–1.

### Step 1: Data Acquisition

Data you acquire through your history and physical exam, sometimes accompanied by preliminary laboratory tests, form the basis for your initial diagnostic reasoning. Your reasoning will be faulty unless you start with accurate data, so the prerequisite for obtaining valid data is well developed interviewing and physical examination skills.

### Step 2: Accurate Problem Representation

This step consists of developing a "problem synthesis statement," a concise, single sentence summary of the main **clinical problem** and its associated **context**.

**Clinical problems** are symptoms, physical findings, test abnormalities, or health conditions for which diagnostic evaluation could be undertaken. The problem synthesis statement is meant to focus on the patient's most important problem, usually the **chief complaint.**

**Context** refers to **pivotal points,** generally one of a pair of opposing descriptors used to compare and contrast diagnoses or clinical characteristics; for example, old versus new headache, unilateral versus bilateral edema, smoker versus nonsmoker. Extracting pivotal points from the history and physical exam enables the clinician to focus a broad differential diagnosis to a more limited set of diagnoses pertinent to that particular patient. The prerequisite for being able to construct an accurate problem representation is knowledge of the pivotal points for specific clinical problems.

### Step 3: Develop a Complete, Framed Differential Diagnosis

The process for developing a differential diagnosis will be discussed later in this chapter; subsequent chapters will present comprehensive, framed differential diagnoses specific for each problem discussed.

### Step 4: Prioritize the Differential Diagnosis

Not all diagnoses in a given differential are equally likely, or equally important. In order to effectively select diagnostic tests and therapies, it is necessary to select a "leading hypothesis," a "must not miss" hypothesis, and other "active alternative hypotheses" (see full discussion later). The prerequisites for this step are knowledge of pivotal points; typical or "textbook" presentations of disease; the variability of disease presentation; and which diseases are life-threatening, very common, or easily treatable. It is also necessary to know how to estimate pretest probability, and which history, physical, or laboratory findings are so specific for a disease they are diagnostic; in other words, such findings are "**fingerprints**" for the disease.

### Step 5: Test Your Hypothesis

Sometimes you are certain about the diagnosis based on the initial data and proceed to treatment. Most of the time, however, you require additional data to confirm your diagnostic hypotheses; in other words, you need to order diagnostic tests. Whenever you do so, you should understand how much the test will change the probability the patient has the disease in question. The prerequisite for this step is knowing the sensitivity, specificity and likelihood ratios (LRs) of the tests you have chosen, knowing how to interpret these test characteristics, and understanding how to determine posttest probability using pretest probabilities and LRs.

### Step 6: Review and Reprioritize the Differential Diagnosis

Remember, ruling out a disease is usually not enough; you must also determine the cause of the patient's symptom. For example, you may have eliminated myocardial infarction (MI) as a cause of chest pain, but you still need to determine whether the pain is due to reflux or muscle strain, etc. Whenever you have not made a diagnosis, or when you encounter data that conflict with your original hypotheses, go back to the complete differential diagnosis and reprioritize it, taking the new data into consideration. Failure to carry out this step is one of the most common diagnostic errors made by clinicians and is called "premature closure."

### Step 7: Test the New Hypotheses

Repeat the process until a diagnosis is reached.

## CONSTRUCTING A DIFFERENTIAL DIAGNOSIS

### Step 1: Data Acquisition

PATIENT ▽1

Mrs. S is a 58-year-old woman who comes to an urgent care clinic complaining of painful swelling of her left calf that has lasted for 2 days. She feels slightly feverish but has no other symptoms such as chest pain, shortness of breath, or abdominal pain. She has been completely healthy except for mild osteoarthritis of her knees, with no history of other medical problems, surgeries, or fractures.

(continued)

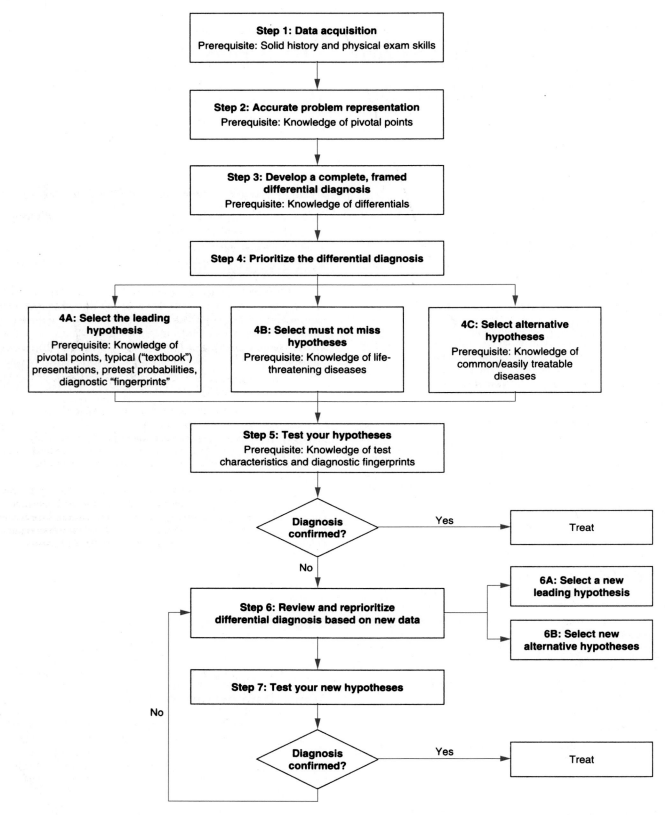

*Figure 1–1.* The clinical reasoning process.

She takes no medications and had a normal pelvic exam and Pap smear 1 month ago. Physical exam shows that the circumference of her left calf is 3.5 cm greater than her right calf, and there is 1+ pitting edema. The left calf is uniformly red and very tender, and there is slight tenderness along the popliteal vein and medial left thigh. There is a healing cut on her left foot. Her temperature is 37.7°C. The rest of her exam is normal.

A. Skin: Stasis dermatitis
B. Soft tissue: Cellulitis
C. Calf veins: Distal deep venous thrombosis (DVT)
D. Knee: Ruptured Baker cyst
E. Thigh veins: Proximal DVT
F. Pelvis: Mass causing lymphatic obstruction

## Step 2: Accurate Problem Representation

Focusing on the chief complaint and identifying pivotal points obtained during data acquisition are key to constructing and prioritizing a differential diagnosis. In this case, the patient's chief complaint is leg swelling, and the pivotal points are acute, unilateral, and erythema. A problem synthesis statement for this patient would be "The patient is a 58-year-old healthy woman with **acute**, **unilateral** leg swelling and **erythema.**

How would you construct a differential diagnosis for Mrs. S's problem, acute, unilateral leg swelling with erythema?

## Step 3: Develop a Complete, Framed Differential Diagnosis

It might be possible to memorize long lists of causes, or differential diagnoses, for multiple specific problems. However, doing so would not necessarily lead to a clinically useful organization of differentials that facilitates clinical reasoning. Instead, it is preferable to use some kind of *framework* to develop, organize, and remember differentials. There are several frameworks that can be useful.

A. An **anatomic** framework.
   1. Works well for problems such as chest pain
   2. Example list for chest pain: chest wall, pleura, lung parenchyma, heart (blood supply, valves, muscle), esophagus
B. An **organ/system** framework.
   1. This works well for symptoms with very broad differential diagnoses, such as fatigue.
   2. Start with broad categories, and then construct a list for each category.
   3. Example list for fatigue: endocrine (hypothyroidism, adrenal insufficiency), psychiatric (depression, anxiety), cardiovascular (ischemia, heart failure), pulmonary, GI, infectious disease, etc.
C. A **pathophysiologic** framework.
D. **Mnemonics.**
E. Be flexible and **combine frameworks** to fit the problem.

An anatomic framework works well for Mrs. S's unilateral swollen and red leg (see Chapter 15 for the full differential diagnosis of peripheral edema). The pivotal points in this case, the swelling being acute and unilateral, lead to this portion of the edema differential:

## Step 4: Prioritize the Differential Diagnosis

There are 4 approaches to organizing and prioritizing the differential diagnosis for a given problem.

A. **Possibilistic approach:** Consider all known causes equally likely and simultaneously test for all of them. This is not a useful approach.
B. **Probabilistic approach:** Consider first those disorders that are more likely; that is, those with the highest **pretest probability**. (Pretest probability is the probability that a disease is present before further testing is done.)
C. **Prognostic approach:** Consider the most serious diagnoses first.
D. **Pragmatic approach:** Consider the diagnoses most responsive to treatment first.

Experienced physicians often simultaneously integrate probabilistic, prognostic, and pragmatic approaches when constructing a differential diagnosis and deciding how to choose tests (Table 1–1). This thought process leads to selecting a leading hypothesis, must not miss hypotheses, and other active alternative hypotheses (see Figure 1–1).

If both the leading hypothesis and active alternatives are disproved, it is extremely important to continue the diagnostic process, prioritizing and testing for other hypotheses. Sometimes the correct diagnosis seems unlikely initially, which is why review and reprioritizing the differential diagnosis based on new data (Step 6) is so crucial.

Mrs. S has a constellation of symptoms and signs supporting the diagnosis of cellulitis as the leading hypothesis: fever; an entry site for infection on her foot; and a red, tender, swollen leg. Even without risk factors for DVT, either proximal or calf vein DVT are the active alternatives, being both common and "must not miss" diagnoses. Ruptured Baker cyst and a pelvic mass would be other hypotheses to be looked for if cellulitis and DVT are not present. Finally, stasis dermatitis is excluded in a patient without a history of chronic leg swelling.

How certain are you that Mrs. S has cellulitis? Should you treat her with antibiotics? How certain are you that she does not have DVT? Should you test for DVT?

***Table 1-1.*** Prioritizing the differential diagnosis.

| Diagnostic Hypotheses | Description | Implications for Choosing Tests |
|---|---|---|
| Leading hypothesis ("working diagnosis") | Single best overall explanation | Choose tests to confirm this disease (those with high specificity and high LR+) |
| Active alternatives ("rule outs") | Not as likely as the leading hypothesis, but serious, treatable, or likely enough to be actively sought in the patient (**"most common"** and **"must not miss"** diagnoses) | Choose tests to exclude these diseases (those with high sensitivity and very low LR–) |
| Other hypotheses | Not excluded, but not serious, treatable, or likely enough to be tested for initially | Test for these only if the leading hypothesis and active alternatives are disproved |
| Excluded hypotheses | Disproved causes | No further tests necessary |

Source: Adapted from Richardson WS et al. How to use an article about disease probability for differential diagnosis. JAMA. 1999;281:1214–1219.

## THE ROLE OF DIAGNOSTIC TESTING

### Step 5: Test Your Hypotheses

 I have a leading hypothesis and an active alternative—how do I know if I need to do a test or if I should start treatment?

Once you have generated a leading hypothesis, with or without active alternatives, you need to decide whether you need further information before proceeding to treatment or before excluding the diagnosis. One way to think about this is in terms of certainty: how certain are you that your hypothesis is correct, and how much more certain do you need to be before starting treatment? Another way to think about this is in terms of **probability**: is **your pretest probability** of disease high enough or low enough that you do not need any further information from a test?

### Determine the Pretest Probability

There are 3 ways to determine the pretest probability of your leading diagnosis and your most important (usually most serious) active alternatives: use a validated clinical decision rule (CDR), use information about the prevalence of certain symptoms in a given disease, and use your overall clinical impression.

A. Use a validated CDR
1. Investigators construct a list of potential predictors of the outcome of interest, and then examine a group of patients to determine if the predictors and outcome are present.
    a. Logistic regression is then used to determine which predictors are most powerful and which can be omitted.
    b. The model is then validated by applying it in other patient populations.
    c. To simplify use, the clinical predictors in the model are often assigned point values, and different point totals correspond to different pretest probabilities (see Box, Validated Clinical Model for Determining Pretest Probability of DVT).
2. CDRs are rarely available but are the most precise way of estimating pretest probability.

3. If you can find a validated CDR, you can come up with an exact number (or a small range of numbers) for your pretest probability.

B. Use information about the prevalence of certain symptoms in a given disease.
1. For example, 73% of patients with pulmonary embolism (PE) have dyspnea.
2. However, this does not tell you how many patients with dyspnea have PE.
3. There is often a lot of information available about symptom prevalence.

C. Use your overall clinical impression.
1. This is a combination of what you know about symptom prevalence and disease prevalence, mixed with your clinical experience, and the ever elusive attribute, "clinical judgment."
2. This is just as imprecise as it sounds, and it has been shown that physicians are disproportionately influenced by their most recent clinical experience.
3. Nevertheless, it has also been shown that the overall clinical impression of experienced clinicians has significant predictive value.
4. Clinicians generally categorize pretest probability as low, moderate, or high.
    a. This rather vague categorization is still helpful.
    b. Do not get distracted thinking a number is necessary.

### Consider the Potential Harms

Consider the potential harms of both a missed diagnosis and the treatment.

A. It is very harmful to miss certain diagnoses, such as MI or PE, while it is not so harmful to miss others, such as mild carpal tunnel syndrome. You need to be very certain that harmful diagnoses are not present (that is, have a very low pretest probability), before excluding them without testing.

B. Some treatments, such as thrombolytics, are more harmful than others, such as oral antibiotics; you need to be very certain that potentially harmful treatments are needed (that is, the pretest probability is very high) before prescribing them without testing.

## THE THRESHOLD MODEL: CONCEPTUALIZING PROBABILITIES

The ends of the bar in the threshold model represent 0% and 100% pretest probability. The **treatment threshold** is the probability above which the diagnosis is so likely you would treat the patient without further testing. The **test threshold** is the probability below which the diagnosis is so unlikely it is excluded without further testing (Figure 1–2).

For example, consider Ms. A, a 19-year-old woman, who complains of 30 seconds of sharp right-sided chest pain after lifting a heavy box. The pretest probability of cardiac ischemia is so low that no further testing is necessary (Figure 1–3).

Now consider Mr. B, a 60-year-old man who smokes and has diabetes, hypertension, and 15 minutes of crushing substernal chest pain accompanied by nausea and diaphoresis, with an ECG showing ST-segment elevations in the anterior leads. The pretest probability of an acute MI is so high you would treat without further testing, such as cardiac enzymes (Figure 1–4).

Diagnostic tests are necessary when the pretest probability of disease is in the middle, above the test threshold and below the treatment threshold. A really useful test shifts the probability of disease so much that the **posttest probability** (the probability of disease after the test is done) crosses one of the thresholds (Figure 1–5).

You are unable to find much information about estimating the pretest probability of cellulitis. You consider the potential risk of starting antibiotics to be low, and your overall clinical impression is that the pretest probability of cellulitis is high enough to cross the treatment threshold, so you start antibiotics.

You consider the pretest probability of DVT to be low, but not so low you can exclude it without testing. You are
*(continued)*

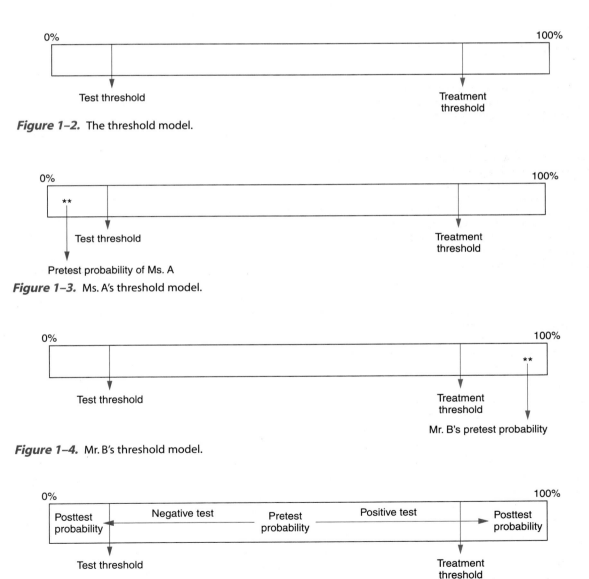

*Figure 1–2.* The threshold model.

*Figure 1–3.* Ms. A's threshold model.

*Figure 1–4.* Mr. B's threshold model.

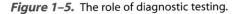

*Figure 1–5.* The role of diagnostic testing.

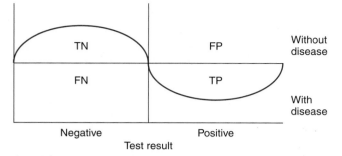

**Figure 1–6.** A perfect diagnostic test.

able to find a clinical decision rule that helps you quantify the pretest probability, and calculate that her pretest probability is 17% (see Box, Validated Clinical Model for Determining Pretest Probability of DVT).

☑ You have read that duplex ultrasonography is the best noninvasive test for DVT. How good is it? Will a negative test rule out DVT?

## UNDERSTANDING TEST RESULTS

☑ How do I know whether a test is really useful— whether it will really shift the probability of disease across a threshold?

A perfect diagnostic test would always be positive in patients with the disease and would always be negative in patients without the disease (Figure 1–6). Since there are no perfect diagnostic tests, some patients with the disease have negative tests (false-negatives {FN}), and some without the disease have positive tests (false-positives) (Figure 1–7).

The **test characteristics** help you to know how often false results occur. They are determined by performing the test in patients known to have or not have the disease, and recording the distribution of results (Table 1–2).

Table 1–3 shows the test characteristics of duplex ultrasonography for the diagnosis of proximal DVT, based on a hypothetical group of 200 patients, 90 of whom have DVT.

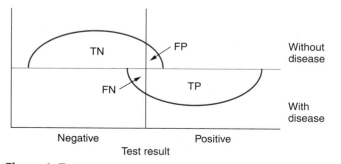

**Figure 1–7.** A pictorial representation of test characteristics.

**Table 1–2.** Test characteristics.

|  | **Disease Present** | **Disease Absent** |
|---|---|---|
| **Test positive** | True-positives | False-positives |
| **Test negative** | False-negatives | True-negatives |

The **sensitivity** is the percentage of patients with DVT who have a true-positive (TP) test result:

$$\text{Sensitivity} = \text{TP/total number of patients with DVT}$$
$$= 86/90 = 0.96 = 96\%$$

Since tests with very high sensitivity have a very low percentage of false-negative results (in Table 1–3, 4/90 = 0.04 = 4%), a negative result is likely a true negative.

The **specificity** is the percentage of patients without DVT who have a true-negative (TN) test result:

$$\text{Specificity} = \text{TN/total number of patients without DVT}$$
$$= 108/110 = 0.98 = 98\%$$

Since tests with very high specificity have a low percentage of false-positive results (in Table 1–3, 2/110 = 0.02 = 2%), a positive result is likely a true positive.

The sensitivity and specificity are important attributes of a test, but they do not tell you whether the test result will change your pretest probability enough to move beyond the test or treatment thresholds, because the shift in probability depends on the interactions between sensitivity, specificity, and pretest probability. The **likelihood ratio (LR),** the likelihood that a given test result would occur in a patient with the disease compared with the likelihood that the same result would not occur in a patient without the disease, enables you to calculate how much the probability will shift.

The LR+ tells you how likely it is that a result is a true-positive (TP), rather than a false-positive (FP):

$$\text{LR+} = \frac{\text{TP/total with DVT}}{\text{FP/total without DVT}} = \frac{\%\text{TP}}{\%\text{FP}} = \frac{\textbf{sensitivity}}{\textbf{1-specificity}} = \frac{0.96}{0.02} = 48$$

**LR+ should be significantly above 1,** indicating that a true-positive is much more likely than a false-positive, pushing you across the treatment threshold. An LR+ > 10 causes a large shift in disease probability; in general, tests with LR+ > 10 are very useful for ruling in disease. An LR+ between 5 and 10 causes a moderate shift in probability,

**Table 1–3.** Results for calculating the test characteristics of duplex ultrasonography.

|  | **Proximal DVT Present** | **Proximal DVT Absent** |
|---|---|---|
| **Abnormal duplex US** | TP = 86 patients | FP = 2 patients |
| **Normal duplex US** | FN = 4 patients | TN = 108 patients |
|  | Total number of patients with DVT = 90 | Total number of patients without DVT = 110 |

US, ultrasound; TP, true-positive; FP, false-positive; FN, false-negative; TN, true-negative.

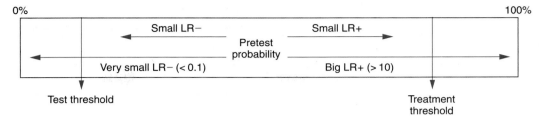

**Figure 1–8.** Incorporating likelihood ratios (LRs) into the threshold model.

and tests with these LRs are somewhat useful. "Fingerprints," findings that rule in a disease, have very high positive LRs.

**The negative LR (LR–)** tells you how likely it is that a result is a false-negative (FN), rather than a true-negative (TN):

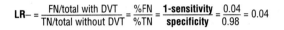

$$LR- = \frac{FN/total\ with\ DVT}{TN/total\ without\ DVT} = \frac{\%FN}{\%TN} = \frac{1-sensitivity}{specificity} = \frac{0.04}{0.98} = 0.04$$

**LR– should be significantly less than 1,** indicating that a false-negative is much less likely than a true-negative, pushing you below the test threshold. An LR– less than 0.1 causes a large shift in disease probability; in general, tests with LR– less than 0.1 are very useful for ruling out disease. An LR– between 0.1 and 0.5 causes a moderate shift in probability, and tests with these LRs are somewhat useful.

The closer the LR is to 1, the less useful the test; tests with an LR = 1 do not change probability at all and are useless.

The following threshold model incorporates LRs and illustrates how tests can change disease probability (Figure 1–8).

When you have a specific pretest probability, you can use the LR to calculate an exact posttest probability (see Box, Calculating an Exact Posttest Probability and Figure 1–9, Likelihood Ratio Nomogram). Table 1–4 shows some examples of how much LRs of different magnitudes change the pretest probability.

If you are using descriptive pretest probability terms such as low, moderate, and high, you can use LRs as follows:

A. A test with an LR– of 0.1 or less will rule out a disease of low or moderate pretest probability.

B. A test with an LR+ of 10 or greater will rule in a disease of moderate or high probability.

C. **Beware if the test result is the opposite of what you expected!**

1. If your pretest probability is high, a negative test rarely rules out the disease, no matter what the LR– is.

2. If you pretest probability is low, a positive test rarely rules in the disease, no matter what the LR+ is.

3. *In these situations, you need to perform another test.*

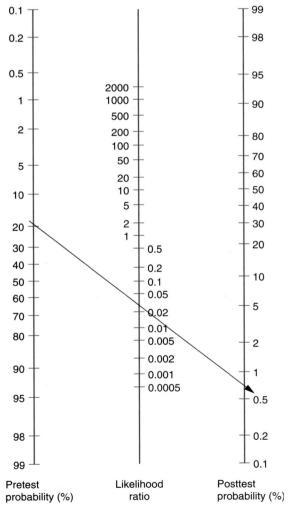

**Figure 1-9.** Likelihood ratio nomogram. Find the patient's pretest probability on the left, and then draw a line through the likelihood ratio of the test to find the patient's posttest probability.

Mrs. S has a normal duplex ultrasound scan. Since your pretest probability was moderate and the LR– is < 0.1, proximal DVT has been ruled out. Since duplex ultrasound is less sensitive for distal than for proximal DVT, clinical follow-up is particularly important. Some clinicians repeat the duplex ultrasound after 1 week to confirm the absence of DVT, and some clinicians order a D-dimer assay. When she returns for reexamination after 2 days, her leg looks much better, with minimal erythema, no edema, and no tenderness. The clinical response confirms your diagnosis of cellulitis, and no further diagnostic testing is necessary. (See Box, Does every patient in whom DVT is being considered need an ultrasound? When should a D-Dimer be ordered?)

***Table 1–4.*** Calculating posttest probabilities using likelihood ratios (LRs) and pretest probabilities.

|  | Pretest Probability = 5% | Pretest Probability = 10% | Pretest Probability = 20% | Pretest Probability = 30% | Pretest Probability = 50% | Pretest Probability = 70% |
|---|---|---|---|---|---|---|
| LR = 10 | 34% | 53% | 71% | 81% | 91% | 96% |
| LR = 3 | 14% | 25% | 43% | 56% | 75% | 88% |
| LR = 1 | 5% | 10% | 20% | 30% | 50% | 70% |
| LR = 0.3 | 1.5% | 3.2% | 7% | 11% | 23% | 41% |
| LR = 0.1 | 0.5% | 1% | 2.5% | 4% | 9% | 19% |

### VALIDATED CLINICAL DECISION RULE FOR DETERMINING PRETEST PROBABILITY OF DVT

| Symptoms or Findings | Score |
|---|---|
| Active cancer | +1 |
| Paralysis, paresis, or recent casting of lower extremity | +1 |
| Recently bedridden > 3 days, major surgery within weeks | +1 |
| Localized tenderness along deep venous system | +1 |
| Swelling of entire leg | +1 |
| Calf swelling > 3 cm compared with asymptomatic leg | +1 |
| Pitting edema greater in symptomatic leg | +1 |
| Nonvaricose collateral superficial veins | +1 |
| Previously documented DVT | +1 |
| Alternative diagnosis as likely or greater than DVT | −2 |

Key:
Score 3 or more = high probability = prevalence 53%.
Score 1 or 2 = moderate probability = prevalence 17%.
Score 0 or less = low probability = prevalence 5%.

Mrs. S has the likely alternative diagnosis of cellulitis (−2), asymmetric calf swelling (+1) and edema (+1), and slight tenderness along the deep venous system (+1), for a total score of 1, suggesting her pretest probability is 17%.

### CALCULATING AN EXACT POSTTEST PROBABILITY

For mathematical reasons, it is not possible to just multiply the pretest probability by the LR to calculate the posttest probability. Instead, it is necessary to convert to odds and then back to probability.

**A. Step 1**
 1. Convert pretest probability to pretest odds.
 2. Pretest odds = pretest probability/(1 − pretest probability).

**B. Step 2**
 1. Multiply pretest odds by the LR to get the posttest odds.
 2. Posttest odds = pretest odds × LR.

**C. Step 3**
 1. Convert posttest odds to posttest probability.
 2. Posttest probability = posttest odds/(1 + posttest odds).

For Mrs. S, the pretest probability of DVT was 17%, and the LR− for duplex ultrasound was 0.04.

A. Step 1: pretest odds = pretest probability/(1 − pretest probability) = 0.17/(1 − 0.17) = 0.17/0.83 = 0.2

B. Step 2: posttest odds = pretest odds × LR = 0.2 × 0.04 = 0.008

C. Step 3: posttest probability = posttest odds/(1 + posttest odds) = 0.008/(1 + 0.008) = 0.008/1.008 = 0.008

So Mrs. S's posttest probability of proximal DVT is 0.8%.

## DOES EVERY PATIENT IN WHOM DVT IS BEING CONSIDERED NEED AN ULTRASOUND? WHEN SHOULD A D-DIMER BE ORDERED?

D-dimer, a fibrin degradation product, is elevated in acute venous thromboembolism and non-thrombotic conditions such as recent major surgery, hemorrhage, trauma, pregnancy, and cancer. D-dimer levels are nonspecific and cannot be used to diagnose DVT. However, very low D-dimer levels can significantly lower the probability the patient has a DVT. High sensitivity ELISA D-dimer assays have an LR– of 0.06–0.10. Moderate sensitivity whole blood or latex agglutination D-dimer assays have an LR- of about 0.20.

A. You need to know what kind of D-dimer assay your lab uses.

B. In patients with a low pretest probability based on the clinical decision rule (CDR), a negative D-dimer assay, regardless of type, rules out DVT.

C. In patients with moderate pretest probability based on the CDR, a negative high sensitivity D-dimer can rule out DVT; a moderate sensitivity D-dimer does not have a sufficiently low LR- and should not be used in patients with moderate pretest probability.

D. All patients with high pretest probabilities, and some with moderate pretest probabilities, should have duplex ultrasound testing instead of D-dimer tests.

E. All patients with positive D-dimer tests need further testing, most often a duplex ultrasound.

## REFERENCES

Bowen JL. Educational strategies to promote clinical diagnostic reasoning. N Engl J Med. 2006;355:2217–25.

Richardson WS, Wilson MC, Guyatt GH, Cook DJ, Nishikawa J; for the Evidence-Based Medicine Working Group. Users' Guides to the Medical Literature: XV. How to use an article about disease probability for differential diagnosis. JAMA. 1999;281:1214–19.

Wells PS, Owen C, Doucette S et al. Does this patient have deep vein thrombosis? JAMA. 2006;295:199–207.

# I have a healthy patient. How do I determine which screening tests to order?

**PATIENT 1**

Mr. S is a healthy 45-year-old white man who wants to be "checked for everything."

> How do you know when it is worthwhile to screen for a disease? Where do you find information on screening guidelines? How do you interpret screening guidelines?

> How do you know when it is worthwhile to screen for a disease?

It seems intuitive that it is best to prevent a disease from occurring at all and next best to diagnose and treat it early. However, there are risks and benefits to every intervention, and it is especially important to make sure an intervention is not going to harm a healthy individual. This chapter focuses on understanding the reasoning behind current screening practices.

**A.** Screening can be used to identify an unrecognized disease or risk factor in a seemingly well person.

**B.** Screening can be accomplished by collecting a thorough history, performing a physical examination, or obtaining laboratory tests.

**C.** Examples of screening include mammography and cholesterol testing.

  **1.** Mammography can detect unrecognized, asymptomatic breast cancer.

  **2.** Cholesterol testing can be used

    **a.** To identify high-risk individuals who do not yet have coronary disease (called primary prevention by clinicians).

    **b.** To prevent complications in patients with known coronary disease (called secondary prevention by clinicians; not actually screening).

**D.** The following criteria are helpful in determining whether screening for a disease is worthwhile:

  **1.** The burden of disease must be sufficient to warrant screening.

    **a.** Screen only for conditions that cause severe disease, disability, or death.

    **b.** Consider prevalence of target disease and ability to identify high-risk group since the yield of screening is higher in high-risk groups.

  **2.** The test used for screening must be of high quality.

    **a.** Screening tests should accurately detect the target disease when it is asymptomatic.

    **b.** Screening tests should have high sensitivity and specificity.

    **c.** Test results should be reproducible in a variety of settings.

    **d.** Screening tests must be safe and acceptable to patients.

    **e.** Ideally, screening tests should be simple and shown to be cost-effective.

  **3.** There should be evidence that screening reduces morbidity or mortality.

    **a.** There must be effective treatment for the target disease.

    **b.** Early detection followed by treatment must improve survival compared with detection and treatment at the usual time of presentation; in other words, people in whom the condition was diagnosed by screening should have better health outcomes than those in whom the condition was diagnosed clinically.

    **c.** The benefits of screening must outweigh any adverse effects of the screening test, treatment, or impact of early diagnosis.

    **d.** Ideally, benefits and harms are evaluated through a randomized trial of screening (Figure 2–1).

      **(1)** The best outcome to measure is either all-cause mortality or disease-specific mortality, such as breast cancer or prostate cancer mortality.

      **(2)** Outcomes such as cancer stage distribution (ie, whether there are more or fewer early-stage cancers found) and length of survival after diagnosis can be misleading because of lead time and length time biases.

        **(a)** Lead time bias: If early treatment is not more effective than later treatment, the duration of time the individual lives with the disease is longer, but the mortality rate is the same (Figure 2–2).

        **(b)** Length time bias: Cancers that progress rapidly from onset to symptoms are less likely to be detected by screening than slow-growing cancers, so that screening tends to identify a more treatment-responsive subgroup.

    **e.** Often must make decisions based on less direct evidence, such as cohort or case-control studies.

> Where do you find information on screening guidelines?

Because of the complexity and rapid evolution of the evidence underlying screening recommendations, most physicians rely on published guidelines to inform them about screening decisions. Guidelines are developed and updated by a variety of

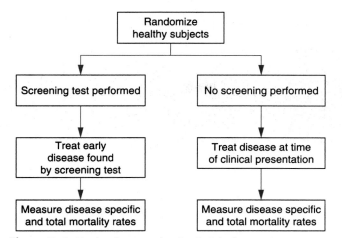

***Figure 2–1.*** Design for a randomized trial of screening.

organizations. It is important to be familiar with different sources of guidelines and to understand how to access the most recent versions of guidelines.

A. The US Preventive Services Task Force (USPSTF)
   1. Web site: http://www.ahrq.gov/clinic/uspstfix.htm
   2. An independent panel of 16 experts in primary care and prevention, now under the aegis of the Agency for Healthcare Research and Quality (AHRQ)
   3. Supported by outside experts and several evidence-based practice centers, university centers that help identify high-priority topics, produce systematic reviews, and draft guidelines.
   4. USPSTF guidelines often form the basis of clinical guidelines developed by professional societies.
   5. Highly evidence-based recommendations on when and how to screen

B. The National Guideline Clearinghouse (NGC)
   1. Web site: http://www.guideline.gov/
   2. A public resource for evidence-based clinical practice guidelines
   3. Sponsored by the AHRQ and US Department of Health and Human Services in partnership with the American Medical Association and America's Health Insurance Plans (AHIP)
   4. A way to access and compare a variety of guidelines, including those written by USPSTF, professional societies, and other private organizations

C. Canadian Task Force on Preventive Health Care
   1. Web site: http://www.ctfphc.org/
   2. Canadian equivalent of the USPSTF

D. Professional/specialty societies
   1. Often do their own independent reviews and issue their own guidelines regarding relevant diseases
   2. Specific guidelines generally available through the society Web site or the NGC
   3. Examples include
      a. Specialty societies (eg, American College of Physicians [internal medicine], American College of Obstetrics and Gynecology, American College of Surgery)
      b. Subspecialty societies (eg, American Thoracic Society, American College of Rheumatology, American Urologic Association, American Gastroenterological Association, American College of Cardiology)
      c. Others (eg, American Cancer Society, American Diabetes Association, National Osteoporosis Foundation, American Heart Association)

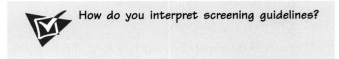

How do you interpret screening guidelines?

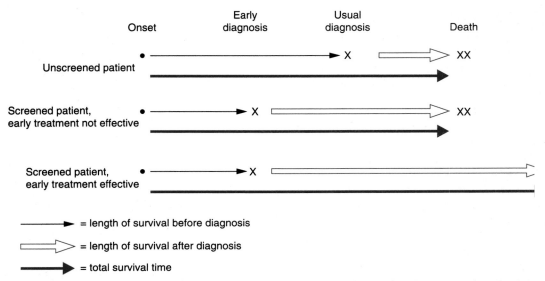

***Figure 2–2.*** Lead time bias. (The total survival times for the unscreened patient and the screened patient in whom early treatment is not effective are the same. The total survival time for the screened patient in whom early treatment is effective is lengthened.)

The USPSTF has developed a standardized system and vocabulary for evaluating the quality of the evidence addressing screening questions and for grading recommendations. The recommendation grade is based on a combination of the quality of the underlying evidence and an assessment of the size of the benefit. This general approach is often adopted by other organizations that make screening recommendations.

A. USPSTF levels of certainty regarding net benefit

1. High: Consistent results from well-designed studies in representative primary care populations that assess the effects of the preventive service on health outcomes; it is unlikely that these conclusions will change based on future studies.

2. Moderate: Evidence sufficient to determine the effects of the preventive service on health outcomes, but methodological issues such as limited generalizability, inconsistent findings, or inadequate size or number of studies exist; these conclusions could change based on future studies.

3. Low: Insufficient evidence to assess effects on health outcomes, due to limited number or size of studies, flaws in study designs, inconsistency of findings, lack of generalizability.

B. Grades of recommendations

1. A: The USPSTF recommends this service. There is high certainty that the net benefit is substantial.

2. B: The USPSTF recommends this service. There is high certainty that the net benefit is moderate or there is moderate certainty that the net benefit is moderate to substantial.

3. C: The USPSTF recommends against routinely providing the service. There may be considerations that support providing the service in an individual patient. There is moderate or high certainty that the net benefit is small.

4. D: The USPSTF recommends against the service. There is moderate or high certainty that the service has no net benefit or that the harms outweigh the benefits.

5. I statement: The USPSTF concludes that the current evidence is insufficient to assess the balance of benefits and harms of the service. Evidence is lacking, of poor quality, or conflicting, and the balance of benefits and harms cannot be determined.

Mr. S feels fine and has no medical history. He takes no medications, does not smoke currently, and drinks occasionally; however, he did smoke occasionally in college, and he estimates he smoked a total of 2–3 packs of cigarettes over 4 years. He exercises regularly by cycling 50–100 miles/week. His family history is notable for high cholesterol, hypertension, and a CVA in his father; his mother was diagnosed with colon cancer at age 54. His physical exam shows a BP of 120/80 mm Hg and pulse of 56 bpm. His body mass index (BMI) is 22 kg/m². HEENT, neck, cardiac, pulmonary, abdominal, and extremity exams are normal. He refuses a rectal exam. Mr. S shows you a list of tests he wants done, derived from research he has done on the Internet: lipid panel, prostate specific antigen (PSA), chest radiograph, and fecal occult blood test. In addition, he shows you a letter from a company offering "vascular screening" with ultrasounds of the carotids and aorta and wants to know if he should have those tests done.

**Should Mr. S be screened for prostate cancer with a PSA?**

A. What is the burden of disease?

1. 218,890 new diagnoses of prostate cancer in 2007, with 27,350 deaths in 2006

2. Second leading cause of cancer death in men in the United States

3. Many more men are diagnosed with prostate cancer (lifetime risk about 1 in 6) than die of it (lifetime risk about 1 in 29).

B. Is it possible to identify a high-risk group that might especially benefit from screening?

1. Older age (200 cases/100,000 white men aged 50–59 compared with 900/100,000 men older than 70 years)

2. African American race

a. Higher prostate cancer incidence than white men: 217.5 vs 134.5 cases per 100,000

b. Higher prostate cancer mortality than white men: 56.1 vs 23.4 deaths per 100,000

3. Family history: RR of about 2 for men with a first-degree relative with prostate cancer; RR about 5 if 2 first-degree relatives affected

C. What is the quality of the screening test?

1. Digital rectal exam (DRE)

a. Sensitivity 59%

b. Specificity unknown, but possibly as high as 94%; reproducibility poor

c. Positive predictive value: 5–30%

d. Neither sensitive nor specific enough to be used as a screening test, although may add to cancer detection when combined with PSA

2. PSA

a. For a PSA $\geq$ 4.0 ng/mL, sensitivity 68–80%, specificity 60–70%

b. Positive predictive values vary with PSA level

(1) For a PSA of 4–10 ng/mL, the PPV is about 25%

(2) For a PSA > 10 ng/mL, the PPV is 42–64%

c. Prostate cancer is found in some men even with very low PSA levels.

(1) PSA $\leq$ 0.5 ng/mL: cancer in 6.6% of men, 12% of which was high grade

(2) PSA 0.6–1.0 ng/mL: cancer in 10%

(3) PSA 1.1–2.0 ng/mL: cancer in 17%

(4) PSA 2.1–3.0 ng/mL: cancer in 24%, 19% of which was high grade

d. PSA velocity (rate of change in PSA), PSA density (PSA per volume of prostate tissue measured on transrectal ultrasound or MRI), and free PSA (ratio of unbound to total PSA) are purported to increase PSA accuracy, but data are insufficient to recommend their use.

D. Does screening reduce morbidity or mortality?

1. Two randomized controlled trials of PSA screening recently published

2. Both found lower grade cancers in screened group

3. PLCO trial of 76,693 American men aged 55–74 years

   a. Annual PSA for 6 years and DRE for 4 years; 97% follow up at 7 years, 67% at 10 years

   b. 50% of control group screened outside of trial

   c. Increased frequency of diagnosis, but no difference in prostate cancer mortality

4. European trial of 182,000 men aged 50–74 years

   a. PSA every 4 years; median follow up 9 years

   b. RR of prostate cancer death in screened group = 0.8 (95% CI, 0.67–0.98)

   c. To prevent 1 prostate cancer death, would need to screen 1400; 224 would have a positive screen and need a biopsy

      (1) 48 would need to be treated

      (2) 7 would develop impotence, 3 incontinence

E. What are the current guidelines?

1. USPSTF (2008)

   a. Evidence is insufficient to recommend for or against routine screening for prostate cancer in men younger than 75 using PSA or DRE.

      (1) Grade I recommendation

      (2) The balance of benefits and harms cannot be determined

   b. Recommends against screening for prostate cancer in men ≥ 75 year of age

      (1) Grade D recommendation

      (2) Moderate certainty that the harms outweigh the benefits

2. American Cancer Society (2008)

   a. DRE and PSA should be offered annually, beginning at age 50, to men who have a life expectancy of at least 10 years.

   b. High-risk men (African American and those with a positive family history of prostate cancer in a first-degree relative diagnosed before age 65) should begin testing at age 45.

   c. Should discuss risks and benefits before testing, and men who ask the doctor to make the decision should be tested.

3. American Urological Association (2009)

   a. Men age 40 or older with a life expectancy of 10 or more years should be regularly screened with DRE and PSA.

   b. The decision to screen should be individualized, accompanied by a complete discussion of risks and benefits.

⟁1

You explain to Mr. S that there are important unresolved issues with regard to PSA screening for prostate cancer: whether early detection through screening actually saves lives, that 75% of men with PSA levels of 4–10 ng/mL do not have cancer but need to have biopsies, and that the treatment for prostate cancer can have significant side effects such as incontinence and erectile dysfunction.

You also explain that there is some evidence that radical prostatectomy for prostate cancer not diagnosed by screening does save lives and reduces the development of metastatic disease, with about 6% fewer deaths from prostate cancer, at the cost of one-third more men having urinary or sexual problems. Finally, you point out that none of the expert guidelines recommend beginning PSA testing before age 50 in white men without an affected first-degree relative.

 **Should Mr. S be screened for colorectal cancer with fecal occult blood testing?**

A. What is the burden of disease?

1. Third most common cancer in the United States and second leading cause of death from cancer

2. About 148,000 diagnoses anticipated in 2008, with about 49,000 deaths

3. 80–95% of colorectal cancers arise from adenomatous polyps

   a. 10% of polyps > 1 cm become malignant in 10 years; 25% do so after 20 years

   b. Adenomas found in 40% of adults by age 60

   c. Advanced adenomas, defined as those ≥ 10 mm or having high-grade dysplasia or a villous component, are the most likely to develop into carcinoma.

B. Is it possible to identify a high-risk group that might especially benefit from screening? (Tables 2–1 and 2–2)

1. 20% of colorectal cancers occur in patients with specific risk factors.

   a. History in a first-degree relative of either colorectal cancer or adenomatous polyps, especially if diagnosed before age 60

   b. Personal history of adenomatous polyps

   c. Long-standing ulcerative colitis

2. 6% occur in patients with rare genetic syndromes, such as familial polyposis or hereditary nonpolyposis colorectal cancer (HNPCC).

   a. Colorectal cancer develops in 80% of patients with HNPCC by age 50 years

**Table 2–1.** Questions that help identify patients at high risk for colorectal cancer.

| |
|---|
| Has the patient had colorectal cancer or an adenomatous polyp? |
| Does the patient have an illness, such as inflammatory bowel disease, that increases the risk of colorectal cancer? |
| Has a family member been diagnosed with colorectal cancer or an adenomatous polyp?<br>    Was it a first-degree relative (parent, sibling, or child)?<br>    At what age was the cancer or polyp first diagnosed?<br>    How many first-degree relatives have been diagnosed? |

**Table 2–2.** Magnitude of risk for colorectal cancer.

| Risk Factor | Approximate Lifetime Risk of Colorectal Cancer |
|---|---|
| None | 6% |
| One first-degree relative with colon cancer | RR 2–3 |
| Two first-degree relatives with colon cancer | RR 3–4 |
| First-degree relative aged ≤ 50 at cancer diagnosis | RR 3–4 |
| One second- or third-degree relative with colon cancer | RR 1.5 |
| Two second-degree relatives with colon cancer | RR 2–3 |
| One first-degree relative > age 60 with an adenoma | RR 1.8 |
| One first-degree relative < age 60 with an adenoma | RR 2.6 |

  **b.** The mutation associated with HNPCC also increases the risk of cancer of the uterus, ovaries, ureter, renal pelvis, stomach, small bowel, and bile duct

  **c.** Familial polyposis patients have diffuse colonic polyps at an early age, and colorectal cancer will develop without intervention.

 **3.** The remaining colorectal cancers occur sporadically.

**C.** What is the quality of the screening test?

 **1.** Fecal occult blood testing (FOBT)

  **a.** Two distinct samples of 3 different stools are applied to 6 test card panels.

  **b.** If Hgb is present, a blue color appears when hydrogen peroxide is added.

  **c.** False-negative tests can occur if the patient has ingested > 250 mg of vitamin C, and false-positive tests occur with use of nonsteroidal antiinflammatory drugs (NSAIDs) and ingestion of red meat.

  **d.** "Low sensitivity" tests, such as Hemoccult II have a sensitivity of 37% and specificity of 98%.

  **e.** "High sensitivity" tests, such as Hemoccult SENSA, have a sensitivity of 79% and specificity of 87%.

  **f.** Annual screening detected 49% of cancers; biannual screening detected 27–39% of cancers.

  **g.** A single panel test after a DRE has a sensitivity of 9% and should never be considered an adequate screening test for colorectal cancer.

 **2.** Flexible sigmoidoscopy

  **a.** Only 20–30% of proximal cancers are associated with a distal adenoma.

  **b.** However, sigmoidoscopy has been found to identify 70–80% of patients with significant findings in the colon, assuming finding a polyp triggers a full colonoscopy.

  **c.** Detects 7 cancers and about 60 large (> 1 cm) polyps/1000 examinations

  **d.** Bowel perforation rate 4.6/100,000 examinations

  **e.** Serious complication rate (deaths or events requiring hospital admission) 3.4/10,000 procedures

 **3.** Combined FOBT and sigmoidoscopy

  **a.** 7 additional cancers/1000 examinations compared with sigmoidoscopy alone

  **b.** Did not improve yield at initial screening exam

 **4.** Colonoscopy

  **a.** Miss rate of 5% for cancers, 6% for adenomas > 1 cm, 13% for adenomas 6–9 mm, and 27% for those < 5 mm (based on study of tandem colonoscopies by 2 examiners)

  **b.** Complication rates

   **(1)** Bowel perforation rate 3.8/10,000 procedures

   **(2)** Bleeding rate 12.3/10,000 procedures

   **(3)** Serious complication rate (deaths or events requiring hospital admission) 25/10,000 procedures

 **5.** Double-contrast barium enema

  **a.** Sensitivity = 48%

  **b.** Specificity = 85%

  **c.** Perforation rate = 1/25,000

 **6.** CT colonography (CTC) (virtual colonoscopy)

  **a.** CT scanning with 2D and 3D image display

  **b.** Requires same bowel preparation as colonoscopy

  **c.** A small rectal catheter is inserted for air insufflation, but no sedation is required

  **d.** Sensitivity for cancer = 96%

  **e.** Sensitivity for polyps ≥ 10 mm = 85–93%, with specificity 97%

  **f.** Sensitivity for polyps 6-9 mm = 70–86%, with specificity 86–93%

 **7.** Summary of relative test characteristics, as assessed by the USPSTF

  **a.** Sensitivity: Hemocccult II < fecal DNA testing ≤ Hemoccult SENSA ≈ flexible sigmoidoscopy < colonoscopy

  **b.** Specificity: Hemoccult SENSA < fecal DNA testing ≈ Hemoccult II < flexible sigmoidoscopy = colonoscopy

**D.** Does screening reduce morbidity or mortality?

 **1.** FOBT

  **a.** 3 large randomized trials show reduced colorectal cancer mortality.

  **b.** Relative RR of colorectal cancer death: 15–33%

  **c.** NNS = 217 for annual screening, 344–1250 for biennial screening

**2.** Flexible sigmoidoscopy

    **a.** Current recommendations are based on several well-done case-control studies.

    **b.** Relative RR of colorectal cancer death = 59%

**3.** Combinations FOBT and sigmoidoscopy

    **a.** No studies of FOBT and flexible sigmoidoscopy

    **b.** 1 nonrandomized controlled trial of FOBT and rigid sigmoidoscopy found the combination detected more cancers than sigmoidoscopy alone, but the mortality benefit did not reach significance (36 deaths/1000/year in the combination group compared with 63 in the sigmoidoscopy alone group, $P = 0.11$)

**4.** Colonoscopy

    **a.** No randomized trial data

    **b.** 1 case-control study showed lower incidence of colon cancer (OR = 0.47) and lower colorectal cancer mortality (OR = 0.43).

    **c.** A 2009 case control study found a reduction in death for colorectal cancers in the left colon (OR = 0.33) but not the right colon (OR = 0.99)

    **d.** Generally assumed that the mortality reductions seen in the FOBT trials is actually due to the follow-up colonoscopies.

**5.** Double-contrast barium enema: no outcome data available

**6.** CTC

    **a.** No randomized trial data available

    **b.** 1 nonrandomized study showed that rates of detection of advanced adenomas + cancers were similar in patients screened with CTC (3.2%) compared with conventional colonoscopy (3.4%)

**7.** Potential harms of screening include the complication rates noted previously, complications of sedation used for colonoscopy, and patient discomfort.

**E.** What are the current guidelines?

**1.** USPSTF (2008)

    **a.** Strongly recommends screening average risk men and women beginning at age 50 years and continuing to age 75 years, using FOBT, sigmoidoscopy, or colonoscopy

       **(1)** Grade A recommendation

       **(2)** Insufficient data to assess the benefits and harms of CT colonography and fecal DNA testing as screening modalities (I recommendation)

    **b.** Recommends against routine screening in adults age 76–85 years (C recommendation)

    **c.** Recommends against screening in adults older than age 85 years (D recommendation)

**2.** American Cancer Society (2008)

    **a.** Average risk men and women

       **(1)** Begin screening at age 50

       **(2)** Acceptable strategies include annual FOBT alone, annual FOBT plus sigmoidoscopy every 5 years, sigmoidoscopy alone every 5 years, colonoscopy every 10 years, CTC every 5 years, or double-contrast barium enema every 5 years

       **(3)** Imaging procedures that can detect both adenomatous polyps and cancer are preferred over stool tests that primarily detect cancer.

**3.** American Gastroenterological Association (2003)

    **a.** Average risk screening: same as American Cancer Society

    **b.** High risk screening

       **(1)** Colorectal cancer or adenomatous polyps in any first-degree relative before age 60 or in ≥ 2 first-degree relatives at any age: colonoscopy at age 40 or at age equivalent to 10 years younger than the relative at the time of diagnosis; repeat colonoscopy every 5 years

       **(2)** Colorectal cancer or adenomatous polyps in any first-degree relative after age 60, or 2 second-degree relatives with colorectal cancer: follow average-risk screening guidelines but begin at age 40

    **c.** Surveillance after polypectomy

       **(1)** Hyperplastic polyps: repeat colonoscopy in 10 years

       **(2)** 1–2 low-risk adenomas (tubular adenomas < 10 mm): repeat colonoscopy in 5–10 years

       **(3)** 3–10 low-risk adenomas, or any high-risk adenoma (≥ 10 mm or high-grade dysplasia or villous features): repeat colonoscopy in 3 years

       **(4)** > 10 adenomas: repeat in < 3 years

       **(5)** Inadequately removed adenoma: repeat in 2–6 months

*You explain to Mr. S that because colon cancer was diagnosed in his mother when she 54 years old, his risk of developing colon cancer during his lifetime is increased from about 6% to somewhere between 12% and 18%. Although fecal occult blood test alone are an acceptable screening strategy for low-risk individuals, all of the expert guidelines recommend screening colonoscopy for patients with his risk profile.*

**Should Mr. S be screened for hyperlipidemia with a lipid panel?**

**A.** What is the burden of disease?

**1.** Coronary heart disease (CHD) is the leading cause of death in the United States.

**2.** Overall costs of CHD and stroke in 2003 estimated to be > 50 billion.

**3.** Lifetime risk of a CHD event, calculated at age 40 years, is 49% for men and 32% for women; nearly one-third of CHD events are attributable to total cholesterol > 200 mg/dL.

**B.** Is it possible to identify a high-risk group that might especially benefit from screening?

**1.** The low-density lipoprotein (LDL) and high-density lipoprotein (HDL) levels themselves are independent risk factors for CHD, with the increased risk being continuous and linear.

    **a.** For every 38 mg/dL increase in LDL above 118 mg/dL, the RR for CHD is 1.42 in men and 1.37 in women.

    **b.** For every 15.5 mg/dL increase in HDL above 40 mg/dL in men, the RR for CHD is 0.64.

    **c.** For every 15.5 mg/dL increase in HDL above 51 mg/dL in women, the RR for CHD is 0.69.

**d.** Total cholesterol–HDL ratio

**(1)** In men, a ratio ≥ 6.4 was associated with a 2–14% greater risk than predicted from total cholesterol or LDL alone.

**(2)** In women, a ratio ≥ 5.6 was associated with a 25–45% greater risk than predicted from total cholesterol or LDL alone.

**2.** Clinical characteristics can be used to classify patients into 3 risk categories.

**a.** Highest risk category

**(1)** Patients with established CHD

**(2)** Patients with CHD risk equivalents

**(a)** Other atherosclerotic disease: peripheral vascular disease, cerebrovascular/carotid disease, abdominal aortic aneurysm

**(b)** Diabetes

**(c)** Multiple risk factors that confer a 10-year risk for CHD > 20%, calculated using Framingham risk model, available at http://hp2010. nhlbihin.net/atpiii/calculator.asp?usertype= pub (Figure 2–3)

**b.** Intermediate risk category

**(1)** Patients with 2 or more risk factors

**(a)** Smoking

**(b)** Hypertension (BP ≥ 140/90 mm Hg or on antihypertensive therapy)

**(c)** HDL < 40 mg/dL (if HDL > 60 mg/dL, decrease risk factor count by 1)

**(d)** Family history of premature coronary artery disease (CAD) (male first-degree relative < 55 years, female first-degree relative < 65 years)

**(e)** Age (men ≥ 45 years, women ≥ 55 years)

**(2)** 10-year CHD risk of 10–20%, calculated using the Framingham risk model

**c.** Lower risk category

**(1)** 0–1 of above risk factors

**(2)** 10-year CHD risk < 10%, calculated using the Framingham risk model

**C.** What is the quality of the screening test?

**1.** Total cholesterol and HDL are minimally affected by eating and can be measured in fasting or nonfasting individuals.

**2.** Triglycerides are increased 20–30% by eating and must be measured in the fasting state.

**3.** LDL can be directly measured but is most commonly estimated using the following equation, which is valid only when the fasting triglycerides are less than 400 mg/dL: total cholesterol − (triglycerides/5 + HDL) = LDL.

**4.** Total cholesterol can vary by 4–11% within an individual; HDL and triglyceride measurements can vary even more. Clinicians should measure twice before starting therapy.

**D.** Does screening reduce morbidity or mortality?

**1.** In primary prevention studies of drug therapy (including only patients without established CAD, primarily men):

**a.** Total CHD events (nonfatal myocardial infarction [MI] plus death from CHD) are reduced by about 30% (95% CI, 20–38%).

**b.** CHD death is reduced by 26% (95% CI, 2–43%).

**c.** NNT over 5 years to prevent 1 CHD event with statin therapy = 42–49.

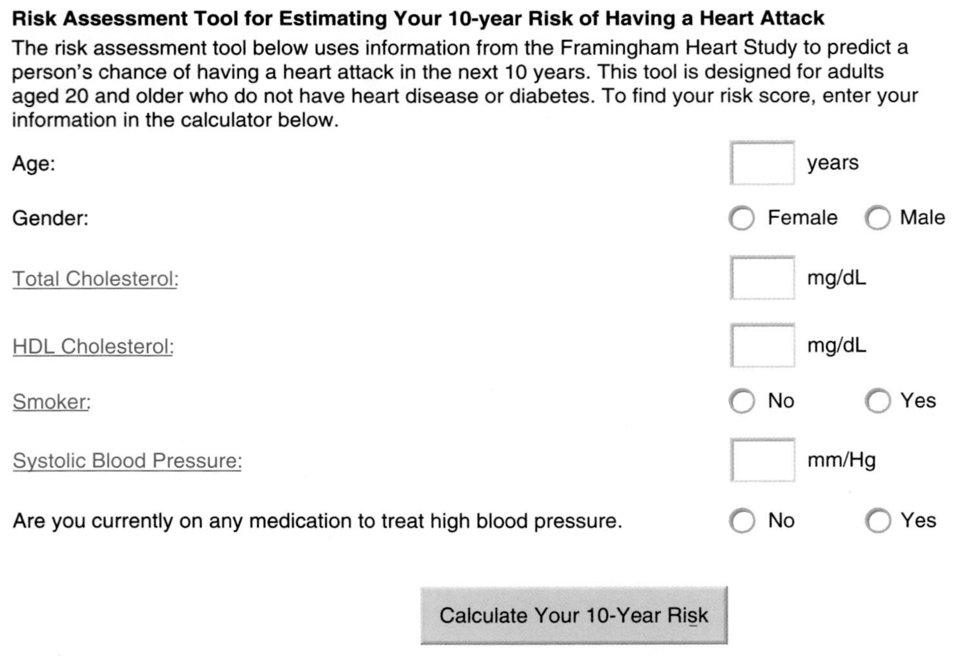

**Risk Assessment Tool for Estimating Your 10-year Risk of Having a Heart Attack**

The risk assessment tool below uses information from the Framingham Heart Study to predict a person's chance of having a heart attack in the next 10 years. This tool is designed for adults aged 20 and older who do not have heart disease or diabetes. To find your risk score, enter your information in the calculator below.

Age: ____ years

Gender: ○ Female  ○ Male

Total Cholesterol: ____ mg/dL

HDL Cholesterol: ____ mg/dL

Smoker: ○ No  ○ Yes

Systolic Blood Pressure: ____ mm/Hg

Are you currently on any medication to treat high blood pressure.  ○ No  ○ Yes

Calculate Your 10-Year Risk

***Figure 2–3.*** Framingham risk calculator: This is the on line risk assessment tool which uses information from the Framingham Heart Study to predict a person's risk of heart attack in the next 10 years. (Source: http://hp2010. nhlbihin.net/atpiii/calculator.asp?usertype=pub)

**2.** There is conflicting evidence for the efficacy of lipid-lowering agents in asymptomatic women; in trials including high-risk women, reductions in CHD events were similar to those seen in men.

**3.** No evidence that diet therapy reduces CHD events in primary prevention populations

   **a.** Maximum expected cholesterol reduction with diet therapy is 10–20%.

   **b.** Most trials achieve an average reduction of about 5%.

**E.** What are the current guidelines?

   **1.** USPSTF (2008)

      **a.** Screen all men at age 35 and women with risk factors at age 45.

         **(1)** Grade A recommendation

         **(2)** Good evidence that screening can identify asymptomatic people at increased risk for CAD and that lipid-lowering drug therapy decreases the incidence of CHD

      **b.** Screen men aged 20–35 and women aged 20–45 if other risk factors present.

         **(1)** Grade B recommendation

         **(2)** Other risk factors include diabetes, family history of cardiovascular disease before age 50 in male relatives or age 60 in female relatives, family history suggestive of familial hyperlipidemia, obesity (BMI $\geq$ 30 kg/m$^2$), presence of multiple other risk factors (eg, hypertension, smoking).

      **c.** No recommendation regarding screening younger adults without risk factors (grade C recommendation).

      **d.** Screening should include measurement of total cholesterol and HDL.

      **e.** Optimal screening interval unclear

   **2.** National Cholesterol Education Program (NCEP) (2001)

      **a.** Fasting cholesterol LDL, HDL, and triglycerides every 5 years for adults aged 20 or older

      **b.** Risk assessment for all patients

   **3.** American Academy of Family Physicians: periodic cholesterol measurement in men aged 35–65 and women aged 45–65

---

⃟1

You agree with Mr. S that a fasting lipid panel is an important screening test to do for men over 45, even in the absence of other risk factors.

✔ **Should Mr. S have a screening chest radiograph?**

---

**A.** What is the burden of disease?

   **1.** Lung cancer is leading cause of cancer death in both men and women.

   **2.** About 150,000 deaths from lung cancer in 2002 compared with about 126,000 for colorectal, breast, and prostate cancer combined

**3.** Prognosis of non-stage I lung cancers poor

**B.** Is it possible to identify a high-risk group that might especially benefit from screening?

   **1.** Cigarette smoking responsible for about 87% of lung cancers

      **a.** Compared with nonsmokers, RR of developing lung cancer is 10–30

      **b.** A 65-year-old who has smoked 1 pack/day for 50 years has a 10% risk of developing lung cancer over the next 10 years.

      **c.** A 75-year-old who has smoked 2 packs/day for 50 years has a 15% risk.

   **2.** Other risk factors include exposure to asbestos, nickel, arsenic, haloethers, polycyclic aromatic hydrocarbons, and environmental cigarette smoke.

**C.** What is the quality of the screening test?

   **1.** Chest radiograph: reported sensitivity ranges from 36% to 84%, with specificity of about 90%; PPV ranges from 41% to 60%

   **2.** CT scan: sensitivity = 93%, specificity = 49–89%

      **a.** Most false-positive abnormalities could be resolved on high-resolution CT (HRCT) scan.

      **b.** 5–15% of patients referred for biopsy after HRCT, with 63–90% of those being diagnosed with cancer

**D.** Does screening reduce morbidity or mortality?

   **1.** All randomized trials reported to date have excluded women.

   **2.** 6 randomized trials of chest radiography, with or without sputum cytology, have failed to demonstrate a decrease in lung cancer mortality; all were limited by the control population undergoing some screening.

   **3.** Low-dose CT scanning

      **a.** A low-resolution image of the entire thorax obtained in a single breath holding with low-radiation exposure

      **b.** Results from cohort studies suggest that low-dose CT does identify more, and earlier stage, lung cancers than chest radiography.

      **c.** One study comparing observed rates of lung cancer diagnoses to expected rates calculated from validated models found no reduction in mortality from CT screening.

**E.** What are the current guidelines?

   **1.** USPSTF (2004)

      **a.** Evidence is insufficient to recommend for or against screening asymptomatic people with low-dose CT scanning, chest radiography, sputum cytology, or some combination of these tests.

      **b.** Grade I recommendation

      **c.** Fair evidence that screening can detect earlier stage lung cancer but poor evidence that screening reduces mortality.

      **d.** There is potential for significant harm because of the high number of false-positive tests and the need for invasive diagnostic testing.

   **2.** American College of Chest Physicians (2007) recommends screening only when done as part of a clinical trial.

   **3.** American Cancer Society (2001, 2004): no recommendation

You explain to Mr. S that there have been no studies showing that screening chest radiographs prevent lung cancer in smokers, much less in nonsmokers. You add that no expert guidelines recommend routine chest radiographs, even in patients who smoke.

**Should Mr. S be screened for abdominal aortic aneurysm and carotid artery stenosis with ultrasonography?**

## Abdominal Aortic Aneurysm (AAA)

A. What is the burden of disease?
  1. 4–8% of older men and 0.5–1.5% of older women have an AAA.
  2. AAA accounts for about 9000 deaths per year in the United States.
    a. 1-year rupture rates are 9% for AAAs 5.5–5.9 cm, 10% for 6–6.9 cm, and 33% for AAAs ≥ 7 cm.
    b. 10–25% of patients with ruptured AAA survive to hospital discharge

B. Is it possible to identify a high-risk group that might especially benefit from screening?
  1. Age > 65, ever smoking (≥ 100 lifetime cigarettes), male sex, and family history are the strongest risk factors for an AAA > 4.0 cm.
    a. The OR increases by 1.7 for each 7-year age interval.
    b. Current or past smoking increases the risk of AAA by 3–5.
    c. The prevalence of AAA increases more rapidly with age in ever smokers than in never smokers.
    d. The prevalence of AAA > 4 cm in never smokers is < 1% for all ages.
    e. The OR is 1.94 for a positive family history.
    f. The OR is ~1.3–1.5 for history of CAD, hypercholesterolemia, or cerebrovascular disease.
    g. The OR is 0.53 for black persons and 0.52 for patients with diabetes.

C. What is the quality of the screening test?
  1. Ultrasonography has a sensitivity of 95% and specificity of 100% for the detection of AAA, defined as an infrarenal aortic diameter > 3.0 cm.
  2. One time screening is sufficient, since cohort studies of repeated screening have shown that over 10 years, the incident rate for new AAAs is 4%, with no AAAs of > 4.0 cm found
  3. Abdominal palpation is not reliable.

D. Does screening reduce morbidity or mortality?
  1. A meta-analysis of 4 randomized controlled trials of screening for AAA in men showed a reduction in mortality from AAA, with a pooled OR of 0.57 (95% CI, 0.45–0.74)
    a. Overall in-hospital mortality for open AAA repair is 4.2%; lower mortality is seen in high volume centers performing > 35 procedures/year (3% mortality vs 5.5% in low volume centers) and when vascular surgeons perform the repair (2.2% for vascular surgeons, 4.0% for cardiac surgeons, 5.5% for general surgeons).
    b. Endovascular repair, when compared with open repair, has reduced 30-day mortality rates, but 4-year mortality rates for the 2 procedures are equal; there are no longer term comparative data.
  2. There was no reduction in all cause mortality, or in AAA specific mortality in women.

E. What are the current guidelines?
  1. USPSTF (2005)
    a. One time screening by ultrasonography in men age 65–75 who have ever smoked
    b. Grade B recommendation, based on good evidence of decreased AAA specific mortality with screening
  2. Society of Vascular Surgery
    a. Screening in all men age 60–85, women age 60–85 with cardiovascular risk factors, and patients age ≥ 50 with a family history of AAA
    b. If aortic diameter < 3.0 cm, no further screening; if 3–4 cm, annual ultrasonography; if 4–4.5 cm, twice yearly ultrasonography; if > 4.5 cm, refer to a vascular specialist

## Carotid Artery Stenosis (CAS)

A. What is the burden of disease?
  1. The estimated prevalence of significant CAS (60–99%) in the general population is about 1%.
  2. The contribution of significant CAS to morbidity or mortality from stroke is not known, nor is the natural progression of asymptomatic CAS.

B. Is it possible to identify a high-risk group that might especially benefit from screening?
  1. CAS is more prevalent in patients with hypertension or heart disease, and in those who smoke.
  2. There are no risk assessment tools that reliably identify patients with clinically important CAS.

C. What is the quality of the screening test?
  1. For the detection of > 70% stenosis, carotid duplex ultrasonography has a sensitivity of 86–90% and a specificity of 87–94%.
  2. For the detection of > 60% stenosis, the sensitivity is 94% and the specificity is 92%.
  3. There is some variability in measurements done in different laboratories.
  4. Screening for bruits on physical exam has poor reliability and sensitivity.

D. Does screening reduce morbidity or mortality?
  1. There have been 2 randomized controlled trials of carotid endarterectomy for asymptomatic CAS, both of which showed about a 5% absolute reduction in stroke or perioperative death in the surgical group (~5.5–6.5%), compared with the medically treated group (~11–12%); the absolute RR for disabling stroke was about 2.5%.
    a. These results may not be generalizable due to the highly selected participants and surgeons.
    b. The medical treatment was not well defined, and did not include current standard care, such as aggressive control of BP and lipids.

**2.** All positive ultrasounds need to be confirmed by digital subtraction angiography, which has a stroke rate of 1%, or by MRA or CTA, both of which are less than 100% accurate.

**3.** 30-day perioperative stroke or death rates in asymptomatic patients range from 1.6% to 3.7%, with rates for women at the higher end of the range; in some states, rates are as high as 6%.

**4.** The perioperative MI rate is 0.7–1.1%, going up to 3.3% in patients with more comorbidities.

**E.** What are the current guidelines?

**1.** USPSTF (2007)

**a.** Recommends against screening for asymptomatic CAS in the general adult population

**b.** Grade D recommendation, based on moderate certainty that the benefits of screening do not outweigh the harms.

**2.** American Heart Association (2006) does not recommend screening.

**3.** American Society of Neuroimaging (2007) recommends against screening unselected populations but does recommend considering screening in adults age ≥ 65 years with 3 or more cardiovascular risk factors.

**4.** Society for Vascular Surgery (2007) recommends screening patients age ≥ 55 years with cardiovascular risk factors.

You explain to Mr. S that he should not invest in the "vascular screening." Screening for CAS is not recommended for the general population, and since he is younger than 65 years with a minimal history of smoking, he does not need to be screened for AAA.

Mr. S has a second list for his wife, a 42-year-old similarly healthy woman who is scheduled to see you next: lipid panel, chest radiograph, bone mineral density (BMD), Pap smear, and mammogram.

Mrs. S also has no medical history, except for 2 normal vaginal deliveries, the first at age 25. Her menses are regular. She does not smoke or drink, and she jogs regularly. She had 1 sexual partner before Mr. S and has been monogamous for 20 years. Her family history is negative, except for osteoporosis in her mother and grandmother. She has had a normal Pap smear every year since her first child was born. She weighs 125 pounds, her BP is 105/70 mm Hg, and her general physical exam, including breast exam, is entirely normal.

**☑ Should Mrs. S be screened for cervical cancer with a Pap smear?**

**A.** What is the burden of disease?

**1.** About 13,000 new cases of cervical cancer and 4100 cervical cancer–related deaths in the United States in 2002; tenth leading cause of cancer death

**2.** Rates considerably higher in countries where cytologic screening is not widely available; worldwide, cervical cancer is the second most common cancer in women and the most common cause of mortality from gynecologic malignancy.

**3.** Women with preinvasive lesions have a 5-year survival of nearly 100%, with a 92% 5-year survival for early-stage invasive cancer; only 13% survive distant disease.

**B.** Is it possible to identify a high-risk group that might especially benefit from screening?

**1.** 93–100% of squamous cell cervical cancers contain DNA from high-risk human papillomavirus (HPV) strains

**a.** Low- and high-risk subtypes

**b.** Cervix especially vulnerable to infection during adolescence when squamous metaplasia is most active

**c.** Most infections cleared by immune system in 1–2 years without producing neoplastic changes.

**(1)** 90% low-risk subtypes resolve over 5 years

**(2)** 70% of high-risk subtypes resolve

**d.** Women older than 30 years with HPV are more likely to have high-grade lesions or cancer than women younger than 30 with HPV.

**2.** Early-onset of intercourse (before age 17) and a greater number of lifetime sexual partners (> 2) are risk factors for acquiring HPV.

**3.** Cigarette smoking increases risk by 2- to 4-fold.

**4.** Immunocompromise and other sexually transmitted infections, such as herpes and HIV, also increase risk.

**C.** What is the quality of the screening test?

**1.** Interpretation of Pap smears: the Bethesda Classification of Cervical Cytology

**a.** Negative for intraepithelial lesion or malignancy

**b.** Epithelial cell abnormalities: squamous cells

**(1)** Atypical squamous cells (ASC)

**(a)** ASC-US: of undetermined significance

**(b)** ASC-H: cannot exclude high-grade squamous intraepithelial lesion (HSIL)

**(2)** Low-grade squamous intraepithelial lesion (LSIL)

**(a)** Cellular changes consistent with HPV

**(b)** Same as mild dysplasia, histologic diagnosis of CIN 1 (cervical intraepithelial neoplasia)

**(3)** HSIL

**(a)** Same as moderate/severe dysplasia, histologic diagnosis of CIN 2, CIN 3, CIS (carcinoma in situ)

**(b)** Should indicate if invasion suspected

**(4)** Squamous cell carcinoma

**c.** Epithelial cell abnormalities: glandular cells

**(1)** Atypical (endocervical, endometrial, or glandular)

**(2)** Atypical, favors neoplastic

**(3)** Endocervical adenocarcinoma in situ (AIS)

**(4)** Adenocarcinoma

**2.** Pap smear techniques

**a.** Conventional Pap smear: cervical cells are spread on a glass slide and treated with a fixative by the examiner

**b.** Liquid-based cytology: cervical cells are suspended in a vial of liquid preservative by the examiner, followed by debris removal and placement onto a slide in the laboratory

**3.** HPV testing

  **a.** A cervical specimen is placed into a transport medium or into the liquid preservative used for the liquid-based cytology Pap smear method

  **b.** Specific RNA probes are added that combine with oncogenic DNA, and the DNA-RNA hybrids are detected by antibodies.

**4.** Test characteristics of conventional Pap smear

  **a.** For LSIL/CIN 1: sensitivity 30–87% (mean 47%), specificity 86–100% (mean 95%)

  **b.** For LSIL/CIN 2,3: sensitivity 44–99%, specificity 91–98%

**5.** Conventional Pap smear vs liquid-based cytology

  **a.** Specimen less likely to be unsatisfactory with liquid based (4.1% vs 2.6% of specimens)

  **b.** Sensitivities for CIN 2 similar: relative sensitivity of liquid-based compared with conventional = 1.17, (95% CI 0.87–1.56)

  **c.** PPV of liquid-based cytology for CIN 2 lower than conventional: relative PPV = 0.58, (95% CI 0.44–0.77)

**6.** Conventional Pap smear vs HPV testing (Table 2–3)

  **a.** Sensitivities of either test alone were similar, with the specificity and PPV somewhat better for Pap alone than HPV testing alone

  **b.** While the sensitivity of reflexive testing (HPV or Pap followed by the other test if first test positive; if both positive, referral for colposcopy) was much lower than that of co-testing (simultaneous testing; colposcopy referral if one is positive), the negative predictive values for both strategies were quite high at over 99%.

  **c.** Co-testing has a lower specificity and PPV, leading to higher rates of referral for colposcopy (7.9% vs 1.4% for reflexive testing).

**D.** Does screening reduce morbidity or mortality?

**1.** No randomized trial data

**2.** Many observational studies show a decrease in both the incidence of cervical cancer (60–90%) and cervical cancer mortality (20–60%).

**3.** Evidence regarding optimal interval between screening tests has been largely indirect and based on modeling; a recent analysis found that, in women with 3 consecutive normal Pap smears, few cases of cervical cancer would be missed by subsequently screening every 3 years rather than annually (excess risk of 3 cases of cervical cancer per 100,000 women screened less often).

**E.** What are the current guidelines?

**1.** USPSTF (2003)

  **a.** Strongly recommends Pap smear screening in sexually active women with a cervix

    **(1)** Grade A recommendation

    **(2)** Good evidence that screening reduces cervical cancer mortality

    **(3)** Indirect evidence that screening should start within 3 years of the onset of sexual activity or age 21 and be done at least every 3 years

  **b.** Recommends against screening women older than 65 with a history of adequate recent screening, who are not otherwise at high risk

    **(1)** Grade D recommendation

    **(2)** Harms likely to outweigh benefits

  **c.** Recommends against routine screening in women who have had a total hysterectomy for benign disease (grade D recommendation)

  **d.** Evidence is insufficient to recommend for or against the routine use of new technologies (liquid-based cytology, computerized rescreening, and algorithm-based screening) to screen (grade I recommendation)

  **e.** Evidence is insufficient to recommend for or against the routine use of HPV testing as a *primary* screening test.

**2.** American Cancer Society (2004)

  **a.** Begin 3 years after becoming sexually active or at age 21

  **b.** Every year with conventional Pap smear or every 2 years with liquid-based cytology

  **c.** Women older than age 30 with 3 normal tests in a row may choose to be screened every 2–3 years.

  **d.** Women older than age 70 with at least 3 normal tests and no abnormal tests within the last 10 years may choose to stop screening.

  **e.** Screening is not indicated for women who have had a total hysterectomy for benign disease.

  **f.** Women who have a history of in utero DES exposure; are HIV-positive; or are immunocompromised by organ transplantation, chemotherapy, or long-term corticosteroid treatment should have annual screening.

**3.** American College of Obstetrics and Gynecology (2003)

  **a.** Level A recommendations

    **(1)** Annual screening beginning 3 years after becoming sexually active or at age 21

**Table 2–3.** Comparing test characteristics of conventional Pap smears with HPV testing.

|  | Sensitivity (%) | Specificity (%) | NPV (%) | PPV (%) |
|---|---|---|---|---|
| Pap | 43 | 97 | 99.6 | 9.1 |
| HPV | 46 | 94 | 99.4 | 8.0 |
| Reflexive testing | 54 | 99 | 99.8 | 18.2 |
| Co-testing | 100 | 93 | 100 | 5.5 |

HPV, human papillomavirus; NPV, negative predictive value; Pap, Papanicolaou; PPV, positive predictive value.

(2) Women older than age 30 with no history of CIN 2 or 3, immunocompromise, HIV, or in utero DES exposure, with 3 normal tests in a row, may choose to be screened every 2–3 years.

(3) Both liquid-based and conventional cytology are acceptable for screening.

(4) Women who have had a total hysterectomy for benign disease and no history of CIN 2 or 3 may stop screening.

  **b.** Level B recommendations

(1) Cervical cytology and HPV screening can be used in women older than age 30; if both are negative, the screening interval should be no less than 3 years.

(2) Women with a history of CIN 2 or 3 should be monitored annually posttreatment until 3 consecutives tests are normal.

(3) Women who have had a hysterectomy, with a history of CIN 2 or 3, should be screened annually until 3 consecutive vaginal smears are normal.

**4.** Table 2–4 summarizes current recommendations regarding follow-up of abnormal Pap smears.

You explain to Mrs. S that the combination of her sexual history and her history of 12 normal Pap smears in a row puts her at extremely low risk for cervical cancer. You point out that all expert guidelines consider it acceptable to perform Pap smears every 2 or 3 years in women with her history.

☑ **Should Mrs. S be screened for breast cancer with a mammogram?**

**A.** What is the burden of disease?

**1.** Incidence rates per 100,000 are 132.5 for white women, 118.3 for African American women, and 89 for Asian American and Hispanic women.

**2.** Breast cancer mortality rates per 100,000 are 25 for white women, 33.8 for African American women, and 12–16 for Asian American and Hispanic women.

**3.** Second leading cause of cancer mortality in women (lung cancer is first).

**B.** Is it possible to identify a high-risk group that might especially benefit from screening?

**1.** Women who have a *BRCA1/BRCA2* mutation are a special high-risk group; certain family history patterns are associated with an increased likelihood of *BRCA* mutations.

  **a.** For women of Ashkenazi Jewish descent: Any first-degree relative, or 2 second-degree relatives on the same side of the family with breast or ovarian cancer

  **b.** For all other women:

  (1) 2 first-degree relatives with breast cancer, at least 1 of whom was diagnosed at age 50 or younger

  (2) 3 or more first- or second-degree relatives with breast cancer

**Table 2–4.** Management of abnormal Pap smears.

| Result | Recommendation |
|---|---|
| ASC-US | **Strategy 1:** HPV testing, followed by referral for colposcopy if high-risk subtype identified; If HPV negative, repeat cytology in 12 months (preferred strategy) OR **Strategy 2:** Repeat cytology every 4–6 months until normal twice, with referral for colposcopy if persistently abnormal OR **Strategy 3:** Refer for colposcopy Adolescents: repeat cytology in 12 months[1] |
| ASC-H | Refer for colposcopy |
| Atypical glandular cells | Refer for colposcopy |
| LSIL | Refer for colposcopy Adolescents: repeat cytology in 12 months[1] |
| HSIL | Refer for colposcopy |

[1]Adolescents have high rates of HPV positivity and transient cytologic abnormalities, but rates of invasive cancer near zero, so repeat Pap testing in 12 months is recommended. ASC-H, atypical squamous cells-cannot exclude HSIL; ASC-US, atypical squamous cells-undetermined significance; HSIL, high-grade squamous intraepithelial lesion; LSIL, Low-grade squamous intraepithelial lesion.

(3) Both breast and ovarian cancer among first- and second-degree relatives

(4) A first-degree relative with bilateral breast cancer

(5) 2 or more first- or second-degree relatives with ovarian cancer

(6) A first- or second-degree relative with both breast and ovarian cancer

(7) Breast cancer in a male relative

**2.** Otherwise, age is the strongest risk factor (RR = 18 for women aged 70–74 compared with women aged 30–34).

**3.** Other risk factors include mother or sister with breast cancer (RR = 2.6), age at menarche younger than 12 years, age at first birth older than 30, age at menopause older than 55, current use of hormone replacement therapy (HRT), excess alcohol use (> 2–5 drinks/day), high breast density on mammography, highest quartile of bone density, history of a breast biopsy.

**4.** Protective factors include > 16 months of breastfeeding, 5 or more pregnancies, exercise, postmenopausal BMI < 23 kg/m², oophorectomy before age 35.

**5.** A Breast Cancer Risk Assessment Tool has been developed

  **a.** Available at http://www.cancer.gov/bcrisktool/

  **b.** Uses statistical methods applied to data from the Breast Cancer Detection and Demonstration Project, a mammography screening project conducted in the 1970s, to assess breast cancer risk

**C.** What is the quality of the screening test?

**1.** Sensitivity (Table 2–5)

**Table 2–5.** Sensitivity of annual screening mammography.

| Age Group | Sensitivity (%) | Positive Predictive Value (%) |
|---|---|---|
| 40–49 | 73–81 | 1–4 |
| 50–59 | 71–96 | 4–9 |
| 60–69 | 85–95 | 10–19 |
| 70–74 | 81–98 | 18–20 |

  a. Reduced by younger patient age, increased breast density, use of HRT, technical factors, lack of skill of radiologist

  b. Increased if radiologist tends to label results abnormal (at expense of reduced specificity)

2. Specificity

  a. Overall specificity of a single mammogram is 94–97%.

  b. However, the PPV is low in young women, increasing with age as risk of breast cancer increases (see Table 2–5).

  c. About 23% of women have at least 1 false-positive mammogram requiring additional evaluation (additional imaging or biopsy).

  d. The false-positive rate tends to be higher in younger women and those taking HRT because of denser breasts.

3. Test characteristics in high-risk women (*BRCA* positive or > 20% lifetime risk as calculated by a validated model)

  a. Mammography alone: sensitivity 25–59%

  b. Mammography + MRI: sensitivity 93–100%

  c. Mammography + ultrasound (+/- clinical breast exam): sensitivity 49–67%

  d. When MRI is added to mammography, specificity drops 1–17%, compared with mammography alone, with a consequent increase in unnecessary recalls for further evaluation (RR of recall = 3.4–4.8, ~71 additional recalls/1000 screening rounds) and unnecessary biopsy (RR of biopsy = 1.2-9.5, 7–46 additional biopsies/1000 screening rounds).

  e. There have been no studies of whether screening with MRI + mammography, compared with screening with mammography alone, reduces breast cancer deaths.

D. Does screening reduce morbidity or mortality?

  1. There are several randomized trials of screening mammography, although all have some methodologic limitations.

  2. For all age groups combined, RR of breast cancer death is 0.74 (95% CI, 0.77–0.91), with a NNS to prevent 1 breast cancer death over 14 years of 1224.

  3. For women older than 50 years, the RR of breast cancer death is 0.78 (95% CI, 0.70–0.87), with an NNS of 838.

  4. For women ages 40–49, the RR of breast cancer death is 0.85 (95% CI, 0.73–0.99), with a NNS of 1792.

  5. Potential harms include anxiety about testing, identifying nonprogressive forms of ductal carcinoma in situ (DCIS), radiation exposure, and false-positive mammograms.

  6. Table 2–6 outlines another approach to calculating the benefit of screening mammography.

E. What are the current guidelines?

  1. USPSTF (2002, update pending)

    a. Screening mammography, with or without clinical breast exam every 1–2 years in women aged 40 and older

      (1) Grade B recommendation

      (2) Fair evidence that mammography every 12–33 months significantly reduces breast cancer mortality

        (a) Evidence stronger for women aged 50–69

        (b) Evidence weaker, and benefit smaller, for women aged 40–49; optimal screening interval for this age group unclear

        (c) Evidence generalizable to women 70 and older if their life expectancy is not compromised by comorbid disease

    b. Evidence insufficient to recommend for or against clinical breast exam alone as a screen for breast cancer (Grade I recommendation)

    c. Evidence insufficient to recommend for or against breast self-exam as a screen for breast cancer (Grade I recommendation)

  2. American Cancer Society (2008)

    a. Begin annual mammography at age 40

    b. Clinical breast exam every 3 years from ages 20–39 and annually beginning at age 40

    c. Women at high risk (> 20% lifetime risk) should have annual mammography and breast MRI.

**Table 2–6.** Number of women with different breast cancer outcomes in 1000 women who undergo annual mammography for 10 years.

| Age | ≥ 1 False-Positive Mammogram | ≥ 1 biopsy | Development of Breast Cancer | Breast Cancer Cured, Regardless of Screening | Diagnosis of DCIS because of Mammography | Lives Saved by Screening Mammography |
|---|---|---|---|---|---|---|
| 40 | 560 | 190 | 15 | 8 | 3 | 2 |
| 50 | 470 | 190 | 28 | 14 | 7 | 4 |
| 60 | 360 | 190 | 37 | 18 | 7 | 6 |

DCIS, ductal carcinoma in situ. Reproduced, with permission, from Fletcher S, Elmore J. Mammographic screening for breast cancer. N Engl J Med. 2003;348:1672–80.

**3.** American College of Obstetrics and Gynecology (2003)

    **a.** Mammography every 1–2 years beginning at age 40; annually beginning at age 50

    **b.** Clinical breast exam beginning at age 19

You explain to Mrs. S that in women with no factors that increase the risk of breast cancer, the chance that she will have a false-positive mammogram is much larger than the chance a breast cancer will be found: For every 1700 women between the ages of 40 and 49 who are screened, 1 life will be saved, but about 425 women will have false-positive mammograms. You add that, despite these statistics, most expert guidelines recommend beginning annual mammography at age 40.

**Should Mrs. S be screened for osteoporosis?**

**A.** What is the burden of disease?

    **1.** More than 10 million people in the United States have osteoporosis, and another 33.6 million have low bone density at the hip.

    **2.** 15% will have a hip fracture, which is associated with loss of independence in up to 60% of patients and excess mortality of 10–20% within 1 year.

**B.** Is it possible to identify a high-risk group that might especially benefit from screening?

    **1.** Low BMD itself is the strongest risk factor for fracture.

    **2.** Increasing age is the strongest risk factor for low BMD; other risk factors include low body weight (< 132 pounds), lack of HRT use, family history of osteoporosis, personal history of fracture, ethnic group (white, Asian, Hispanic), current smoking, 3 or more alcoholic drinks/day, long-term corticosteroid use (≥ 5 mg of prednisone daily for ≥ 3 months).

    **3.** A new tool, the WHO Fracture Risk Algorithm (FRAX), calculates the 10-year probability of hip or major osteoporotic fracture using femoral neck BMD and clinical risk factors.

        **a.** It should be used in untreated postmenopausal women and men over age 50.

        **b.** The tool is available at http://www.shef.ac.uk/FRAX/

        **c.** Depending on the dual-energy x-ray absorptiometry (DEXA) scanner used, it is sometimes necessary to adjust the T score before using the tool; this can be done at http://www.nof.org/frax_patch_full.htm

**C.** What is the quality of the screening test?

    **1.** Background

        **a.** Can measure bone density with a variety of methods (DEXA, single-energy x-ray absorptiometry, ultrasonography, quantitative CT) at a variety of sites (hip, lumbar spine, heel, forearm)

        **b.** Current bone density is compared with peak predicated bone density and then reported as number of SD above or below peak predicted bone density.

        **c.** Osteoporosis is defined as a bone density "T score" at least 2.5 SD below peak predicted bone density (T score = −2.5 or more negative).

        **d.** Osteopenia is defined as a T score between −1.0 and −2.5.

        **e.** Normal is within 1 SD of peak predicted bone density.

    **2.** DEXA is the gold standard test.

        **a.** Has been shown to be a strong predictor of hip fracture risk; femoral neck is best site to measure

        **b.** The RR of hip fracture is 2.6 for each decrease of 1 SD in bone density at the femoral neck.

    **3.** Some evidence that measuring BMD at the heel is similarly predictive of fracture risk (women with osteoporosis had RR of 2.7 for all fractures compared with those with normal BMD)

**D.** Does screening reduce morbidity or mortality?

    **1.** No studies of the effectiveness of screening in reducing osteoporotic fractures

    **2.** Many studies show treatment substantially reduces fracture risk.

    **3.** Potential harms of screening include misinterpretation of test results, increasing anxiety in patients, side effects of medications, and cost.

    **4.** If 10,000 women aged 65–69 are screened (assuming 37% relative RR for hip fracture, 50% relative RR for vertebral fracture, and 70% adherence rate)

        **a.** Will prevent 14 hip fractures and 40 vertebral fractures over 5 years

        **b.** NNS to prevent 1 hip fracture = 731; NNS to prevent 1 vertebral fracture = 248

    **5.** If 10,000 women aged 60–64 are screened

        **a.** Will prevent 5 hip fractures over 5 years, with NNS ≈ 2000

        **b.** If these women have 1 of 3 risk factors (increasing age, weight < 132 pounds, or nonuse of HRT), will prevent 9 hip fractures, with NNS = 1092

**E.** What are the current guidelines?

    **1.** USPSTF (2002)

        **a.** Women 65 years of age and older should be screened routinely for osteoporosis; screening should begin at age 60 for women at increased risk for osteoporotic fractures.

            **(1)** Grade B recommendation

            **(2)** Good evidence that the risk of osteoporosis increases with age, that bone density measurements accurately predict fracture risk, and that treating asymptomatic women reduces fracture risk

        **b.** No recommendation for or against routine screening in postmenopausal women younger than 60 or those aged 60–64 without increased risk (grade C recommendation)

    **2.** National Osteoporosis Foundation (NOF) (2008)

        **a.** BMD testing for all women aged ≥ 65, and men ≥ 70

        **b.** BMD testing for younger postmenopausal women and men age 50–69 if concerned for low BMD based on clinical risk factors

        **c.** BMD testing for adults who experience a fracture after age 50 and for adults with a condition (such as rheumatoid arthritis) or taking a medication associated with low bone density

***Table 2–7.*** Numbers needed to screen.

| Test/Disease | Population | NNS |
|---|---|---|
| Ultrasonography/AAA | Ever smoking men, age 65–74 | 500 to prevent 1 AAA specific death over 5 years |
| Ultrasonography/CAS | Primary care | 4348 to prevent 1 stroke over 5 years; 8696 to prevent 1 disabling stroke over 5 years |
| DEXA/Osteoporosis | Women 65–69<br>Women 60–64<br>Women 60–64 with additional risk factors | 731 to prevent 1 hip fracture over 5 years; 248 to prevent 1 vertebral fracture<br>2000 to prevent 1 hip fracture<br>1092 to prevent 1 hip fracture |
| Mammography/Breast Cancer | Women 40–70<br>Women 50–70<br>Women 40–49 | 1224 to prevent 1 breast cancer death over 14 years<br>838 to prevent 1 breast cancer death over 14 years<br>1792 to prevent 1 breast cancer death over 14 years |
| Fecal occult blood testing/Colorectal Cancer | Annual screening, patients over 50<br>Biennial screening | 217 to prevent 1 colorectal cancer death<br>344–1250 to prevent 1 colorectal cancer death |

***Table 2–8.*** Summary of USPSTF screening recommendations in 2008.

| Recommendation | Men | Women |
|---|---|---|
| Abdominal aortic aneurysm screening | One time screening with ultrasound in men 65- to 75-years-old who have ever smoked (≥ 100 cigarettes) | Screening not recommended |
| Alcohol misuse screening and behavioral counseling | All | All |
| Aspirin for the primary prevention of CV events | If increased risk for CAD | If increased risk for CAD |
| Breast cancer screening | NA | Mammography every 1–2 years beginning at age 40 |
| Breast cancer, genetic risk assessment | NA | In women with characteristic family histories |
| Cervical cancer screening | NA | In sexually active women with a cervix |
| Chlamydia infection screening | Screening not recommended | Sexually active women ≤ 25 and others at increased risk |
| Colorectal cancer screening | ≥ age 50 | ≥ age 50 |
| Depression screening | When systems for treatment in place | When systems for treatment in place |
| Type 2 DM screening | If hypertension or hyperlipidemia present | If hypertension or hyperlipidemia present |
| Gonorrhea screening | Screening not recommended | Sexually active women |
| Hypertension screening | All | All |
| HIV screening | If increased risk | If increased risk |
| Lipid disorders screening | ≥ age 35, or younger if other CV risk factors | ≥ age 45, or younger if other CV risk factors |
| Obesity screening | All | All |
| Osteoporosis | Screening not recommended | ≥ age 65, or ≥ 60 if risk factors |
| Syphilis screening | If increased risk | If increased risk |
| Tobacco use screening | All | All |

CAD, coronary artery disease; DM, diabetes mellitus.

⚠️1

You agree with Mrs. S that she is at increased risk for osteoporosis, but you explain that there are no data regarding testing before menopause. You discuss the importance of maintaining adequate calcium and vitamin D intake (1200 mg daily of calcium and 800-1000 international units daily of vitamin D).

## CASE RESOLUTION

⚠️1

Based on your discussion, Mr. S decides to forego the chest radiograph and PSA level. He agrees to be scheduled for a fasting lipid panel and a colonoscopy.

You discuss with Mrs. S that, because she has no additional risk factors for coronary disease, expert guidelines recommend waiting until age 45 before screening for hyperlipidemia.

Mrs. S opts to have a mammogram but is happy to let a Pap smear and a lipid panel wait a couple of years. She leaves with a handout about the role of calcium and vitamin D intake in the prevention and treatment of osteoporosis.

Tables 2–7 and 2–8 provide summary information regarding numbers needed to screen and current screening recommendations.

## REFERENCES

Andriole GL, Crawford ED, Grubb RL, et al. Mortality results from a randomized prostate cancer screening trial. NEJM. 2009;360:1310–1319.

Armstrong K, Moye E, Williams S et al. Screening mammography for women 40–49 years of age: a systematic review for the American College of Physicians. Ann Intern Med. 2007;146:516–26.

Bach PB, Jett JR, Pastorino U et al. Computed tomography screening and lung cancer outcomes. JAMA. 2007;297:953–61.

Baxter NN, Goldwasser MA, Paszat LF et al. Association of colonoscopy and death from colorectal cancer. Ann Intern Med. 2009;150:1–8.

Eisen GM, Weinberg DS. Narrative review: screening for colorectal cancer in patients with a first degree relative with colonic neoplasia. Ann Intern Med. 2005;143:190–98.

Lederle F, Kane RL, MacDonald R, Wilt T. Systematic review: repair of unruptured abdominal aortic aneurysm. Ann Intern Med. 2007;146:735–41.

Levin B, Lieberman DA, McFarland B et al. Screening and surveillance for the early detection of colorectal cancer and adenomatous polyps 2008: A joint guideline from the American Cancer Society, the Us Multi-society Talk Force on Colorectal Cancer, and the American College of Radiology. CA Cancer J Clin. 2008;58 (http://CAonline.AmCancer.Soc.org)

Levine J, Ahnen D. Adenomatous Polyps of the Colon. N Engl J Med. 2006;355:2551–7.

Lord SJ, Craft P, Cawson JN et al. A systematic review of the effectiveness of MRI as an addition to mammography and ultrasound in screening young women at high risk of breast cancer. Eur J Cancer. 2007;43:1905–17.

Mayrand MH, Duarte-France E, Rodrigues I et al. Human papillomavirus DNA versus Papanicolaou screening tests for cervical cancer. N Engl J Med. 2007;357:1579–88.

National Osteoporosis Foundation. Clinician's guide to prevention and treatment of osteoporosis. 2008 (http://www.nof.org/professionals/NOF_Clinicians_Guide.pdf)

Qaseem A, Snow V, Sherif K et al. Screening mammography for women 40–49 years of age: a clinical practice guideline from the American College of Physicians. Ann Intern Med. 2007;146:511–15.

Ronco G, Cuzick J, Pierotti P et al. Accuracy of liquid based versus conventional cytology: overall results of new technologies for cervical cancer screening: randomized controlled trial. BMJ. 2007;335:28.

Schroder FH, Hugosson J, Roobol MJ, et al. Screening and prostate cancer mortality in a randomized European study. 2009;360:1320–1328.

U.S. Preventive Services Task Force. http://www.ahrq.gov/clinic/uspstfix.htm

# I have a patient with abdominal pain.
# How do I determine the cause?

## CHIEF COMPLAINT

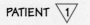

PATIENT ⋁1⃥

Mr. C is a 22-year-old man who complains of diffuse abdominal pain.

 **What is the differential diagnosis of abdominal pain? How would you frame the differential?**

## CONSTRUCTING A DIFFERENTIAL DIAGNOSIS

Abdominal pain is the most common cause for hospital admission in the United States. Diagnoses range from benign entities (eg, irritable bowel syndrome [IBS]) to life-threatening diseases (eg, ruptured abdominal aortic aneurysms [AAAs]). The first pivotal step in diagnosing abdominal pain is to identify the **location** of the pain. The differential diagnosis can then be narrowed to a subset of conditions that cause pain in that particular quadrant of the abdomen (Figure 3–1 and Summary table of abdominal pain by location at the end of the chapter). The **character** and **acuity** of the pain are also pivotal features that help prioritize the differential diagnosis.

Other important historical points include factors that make the pain better or worse (eg, eating), radiation of the pain, duration of the pain, and associated symptoms (nausea, vomiting, anorexia, inability to pass stool and flatus, melena, hematochezia, fever, chills, weight loss, altered bowel habits, orthostatic symptoms, or urinary symptoms). Pulmonary symptoms or a cardiac history can be clues to pneumonia or myocardial infarction (MI) presenting as abdominal pain. In women, sexual and menstrual histories are important. The patient should be asked about alcohol consumption.

A few points about the physical exam are worth emphasizing. First, vital signs are just that, vital. Hypotension, fever, tachypnea, and tachycardia are pivotal clinical clues that must not be overlooked. The HEENT exam should look for pallor or icterus. Careful heart and lung exams can suggest pneumonia or other extra-abdominal causes of abdominal pain.

 The physical exam of a patient with abdominal pain includes more than just the abdominal exam.

Of course, the abdominal exam is key. Inspection assesses for distention (often associated with bowel obstruction or ascites). Auscultation evaluates whether bowel sounds are present. Absent bowel sounds may suggest an intra-abdominal catastrophe; high-pitched tinkling sounds and rushes suggest an intestinal obstruction. Palpation should be done last. *It is useful to distract the patient by continuing to talk with him or her during abdominal palpation.* This allows

the examiner to get a better appreciation of the location and severity of maximal tenderness. The clinician should palpate the painful area last. The rectal exam should be performed, and the stool tested for occult blood. Finally, the pelvic exam should be performed in adult women and the testicular exam in men.

⋁1⃥

Mr. C felt well until the onset of pain several hours ago. He reports that the pain is a pressure-like sensation in the mid-abdomen, which is not particularly severe. He reports no fever, nausea, or vomiting. His appetite is diminished, and he has not had a bowel movement since the onset of pain. He reports no history of urinary symptoms such as frequency, dysuria, or hematuria. His past medical history is unremarkable. On physical exam, his vital signs are temperature 37.0°C, RR 16 breaths per minute, BP 110/72 mm Hg, and pulse 85 bpm. His cardiac and pulmonary exams are normal. Abdominal exam reveals a flat abdomen with hypoactive but positive bowel sounds. He has no rebound or guarding; although he has some mild diffuse tenderness, he has no focal or marked tenderness. There is no hepatosplenomegaly. Rectal exam is nontender, and stool is guaiac negative.

 **At this point, what is the leading hypothesis, what are the active alternatives, and is there a must not miss diagnosis? Given this differential diagnosis, what tests should be ordered?**

## PRIORITIZING THE DIFFERENTIAL DIAGNOSIS

The patient's history is not particularly suggestive of any diagnosis. Focus your attention on diseases associated with mid-abdominal pain. Appendicitis should always be considered in young, otherwise healthy patients with unexplained abdominal pain. Peptic ulcer disease (PUD) and pancreatitis may also present with epigastric or mid-abdominal pain. Table 3–1 lists the differential diagnosis.

⋁1⃥

Mr. C reports no history of nonsteroidal antiinflammatory drug (NSAID), aspirin, or alcohol ingestion. He has no known gallstones and no prior history of abdominal surgery. He reports that he is passing flatus and denies vomiting.

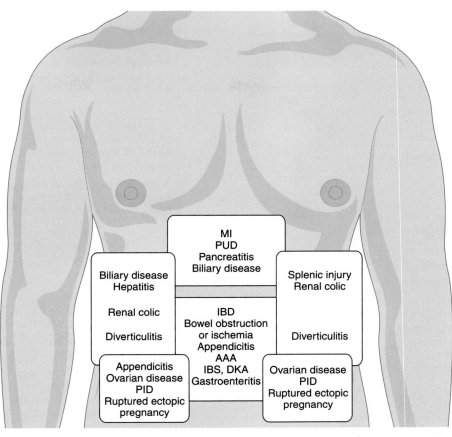

AAA, abdominal aortic aneurysm; DKA, diabetic ketoacidosis; IBD, inflammatory bowel disease;
IBS, irritable bowel syndrome; MI, myocardial infarction; PID, pelvic inflammatory disease;
PUD, peptic ulcer disease.

*Figure 3–1.* The differential diagnosis of abdominal pain by location.

 **Is the clinical information sufficient to make a diagnosis? If not, what other information do you need?**

## Leading Hypothesis: Appendicitis

### Textbook Presentation

The classic presentation of appendicitis is abdominal pain that is initially diffuse and then intensifies and migrates toward the right lower quadrant (RLQ) to McBurney point (1.5–2 inches from the anterior superior iliac crest toward umbilicus). Patients often complain of bloating and anorexia.

### Disease Highlights

A. Appendicitis is one of most common causes of an acute abdomen, with a 7% lifetime occurrence rate.

B. It develops secondary to obstruction of the appendiceal orifice with secondary mucus accumulation, swelling, ischemia, necrosis, and perforation.

C. Initially, the pain is poorly localized. However, progressive inflammation eventually involves the parietal peritoneum, resulting in pain localized to the RLQ.

D. The risk of perforation increases steadily with age (ages 10–40, 10%; age 60, 30%; and age > 75, 50%).

### Evidence-Based Diagnosis

A. Most individual clinical findings have a low sensitivity for appendicitis making it difficult to rule out the diagnosis.

1. In one study, guarding was completely absent in 22% of patients, and rebound was completely absent in 16% of patients with appendicitis.

2. Fever was present in only 40% of patients with perforated appendices.

**Fever, severe tenderness, guarding, and rebound may be absent in patients with appendicitis.**

B. Nonetheless, certain classic findings increase the likelihood of appendicitis when present (ie, rebound, guarding) (Table 3–2).

C. History is particularly important in women to differentiate other causes of RLQ pain (eg, pelvic inflammatory disease [PID], ruptured ectopic pregnancy, ovarian torsion, and ruptured ovarian cyst). The most useful clinical clues that suggest PID include the following:

***Table 3–1.*** Diagnostic hypotheses for Mr. C.

| Diagnostic Hypothesis | Clinical Clues | Important Tests |
|---|---|---|
| **Leading Hypothesis** | | |
| Appendicitis | Migration of pain from periumbilical region to right lower quadrant | Clinical exam CT scan |
| **Active Alternatives-Most Common** | | |
| Peptic ulcer | NSAID use *Helicobacter pylori* infection Melena Pain relieved by eating | Esophagogastroduodenoscopy Urea breath test for *H pylori* |
| Pancreatitis | Alcohol abuse Gallstones | Serum lipase |
| **Active Alternatives-Must Not Miss** | | |
| Early bowel obstruction | Inability to pass stool or flatus Nausea, vomiting Prior abdominal surgery | Abdominal radiographs, CT scan Small bowel study Barium enema |

1. History of PID
2. Vaginal discharge
3. Cervical motion tenderness on pelvic exam

 Rule out ectopic pregnancy in women of childbearing age who complain of abdominal pain by testing urine for β-HCG.

***Table 3–2.*** Classic clinical and laboratory findings in appendicitis.

| Finding | Sensitivity | Specificity | LR + | LR − |
|---|---|---|---|---|
| **Clinical Findings** | | | | |
| Fever > 38.1°C | 15–67% | 85% | 1 | 1 |
| Vomiting | 49% | 76% | 2.0 | 0.7 |
| Pain migration to RLQ | 54% | 63% | 1.5 | 0.7 |
| RLQ tenderness | 88% | 33% | 1.3 | 0.4 |
| Guarding (moderate to severe) | 46% | 92% | 5.5 | 0.59 |
| Rebound (moderate to severe) | 61% | 82% | 3.5 | 0.47 |
| **Laboratory Findings** | | | | |
| WBC > 7000/mcL | 98% | 21% | 1.2 | 0.1 |
| WBC > 11,000/mcL | 76% | 74% | 2.9 | 0.3 |
| WBC > 17,000/mcL | 15% | 98% | 7.5 | 0.9 |

D. Symptoms are different in octogenerians than in patients aged 60–79 years.
   1. The duration of symptoms is longer prior to evaluation (48 vs 24 hours).
   2. They are less likely to report pain that migrated to the RLQ (29% vs 49%).

E. WBC
   1. Very low WBCs (< 7000/mcL) and very high WBCs (> 17,000/mcL) substantially decrease or increase the likelihood of appendicitis respectively (see Table 3–2). Moderate elevations are less predictive.
   2. A low WBC does not exclude appendicitis in patients who have severe rebound or guarding; 80% of such patients had appendicitis even when WBC < 8000/mcL.

 The WBC is not reliably elevated in patients with acute appendicitis.

F. Urinalysis may be confusing and reveal pyuria and hematuria due to bladder inflammation from an adjacent appendicitis.

G. Plain radiography is useful only to detect free air or signs of another process (ie, small bowel obstruction [SBO]).

H. CT scanning is an accurate imaging method that is helpful when the diagnosis is uncertain. Studies have shown that it is more sensitive than ultrasonography in adults.
   1. CT scanning: 94% sensitive, 94% specific; LR+, 15.6; LR−, 0.06
   2. Ultrasonography: 83% sensitive, 93% specific; LR+, 11.9; LR−, 0.18
   3. One study showed that only 3% of patients who had a CT scan performed preoperatively underwent unnecessary appendectomy versus 6–13% of patients who did not have a CT scan performed. CT scanning resulted in lower overall costs.
   4. Although ultrasonography is inferior to CT scanning, it should be substituted for CT scanning in pregnant patients.

**Treatment**

A. Observation is critical
B. Monitor urinary output, vital signs
C. IV fluid resuscitation
D. Broad-spectrum antibiotics, including gram-negative and anaerobic coverage
E. Urgent appendectomy

## MAKING A DIAGNOSIS

Mr. C's symptoms are consistent with—but certainly not diagnostic of—appendicitis. None of the historical features (ie, no alcohol use, NSAID ingestion, or prior abdominal surgery) suggest any of the alternative diagnoses of pancreatitis, PUD, or bowel obstruction. Diagnostic options include obtaining a CBC (clearly of limited value), continued observation and reexamination, surgical consultation, and obtaining a CT scan. Given the lack of evidence for any of the less concerning possibilities you remain concerned that the patient has early appendicitis. You elect to observe the patient, obtain a CBC and lipase, and ask for a surgical consult.

Frequent clinical observations are exceptionally useful when evaluating a patient with possible appendicitis.

The CBC reveals a WBC of 8700/mcl (86% neutrophils, 0% bands) and a Hct of 44%. The lipase is normal. The surgical resident evaluates the patient who complains that the pain is now more severe in the RLQ. On exam, the patient's abdomen is moderately tender but still without rebound or guarding. The surgical resident agrees that the normal CBC and absence of fever do not exclude appendicitis and recommends an abdominal CT scan.

The migration of pain to the RLQ is suggestive of appendicitis. Less likely considerations might include Crohn ileitis as well as diverticulitis or colon cancer (both unlikely in this age group). If our patient were a woman, PID and ovarian pathology (ruptured ectopic pregnancy, ovarian torsion, or ruptured ovarian cyst) would also need to be considered.

Diffuse abdominal pain that subsequently localizes and becomes more constant, suggests parietal peritoneal inflammation.

The CT scan reveals a hypodense fluid collection on the right side inferior to the cecum. An appendolith is seen. The interpretation is possible appendiceal perforation versus Crohn disease.

## CASE RESOLUTION

The patient's symptom complex, particularly the pain's migration, localization, and intensification are highly suggestive of appendicitis. CT findings make this diagnosis likely. At this point, surgical exploration is appropriate.

The patient undergoes surgery and purulent material is found in the peritoneal cavity. A necrotic appendix is removed, and the peritoneal cavity is irrigated. The patient is treated with broad-spectrum antibiotics and does well postoperatively.

## CHIEF COMPLAINT

PATIENT 2

Ms. R is a 50-year-old woman who comes to the office complaining of abdominal pain. The patient reports that she has been having "episodes" or "attacks" of abdominal pain over the last several months. She reports that the attacks of pain are in the epigastrium, last up to 4 hours, and often awaken her at night. The pain is described as a severe cramping-like sensation that is very intense and steady for hours. Occasionally, the pain radiates to the right back. The pain is associated with emesis. She may get several attacks in a week or go weeks or months without them. She reports that the color of her urine and stool are normal. On physical exam, her vital signs are stable. She is afebrile. On HEENT exam, she is anicteric. Her lungs are clear, and cardiac exam is unremarkable. Abdominal exam is soft with only mild epigastric discomfort to deep palpation. Murphy sign (tenderness in the right upper quadrant [RUQ] with palpation during inspiration) is negative. Rectal exam reveals guaiac-negative stool.

**At this point, what is the leading hypothesis, what are the active alternatives, and is there a must not miss diagnosis? Given this differential diagnosis, what tests should be ordered?**

## PRIORITIZING THE DIFFERENTIAL DIAGNOSIS

The pivotal features of Ms. R's abdominal pain are its epigastric location, episodic frequency, colicky quality, and its severe intensity. Epigastric pain is commonly caused by PUD, biliary colic, and pancreatitis. Well-defined discrete episodes of abdominal pain are more typical of biliary colic than either PUD or pancreatitis. Other causes of intermittent abdominal pain include IBS and chronic mesenteric ischemia. Finally, the severe intense crampy quality (colic) suggests obstruction of a hollow viscera, which can be caused by biliary colic, bowel obstruction, or ureteral obstruction (eg, due to nephrolithiasis). Given the epigastric location, recurring episodic nature, quality and intensity of the pain, biliary colic is most likely. Table 3–3 lists the differential diagnosis.

Ms. R reports no history of alcohol bingeing, NSAID use, or known PUD. The pain does not improve with food or antacids. She denies any history of flank pain or hematuria. The pain is not relieved by defecation. There is no history of coronary artery disease (CAD) or peripheral vascular disease.

**Is the clinical information sufficient to make a diagnosis? If not, what other information do you need?**

***Table 3–3.*** Diagnostic hypotheses for Ms. R.

| Diagnostic Hypotheses | Clinical Clues | Important Tests |
| --- | --- | --- |
| **Leading Hypothesis** | | |
| Biliary colic | Episodic and crampy pain may radiate to back | Ultrasonography |
| **Active Alternatives-Most Common** | | |
| Peptic ulcer disease | NSAID use *Helicobacter pylori* infection Melena Pain relieved by eating or by antacids | EGD *Urea breath test for H pylori* |
| Pancreatitis | Alcohol abuse Gallstones | Serum lipase |
| Renal colic | Hematuria Radiation to flank, groin, genitals | Urinalysis Renal CT scan |
| Irritable bowel syndrome | Long history (years) of intermittent pain relieved by defecation or associated with diarrhea | Rome criteria and absence of alarm symptoms (eg, anemia, fever, weight loss, positive fecal occult blood test) Exclusion of other diagnoses |
| **Active Alternatives-Must Not Miss** | | |
| Chronic mesenteric ischemia | Postprandial pain Weight loss CAD or PVD | Mesenteric duplex ultrasonography Angiogram |

CAD, coronary artery disease; EGD, esophagogastroduodenoscopy; NSAID, nonsteroidal antiinflammatory drug; PVD, peripheral vascular disease.

## Leading Hypothesis: Biliary Colic

### Textbook Presentation

Gallstone disease may present as incidentally discovered asymptomatic cholelithiasis, biliary colic, cholecystitis, cholangitis, or pancreatitis. The pattern depends on the location of the stone and its chronicity (Figure 3–2). Biliary colic typically presents with episodes of intense abdominal pain that begin 1 hour or more after eating. The pain is usually located in the RUQ, although epigastric pain is also common. The pain may radiate to the back and may be associated with nausea and vomiting. The pain usually lasts for more than 30 minutes and may last for hours.

### Disease Highlights

A. Asymptomatic cholelithiasis

1. Predisposing factors

   a. Increasing age is the predominant risk factor. The prevalence is 8% in patients older than 40 years and 20% in those older than 60 years (Figure 3–3).

   b. Obesity

   c. Gender: more women are affected than men (risk increased during pregnancy)

   d. Gallbladder stasis (due to rapid weight loss, which may occur in patients on very low calorie diets, on total parenteral nutrition, and after surgery)

   e. Family history

   f. Crohn disease

   g. Hemolytic anemias can lead to increased bilirubin excretion and bilirubin stones (eg, thalassemia, sickle cell disease)

2. Cholecystectomy not advised for patients with asymptomatic cholelithiasis.

 Make sure the gallstones are *causing the pain* before advising cholecystectomy.

3. Annual risk of biliary colic developing in patients with asymptomatic gallstones is 1–4%.

B. Biliary colic

1. Occurs when gallstone becomes lodged in cystic duct and the gallbladder contracts against the obstruction

2. Presents as one of the classic visceral obstructive syndromes with severe, constant, and crampy waves of pain that incapacitate the patient

3. The pain usually lasts < 2–4 hours. An episode longer than 4–6 hours, fever, or marked tenderness, suggest cholecystitis.

4. Characterized by episodes of pain with pain free intervals of weeks to years.

5. Pain begins 1–4 hours after eating or may awaken the patient during the night. May be precipitated by fatty meals.

6. The pain is usually associated with nausea and vomiting.

7. Resolution occurs if the stone comes out of the gallbladder neck. The intense pain improves fairly rapidly, although mild discomfort may persist for 1 to 2 days.

8. Biliary colic recurs in 50% of symptomatic patients.

9. Complications (eg, pancreatitis, acute cholecystitis, or ascending cholangitis) occur in 1–2% of patients with biliary colic per year.

10. Colic occasionally develops in patients without stones secondary to sphincter of Oddi dysfunction or scarring leading to obstruction.

### Evidence-Based Diagnosis

A. Pain is located in RUQ in 54% of cases and in the epigastrium in 34% of cases. It may occur as a band across the entire upper abdomen, or rarely in the mid-abdomen. Pain may radiate to back, right scapula, right flank, or chest.

B. Laboratory tests (liver function tests [LFTs]), lipase, urinalysis) should be normal in uncomplicated biliary colic. Abnormalities suggest other diagnoses.

C. Ultrasonography is the test of choice; sensitivity 89%, specificity 97%, LR+ 30, LR− 0.11 (CT scan is only 79% sensitive.)

D. Endoscopic ultrasound is 100% sensitive and is useful in patients with a negative transabdominal ultrasound but in whom biliary colic is still strongly suspected.

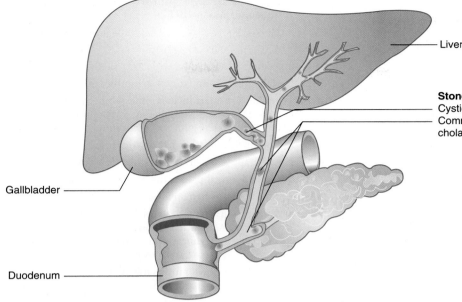

*Figure 3–2.* Common sites of calculus formation. (Modified, with permission, from Wrong Diagnosis.com)

## Treatment

A. Cholecystectomy is recommended.

B. Lithotripsy is not advised.

C. Dissolution therapies (eg, ursodiol) are reserved for nonsurgical candidates.

## MAKING A DIAGNOSIS

Ms. R's history suggests biliary colic. You order an ultrasound of the RUQ.

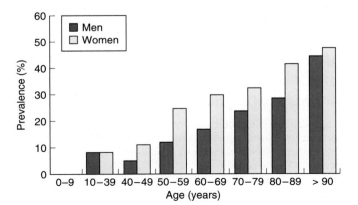

② A RUQ ultrasound reveals multiple small gallstones within the gallbladder. The common bile duct (CBD) is normal, and no other abnormalities are seen. A serum lipase and LFTs are normal, and urea breath test for *Helicobacter pylori* is negative.

Have you crossed a diagnostic threshold for the leading hypothesis, biliary colic? Have you ruled out the active alternatives? Do other tests need to be done to exclude the alternative diagnoses?

## Alternative Diagnosis: IBS

### Textbook Presentation

Patients often complain of intermittent abdominal pain accompanied by diarrhea or constipation or both of *years* duration. The diarrhea is often associated with cramps that are relieved by defecation. Pain cannot be explained by structural or biochemical abnormalities. Weight loss or anemia should alert the clinician to other possibilities.

*New* persistent *changes* in bowel habits (either diarrhea or constipation) should be thoroughly evaluated to exclude colon cancer, inflammatory bowel disease (IBD), or other process. An assumption of IBS in such patients is inappropriate.

### Disease Highlights

A. Affects 10–15% of adults, women 2 times more than men.

B. Etiology is a combination of altered motility, visceral hypersensitivity, autonomic function, and psychological factors.

*Figure 3–3.* Prevalence of asymptomatic gallstones by age. (Reproduced, with permission, from the BMJ Publishing Group, Bateson MC. Gallbladder disease. *BMJ.* 1999;318:1745–48.)

**C.** Symptoms often exacerbated by psychological or physical stressors

### Evidence-Based Diagnosis

**A.** There are no known biochemical or structural markers for IBS.

**B.** The diagnosis is usually made by a combination of (1) fulfilling the Rome criteria, (2) the absence of alarm features, and (3) a limited work-up to exclude other diseases.

  **1.** Rome criteria: Recurrent abdominal pain or discomfort (of ≥ 6 months duration) at least 3 days per month for the past 3 months, associated with two or more of the following:

    **a.** Improvement with defecation

    **b.** Onset associated with a change in frequency of stool

    **c.** Onset associated with a change in form (appearance) of stool

  **2.** Alarm symptoms (suggest alternative diagnosis and necessitate evaluation)

    **a.** Positive fecal occult blood test or rectal bleeding

    **b.** Anemia

    **c.** Weight loss > 10 lbs

    **d.** Fever

    **e.** Persistent diarrhea causing dehydration

    **f.** Severe constipation or fecal impaction

    **g.** Family history of colorectal cancer

    **h.** Onset of symptoms at age 50 years or older

    **i.** Major change in symptoms

    **j.** Nocturnal symptoms

    **k.** Recent antibiotic use

  **3.** Work-up

    **a.** Common recommendations for patients fulfilling Rome criteria without alarm symptoms include the following:

      **(1)** Obtain a CBC

      **(2)** Test stool for occult blood

      **(3)** Perform serologic tests for celiac sprue (eg, IgA tGT or IgA EMA) in patients with diarrhea as the predominant symptom

      **(4)** Routine chemistries are recommended by some experts.

    **b.** Colonoscopy with biopsy (to rule out microscopic colitis) is recommended in patients with alarm symptoms, in those aged ≥ 50 years, and in patients with a marked change in symptoms.

    **c.** There is no evidence that routine flexible sigmoidoscopy or colonoscopy is necessary in young patients without alarm symptoms.

    **d.** In addition to the above testing, the following should be evaluated in patients with alarm symptoms:

      **(1)** TSH levels

      **(2)** Basic chemistries

      **(3)** Stool for *Clostridium difficile* toxin and presence of ova and parasites

    **e.** A variety of serum and fecal markers, including ASCA, pANCA, fecal calprotectin, and fecal lactoferrin, are useful in selected patients and can suggest bowel inflammation or IBD.

### Treatment

**A.** Nonspecific management

  **1.** Certain foods may worsen symptoms in some patients.

  **2.** Common offenders include milk products, caffeine, alcohol, fatty foods, gas-producing vegetables, and sorbitol products (sugarless gum and diet candy).

  **3.** A food diary can help identify triggers.

**B.** Specific therapy is based on predominant syndrome.

  **1.** When abdominal pain is the predominant symptom

    **a.** Modify diet when applicable

    **b.** Medications include anticholinergics (dicyclomine, hyoscyamine), nitrates, low-dose tricyclic antidepressants (amitriptyline or nortriptyline) or smooth muscle relaxants (effective but not available in United States).

    **c.** Cognitive behavioral therapy appears to be as effective as pharmacologic therapy.

  **2.** When diarrhea is the predominant symptom

    **a.** Change diet when applicable

    **b.** Medications include loperamide, diphenoxylate, and cholestyramine.

    **c.** Alosetron is a 5-HT3 receptor antagonist that is useful in women with diarrhea-predominant IBS.

      **(1)** However, rare but serious complications have occurred including bowel obstruction and ischemic colitis.

      **(2)** Alosetron is recommended only in women with severe diarrhea-predominant IBS who have not responded to other antidiarrheal therapies.

  **3.** When constipation is the predominant symptom

    **a.** Change in diet (fiber, psyllium)

    **b.** Osmotic laxative: Lactulose, polyethylene glycol, or other

**C.** Treat underlying lactose intolerance. Such treatment in lactase deficient individuals with IBS markedly reduces outpatient visits.

## Alternative Diagnosis: PUD

See Chapter 27, Involuntary Weight Loss.

## Alternative Diagnosis: Acute Pancreatitis (see below)

## Alternative Diagnosis: Ischemic Bowel

Three distinct clinical subtypes of ischemic bowel include chronic mesenteric ischemia (chronic small bowel ischemia), acute mesenteric ischemia (acute ischemia of small bowel) and ischemic colitis (ischemia of the large bowel).

## 1. Chronic Mesenteric Ischemia

### Textbook Presentation

Patients with chronic mesenteric ischemia typically complain of recurrent postprandial abdominal pain (often in the first hour and diminishing 1–2 hours later), food fear, and weight loss. Patients often have a history of tobacco use, peripheral vascular disease or CAD.

### Disease Highlights

A. Secondary to near obstructive atherosclerotic disease of the superior mesenteric artery (SMA) or celiac artery or both

B. Arterial stenosis results in an imbalance between intestinal oxygen supply and demand that is accentuated after eating leading to intestinal angina resulting in food fear and weight loss

C. Two or more vessels (ie, SMA *and* celiac artery) are involved in 91% of affected patients.

### Evidence-Based Diagnosis

A. Weight loss occurs in 80% of patients and is due to food aversion.

B. Although stenoses are common (18% of population over age 65 years), symptomatic chronic ischemia is rare, and documented stenosis does *not* confirm the diagnosis of mesenteric ischemia. It is important to exclude more common disorders (ie, PUD and gallstone disease).

C. Duplex ultrasonography is very sensitive (> 90%) and can be used as the initial diagnostic tool. Normal results make the diagnosis very unlikely.

D. CT angiography and magnetic resonance angiography have also been used. Angiography should be considered if the results of noninvasive testing suggest vascular obstruction.

### Treatment

Revascularization (surgical repair or angioplasty [with stent]) is the only treatment.

## 2. Acute Mesenteric Ischemia

### Textbook Presentation

Acute mesenteric ischemia is a life-threatening condition that virtually always presents with the abrupt onset of acute severe abdominal pain that is typically out of proportion to a relatively benign physical exam. Acute mesenteric ischemia usually occurs in patients with risk factors of arterial thrombosis or systemic embolization.

### Disease Highlights

A. Usually due to SMA or celiac artery embolism (50%). Other causes include thrombosis (15–25%), low flow states without obstruction 20–30% (nonobstructive mesenteric ischemia [NOMI]), and mesenteric venous thrombosis (5%).

   1. Embolism

      a. Risk factors include atrial fibrillation, acute MI, valvular heart disease, heart failure (HF), ventricular aneurysms, angiography of abdominal aorta, and hypercoagulable states.

      b. The onset is often sudden without prior symptoms.

   2. Thrombosis

      a. Usually occurs in patients with atherosclerotic disease of the involved artery.

      b. Approximately half of such patients have a prior history of chronic mesenteric ischemia with intestinal angina.

   3. Nonobstructive mesenteric ischemia

      a. Often occurs in elderly patients with mesenteric atherosclerotic disease and superimposed hypotension (due to MI, HF, cardiopulmonary bypass, dialysis, or sepsis)

      b. May also occur after cocaine use and following endurance exercise activities (eg, marathon, cycling).

   4. Mesenteric venous thrombosis is often secondary to portal hypertension, hypercoagulable states, and intra-abdominal inflammation.

B. Patients have acute abdominal pain that is often out of proportion to their abdominal exam. If left untreated, bowel infarction and peritoneal findings will develop.

C. Incidence: 0.1–0.3% of hospital admissions

D. Mortality is high at 30–65%.

### Evidence-Based Diagnosis

A. Common presenting symptoms are abdominal pain (94%), nausea (56%), vomiting (38%), and diarrhea (31%).

B. 50% of patients have a prior history of intestinal angina

C. The WBC is abnormal in 90% of patients and often markedly elevated. (Mean WBC $21.4 \times 10^9$/mL)

D. Lactate level was elevated in 77–89% of patients (mean 3.3 mmol/L (normal < 2.0 mmol/L)

 A normal lactate level does not rule out acute mesenteric ischemia.

E. Plain abdominal radiographs may reveal thickening of bowel loops or thumbprinting but are insensitive (40%).

F. Doppler ultrasonography is insensitive due to distended bowel.

G. Standard CT scanning may demonstrate SMA occlusion or findings suggesting ischemic and necrosis such as segmental bowel wall thickening or pneumatosis but is insensitive (64%).

H. Although CT angiography and magnetic resonance angiography have been used, direct angiography is the gold standard and recommended.

### Treatment

A. Emergent revascularization (via thromboembolectomy, thrombolysis, vascular bypass or angioplasty) and surgical resection of necrotic bowel are the mainstays of therapy. Prompt surgical intervention (< 12 hours) reduces mortality compared with delayed intervention (> 12 hours) (14% vs 75%).

B. Broad-spectrum antibiotics

C. Volume resuscitation

D. Preoperative and postoperative anticoagulation to prevent thrombus propagation

E. For patients with NOMI, improved perfusion is paramount.

F. Intra-arterial papaverine has been used to block reactive mesenteric arteriolar vasoconstriction and improve blood flow.

## 3. Ischemic Colitis

### Textbook Presentation

Ischemic colitis typically presents with left-sided abdominal pain. Patients frequently have bloody or maroon stools or diarrhea. Profuse bleeding is unusual.

### Disease Highlights

A. Usually due to nonocclusive decrease in colonic perfusion

B. Typically involves the watershed areas of the colon, most commonly the splenic flexure, descending colon, and rectosigmoid junction

C. Precipitating events may include hypotension, MI, sepsis, or HF, but the cause is not usually identified.

D. Uncommon causes include vasculitis, hypercoagulable states, vasoconstrictors, vascular surgery, drugs (eg, alosetron) and long distance running or bicycling (presumably due to shunting and hypoperfusion).

### Evidence-Based Diagnosis

A. Abdominal pain (not usually severe) is reported by 84% of patients.

B. Hematochezia is a helpful diagnostic clue when present but not diagnostic when absent. Sensitivity 46%, specificity 90.9%; LR+ 5.1, LR− 0.6

C. Diarrhea is seen in approximately 40% of patients.

D. Abdominal tenderness is common (81%), but rebound tenderness is rare (15%).

E. Risk factors that increase the likelihood of ischemic colitis include age > 60 years, hemodialysis, hypertension, diabetes, hypoalbuminemia, and medications that induce constipation.

F. Features that distinguish acute mesenteric ischemia (small bowel) from ischemic colitis are summarized in Table 3–4.

G. Colonoscopy is the preferred test to evaluate ischemic colitis.

H. Plain radiographs rarely demonstrate free air (perforation) or thumbprinting (specific for ischemia).

I. CT scanning may demonstrate segmental circumferential wall thickening (which is nonspecific) or be normal.

J. Vascular studies are usually normal and not indicated except in the unusual case of isolated right-sided ischemic colitis.

### Treatment

A. Therapy is primarily supportive with bowel rest, IV hydration, and broad-spectrum antibiotics.

B. Colonic infarction occurs in a small percentage of patients (15–20%) and requires segmental resection.

C. Indications for surgery include peritonitis, sepsis, free air on plain radiographs, clinical deterioration (persistent fever, increasing leukocytosis, lactic acidosis), or strictures.

## CASE RESOLUTION

Ms. R discussed her case with her primary care physician and surgeon. Both agree that her symptom complex and ultrasound suggest biliary colic. Furthermore, there was no evidence of any of the alternative diagnoses. The normal lipase effectively rules out pancreatitis, and the combination of no NSAIDs and a negative urea breath test for H pylori makes PUD very unlikely. She also lacked any risk factors for mesenteric ischemia. They recommend surgery, which she schedules for the end of the summer.

## FOLLOW-UP

Ms. R returns 3 weeks later (and prior to her scheduled surgery) in acute distress. She reports that her pain began last evening, is in the same location as her previous bouts of pain, but unlike her previous episodes, the pain has persisted. She is very uncomfortable. She reports that her urine has changed color and is now quite dark, "like tea." In addition, she complains of "teeth chattering" chills. On physical exam, Ms. R is febrile (38.5°C). Her other vital signs are stable. Sclera are anicteric and cardiac and pulmonary exams are all completely normal. Abdominal exam reveals moderate tenderness in the epigastrium and RUQ. Murphy sign is positive.

 At this point, what is the leading hypothesis, what are the active alternatives, and is there a must not miss diagnosis? Given this differential diagnosis, what tests should be ordered?

**Table 3–4.** Features that distinguish ischemic colitis from acute mesenteric ischemia.

| Ischemic Colitis | Acute Mesenteric Ischemia |
| --- | --- |
| Usually due to nonocclusive decrease in colonic perfusion | Usually due to acute arterial occlusion of SMA or celiac artery |
| Precipitating cause often not identified | Precipitating cause typical (MI, atrial fibrillation etc) |
| Patients are usually not severely ill | Patients appear severely ill |
| Abdominal pain usually mild | Abdominal pain usually severe |
| Abdominal tenderness usually present | Abdominal tenderness not prominent early |
| Hematochezia common | Hematochezia uncommon until very late |
| Colonoscopy procedure of choice, angiography *not* usually indicated | Angiography indicated |

MI, myocardial infarction; SMA, superior mesenteric artery.

## PRIORITIZING THE DIFFERENTIAL DIAGNOSIS

This episode of abdominal pain raises several possibilities. The first is that the current symptom complex is in some way related to her known cholelithiasis. Although the persistent pain may suggest cholecystitis (due to a stone lodged in the cystic duct), the dark urine is a pivotal clinical clue, which suggests a different complication. One cause of dark urine is bilirubin in the urine (bilirubinuria). Bilirubinuria only occurs in patients with conjugated hyperbilirubinemia which, in turn, is due to either CBD obstruction or hepatitis. In our patient, the preexistent biliary colic, persistent RUQ pain, and dark urine make the most likely diagnosis CBD obstruction due to migration of a stone into the CBD (choledocholithiasis) (Figure 3–2). On the other hand, in patients with cholecystitis, only the cystic duct is obstructed. The CBD remains open and therefore cholecystitis does not cause hyperbilirubinemia, dark urine, or significant increases in ALT (SGPT) or AST (SGOT). Finally, Ms. R's fever suggests that the CBD obstruction has been complicated by ascending infection (ascending cholangitis), a life-threatening condition (Figure 3–4).

Dark urine suggests bilirubinuria and may precede icterus.

Rigors (defined as visible shaking or teeth chattering chills) suggests bacteremia and should increase the suspicion of a life-threatening bacterial infection.

Other considerations include hepatitis or pancreatitis, which may be caused by CBD obstruction. While hepatitis can cause RUQ pain, hyperbilirubinemia, and bilirubinuria, it would also require giving Ms. R. another unrelated diagnosis and is therefore less likely. Table 3–5 lists the differential diagnosis.

Laboratory results include WBC 17,000/mcL (84% neutrophils, 10% bands). Hct is 38%, lipase 17 units/L (nl 11–65 units/L), alkaline phosphatase 467 units/L (nl 30–120), bilirubin 4.2 mg/dL, conjugated bilirubin 3.0 mg/dL (nl 0 – 0.3), GGT 246 units/L (nl 8–35), ALT 100 units/L (nl 15–59). Ultrasound shows sludge and stones within the gallbladder. No CBD dilatation or CBD stone is seen. Blood cultures are ordered and you initiate broad-spectrum IV antibiotics (ie, piperacillin/tazobactam).

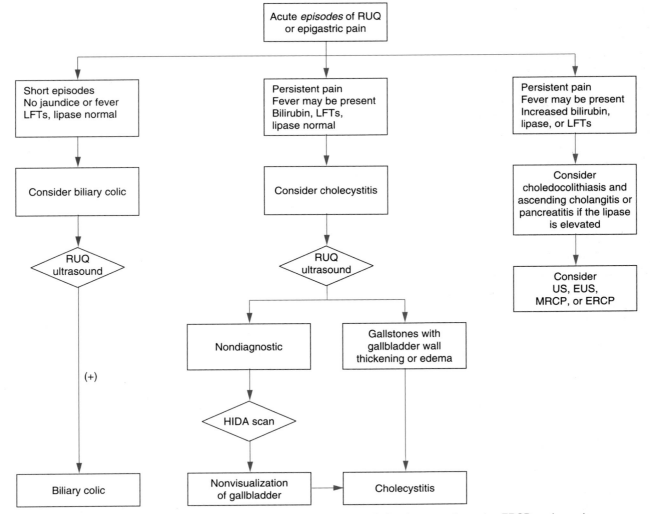

US, ultrasound; EUS, endoscopic ultrasound; MRCP, magnetic resonance cholangiopancreatography; ERCP, endoscopic retrograde cholangiopancreatography

***Figure 3–4.*** Diagnostic approach: biliary disease.

**Table 3–5.** Diagnostic hypotheses for Ms. R on follow-up.

| Diagnostic Hypothesis | Clinical Clues | Important Tests |
|---|---|---|
| **Leading Hypothesis** | | |
| Ascending cholangitis | Right upper quadrant or epigastric pain<br>Dark urine<br>Fever<br>Rigors | Ultrasound<br>Endoscopic ultrasound<br>ERCP<br>MRCP<br>CBC<br>Blood cultures |
| **Active Alternatives-Most Common** | | |
| Acute cholecystitis | Right upper quadrant pain<br>Fever | Ultrasound |
| Pancreatitis | Alcohol abuse<br>Gallstones | Serum lipase |
| Hepatitis | Alcohol abuse<br>Right upper quadrant pain<br>Nausea<br>Dark urine | Elevated ALT and AST<br>Viral serologies |

ERCP, endoscopic retrograde cholangiopancreatography; MRCP, magnetic resonance cholangiopancreatography.

Is the clinical information sufficient to make a diagnosis of ascending cholangitis? If not, what other information do you need?

## Leading Hypothesis: Choledocholithiasis & Ascending Cholangitis

### Textbook Presentation

Patients typically have some form of CBD obstruction (most often from gallstones); RUQ pain, fever, and jaundice are presenting symptoms.

### Disease Highlights

A. 10–20% of patients with symptomatic gallstones have stones within the CBD (choledocholithiasis).

B. Patients with choledocholithiasis may be asymptomatic.

C. Complications of choledocholithiasis may be the presenting manifestations:

1. Obstruction and jaundice

2. Fever, jaundice, and leukocytosis may be present due to ascending infection from the duodenum (ascending cholangitis).

3. Pancreatitis

### Evidence-Based Diagnosis

A. Ascending cholangitis

1. Clinical findings in patients with cholangitis include jaundice, 79%; temperature ≥ 38.0 °C, 77%; and RUQ pain, 68%. In various studies 42–75% of patients had all three (Charcot triad).

2. There is leukocytosis in 73% of patients and elevated alkaline phosphatase and bilirubin in 91% and 87%, respectively.

3. 74% of patients were bacteremic

B. Choledocholithiasis

1. Any of the following suggests choledocholithiasis and warrants CBD evaluation (Table 3–6):

a. Cholangitis

b. Jaundice

c. Dilated CBD on ultrasound

d. Elevated alkaline phosphatase

e. Elevated amylase

2. CBD stones are present in 5–8% of patients without any of the aforementioned risk factors.

3. Transabdominal ultrasound is noninvasive but *not* consistently sensitive for choledocholithiasis as opposed to its performance in cholelithiasis (sensitivity 25–81%, specificity 88–91%). A dilated CBD is seen in only 25% of patients.

4. Endoscopic retrograde cholangiopancreatography (ERCP), magnetic resonance cholangiopancreatography (MRCP), and endoscopic ultrasound (EUS) are highly accurate in detecting CBD stones. These techniques share high sensitivity (90–100%) and specificity (90–100%).

a. ERCP

(1) Invasive procedure that allows direct cannulation of CBD *and* relieves obstruction via simultaneous stone extraction and sphincterotomy

(2) > 90% sensitive, 99% specific for diagnosis

(3) Requires sedation

(4) Complicated by pancreatitis in 1–5% of patients

(5) Preferred procedure in patients with a high pretest probability of CBD stones particularly those with jaundice and fever who need prompt relief of obstruction

**Table 3–6.** Test characteristics for choledocholithiasis.

| Finding | Sensitivity | Specificity | LR+ | LR– |
|---|---|---|---|---|
| Cholangitis | 11% | 99% | 18.3 | 0.93 |
| Jaundice | 36% | 97% | 10.1 | 0.69 |
| Dilated CBD on ultrasound | 42% | 96% | 6.9 | 0.77 |
| Elevated alkaline phosphatase | 57% | 86% | 2.6 | 0.65 |
| Elevated amylase | 11% | 95% | 1.5 | 0.99 |

CBD, common bile duct.
Modified, with permission, from Springer. Paul A. Diagnosis and treatment of common bile duct stones. Surg Endosc. 1998;12:856–64.

**(6)** In patients less likely to have a CBD stone (ie, those with cholelithiasis and isolated elevation in alkaline phosphatase), a less invasive test (eg, MRCP or EUS) is an appropriate initial study.

**b.** MRCP

**(1)** Noninvasive scan visualizes CBD and adjacent structures

**(2)** Highly accurate for CBD stones: 90–100% sensitive, 88–100% specific

**c.** EUS is both sensitive (89–98%) and specific (94–98%) for CBD stones.

**(1)** One study reported that EUS was more sensitive than ERCP (97% vs 67%).

**(2)** EUS can be converted to ERCP in patients discovered to have CBD stones.

**(3)** A negative EUS or MRCP would obviate the need for a more invasive ERCP.

**d.** CT scanning is only 75% sensitive for choledocholithiasis. Two studies suggest that multi-detector CT using iotroxate (which is excreted in the biliary system) is highly accurate for choledocholithiasis (85–96% sensitive, 88–94% specific).

## Treatment

**A.** IV broad-spectrum antibiotics and IV hydration

**B.** Decompression of the biliary system, preferably via ERCP, is vital.

**1.** This should be performed emergently in patients with persistent pain, hypotension, altered mental status, persistent high fever, WBC ≥ 20,000/mcL, bilirubin ≥ 10 mg/dL and electively in more stable patients.

**2.** Transhepatic stent or surgical decompression is rarely used.

**C.** Cholecystectomy

## MAKING A DIAGNOSIS

Neither dilation of the CBD nor CBD stone can be seen on ultrasound (but is only 25% sensitive). You still suspect choledocholithiasis because of the jaundice and increased transaminases.

> ⟨2⟩
>
> Twenty-four hours later, blood cultures are positive for *Escherichia coli* (consistent with ascending cholangitis).
>
> ☑ Have you crossed a diagnostic threshold for the leading hypothesis, ascending cholangitis? Have you ruled out the active alternatives? Do other tests need to be done to exclude the alternative diagnoses?

## Alternative Diagnosis: Acute Hepatitis

See Abnormal liver tests in Chapter 22, Jaundice and Abnormal Liver Enzymes.

## Alternative Diagnosis: Acute Cholecystitis

### Textbook Presentation

Typical symptoms of acute cholecystitis include *persistent* RUQ or epigastric pain, fever, nausea, and vomiting.

### Disease Highlights

**A.** Secondary to prolonged cystic duct obstruction (> 12 hours)

**B.** Persistent obstruction results in increasing gallbladder inflammation and pain. Necrosis, infection, and gangrene may occur.

**C.** Jaundice and marked elevation of liver enzymes are seen only if the stone migrates into the CBD and causes obstruction.

### Evidence-Based Diagnosis

**A.** No clinical finding is sufficiently sensitive to rule out cholecystitis.

**1.** Fever: present in 35% of patients

**2.** Murphy sign

**a.** Sensitivity, 65%; specificity, 87%

**b.** LR+ = 5.0, LR− = 0.4

**B.** Laboratory findings

**1.** Leukocytosis (> 10,000/mcL) is present in 63% of patients.

**2.** Cholecystitis does *not* typically cause significant increases in lipase or LFTs. Such findings suggest complications of pancreatitis and choledocholithiasis.

**C.** Ultrasound

**1.** Findings that suggest acute cholecystitis include gallstones *with* gallbladder wall thickening, pericholecystic fluid, sonographic Murphy sign, or gallbladder enlargement > 5 cm

**2.** Sensitivity, 88%; specificity, 80%

**3.** LR+, 4.4; LR−, 0.15

**D.** Cholescintigraphy (HIDA) scans

**1.** Radioisotope is excreted by the liver into the biliary system. In normal patients, the gallbladder concentrates the isotope and is visualized.

**2.** Nonvisualization of the gallbladder suggests cystic duct obstruction and is highly specific for acute cholecystitis (97% sensitive, 90% specific).

**3.** Nonvisualization can also be seen in prolonged fasting, hepatitis, and alcohol abuse.

**4.** Useful when the pretest probability is high and the ultrasound is nondiagnostic (ie, the ultrasound demonstrates stones within the gallbladder) but no clear evidence of cholecystitis is seen (eg, no stones within the cystic duct nor evidence of gallbladder wall thickening or pericholecystic fluid).

**5.** Visualization of the gallbladder essentially excludes acute cholecystitis.

**E.** Ultrasound is the test of choice for following reasons:

**1.** Less expensive

**2.** Faster

**3.** Avoids radiation

**4.** Can image adjacent organs

**F.** If ultrasound is normal, consider HIDA.

**G.** An algorithm to the diagnosis is shown in Figure 3–4.

### Treatment

Patients with acute cholecystitis should be admitted, administered parenteral antibiotics, and undergo cholecystectomy.

# Alternative Diagnosis: Acute Pancreatitis

## Textbook Presentation

Patients with acute pancreatitis often complain of a constant and boring abdominal pain of moderate to severe intensity that develops in the epigastrium and may radiate to the back. Associated symptoms may include nausea, vomiting, low-grade fever, and abdominal distention.

## Disease Highlights

A. Etiology

1. Alcohol abuse (typically binge drinking) and choledocholithiasis cause 80% of acute pancreatitis cases.

2. 15–25% of cases are idiopathic (67% of patients with idiopathic pancreatitis were found to have small gallstones at ERCP)

3. Post ERCP

4. Drugs commonly associated with pancreatitis include azathioprine, didanosine (DDI), estrogens, furosemide, hydrochlorothiazide, L-asparaginase, metronidazole, opioids, pentamidine, sulfonamides, corticosteroids, tamoxifen, tetracycline, valproate, and many others.

5. Less common causes include trauma, marked hypertriglyceridemia (> 1000 mg/dL), hypercalcemia, ischemia, HIV infection, other infection, trauma, pancreatic carcinoma, pancreatic divisum and organ transplantation.

6. Regardless of the inciting event, trypsinogen is activated to trypsin, which activates other pancreatic enzymes resulting in pancreatic autodigestion and inflammation (which may become systemic and lethal). Interleukins contribute to the inflammation.

B. Complications may be local or systemic. Severe, potentially fatal pancreatitis develops in about 20% of patients.

1. Local complications

   a. Pancreatic pseudocyst

   b. Pancreatic necrosis

   c. Infections

      (1) Infected pancreatic pseudocyst (abscess)

      (2) Infected pancreatic necrosis

      (3) Ascending cholangitis (in patients with gallstone-associated pancreatitis)

2. Systemic complications

   a. Hyperglycemia

   b. Hypocalcemia

   c. Acute respiratory distress syndrome

   d. Acute renal failure

   e. Disseminated intravascular coagulation

3. Death

   a. Usually occurs in patients with infected pancreatic necrosis and in patients in whom multiple organ dysfunction develops.

   b. Several predictive scores have been developed including the Ranson criteria and Apache II score. These are fairly complex to use.

   c. Hemoconcentration (Hct ≥ 50%) on admission predicts severe pancreatitis; LR+ 7.5 (vs 0.4 for patients with Hct ( 45%).

   d. C-reactive protein > 150 mg/L at 48 hours can also predict severe pancreatitis; sensitivity 85%, specificity 74%; LR+ 3.2, LR– 0.2

## Evidence-Based Diagnosis

A. History and physical

1. Low-grade fevers (< 38.3°C) are common (60%).

2. Pain may radiate to the back (50%) and may be exacerbated in the supine position.

3. Nausea and vomiting are usually present (75%).

4. Rebound is rare on presentation; guarding is common (50%).

5. Periumbilical bruising (Cullen sign) is rare.

6. Flank bruising (Turner sign) is rare.

B. Laboratory studies

1. Lipase

   a. 94% sensitive, 96% specific; LR+ = 23, LR– = .06

   b. Remains elevated longer than serum amylase

   c. Marked elevations suggest pancreatitis secondary to gallstones.

2. Amylase

   a. Less sensitive and specific than lipase

   b. Should not be routinely ordered if lipase available

3. LFTs

   a. Useful in detecting gallstone-associated pancreatitis (GAP); patients with GAP have high risk of recurrent pancreatitis and require cholecystectomy.

   b. Studies suggest that *significant* elevations of the bilirubin, alkaline phosphatase, ALT, or AST predict GAP. (These enzymes increase due to concomitant obstruction of the CBD.)

      (1) ALT or AST elevations > 100 suggest GAP (sensitivity ≈ 55%, specificity ≈ 93%; LR+ 8–9)

      (2) AST levels < 50 make GAP unlikely. (sensitivity 90%, specificity 68%; LR– 0.15)

      (3) 10% of patients with GAP have normal levels of alkaline phosphatase, bilirubin, AST, and ALT.

4. Plain radiography is useful to rule out free air or SBO.

5. Imaging: A variety of imaging techniques can be used in patients with acute pancreatitis.

   a. Transabdominal ultrasound is noninvasive and should be performed in *all* patients with pancreatitis to determine if they have gallstones or CBD dilatation suggesting GAP.

   b. CT scanning is 87–90% sensitive and 90–92% specific for the diagnosis of acute pancreatitis but insensitive for determining whether or not patients have GAP.

      (1) Should be performed when the diagnosis is unclear or complications are suspected (pseudocysts or pancreatic necrosis)

      (2) Pancreatic necrosis should be suspected in patients with severe pancreatitis, when signs of sepsis are present, and in patients in patients who do not improve in the first 72 hours.

      (3) IV contrast is required to demonstrate necrosis.

   c. Detecting GAP

**(1)** Neither transabdominal ultrasound nor CT are sensitive at detecting choledocholithiasis (21% and 40% respectively).

**(2)** MRCP is highly accurate for choledocholithiasis (80–94% sensitive) as are EUS and ERCP (≈ 98% sensitive)

**(3)** ERCP can relieve CBD obstruction and is recommended in patients with persistent obstruction or cholangitis. Some authorities also recommend ERCP for patients with severe pancreatitis. ERCP can *precipitate* pancreatitis and is therefore not recommended for *all* patients with GAP. ERCP with sphincterotomy can be therapeutic but is invasive.

**(4)** Figure 3–5 outlines an approach to GAP.

### Treatment

**A.** Vital signs, orthostatic BPs, and urinary output should be carefully monitored to assess intravascular volume.

**B.** IV fluid is critical to maintain appropriate BP and urinary output (> 0.5 mL/kg/h)

**C.** No oral intake

**D.** Parenteral pain medication

**E.** Nasogastric (NG) tube if recurrent vomiting

**F.** ICU admission for severe pancreatitis

**G.** *Prophylactic* antibiotics for patients with pancreatic necrosis are controversial.

**H.** If infection is suspected (due to increasing fever, leukocytosis or deterioration) evaluate with fine-needle aspiration and culture. If infection is confirmed, broad-spectrum antibiotics should be administered and surgical debridement considered.

**I.** ERCP and sphincterotomy (see above)

**J.** Patients with GAP are at high risk for recurrent pancreatitis (≈ 30%), cholangitis, and biliary colic. Cholecystectomy should be performed after recovery and prior to discharge to prevent recurrences. Intraoperative cholangiogram or ERCP is required to ensure that the CBD is clear of stones.

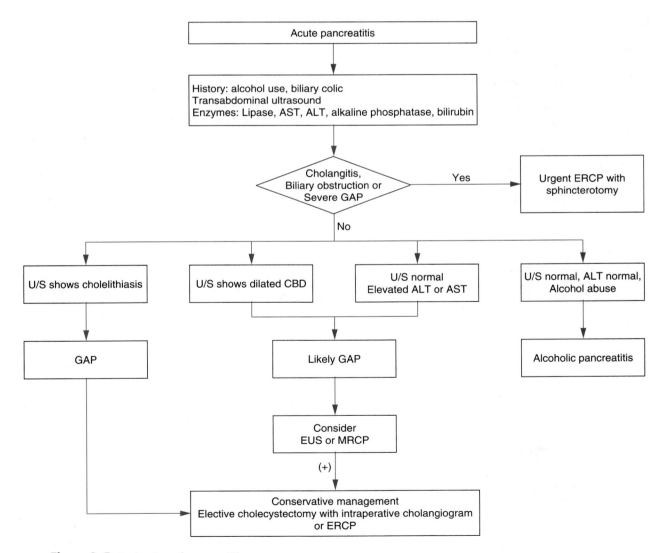

***Figure 3–5.*** Evaluation of pancreatitis.

K. Alcohol abstinence

L. Enteral feeding via nasoenteric feeding tubes, preferably placed in the jejunum, is recommended in patients with severe or complicated pancreatitis.

## Alternative Diagnosis: Chronic Pancreatitis

See Chapter 27, Involuntary Weight Loss.

## CASE RESOLUTION

▽2

An ERCP demonstrates multiple small stones within the CBD, which are extracted. Ms. R underwent cholecystectomy and recovered without incident.

## CHIEF COMPLAINT

PATIENT ▽3

Mr. J is a 63-year-old man with severe abdominal pain for 48 hours. The pain is periumbilical with severe crampy exacerbations that last for several minutes and then subside. He notes loud intestinal noises (borborygmi) during the periods of increased pain. The pain is associated with nausea and vomiting. He reports decreased appetite with no oral intake in the last 48 hours.

☑ At this point, what is the leading hypothesis, what are the active alternatives, and is there a must not miss diagnosis? Given this differential diagnosis, what tests should be ordered?

## PRIORITIZING THE DIFFERENTIAL DIAGNOSIS

Mr. J's severe crampy abdominal pain suggests some type of visceral obstruction. The syndromes associated with pain of this quality include ureteral obstruction secondary to kidney stones, biliary obstruction, or intestinal obstruction (large or small bowel). The associated nausea and vomiting can be seen with any of those diseases. However, the loud intestinal sounds associated with exacerbations of the pain suggest some form of intestinal obstruction. In addition, the periumbilical location is more suggestive of intestinal obstruction than renal or biliary colic.

Table 3–7 lists the differential diagnoses for Mr. J.

▽3

Three weeks ago, Mr. J noted a small amount of blood on the stool. He reports no other change in bowel habits until 4 days ago. Since that time, he has been constipated and has not passed stool or flatus. He has no prior history of intra-abdominal surgeries, hernias, or diverticulitis. He reports no history of flank pain, groin pain, or hematuria. He has no history of gallstones and has not noticed any tea-colored urine. On physical exam, he is intermittently very uncomfortable with episodes of severe diffuse cramping pain. Vital signs reveal orthostatic hypotension: supine BP, 110/75 mm Hg; pulse, 90 bpm; upright BP, 85/50 mm Hg; pulse, 125 bpm; temperature, 37.0°C; RR, 18 breaths per minute. He is anicteric.

**Table 3–7.** Diagnostic hypotheses for Mr. J.

| Diagnostic Hypothesis | Clinical Clues | Important Tests |
|---|---|---|
| **Leading Hypothesis** | | |
| Bowel obstruction | Inability to pass stool or flatus<br>Nausea, vomiting<br>Prior abdominal surgery or altered bowel habits,<br>Hematochezia,<br>Abdominal distention,<br>hyperactive bowel sounds (with tinkling) or hypoactive bowel sounds<br>Prior abdominal surgery | Abdominal radiographs<br>CT scan |
| **Active Alternatives—Most Common** | | |
| Biliary colic | Episodic, crampy pain<br>Dark urine | Ultrasound |
| Renal colic | Flank or groin pain<br>Hematuria | Urinalysis<br>Renal CT scan |

Cardiac and lung exams are unremarkable. Abdominal exam reveals prominent distention. Bowel sounds show intermittent rushes. He has mild diffuse tenderness to exam without rebound or guarding. Stool is brown and heme positive.

The constipation, absence of flatus, abdominal distention, and rushing bowel sounds further increase the suspicion of bowel obstruction. Most *small* bowel obstructions (SBO) are due to adhesions from prior surgery. Mr. J's negative surgical history makes this unlikely. However, the hematochezia raises the possibility of a malignant obstruction. The orthostatic hypotension suggests significant dehydration.

▽3

Laboratory findings are WBC 10,000/mcL (70% neutrophils, 0% bands); Hct, 41%. Electrolytes: Na, 141; K, 3.0; $HCO_3$, 32; Cl, 99; BUN, 45; Creatinine 1.0 mg/dL. An abdominal upright radiograph is shown Figure 3–6.

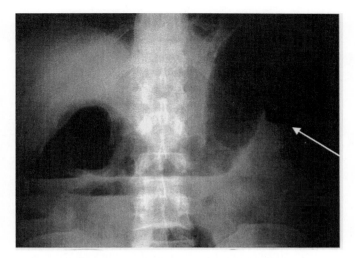

**Figure 3–6.** Plain radiography reveals grossly distended ascending colon, multiple air-fluid levels and an abrupt termination of air in the transverse colon (arrow) suggestive of large bowel obstruction.

**Table 3–8.** Test characteristics for predicting bowel obstruction.

| Finding | Sensitivity | Specificity | LR+ | LR– |
|---|---|---|---|---|
| Visible peristalsis | 6% | 99.7% | 20 | 0.94 |
| Prior abdominal surgery | 69% | 94% | 11.5 | 0.33 |
| Constipation | 44% | 95% | 8.8 | 0.59 |
| Abdominal distention | 63% | 89% | 5.7 | 0.42 |
| Increased bowel sounds | 40% | 89% | 3.6 | 0.67 |
| Reduced bowel sounds | 23% | 93% | 3.3 | 0.83 |
| Colicky pain | 31% | 89% | 2.8 | 0.78 |
| Vomiting | 75% | 65% | 2.1 | 0.38 |

LR, likelihood ratio.
Modified, with permission, from Taylor & Francis Ltd. Böhmer H. Simple Data from History and Physical Examination Help to Exclude Bowel Obstruction and to Avoid Radiographic Studies in Patients with Acute Abdominal Pain. http://www.tandf.co.UK/journals.

Is the clinical information sufficient to make a diagnosis? If not, what other information do you need?

## Leading Hypothesis: Large Bowel Obstruction (LBO)

### Textbook Presentation

Bowel obstructions present with severe crampy abdominal pain that is accentuated in waves, which the patient finds incapacitating. Vomiting is common. The pain is often diffuse and poorly localized. Initially, the patient may have several bowel movements as the bowel *distal* to the obstruction is emptied. Bowel sounds are hyperactive early in the course. Abdominal distention is often present. (Distention is less marked in proximal SBOs.) At first, the pain is intermittent; later, the pain often becomes more constant, bowel sounds may diminish and become absent, constipation progresses and the patient becomes unable to pass flatus. If bowel infarction occurs, peritoneal findings may be seen.

In patients with abdominal pain, the absence of bowel movements or flatus suggests bowel obstruction.

### Disease Highlights

Etiology and related prevalence is as follows:

1. Cancer, 53%

2. Sigmoid or cecal volvulus, 17%

3. Diverticular disease, 12%

4. Extrinsic compression from metastatic cancer, 6%

5. Other, 12% (adhesions rarely cause LBO)

### Evidence-Based Diagnosis

A. History and physical exam (Table 3–8)

   1. None of the expected clinical findings are very sensitive

      a. Vomiting, 75%

      b. Abdominal distention, 63%

   2. Certain findings are fairly specific

      a. Constipation, 95%; LR+, 8.8

      b. Prior abdominal surgery, 94%; LR+, 11.5

      c. Abdominal distention, 89%; LR+, 5.7

   3. Certain combinations are insensitive (27–48%) but highly specific.

      a. Distention associated with any of the following highly suggestive (LR+ ≈ 10): increased bowel sounds, vomiting, constipation, or prior surgery

      b. Increased bowel sounds with prior surgery or vomiting also very suggestive of obstruction (LR+ of 11 and 8, respectively)

B. A CBC and electrolytes should be obtained: Anion gap acidosis suggests bowel infarction or sepsis.

Marked leukocytosis, left shift or anion gap acidosis in a patient with bowel obstruction is a *late* finding and suggests bowel infarction.

C. Plain radiography may show air-fluid levels and distention of large bowel (> 6 cm).

   1. 84% sensitive, 72% specific for presence of LBO (not etiology)

   2. Small bowel distention also occurs if ileocecal valve is incompetent.

D. Barium enema (water soluble) or colonoscopy

   1. Barium enema is highly accurate for LBO.

a. 96% sensitive, 98% specific

b. LR+ 48, LR– 0.04

2. Can determine etiology preoperatively (if patient stable)

3. Can exclude acute colonic pseudo-obstruction (distention of the cecum and colon without mechanical obstruction)

4. Colonoscopy can decompress pseudo-obstruction and prevent cecal perforation.

E. CT scan is also accurate in the diagnosis of LBO.

1. 91% sensitive, 91% specific

2. LR+ 10.1, LR– 0.1

## Treatment of LBO

A. Aggressive rehydration and monitoring of urinary output is vital.

B. Broad-spectrum antibiotics advised: 39% of patients have microorganisms in the mesenteric nodes

C. Surgery

D. For patients with sigmoid volvulus, and no evidence of infarction, sigmoidoscopy allows decompression and elective surgery at a later date to prevent recurrence.

1. Emergent indications: perforation or ischemia

2. Nonemergent indications: increasing distention, failure to resolve

# MAKING A DIAGNOSIS

3

After reviewing the plain films, you order a barium enema.

**Have you crossed a diagnostic threshold for the leading hypothesis, large bowel obstruction? Have you ruled out the active alternatives? Do other tests need to be done to exclude the alternative diagnoses?**

## Alternative Diagnosis: SBO

### Textbook Presentation

The presentation is similar to that for LBO with the exception that more patients have a history of prior abdominal surgery.

### Disease Highlights

A. Bowel obstruction accounts for 4% of patients with abdominal pain.

B. SBO accounts for 80% of all bowel obstructions.

C. Etiology

1. Adhesions present in 70% of cases

a. Usually postsurgical

b. 93% of patients with prior abdominal surgery have adhesions

c. Up to 14% of patients with prior surgery require readmission for adhesions over the next 10 years.

2. Malignant tumor 10–20%; usually metastatic. 39% of SBOs in patients with a prior malignancy are due to adhesions or benign causes.

3. Hernia (ventral, inguinal, or internal) 10%

4. IBD (with stricture) 5%

5. Radiation

6. Less common causes of SBO include gallstones, bezoars, and intussusception.

D. SBOs may be partial or complete.

1. Complete SBO

a. 20–40% progress to strangulation and infarction

b. Clinical signs do *not* allow for identification of strangulation prior to infarction: Fever, leukocytosis, and metabolic acidosis are late signs of strangulation and suggest infarction.

c. 50–75% of patients admitted for SBO require surgery

2. Partial SBO

a. Rarely progresses to strangulation or infarction

b. Characterized by continuing ability to pass stool or flatus (> 6–12 hours after symptom onset) or passage of contrast into cecum

c. Resolves spontaneously (without surgery) in 60–85% of patients

d. Enteroclysis (an air-contrast study of the small bowel) is test of choice.

e. CT scan only 48% sensitive for partial SBO

### Evidence-Based Diagnosis

A. Ideally, tests for SBO should identify obstruction *and* ischemia or infarction, if present (since ischemia and infarction are indications for emergent surgery rather than further observation.) Unfortunately, even tests that successfully predict SBO do not reliably determine whether there is ischemia and infarction.

B. See test characteristics of history and physical exam under LBO.

C. WBC may be normal even in presence of ischemia.

D. Plain radiographs may show ≥ two air-fluid levels or dilated loops of bowel proximal to obstruction (> 2.5 cm diameter of small bowel).

1. Sensitivity for obstruction 59–93%, specificity 83%

2. Rarely determines etiology

3. Complete obstruction is unlikely in patients with air in the colon or rectum

E. Ultrasound is seldom used for this indication but may be useful in pregnant patients.

F. CT scanning

1. Moderately sensitive at determining high-grade obstruction (80–93%).

a. Obstruction is suggested by a transition point between bowel proximal to the obstruction, which is dilated, and bowel distal to the obstruction, which is collapsed.

b. CT scanning should be performed prior to NG suction, which may decompress the proximal small bowel and thereby decreases the sensitivity of the CT scan for SBO.

2. May delineate etiology of obstruction

3. Test of choice to diagnose *SBO* (not ischemia)

4. Not reliably sensitive at determining the presence of ischemia and infarction (and the need for immediate surgery). Different studies have reported sensitivities ranging from 15% to 100% (specificity 85–94%).

 The absence of CT signs of ischemia in patients with SBO does not in fact rule out ischemia.

G. Small bowel series

1. Accurate in the diagnosis of SBO and useful to predict nonoperative resolution; 45–96% sensitive, 92–96% specific. (Spontaneous resolution likely in patients in whom contrast reaches the colon)

2. Unlike CT scanning, small bowel series cannot delineate etiology of SBO or demonstrate ischemic changes.

3. Typically used when CT scanning not diagnostic and concern for SBO remains

4. Water-soluble contrast and barium have been used

   a. Barium is superior because it is not diluted by intraluminal water.

   b. Barium can become inspissated in the colon and is contraindicated in LBO.

**Treatment**

A. Fluid resuscitation

1. Intravascular dehydration is often prominent due to decreased oral intake, vomiting, *and* third spacing of fluid within the bowel.

2. Monitor urinary output carefully.

B. Careful, frequent observation and repeated physical exam over the first 12–24 hours

C. NG suction

D. Broad-spectrum antibiotics (59% of patients have bacterial translocation to mesenteric lymph nodes)

E. Frequent plain radiographs and CBC

F. Indications for surgery include any of the following

1. Signs of ischemia (increased pain, fever, tenderness, peritoneal findings, acidosis, or worsening leukocytosis)

2. CT findings of infarction

3. SBO secondary to hernia

4. SBO clearly not secondary to adhesion (no prior surgery)

5. Some clinicians recommend surgery when bowel obstruction fails to resolve in 24 hours. Others suggest a small bowel study.

## CASE RESOLUTION

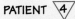

The barium enema reveals an obstructive apple core lesion in the sigmoid colon suggestive of carcinoma of the colon. Mr. J underwent surgical exploration, which confirmed an obstructing colonic mass. The mass was resected and a colostomy created. Pathologic evaluation revealed adenocarcinoma of the colon.

## CHIEF COMPLAINT

PATIENT 4

Mr. L is a 65-year-old man who arrives in the emergency department complaining of 1 hour of excruciating constant abdominal pain radiating to his flank. He has suffered 1 episode of vomiting and feels light headed. The emesis was yellow. He has moved his bowels once this morning. There is no change in his bowel habits, melena, or hematochezia. Nothing seems to make the pain better or worse. He was without any pain until this morning. His past medical history is remarkable for hypertension and tobacco use. On physical exam, he is diaphoretic and in obvious acute distress. Vital signs are BP, 110/65 mm Hg; pulse, 90 bpm; temperature, 37.0°C; RR, 20 breaths per minute. HEENT, cardiac, and pulmonary exams are all within normal limits. Abdominal exam reveals moderate diffuse tenderness, without rebound or guarding. Bowel sounds are present and hypoactive. Stool is guaiac negative.

At this point, what is the leading hypothesis, what are the active alternatives, and is there a must not miss diagnosis? Given this differential diagnosis, what tests should be ordered?

## PRIORITIZING THE DIFFERENTIAL DIAGNOSIS

Given Mr. L's extreme distress, life-threatening diagnoses must be considered carefully. The location of the pain is not terribly helpful in this case although the radiation of the pain to the flank raises the possibilities of renal colic, biliary colic, pancreatitis, or AAA. Clearly, AAA is a must not miss diagnosis. The acuity of the pain is consistent with renal colic, biliary colic, pancreatitis, AAA, or bowel obstruction (although the rapidity is somewhat unusual for bowel obstruction). Diverticular rupture can result in severe sudden onset of pain, although the pain is more often in the left lower quadrant (LLQ) than diffuse. PUD rarely causes such severe pain unless associated with perforation, and the abdominal exam does not suggest peritonitis.

Table 3–9 lists the differential diagnoses for Mr. L.

Mr. L has no history of renal stones or hematuria, gallstones, dark urine, or light stools. He has never had this pain before. He does not drink alcohol. On reexamination, orthostatic maneuvers reveal profound orthostatic hypotension. Supine BP and pulse were 110/65 mm Hg and 90 bpm. Upon standing his BP falls to 65/40 mm Hg

***Table 3–9.*** Diagnostic hypotheses for Mr. L.

| Diagnostic Hypotheses | Clinical Clues | Important Tests |
|---|---|---|
| **Leading Hypothesis** | | |
| Renal colic | Flank pain<br>Radiation to groin<br>Hematuria<br>Costovertebral angle<br>tenderness | Urinalysis<br>Renal CT |
| **Active Alternatives—Most Common** | | |
| Biliary colic | Episodic, crampy pain<br>Dark urine | Ultrasound |
| Diverticulitis | Left lower quadrant<br>pain (usually)<br>Diarrhea<br>Fever | CT scan |
| Pancreatitis | Alcohol abuse<br>Gallstones | Serum lipase |
| **Active Alternatives—Must Not Miss** | | |
| AAA | Orthostatic hypotension<br>Pulsatile abdominal mass<br>Decreased lower extremity<br>pulses | Abdominal<br>CT scan |

with a pulse of 140 bpm. He remains afebrile. Again, you find that he lacks rebound or guarding and is not particularly tender in the LLQ. He has moderate flank and back tenderness to percussion. His abdominal aorta cannot be palpated due to his abdominal girth. Lower extremity pulses are intact. Plain abdominal radiographs do not demonstrate free air.

 **Is the clinical information sufficient to make a diagnosis? If not, what other information do you need?**

The most dramatic and important physical finding is the presence of profound orthostatic hypotension. This suggests significant intravascular depletion and is a pivotal clinical clue. It is unlikely that dehydration is responsible for the profound orthostasis given the absence of significant emesis, diarrhea, or prolonged period of no oral intake. Therefore, the profound orthostasis suggests acute blood loss; either within the GI tract or intra-peritoneal hemorrhage. Large volume GI hemorrhage always exits the bowel quickly resulting in either hematemesis, melena, or hematochezia and is rarely subtle. Therefore, you are more concerned about intra-peritoneal hemorrhage. Causes of massive intra-peritoneal hemorrhage include rupture of an AAA, splenic rupture, or rupture of an ectopic pregnancy. The patient's history is most suggestive of AAA rupture. You revise your leading diagnosis to AAA rupture. You call for a stat vascular surgery consult.

 Orthostatic hypotension is always important. It significantly influences the differential diagnosis and the diagnostic and management decisions, and it may be marked despite a normal supine BP and pulse.

## Leading Hypothesis: AAA

### Textbook Presentation
Classically, patients are men with a history of hypertension who have the triad of severe abdominal pain, a pulsatile abdominal mass, and hypotension.

### Disease Highlights
A. 10,000 deaths per year in United States

B. Misdiagnosis (most commonly renal colic) occurs in 16% of cases.

C. Subtypes of AAA

1. Asymptomatic: Rupture rates rise as aneurysm increases in diameter
   a. AAA 5.5–6.5 cm: 10%/y
   b. AAA 6.5–7.0 cm: 20%/y
   c. AAA > 7 cm: 30%/y

2. Ruptured
   a. Hypotension is a late finding, and palpable mass is often not present.
   b. Mortality with rupture is 70–90%.
   c. Syncope may be present.
   d. Patient may live for days if rupture is contained.
   e. Rupture into the duodenum is a rare complication, is more common in patients with prior AAA graft, and may result in GI bleeding over weeks.

3. Symptomatic, contained
   a. Although rarely considered, some patients present non-emergently with symptomatic contained rupture of the abdominal aorta. Symptoms are primarily secondary to retroperitoneal hemorrhage and are occasionally present for weeks or even months.
   b. Manifestations include
      (1) Abdominal pain 83%
      (2) Flank or back pain 61%
      (3) Syncope 26%
      (4) Abdominal mass on careful exam 52% (only 18% had abdominal mass noted on routine abdominal exam)
      (5) Hypotension or orthostasis 48%
      (6) Leukocytosis (> 11,000/mcL) 70%
      (7) Anemia (unusual)

4. Inflammatory AAA
   a. Comprise about 5–10% of AAAs and usually occurs at a slightly younger age.
   b. Distinguishing characteristic is marked inflammation of aortic adventia
   c. Back pain or abdominal pain is usual presentation (80% of patients); rupture is rarely presenting manifestation.
   d. Symptoms of inflammation (fever, weight loss) present in 20–50% of patients)
   e. Erythrocyte sedimentation rate elevated in 40–90% of cases.
   f. CT or MRI reveal the aneurysm and marked thickening of the aortic wall. Periaortic fat stranding may be seen.

**g.** Therapy includes smoking cessation and repair of aneurysms ≥ 5.5 cm. Immunosuppressants (ie, corticosteroids) have been used.

**D.** Risk factors

**1.** Smoking is the most significant risk factor (OR 5).

**2.** Men are affected 4 to 5 times more often than women.

**3.** Family history of AAA (OR 4.3)

**4.** Increased age

**5.** Hypertension (OR 1.2)

### Evidence-Based Diagnosis

**A.** Physical exam is *not* sufficiently sensitive to rule out AAA.

**B.** Bruits do not contribute to diagnosis.

**C.** Sensitivity of *focused* exam for *asymptomatic* AAA is poor overall (39%) and only 76% among patients with large AAA (≥ 5 cm.) The sensitivity of the physical exam is less in obese patients.

**D.** Sensitivity of abdominal exam *in symptomatic AAA*

**1.** Abdominal pain, distention, and rupture all limit sensitivity.

**2.** Distention was reported in 52–100% in different series.

**3.** Palpable mass was found in 18%.

 A palpable mass is *unusual* in patients with a ruptured AAA.

**E.** Laboratory and radiologic tests

**1.** Bedside emergency ultrasound has been demonstrated to be highly accurate; sensitivity 96–100%, specificity 98–100%.

**2.** For screening, ultrasound is preferred; sensitivity 95%, specificity 100%.

**3.** Preoperative evaluation prior to repair of asymptomatic AAA may include CT scanning, CT angiography, or aortography.

### Treatment

**A.** For ruptured AAA, proceed directly to the operating room.

**B.** Asymptomatic AAA

**1.** Screening men aged 65–75 years with one-time ultrasound has been demonstrated to reduce mortality and be cost effective.

**2.** Although the relative risk reduction was 43%, the absolute reduction in AAA mortality is small (0.14%).

**3.** Operative mortality for elective repair was 3.1–4.6% and substantial operative morbidity occurs in 32% of patients.

**4.** The United States Preventive Services Task Force (USPSTF) recommends one-time screening with ultrasound for AAA in men 65 to 75 years old who have ever smoked cigarettes.

**a.** Repair is recommended when an aneurysm is ≥ 5.5 cm diameter or is tender or has increased in size by ≥ 1 cm in 1 year.

**(1)** Options include open surgical repair versus endovascular stent placement.

**(2)** 30-day mortality is lower with stent placement than open repair (1.7 vs 4.7%) but reinterventions are more common with stent placement.

**b.** For AAA 4.0–5.4 cm, monitor every 6 months with ultrasonography. One report suggested increasing the frequency to every 3 months in patients with aneurysms ≥ 5.0 cm.

**5.** Medical management includes smoking cessation, statin therapy, and blood pressure control.

## MAKING A DIAGNOSIS

 Further evaluation at this point depends on the index of suspicion. If AAA is very likely and the patient is unstable, many vascular surgeons proceed directly to the operating room without further studies in order to avoid the potential lethal delay of obtaining a CT scan. Bedside ultrasonography is a useful option if available. If AAA is less likely and the patient is stable, CT scanning is appropriate.

 **Have you crossed a diagnostic threshold for the leading hypothesis, AAA? Have you ruled out the active alternatives? Do other tests need to be done to exclude the alternative diagnoses?**

## Alternative Diagnosis: Nephrolithiasis

### Textbook Presentation

Patients typically experience rapid onset of excruciating back and flank pain, which may radiate to the abdomen or groin. The intensity of the pain is often dramatic as patients writhe and move about constantly in an unsuccessful attempt to get comfortable. The pain may be associated with nausea, vomiting, or dysuria.

Abdominal *tenderness* is unusual in patients with nephrolithiasis and should raise the possibility of other diagnoses.

### Disease Highlights

**A.** Incidence: Symptomatic stones develop in 5% of people in the United States

**1.** 50% recurrence at 10 years

**2.** Men affected 2 to 3 times more often than women

**3.** Positive family history (RR 2.6)

**B.** Etiology

**1.** Caoxalate stones 75%

**2.** Calcium phosphate stones ($CaPO_4$) 5%

**3.** Uric acid stones 5–10%

**4.** Struvite stones ($MgNH_4PO_4$) 5–15%

**5.** Other: cystine and indinavir stones

**C.** Pathophysiology

**1.** Stones form when the concentration of salts (ie, calcium, oxalate, or uric acid) becomes supersaturated in the urine resulting in precipitation and crystallization.

2. Supersaturation is secondary to a combination of increased urinary salt excretion combined with inadequate diluting urinary volume. Numerous mechanisms can contribute to an increase in urinary mineral excretion including:

   a. Calcium: idiopathic hypercalcuria, primary hyperparathyroidism, immobilization, excessive sodium intake (which increases calcium excretion), systemic acidosis, hypocitraturia (a factor in 20–60% of calcium stones), and excessive vitamin D supplementation

   b. Uric acid: Excessive dietary purines, myeloproliferative disorders, uricosuric agents (for the treatment of gout), and metabolic syndrome. Low urine pH also contributes to uric acid stone formation. Hyperuricosuria can lead to uric acid stones or calcium stones due to heterogeneous ossification.

   c. Oxalate: Causes include excessive dietary oxalates (rhubarb, spinach, chocolate, nuts, vitamin C) and increased oxalate absorption (fat malabsorption complexes calcium and leads to increased oxalate absorption and excretion).

3. In some patients, a decrease in urinary stone inhibitors (urinary citrate) also contribute to stone formation.

4. Infection with urea splitting organisms (ie, *Proteus*) plays a key role in the formation of struvite stones ($MgNH_4PO_4$).

5. Renal colic develops when stones dislodge from the kidney and obstruct urinary flow.

D. Complications

1. Ureteral obstruction

2. Pyelonephritis

3. Sepsis

4. Renal failure is rare, occurring in patients with bilateral obstruction or obstruction of a solitary functioning kidney.

### Evidence-Based Diagnosis

A. The evaluation is directed at establishing the diagnosis of nephrolithiasis *and* its underlying etiology so that measures to prevent its recurrence can be implemented.

B. Establishing the diagnosis

1. Hematuria is present in 80% of patients, LR– is 0.57.

 The absence of hematuria does not rule out nephrolithiasis.

2. Radiographs (kidneys, ureters, bladder [KUB]) or ultrasound are not sufficiently sensitive to rule out nephrolithiasis (sensitivity 29–68% and 32–57%, respectively).

3. Noncontrast helical renal CT is the test of choice.

   a. Sensitivity 95%; specificity 98%

   b. LR+, 48; LR–, 0.05

   c. Importantly, CT scan revealed alternative diagnoses in 33% of patients *clinically* diagnosed with a first episode of nephrolithiasis.

C. Evaluation of documented nephrolithiasis

1. All patients should have a urinalysis and culture and basic serum chemistries, including several measurements of serum calcium.

2. A more comprehensive evaluation, including several 24-hour urine specimens for analysis of calcium, oxalate, uric acid, sodium, creatinine and citrate as well as submission of retrieved stones for chemical analysis, is recommended for patients with recurrent stones. Some experts recommend this for patients with their first stone.

### Treatment

A. Pain control

1. NSAIDS

   a. Treat pain and diminish spasm

   b. Create less dependence than opioids

   c. To be avoided 3 days before lithotripsy due to antiplatelet effects

2. Opioids

B. Hydration (oral if tolerated, otherwise IV)

C. Sepsis or renal failure

1. Necessitate emergent drainage (via percutaneous nephrostomy tube or ureteral stent)

2. For sepsis, broad-spectrum IV antibiotics to cover gram-negative organisms and enterococcus should be administered

D. Stone passage

1. Nifedipine and tamsulosin have been demonstrated to significantly increase the likelihood of stone passage by 65%.

2. Lithotripsy or ureteroscopy are used to remove persistent ureteral stones.

E. Secondary prevention

1. General measures include increasing fluid intake ($\geq 2$ L/d), and moderating sodium and protein intake.

2. More specific management (ie, dietary modification) is complex and depends on the underlying etiology of the patient's nephrolithiasis.

3. Thiazide diuretics decrease urinary calcium excretion (especially when combined with potassium supplementation) and can be useful in patients with recurrent nephrolithiasis and hypercalciuria.

4. Allopurinol can be useful in patients with nephrolithiasis and hyperuricosuria.

## Alternative Diagnosis: Diverticulitis

### Textbook Presentation

Patients typically complain of a constant gradually increasing LLQ abdominal pain, usually present for several days. Fever and diarrhea or constipation are often present. Guarding and rebound may be seen.

### Disease Highlights

A. Diverticula are outpouchings of the colonic wall that may be asymptomatic (diverticulosis), become inflamed (diverticulitis), or hemorrhage.

B. Diverticulosis

1. Develops in 5–10% of patients aged > 45 years, 50% in persons aged > 60 years, and 80% in those aged > 85 years.

2. Low-fiber diets are believed to cause diverticula by decreasing stool bulk, resulting in increased intraluminal pressure creating diverticula as the mucosa and submucosa herniate

through weakness in the colonic wall where vessels penetrate.

C. Diverticulitis

1. Develops secondary to microscopic or frank perforation of diverticula.

2. 85–95% of diverticulitis occurs in sigmoid or descending colon

3. Complications of diverticulitis

   a. Abscess

   b. Peritonitis

   c. Sepsis

   d. Colonic obstruction

   e. Fistula formation (colovesicular fistula most common)

4. Simultaneous diverticular hemorrhage and *diverticulitis* are unusual; diverticular hemorrhage is discussed in Chapter 17, GI Bleeding.

### Evidence-Based Diagnosis (Diverticulitis)

A. Neither fever nor leukocytosis are very sensitive for diverticulitis or diverticular abscess.

1. In patients with uncomplicated diverticulitis, only 45% had temperature of ≥ 38.0°C or WBC > 11,000/mcL.

2. In patients with diverticular abscess, only 64% of patients had temperature of ≥ 38.0°C and 62% had WBC > 11,000/mcL.

B. Plain radiographs may demonstrate free air or obstruction.

C. CT scan is test of choice.

1. May demonstrate diverticula, thickened bowel wall, pericolonic fat stranding, or abscess formation

2. 93-97% sensitive

3. Colon cancer can lead to bowel wall thickening and perforation and be difficult to distinguish from diverticulitis.

D. Acute colonoscopy is not advised due to concern of perforation.

### Treatment

A. Outpatient management is appropriate for patients with a mild attack (ie, patients without marked fever or marked leukocytosis, pain manageable with oral analgesics, tolerating oral intake) and without significant comorbidities, immunocompromise, or advanced age.

1. Ciprofloxacin and metronidazole for 7–10 days

2. Liquid diet

3. High-fiber diet after attack resolves

4. Follow-up colonoscopy (see below)

B. Moderate to severe attack (unable to tolerate oral intake, more severe pain) necessitates inpatient treatment.

1. Broad-spectrum IV antibiotics

2. No oral intake

3. CT guided drainage for abscesses > 5 cm

4. Emergent surgery is recommended in patients with

   a. Frank peritonitis

   b. Uncontrolled sepsis

   c. Clinical deterioration despite medical management

   d. Obstruction or large abscesses that cannot be drained or are contaminated with frank fecal contents

5. The threshold for surgery should be lower in immunocompromised patients.

6. High-fiber diet once the attack has resolved

7. Follow-up colonoscopy is advised 4–6 weeks after resolution of symptoms to exclude carcinoma in patients without a recent colonoscopy. (Colon cancer is found in 17% of patients thought to have complicated diverticular disease.)

## CASE RESOLUTION

**4**

The surgical resident evaluates the patient and agrees with your concern about an AAA. He orders a stat CT scan and contacts his attending. The attending immediately evaluates the patient and redirects the patient directly to the operating room bypassing the CT scan. Surgery reveals a leaking AAA that ruptures during the surgery. The aorta is cross clamped, repaired, and the patient is stabilized.

## REFERENCES

Andersson RE, Hugander AP, Ghazi SH et al. Diagnostic value of disease history, clinical presentation, and inflammatory parameters of appendicitis. World J Surg. 1999;23(2):133–40.

Cardall T, Glasser J, Guss DA. Clinical value of the total white blood cell count and temperature in the evaluation of patients with suspected appendicitis. Acad Emerg Med. 2004;11(10):1021–7.

Dholakia K, Pitchumoni CS, Agarwal N. How often are liver function tests normal in acute biliary pancreatitis? J Clin Gastroenterol. 2004;38(1):81–3.

Frossard JL, Steer ML, Pastor CM. Acute pancreatitis. Lancet. 2008;371(9607):143–52.

Gan SI, Romagnuolo J. Admission hematocrit: a simple, useful and early predictor of severe pancreatitis. Dig Dis Sci. 2004;49(11-12):1946–52.

Gurleyik G, Emir S, Kilicoglu G, Arman A, Saglam A. Computed tomography severity index, APACHE II score, and serum CRP concentration for predicting the severity of acute pancreatitis. JOP. 2005;6(6):562–7.

Ha M, MacDonald RD. Impact of CT scan in patients with first episode of suspected nephrolithiasis. J Emerg Med. 2004;27(3):225–31.

Huguier M, Barrier A, Boelle PY, Houry S, Lacaine F. Ischemic colitis. Am J Surg. 2006;192(5):679–84.

Jacobs DO. Clinical practice. Diverticulitis. N Engl J Med. 2007;357(20):2057–66.

Lederle FA, Simel DL. The rational clinical examination. Does this patient have abdominal aortic aneurysm? JAMA. 1999;281(1):77–82.

Liu CL, Fan ST, Lo CM et al. Clinico-biochemical prediction of biliary cause of acute pancreatitis in the era of endoscopic ultrasonography. Aliment Pharmacol Ther. 2005;22(5):423–31.

Mayer EA. Clinical practice. Irritable bowel syndrome. N Engl J Med. 2008;358(16):1692–9.

Park CJ, Jang MK, Shin WG et al. Can we predict the development of ischemic colitis among patients with lower abdominal pain? Dis Colon Rectum. 2007;50(2):232–8.

Rao PM, Rhea JT, Novelline RA, Mostafavi AA, McCabe CJ. Effect of computed tomography of the appendix on treatment of patients and use of hospital resources. N Engl J Med. 1998;338(3):141–6.

Shea JA, Berlin JA, Escarce JJ et al. Revised estimates of diagnostic test sensitivity and specificity in suspected biliary tract disease. Arch Intern Med. 1994;154(22):2573–81.

Snyder BK, Hayden SR. Accuracy of leukocyte count in the diagnosis of acute appendicitis. Ann Emerg Med. 1999;33(5):565–74.

Tenner S, Dubner H, Steinberg W. Predicting gallstone pancreatitis with laboratory parameters: a meta-analysis. Am J Gastroenterol. 1994;89(10):1863–6.

Zakko SF, Afdhal NH. Clinical features and diagnosis of acute cholecystitis. In: UpToDate; 2007.

Summary table of abdominal pain by location.

| Location | Differential Diagnosis | Quality and Frequency | Radiation and Associated Symptoms | Clinical Clues |
|---|---|---|---|---|
| RUQ | Biliary disease | Obstructive Episodic | Back, right shoulder; N & V | Postprandial or nocturnal pain Dark urine |
| | Pancreatitis | See "Epigastrium" below | | |
| | Renal colic: Usually flank pain | Obstructive Episodic | Groin; N & V | Hematuria (usually microscopic) Writhing, unable to get comfortable |
| LUQ | Splenic infarct or rupture | Constant | Left shoulder pain | Endocarditis, trauma, orthostatic hypotension, shoulder pain |
| Epigastrium | Peptic ulcer | Hunger like, intermittent, gradual changes | Back; early satiety, | Melena, history of NSAIDs; Food may increase or decrease pain |
| | Pancreatitis | Boring, constant | Back; N & V | Worse supine; history of alcohol abuse or gallstones |
| | Biliary disease | See above | | |
| Diffuse periumbilical | Appendicitis | Steady, worsening; Migrates to RLQ | Groin; Occasionally back; N & V anorexia | Migration and progression No prior similar episodes |
| | Bowel Obstruction | Obstructive | N & V anorexia | Inability to pass stool or flatus, prior surgery |
| | Mesenteric ischemia | Severe | Weight loss | Out of proportion to exam, brought on by food, bruit |
| | AAA | Excruciating | Back | Hypotension, syncope or pulsatile abdominal mass |
| | Irritable bowel syndrome | Crampy, recurring | Intermittent diarrhea, constipation | Absence of weight loss or alarm symptoms, recurring nature of symptoms |
| RLQ | Appendicitis | See "Diffuse periumbilical" above | | |
| | Diverticulitis | Usually LLQ; see below | | |
| | Cecal volvulus | Similar to bowel obstruction; see above | | |
| | Ovarian disease | Differential includes ovarian torsion, Mittelschmerz, ectopic pregnancy and PID. | | |
| LLQ | Diverticulitis | Persistent, increasing | Back; Fever, N & V, diarrhea | May have prior episodes, localized tenderness |
| | Ovarian disease | See above | | |
| | Sigmoid Volvulus | Similar to bowel obstructions; see above | | |

AAA, abdominal aortic aneurysm; LLQ, left lower quadrant; LUQ, left upper quadrant; NSAIDs, nonsteroidal antiinflammatory drugs; N & V, nausea and vomiting; PID, pelvic inflammatory disease; RLQ, right lower quadrant; RUQ, right upper quadrant.

# I have a patient with an acid-base abnormality. How do I determine the cause?

## CHIEF COMPLAINT

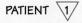

PATIENT 1

Mr. L is a 42-year-old man who complains of weakness, anorexia, abdominal pain, and vomiting. Laboratory studies demonstrate a $HCO_3^-$ of 6 mEq/L.

What is the differential diagnosis of acid-base disorders? How would you frame the differential?

## CONSTRUCTING A DIFFERENTIAL DIAGNOSIS

Listed below are the steps to analyze an acid-base disorder.

### Step 1: Generate Clinical Hypotheses

A. Each clinical scenario suggests a few possible acid-base disorders.
B. The first step considers those possibilities before analyzing the laboratory results.

### Step 2: Check the pH

A. pHs < 7.4 indicates the *primary* disorder is an acidosis.
B. pHs > 7.4 indicates the *primary* disorder is an alkalosis.

### Step 3: Determine Whether the Primary Disorder Is Due to a Metabolic or Respiratory Process

A. Check $HCO_3^-$ and $PaCO_2$
B. $CO_2 + H_2O \Leftrightarrow H_2CO_3 \Leftrightarrow HCO_3^- + H^+$; therefore
C. $HCO_3^-$ changes drive pH as follows:
   1. Increased $HCO_3^-$ drives the reaction to left: This consumes $H^+$ which raises the pH, resulting in a metabolic alkalosis.
   2. Decreased $HCO_3^-$ drives the reaction to the right: This increases $H^+$ which lowers the pH, resulting in a metabolic acidosis. This occurs in two situations:
      a. Processes that produce $H^+$ ion (and consume $HCO_3^-$) (ie, ketoacidosis, lactic acidosis)
      b. Processes that lose $HCO_3^-$ (ie, diarrhea)
D. $PaCO_2$ changes drive pH as follows:
   1. Increased $PaCO_2$ drives reaction to right: This increases $H^+$ which lowers the pH, resulting in a respiratory acidosis.

   2. Decreased $PaCO_2$ drives reaction to left: This decreases $H^+$ which raises pH, resulting in a respiratory alkalosis.

### Step 4: Calculate Whether Compensation Is Appropriate

A. The acid-base system attempts to maintain homeostasis. Alterations in one system (respiratory or metabolic) trigger compensatory changes in the other system to minimize the impact on pH.
B. Formulas predict the expected degree of compensation (Table 4–1).
C. Compensation that is greater or less than expected suggests that an *additional* disease process is affecting the compensating system.

### Step 5: Calculate the Anion Gap

A. Anion gap = $Na^+ - (HCO_3^- + Cl^-)$
B. An increased anion gap suggests that an anion gap metabolic acidosis is present.

Always check the anion gap. An elevated gap suggests an anion gap metabolic acidosis even when the $HCO_3^-$ is above normal.

### Step 6: Reach Final Diagnosis

Figure 4–1 outlines the stepwise approach to acid-base disorders.

### Differential Diagnosis of Acid-Base Disorders

A. Metabolic acidosis
   1. Distinguishing between the 2 types of acidoses **anion gap acidosis** (associated with a elevated anion gap) and the non-**anion gap acidosis** (associated with an normal anion gap) is *pivotal*.
      a. Anion gap metabolic acidosis
         (1) Occurs when an acid is produced and the associated unmeasured anion accumulates (ie, ketones, lactate, sulfates, phosphates, or organic anions), increasing the anion gap.
         (2) Affected by the serum albumin level
            (a) Albumin is negatively charged so that lower serum albumin levels are associated with a lower anion gap.

*Table 4–1.* Compensation in acid-base disorders.[1,2]

| Primary Disorder | Duration | Expected Compensation |
|---|---|---|
| Metabolic acidosis | Acute/Chronic | $PaCO_2 \downarrow$ 1.2 mm Hg per 1 mEq/L $\downarrow HCO_3^-$ (To a minimum $PaCO_2$ of 10–15 mm Hg) |
| Metabolic alkalosis | Acute/Chronic | $PaCO_2 \uparrow$ 0.7 mm Hg per 1 mEq/L $\uparrow HCO_3^-$ |
| Respiratory acidosis | Acute | $HCO_3^- \uparrow$ 1 mEq/L per 10 mm Hg $\uparrow PaCO_2$ |
| | Chronic | $HCO_3^- \uparrow$ 3.5 mEq/L per 10 mm Hg $\uparrow PaCO_2$ |
| Respiratory alkalosis | Acute | $HCO_3^- \downarrow$ 2 mEq/L per 10 mm Hg $\downarrow PaCO_2$ |
| | Chronic | $HCO_3^- \downarrow$ 4 mEq/L per 10 mm Hg $\downarrow PaCO_2$ |

[1]Metabolic compensation is slower than respiratory compensation and becomes more complete with time.
[2]Normal baseline is assumed to be $PaCO_2$ 40 mm Hg, $HCO_3^-$ 24 mEq/L.
Reproduced, with permission, from the McGraw-Hill Companies. Rose BD. *Clinical Physiology of Acid-Base and Electrolyte Disorders,* 2000.

    **(b)** The expected drop in the normal value for the anion gap is 2.5 mEq/L for every 1 g/dL drop in the serum albumin (below 4.4 g/dL).

  **b.** Non-anion gap metabolic acidosis

    **(1)** Occurs when $HCO_3^-$ is lost in the urine or stool.

    **(2)** Since no unmeasured anion accumulates, the anion gap is normal.

    **(3)** The normal anion gap is due to negatively charged proteins such as albumin, phosphates, and sulfates.

    **(4)** The upper limit of normal varies between institutions due to differing technologies.

      **(a)** Although 12 ± 4 is often sited as an ideal cutoff, in some institutions, a normal anion gap is only 7–9 mEq/L.

      **(b)** The reference range at the institution performing the tests should be used.

**2.** Etiologies of metabolic acidosis

  **a.** Anion gap acidoses

    **(1)** Ketoacidosis

      **(a)** Diabetic ketoacidosis (DKA)

      **(b)** Starvation ketoacidosis

      **(c)** Alcoholic ketoacidosis

    **(2)** Lactic acidosis

      **(a)** Secondary to any impairment of aerobic metabolism

      **(b)** The differential diagnosis of lactic acidosis includes any disease that interrupts oxygen transport from the environment to the cell's mitochondria. Common causes include hypoxia or hypotension (due to cardiogenic shock, septic shock, or hypovolemic shock) (Table 4–2).

    **(3)** Uremia (associated with sulfate and phosphate accumulation)

    **(4)** Toxin, drugs, and miscellaneous

      **(a)** Salicylate toxicity

      **(b)** Methanol ingestion

      **(c)** Ethylene glycol ingestion

      **(d)** Rhabdomyolysis

      **(e)** D-Lactic acidosis

  **b.** Non-anion gap metabolic acidosis

    **(1)** Diarrhea

    **(2)** Renal tubular acidosis (RTA) (type IV most common in adults)

    **(3)** Carbonic anhydrase inhibitor

*Table 4–2.* Differential diagnosis of lactic acidosis.

| Pathophysiology of Disorder | Examples |
|---|---|
| **Common Causes** | |
| **Hypoxemia** | Lung disease (eg, pneumonia, COPD, pulmonary embolism), CHF |
| **Shock** (inadequate tissue perfusion; demand > supply) | Cardiogenic shock<br>Hypovolemic shock<br>Septic shock<br>Regional blood flow obstruction (eg, mesenteric ischemia) |
| **Less Common Causes** | |
| Low environmental oxygen | High altitude |
| Severe anemia | |
| Low oxygen saturation ($SaO_2$) (despite normal $PaO_2$) | Carbon monoxide poisoning |
| Cellular inability to utilize oxygen | Cyanide poisoning |
| Increased demand | Intense anaerobic activity<br>Seizures |

CHF, congestive heart failure; COPD, chronic obstructive pulmonary disease.

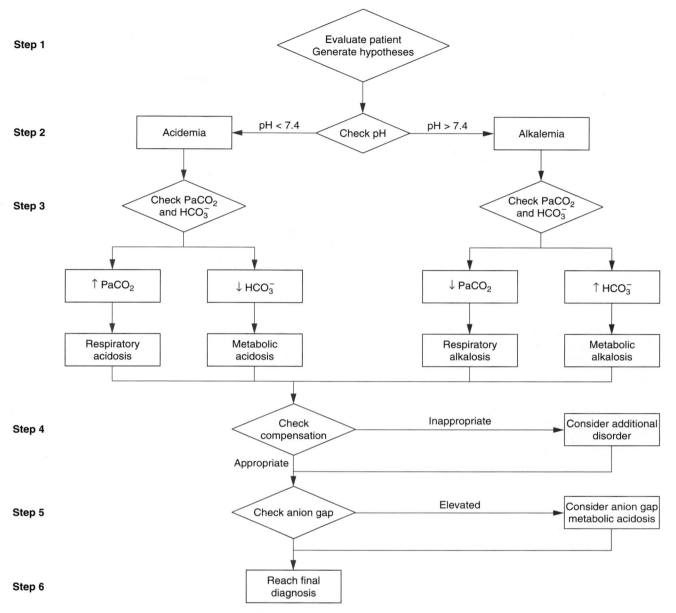

*Figure 4–1.* Stepwise approach to the diagnosis of acid-base disorders.

    **(4)** Dilutional (large volume normal saline administration)

    **(5)** Early renal failure

**B.** Metabolic alkalosis: etiologies

  **1.** Vomiting or nasogastric drainage

  **2.** Volume depletion

    **a.** Diuretics

    **b.** Vomiting

  **3.** Hypokalemia

  **4.** Increased mineralocorticoid activity

    **a.** Primary hyperaldosteronism

    **b.** Hypercortisolism

    **c.** Excessive licorice ingestion

**C.** Respiratory acidosis

  **1.** Any process that participates in normal ventilation (from brain to brainstem, spinal cord, nerve, neuromuscular junction, muscle, chest wall, or lung) can be deranged and cause ventilatory failure and respiratory acidosis.

  **2.** Etiologies of respiratory acidosis

    **a.** Brain

      **(1)** Stroke

      **(2)** Drugs and intoxicants

      **(3)** Hemorrhage

      **(4)** Trauma

      **(5)** Sleep apnea

    **b.** Brainstem: herniation

c. Spinal cord
   (1) Trauma
   (2) Amyotrophic lateral sclerosis
   (3) Polio
d. Nerve: Guillain-Barré syndrome
e. Neuromuscular junction: Myasthenia gravis
f. Chest wall or muscle
   (1) Flail chest
   (2) Muscular dystrophy
g. Pleural disease
   (1) Effusions
   (2) Pneumothorax
h. Lung diseases are the most common etiology.
   (1) Chronic obstructive pulmonary disease (COPD)
   (2) Asthma
   (3) Pulmonary edema
   (4) Pneumonia

D. Respiratory alkalosis: etiologies
   1. Hypoxemia
   2. Pulmonary disorders (via both hypoxic and vagal mechanisms)
      a. Pneumonia
      b. Asthma
      c. Pulmonary embolism
      d. Pulmonary edema
      e. Interstitial lung disease
      f. Mechanical ventilation
   3. Extrapulmonary disorders
      a. Anxiety
      b. Pain
      c. Fever
      d. Pregnancy
      e. CNS insult
      f. Drugs (salicylates, nicotine, catecholamines)
      g. Cirrhosis

---

Mr. L reports that he has had diabetes since he was 10 years old. His diabetes has been complicated by peripheral vascular disease requiring a below the knee amputation and laser surgeries for retinopathy. Two days ago, he began experiencing nausea and some vomiting. He continued to take his insulin. Physical exam reveals supine BP of 90/50 mm Hg and pulse of 100 bpm. Upon standing, his vital signs are BP, 60/30 mm Hg; pulse, 150 bpm; RR, 24 breaths per minute; and temperature, 37.0°C. Retinal exam reveals dot-blot hemorrhages and multiple laser scars. Lungs are clear to percussion and auscultation. Cardiac exam reveals a regular rate and rhythm with a grade I/VI systolic murmur at the upper left sternal border. Abdominal exam is soft and nontender. Stool is guaiac-negative. Lab studies reveal $Na^+$, 138 mEq/L; $K^+$, 6.2 mEq/L; $HCO_3^-$, 6 mEq/L; $Cl^-$, 100 mEq/L; BUN, 40 mg/dL;

creatinine, 1.8 mg/dL; glucose, 389 mg/dL; WBC, 10,500/mcL; Hct, 42%; ALT (SGPT), AST (SGOT), and lipase are normal.

 At this point what is the leading hypothesis, what are the active alternatives, and is there a must not miss diagnosis? Given this differential diagnosis, what tests should be ordered?

## PRIORITIZING THE DIFFERENTIAL DIAGNOSIS

Although an arterial pH has not yet been obtained, the patient's very low $HCO_3^-$ strongly suggests a metabolic acidosis.

### Step 1: Generate Clinical Hypotheses

The history of childhood-onset diabetes mellitus strongly suggests insulin-dependent diabetes mellitus. This form of diabetes is associated with total or near total insulin deficiency increasing the risk of DKA. This is the leading hypothesis. Active alternative hypotheses include type IV RTA (a non-anion gap acidosis), which is common in patients with long-standing diabetes and renal insufficiency. Yet, another possibility is renal failure with uremic acidosis secondary to long-standing diabetes. Finally, lactic acidosis from sepsis is a "must not miss diagnosis" that should always be considered in sick patients with metabolic acidosis. (The hypotheses are listed in Table 4–3).

### Step 2: Check the pH

ABG: pH of 7.15, $PaO_2$ of 80 mm Hg, and $PaCO_2$ of 20 mm Hg. The low pH confirms that the primary disorder is an acidosis.

### Step 3: Determine Whether the Primary Disorder Is Due to a Metabolic or Respiratory Process

$HCO_3^- = 6$ mEq/L and $PaCO_2 = 20$ mm Hg.

A low $HCO_3^-$ is associated with metabolic acidosis, which drives the pH down whereas a low $PaCO_2$ drives the pH up (see above). Since the patient's pH is low (acidemic) the primary disorder must be a metabolic acidosis.

### Step 4: Calculate Whether Compensation Is Appropriate

As shown in Table 4–1 the expected compensation for a metabolic acidosis is the $PaCO_2$ drops by 1.2 mm Hg per 1 mEq/L fall in $HCO_3^-$. The patient's $HCO_3^-$ is 6 mEq/L (normal is 24 mEq/L),

*Table 4–3.* Diagnostic hypotheses for Mr. L.

| Diagnostic Hypothesis | Clinical Clues | Important Tests |
|---|---|---|
| **Leading Hypothesis** | | |
| Diabetic ketoacidosis (DKA) | History of insulin-dependent diabetes mellitus<br>Noncompliance with insulin<br>Precipitating illness (eg, infection or stress) | Increased anion gap<br>Increased serum or urine ketones<br>Tests to identify precipitant (urinalysis, chest radiograph, ECG, lipase, abdominal imaging as indicated) |
| **Active Alternatives—Most Common** | | |
| Uremic acidosis | Oliguria | Elevated BUN, creatinine, and anion gap<br>Elevated $FE_{Na}$<br>Urinalysis<br>Renal ultrasound |
| Type IV renal tubular acidosis | Long-standing diabetes mellitus<br>Nonanion gap acidosis<br>Hyperkalemia | Basic metabolic panel |
| **Active Alternatives—Must Not Miss** | | |
| Lactic acidosis from sepsis | Fever<br>Rigors<br>Urinary frequency<br>Dysuria<br>Cough<br>Diarrhea<br>Abdominal pain | Elevated WBC, anion gap, and serum lactate<br>Urinalysis<br>Chest radiograph (imaging as indicated)<br>Blood cultures |

$FE_{Na}$, fractional excretion of sodium.

which is an 18 mEq/L fall from normal. The $PaCO_2$ should fall by $1.2 \times 18 = 21.6$ mm Hg. Since the normal $PaCO_2$ is approximately 40 mm Hg, we would expect the $PaCO_2$ to be approximately $40 - 21.6 \approx 18$. The actual $PaCO_2$ is close to the predicted value suggesting that respiratory compensation is indeed appropriate. Therefore, Mr. L is suffering from a metabolic acidosis with appropriate respiratory compensation.

## Step 5: Calculate the Anion Gap

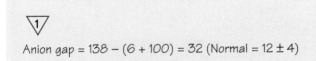

Anion gap = 138 − (6 + 100) = 32 (Normal = 12 ± 4)

Clearly, Mr. L is suffering from an anion gap metabolic acidosis. This excludes RTA and focuses our attention on the remaining possibilities of DKA, lactic acidosis from sepsis, or uremia.

Is the clinical information sufficient to make a diagnosis? If not, what other information do you need?

## Leading Hypothesis: DKA

### Textbook Presentation

DKA often begins with an acute illness (ie, pneumonia, urinary tract infection, myocardial infarction [MI]) in a type 1 diabetic.

Patients often complain of symptoms related to hyperglycemia (polyuria, polydipsia, and polyphagia) and to the precipitating illness (eg, fever, cough, dysuria, chest pain). Nonspecific complaints are common (nausea, vomiting, abdominal pain, and weakness). Patients are profoundly dehydrated and exhibit orthostatic changes or frank hypotension. Confusion, lethargy, and coma may occur secondary to dehydration, hyperglycemia, acidosis, or the underlying precipitating event.

### Disease Highlights

A. Occurs primarily in patients with complete or near complete insulin deficiency

   1. Type 1 autoimmune insulin-dependent diabetes mellitus

   2. DKA occasionally occurs in patients with type 2 diabetes mellitus

      a. Precipitants include

         (1) Severe stress

         (2) Marked hyperglycemia that may transiently impair insulin secretion

      b. Many such patients do not require lifelong insulin for management of their diabetes.

   3. Diabetes secondary to severe chronic pancreatitis and near complete islet cell obliteration

B. Incidence is 4.6–8.0 cases/1000 person years in patients with diabetes

C. Precipitated by low insulin levels or a rise in insulin's counter-regulatory hormones (cortisol, epinephrine, glucagon, and growth hormone), or both.

1. Most common precipitants
   a. New-onset type 1 diabetes mellitus
   b. Noncompliance with insulin
   c. Infection (Urinary tract infections and pneumonia are most common. Patients may be afebrile.)
2. Other precipitants
   a. Other infections
   b. MI
   c. Cerebrovascular accident
   d. Acute pancreatitis
   e. Pulmonary embolism
   f. GI hemorrhage
   g. Severe emotional stress
   h. Drugs (eg, corticosteroids, thiazides, cocaine)
3. The precipitant is the most frequent cause of mortality in DKA.

D. Pathogenesis: A *marked* decrease in insulin levels together with an increase in counterregulatory hormones lead to the following events:

1. Hyperglycemia
   a. Reduced glucose uptake by cells leads to hyperglycemia.
   b. Increased hepatic glycogenolysis and gluconeogenesis augment hyperglycemia.
   c. Glucosuria helps prevent extreme hyperglycemia (> 500–600 mg/dL).
   d. More extreme hyperglycemia occurs if urinary output falls.
2. Ketoacidosis
   a. Marked insulin deficiency increases acetyl CoA production within liver.
   b. Massive production of acetyl CoA overwhelms Krebs cycle resulting in ketone production and ketonemia (primarily β hydroxybutyric acid and to a lesser extent acetoacetic acid).
   c. Ketonemia leads to anion gap metabolic acidosis.
3. Volume depletion: Ketonemia and hyperglycemia result in osmotic diuresis, which results in profound dehydration and typical fluid losses of 3–6 L.
4. Hypokalemia
   a. The osmotic diuresis also causes significant potassium losses.
   b. Dehydration-induced hyperaldosteronism aggravates potassium loss.
   c. Typical potassium deficit is 3–5 mEq/kg body weight.
5. Hyperkalemia
   a. Despite the total body potassium deficit *hyper*kalemia is frequent.
   b. The etiology is multifactorial.
      (1) Insulin normally drives glucose *and potassium* into the cells. Insulin deficiency causes hyperkalemia.
      (2) Plasma hypertonicity drives water and potassium out of the cells and into the intravascular compartment accentuating the hyperkalemia.
      (3) Acidosis shifts potassium out of cells, aggravating *hyperkalemia* despite the total body potassium deficit.

6. Hyponatremia: Hyperglycemia leads to an osmotic shift of water from the intracellular space to intravascular space, resulting in hyponatremia.

E. Mortality rate of DKA is 5–15%. Risk factors for death include:
1. Severe coexistent disease (adjusted OR 16.3)
2. pH < 7.0 at presentation (adjusted OR 8.7)
3. > 50 units of insulin required in first 12 hours (adjusted OR 7.9)
4. Glucose > 300 mg/dL after 12 hours (adjusted OR 8.3)
5. Depressed mental status after 24 hours (adjusted OR 8.6)
6. Fever (axillary temperature ≥ 38.0°C) after 24 hours (adjusted OR 5.8)
7. Increasing age
   a. Mortality rate < 1.25% in persons younger than 55 years
   b. Mortality rate of 11.8% in persons older than 55 years

### Evidence-Based Diagnosis

A. Diagnostic criteria established by the American Diabetes Association (ADA)
1. Glucose > 250 mg/dL
2. pH ≤ 7.3
3. $HCO_3^- ≤ 18$ mEq/L
4. Positive serum ketones

B. Signs and symptoms
1. Polyuria and increased thirst are common.
2. Lethargy and obtundation may be seen with markedly increased effective osmolality (> 320 mOsm/L)
   a. Effective osmolality can be calculated:
      (1) $(2 × Na^+) + Glucose/18$[1]
      (2) That is, $Na^+$ of 140 mEq/L and glucose of 720 mg/dL = osmolality of 320 mOsm/L
   b. Consider neurologic insult (ie, cerebrovascular accident, drug intoxication) if neurologic changes are present in patients with a serum osmolality < 320 mOsm/L or if the neurologic abnormalities fail to resolve with therapy.
3. Abdominal pain
   a. Present in 50–75% of DKA cases
   b. May be secondary to the DKA or another process precipitating DKA (ie, appendicitis, pancreatitis, cholecystitis, abscess)
   c. Abdominal pain is increasingly common with increasing severity of DKA (Table 4–4).

 Always consider an intra-abdominal cause of abdominal pain in patients with DKA, especially if the abdominal pain persists, occurs in patients with mild acidosis ($HCO_3^- > 10$ mEq/L), or in patients older than 40 years.

---

[1]Normally urea's contribution to osmolality is included in the calculation. In this situation, urea is ignored because urea is freely permeable to membranes and does not cause osmotic shifts.

**Table 4–4.** Frequency and etiology of abdominal pain in patients with DKA.

| Serum HCO₃⁻ | Frequency of Abdominal Pain | Patients with DKA as Etiology of Pain | Patients with Other Etiology of Pain |
|---|---|---|---|
| 0–10 mEq/L | 25–75% | 70% | 30% |
| > 10 mEq/L | 12% | 16% | 84% |

DKA, diabetic ketoacidosis.

4. Nausea and vomiting are common and nonspecific.

C. Hyperglycemia

1. Glucose level is variable.

2. 15% of patients with DKA have glucose levels < 350 mg/dL (particularly in pregnancy or in patients with poor oral intake).

3. Glucose > 250 mg/dL has poor specificity for DKA (11%).

D. Ketones

1. 3 ketones: β hydroxybutyrate, acetoacetate, acetone

2. Standard ketone test uses the nitroprusside reaction, which detects acetoacetate but is insensitive for β hydroxybutyrate. In severe DKA, β hydroxybutyrate is the prominent ketone, and the nitroprusside test may be falsely negative. In addition, captopril causes a false-positive nitroprusside reaction.

3. β hydroxybutyrate can be measured directly and rapidly. It is highly accurate for diagnosis of DKA: 98% sensitive, 85% specific, LR+ 6.5, LR- 0.02 (cutoff β > 1.5 mmol/L).

4. Urine ketones are sensitive for DKA but not specific (69%). Blood measurements are preferred.

E. Anion gap

1. Anion gap is elevated in most patients with DKA (even when nitroprusside reaction is negative).

2. In patients evaluated in the emergency department with glucose > 250 mg/dL, the anion gap is 84–90% sensitive and 85–99% specific; LR+, 6–84; LR–, 0.11–0.16.

3. If anion gap is elevated and ketones are negative, βOHB measurements should be measured. If βOHB measurements are not available (or negative), lactic acid should be measured to rule out lactic acidosis.

F. Nonspecific findings

1. Amylase: Nonspecific elevations in amylase are common.

2. Leukocytosis

a. Mild leukocytosis (10,000–15,000/mcL) is common and may occur secondary to stress or infection.

b. One study documented higher WBCs in patients with major infection than in patients without infection (17,900/mcL vs 13,700/mcL).

c. Band counts were also higher in patients with infection (23% vs 6%).

## Treatment

A. Treatment of DKA must include the following:

1. Initial evaluation and frequent monitoring

2. Detection and therapy of the underlying precipitant

 The most common cause of death in patients with DKA is the underlying precipitant. It must be discovered and treated.

3. Fluid resuscitation

4. Insulin

5. Potassium replacement

B. Initial evaluation and monitoring

1. Check electrolytes, glucose, serum ketones, ABG, anion gap, and renal function.

2. Serum creatinine may be artificially elevated due to interference of assay by ketones.

3. The serum glucose should be checked hourly and the electrolytes should be measured frequently (every 2–4 hours) and the anion gap calculated.

C. Detection and therapy of the underlying precipitant

a. Urinalysis, chest film, CBC with differential, blood cultures, lipase, ECG, troponin levels.

b. β-HCG should be measured in women of childbearing age.

D. Fluid resuscitation

1. Evaluate dehydration: check BP, orthostatic BP and pulse, monitor hourly urinary output

2. IV normal saline 0.5–1.5 L bolus initially.

a. Higher rates (1–1.5 L) are useful for patients with significant hypotension.

b. Lower rates (500 mL/h) may allow for more rapid correction of acidosis in patients without marked volume depletion.

3. Reevaluate after each liter by checking BP, orthostatic BP and pulse, urinary output, cardiac and pulmonary exams. Repeat boluses until hypotension and oliguria resolve.

4. Normal saline should be switched to 0.45% normal saline when intravascular volume improves to restore free water deficit.

E. Insulin

1. The ADA recommends an IV bolus of regular insulin (0.1 units/kg) followed by IV regular insulin at 0.1 units/kg/h

2. Marked hypokalemia (< 3.3 mEq/L) should be excluded before insulin therapy is administered (see below).

3. Administer in monitored setting.

4. Monitor glucose levels hourly: target reduction 75–90 mg/dL/h and adjust insulin dose accordingly.

5. Insulin should be continued until the anion gap normalizes and the serum HCO₃⁻ is ≥ 18 mEq/L.

a. Premature discontinuation of IV insulin may result in rebound ketoacidosis.

b. If patient's glucose normalizes (< 200 mg/dL) before the anion gap normalizes and before the HCO₃⁻ is ≥ 18 mEq/L, the insulin dose may be reduced by 50% and glucose (D5W) added to the IV to prevent hypoglycemia.

c. Patients should receive their first dose of SQ insulin 1–2 hours before IV insulin is discontinued in order to prevent an insulin free window and recurrent ketoacidosis.

In DKA, it is important to continue IV insulin until the anion gap returns to normal. Administer glucose as necessary to prevent hypoglycemia.

**F.** Potassium replacement

**1.** Treatment of the insulin deficiency and acidosis shifts potassium back into the intracellular compartment.

**2.** Profound *hypokalemia* is a common complication of therapy and often develops within the first few hours.

**3.** Potassium levels should be monitored hourly, and replacement should be initiated when urinary output resumes and potassium is < 5.3 mEq/L.

**4.** Potassium therapy should be initiated immediately in patients who present with hypokalemia. In addition, insulin therapy should be delayed until the serum potassium > 3.3 mEq/L to prevent life-threatening exacerbation of hypokalemia induced by insulin therapy.

**G.** $HCO_3^-$ therapy

**1.** Use is controversial; if used, monitor patient for hypokalemia.

**2.** $HCO_3^-$ has not been shown to improve outcomes in patients with serum pH > 6.9. It may also paradoxically lower CNS pH.

**3.** The ADA recommends $HCO_3^-$ therapy in patients with a pH < 7.0.

**H.** Phosphate therapy

**1.** Hypophosphatemia is common and may develop during therapy.

**2.** Replacement should be considered in patients with marked hypophosphatemia (< 1.0 mg/dL) or with respiratory depression, cardiac dysfunction, or anemia.

Careful, frequent observation and evaluation of patients with DKA is critical to success.

## MAKING A DIAGNOSIS

Have you crossed a diagnostic threshold for the leading hypothesis, DKA? Have you ruled out the active alternatives or uremia or lactic acidosis (from sepsis)? Do other tests need to be done to exclude the alternative diagnoses?

## Alternative Diagnosis: Uremic Acidosis

### Textbook Presentation

Typically, patients with chronic renal failure have low $HCO_3^-$ levels, high creatinine levels (often > 4–5 mg/dL), and elevated BUN and phosphate levels. Patients often complain of a variety of constitutional symptoms secondary to their renal failure including fatigue, nausea, vomiting, anorexia, and pruritus.

### Disease Highlights

**A.** Pathophysiology

**1.** Each day, ingested nonvolatile acids neutralize $HCO_3^-$.

**2.** In health, the kidneys regenerate the $HCO_3^-$ and maintain the acid-base equilibrium.

**3.** Renal impairment results in failed $HCO_3^-$ regeneration and a metabolic acidosis develops.

**B.** Acidosis in patients with renal failure may be of the anion gap type or non-anion gap type.

**1.** In early renal failure, ammonia-genesis is impaired, resulting in reduced acid secretion and a non-anion gap metabolic acidosis.

**2.** In more advanced chronic renal failure, the kidney remains unable to excrete the daily acid load and also becomes unable to excrete anions such as sulfates, phosphates, and urate. Therefore, an anion gap acidosis develops. $HCO_3^-$ levels stabilize between 12 mEq/L and 20 mEq/L.

**C.** The acidosis has several adverse effects.

**1.** Increased calcium loss from bone

**2.** Increased skeletal muscle breakdown

## Treatment

**A.** $NaHCO_3^-$ replacement

**B.** Hemodialysis

## CASE RESOLUTION

Mr. L's serum ketones are large. Lactate level is 1 mEq/L (normal 0.5–1.5 mEq/L).

The high serum ketones confirm DKA. The normal lactate effectively rules out lactic acidosis, and uremic acidosis is very unlikely with mild renal insufficiency. Evaluation and treatment identifies the precipitant of DKA and treats the acidosis, hyperglycemia, and profound dehydration.

Mr. L confirms he has been taking his insulin. He reports no fever, rigors, dysuria, cough, shortness of breath, diarrhea, or abdominal pain. Urinalysis, chest radiograph, and lipase were sent to search for the precipitating event. All of the results were normal. An ECG revealed T–wave inversion in leads V1–V4, suggesting anterior myocardial ischemia. Troponin T levels were elevated consistent with an acute MI (believed to be the precipitant of his DKA). He was transferred to the ICU for monitoring. He received fluid resuscitation, IV insulin until his ketoacidosis resolved, and supplemental potassium (when his potassium fell below 5.3 mEq/L). His MI was treated with β-blockers and aspirin. Subsequent cardiac catheterization revealed triple vessel disease. After stabilization, he underwent coronary artery bypass grafting and did well.

# CHIEF COMPLAINT

PATIENT 2

Ms. S is a 32-year-old woman who complains of nausea and vomiting. She reports that she felt well until 5 days ago when she noticed urinary frequency and burning on urination. She increased her intake of fluids and cranberry juice but noticed some increasing right back pain 2 days ago. Yesterday, she felt warm and noticed that she had a fever of 38.8°C and teeth-chattering chills. Subsequently, she has been unable to keep down any food or liquids and has persistent nausea and vomiting. She feels weak and dizzy. Physical exam: supine BP, 95/62 mm Hg; pulse, 120 bpm; temperature, 38.9°C; RR, 24 breaths per minute. On standing, her BP falls to 72/40 mm Hg with a pulse of 145 bpm. Cardiac and pulmonary exam are notable only for the tachycardia. She has 2+ right costovertebral angle tenderness. Abdominal exam is soft without rebound, guarding, or focal tenderness.

 At this point, what is the leading hypothesis, what are the active alternatives, and is there a must not miss diagnosis? Given this differential diagnosis, what tests should be ordered?

## PRIORITIZING THE DIFFERENTIAL DIAGNOSIS

### Step 1: Generate Clinical Hypotheses

Ms. S's history of fever, dysuria, and flank pain suggest urinary tract infection and pyelonephritis. Furthermore, her teeth-chattering chills suggest bacteremia, which combined with her hypotension suggests severe sepsis. Septic shock can cause lactic acid production and thereby generate an anion gap metabolic acidosis. This is the leading hypothesis and must not miss diagnosis. Ms. S's history of persistent vomiting combined with her volume depletion (as evidenced by her orthostatic hypotension) could also cause a metabolic alkalosis. This is an alternative hypothesis (Table 4–5).

### Step 2: Check the pH

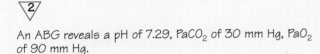

An ABG reveals a pH of 7.29, PaCO₂ of 30 mm Hg, PaO₂ of 90 mm Hg.

The low pH on the ABG confirms the primary process is an acidosis.

### Step 3: Determine Whether the Primary Disorder Is Due to a Metabolic or Respiratory Process

2

Other initial laboratory results include Na⁺, 138 mEq/L; K⁺, 5.4 mEq/L; HCO₃⁻, 14 mEq/L; Cl⁻, 102 mEq/L; BUN, 30 mg/dL; creatinine, 1.2 mg/dL. Glucose, 90 mg/dL; WBC, 18,500 cells/mcL with 62% granulocytes and 30% bands. Urinalysis reveals > 20 WBC/hpf.

*Table 4–5.* Diagnostic hypotheses for Ms. S.

| Diagnostic Hypothesis | Clinical Clues | Important Tests |
|---|---|---|
| **Leading Hypothesis** | | |
| Sepsis causing lactic acidosis | Fever<br>Shaking chills<br>Hypotension<br>Localized symptoms and signs of infection (eg, cough, dysuria, skin redness) | Elevated anion gap and lactate<br>Leukocytosis<br>Left shift<br>Blood cultures<br>Urinalysis<br>Chest radiograph |
| **Active Alternatives—Most Common** | | |
| Metabolic alkalosis | Vomiting<br>Dehydration<br>Nasogastric tube drainage<br>Diuretics | Elevated HCO₃⁻<br>Hypokalemia |

Ms. S's $HCO_3^-$ *and* $PaCO_2$ are both low. Only the low $HCO_3^-$ would create an acidosis. (A low $PaCO_2$ would drive the pH up and cause an alkalosis.) Since her pH is low the primary process is a metabolic acidosis.

### Step 4: Calculate Whether Compensation Is Appropriate

In a metabolic acidosis, the $PaCO_2$ is expected to fall by 1.2 mm Hg per 1 mEq/L fall in $HCO_3^-$ (see Table 4–1). The patient's $HCO_3^-$ is 14 mEq/L (10 mEq/L below normal). The $PaCO_2$ should fall by 1.2 × 10 = 12. Since normal $PaCO_2$ is approximately 40 mm Hg, we would expect the $PaCO_2$ to be approximately 40 − 12 = 28 mm Hg. The actual $PaCO_2$ is 30 mm Hg, quite close to the prediction. This suggests that respiratory compensation is appropriate. Therefore, Ms. S is suffering from a metabolic acidosis with appropriate respiratory compensation.

### Step 5: Calculate the Anion Gap

The next vital step in the differential diagnosis is to calculate the anion gap. Her anion gap = 138 − (102 + 14) = 22.

Clearly, Ms. S is suffering from an anion gap metabolic acidosis. This is alarming. It excludes the possibility of metabolic alkalosis and focuses our attention on the remaining possibility of lactic acidosis due to sepsis. (The clinical history and laboratory results suggest neither DKA nor uremic acidosis.)

 Is the clinical information sufficient to make a diagnosis? If not, what other information do you need?

### Leading Hypothesis: Lactic Acidosis Secondary to Sepsis

#### Textbook Presentation

Patients with septic shock typically have fever, tachypnea, tachycardia, and hypotension. Whereas patients with cardiogenic or hemorrhagic shock often have cold extremities, patients with septic shock often have warm extremities and bounding pulses after fluid resuscitation. (Pulses are bounding due to a widened pulse pressure.) Mentation may be impaired and urinary output decreased.

## Disease Highlights

A. Epidemiology

1. The annual incidence of sepsis has increased 4 times since the 1970s.

2. Sepsis is more common among non-white compared with white populations in the United States (RR 1.90).

3. Most common sources of infection are the lung, intra-abdominal infections, urine, and IV catheters. Commonly overlooked sources include sinusitis (associated with nasogastric tubes), acalculous cholecystitis and *Clostridium difficile* colitis.

 Certain life-threatening infections may produce characteristic rashes (ie meningococcemia, Rocky Mountain spotted fever, or staphylococcal toxic shock syndrome). Rapid recognition and treatment is vital.

B. Pathophysiology

1. Sepsis

a. Occurs when an infection (bacterial, fungal, mycobacterial, or viral) triggers a proinflammatory reaction that is poorly regulated and becomes systemic

b. A noninfectious process (eg, acute pancreatitis) may also trigger a similarly dysregulated immune response called SIRS (systemic inflammatory response syndrome).

2. In early stages of sepsis, hyperimmune responses may play a role in the organ dysfunction and cause multiple organ dysfunction syndrome (MODS), hypotension, disseminated intravascular coagulation, and death.

3. In later stages of sepsis, patients may be hypoimmune. Hypoimmunity may also contribute to infection and death.

4. Mechanisms of hypotension include

a. Vasodilatation (decreased systemic vascular resistance [SVR]) mediated by elevated nitrous oxide levels, increased prostacyclin levels, and low vasopressin levels, lowers BP.

b. Cardiac output (CO) can be increased or decreased in sepsis.

(1) The drop in SVR decreases afterload, which often results in an increase in CO.

(2) On the other hand, leakage of fluid out of intravascular space can decrease venous return and thereby decrease CO.

(3) In addition, myocardial function can be reduced and also decrease CO.

c. Typically, the *initial* hemodynamic response is decreased SVR and increased CO (particularly after fluid resuscitation).

5. MODS

a. Lung involvement: acute respiratory distress syndrome secondary to increased permeability with subsequent pulmonary edema

b. Renal failure secondary to

(1) Hypotension

(2) Renal vasoconstriction

(3) Increased tumor necrosis factor

c. Disseminated intravascular coagulation: Multiple mediators are involved, including decreased protein C.

6. Lactic acidosis multifactorial

a. Microcirculatory lesion impairs oxygen delivery.

(1) Dysregulation of supply and demand

(2) Microvascular occlusion

b. Hypotension impairs oxygen delivery.

c. Mitochondrial injury impairs oxygen utilization.

d. Decreased hepatic clearance of lactate contributes to lactic acidosis.

C. The definitions of sepsis, severe sepsis, and septic shock and their associated mortality rates are shown in Table 4–6.

D. There is an increased risk of septic shock in patients with bacteremia (21%), advanced age (≥ 65), impaired immune system, community-acquired pneumonia, abdominal infection, and markedly elevated WBC.

E. The mortality rate associated with sepsis ranges from 20% to 50%. Predictors of mortality include

1. Age > 40 years

2. Comorbidities: AIDS, hepatic failure, heart failure (HF), diabetes mellitus, cancer, or immunosuppression

3. Temperature < 35.5°C

4. Leukopenia < 4000 cells/mcL

5. Hospital-acquired infection

**Table 4–6.** Definitions of stages of sepsis.

| Category | Definition | Mortality |
|---|---|---|
| Sepsis | Infection and ≥ 2 of following:<br>Temperature > 38.5°C or < 35.0°C<br>Pulse > 90 bpm<br>RR > 20/min or PaCO₂ < 32 mm Hg<br>WBC > 12,000/mcL or < 4000/mcL or > 10% bands | 16% |
| Severe sepsis | Sepsis and at least 1 of the following signs of inadequate tissue perfusion:<br>Altered mental status<br>Oliguria<br>Lactic acidosis<br>Platelet count < 100,000<br>ALI/ARDS | 20% |
| Septic shock | Severe sepsis with mean BP < 60 mm Hg (or < 80 mm Hg if the patient has baseline hypertension) after fluid resuscitation or the need for vasopressors | 46% |

ALI/ARDS, acute lung injury/acute respiratory distress syndrome.

| Mortality in Emergency Department Sepsis (MEDS) Score | |
| --- | --- |
| | **Points** |
| Age > 65 years | 3 |
| Nursing home resident | 2 |
| Rapidly terminal comorbid illness | 6 |
| Lower respiratory infection | 2 |
| Bands > 5% | 3 |
| Tachypnea or hypoxemia | 3 |
| Shock | 3 |
| Platelet count < 150,000/mcL | 3 |
| Altered mental status | 2 |

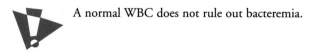

***Figure 4–2.*** Mortality in Emergency Department Sepsis (MED) Score Observed mortality vs. score (error bars are 95% confidence intervals). (Reproduced, with permission, from Howell MD et al. Performance of severity of illness scoring systems in emergency department patients with infection. Acad Emerg Med. 2007;14(8):709–14. )

6. *Candida, Pseudomonas,* or *Staphylococcus aureus* infection
7. Inappropriate antibiotics: appropriate antibiotics associated with 50% decrease in mortality
8. Multiple organ failure
9. Mortality in Emergency Department Sepsis (MED) Score is a validated scoring index that predicts mortality in patients arriving at emergency departments with suspected infection (Figure 4–2).

## Evidence-Based Diagnosis

A. Fever

1. In emergency department patients, fever was higher among bacteremic patients (38.8°C) than nonbacteremic patients 38.1°C.
2. 5% of patients with gram-negative bacteremia are normothermic (temperature < 37.6°C).
3. 13% of patients with bacteremia were hypothermic (< 36.4°C).
4. Among patients with bacteremia, the absence of fever was associated with increased mortality.

B. Chills

1. Chills can vary from mild to moderate to shaking chills (ie, teeth chattering, bed shaking chills).
2. Chills of some kind (mild, moderate, or severe) are common in bacteremic patients (sensitivity 88%).

 3. Shaking chills (rigors) are less sensitive but more specific for bacteremia (sensitivity, 45%; specificity, 90%; LR+, 4.7, LR-, 0.61).

> Providers should consider bacteremia in older patients with significant fever or rigors (teeth-chattering or physically shaking chills). All patients evaluated for sepsis or presenting with rigors should have blood cultures drawn and antibiotics administered.

***Table 4–7.*** Predictors of bacteremia.

| Finding | Sensitivity | Specificity | LR+ | LR– |
| --- | --- | --- | --- | --- |
| Shaking chills | 45% | 90% | 4.7 | 0.61 |
| Injection drug use | 7% | 98% | 2.9 | 0.95 |
| Central venous catheter | 23% | 90% | 2.4 | 0.85 |
| Acute abdomen | 20% | 91% | 2.2 | 0.9 |
| WBC > 15,000/mcL | 28% | 87% | 2.2 | 0.8 |
| WBC < 1000/mcL | 14% | 94% | 2.3 | 0.9 |
| Bandemia ≥ 1500/mcL | 44% | 69% | 1.4 | 0.8 |
| Chills (any type) | 88% | 52% | 1.7 | 0.23 |
| Comorbidity | 86% | 37% | 1.4 | 0.14 |

C. Predictors of bacteremia (Table 4–7)

1. WBC > 15,000/mcL is only 28% sensitive for bacteremia.

> A normal WBC does not rule out bacteremia.

2. Any of the following increase the risk of bacteremia:
   a. Shaking chills
   b. History of injection drug use
   c. Acute abdomen
   d. WBC > 15,000/mcL
   e. Presence of a central venous catheter

**3.** Incidence of bacteremia is low (2%) in patients without *any* of the following risk factors:

    **a.** Temperature > 38.3°C

    **b.** Shaking chills

    **c.** Injection drug use

    **d.** Acute abdomen on exam

    **e.** Major comorbidity

**D.** Catheter site infections

    **1.** Signs of inflammation at the insertion site are *uncommon* in patients with central venous catheter infections (sensitivity 27%). Erythema is present in only 3% of patients with catheter-related bloodstream infections.

    **2.** Certain findings are highly specific of catheter infection including gross pus at the catheter insertion site, cellulitis > 4 mm around the site, or tunnel tract infection.

Consider central catheter line infection in septic patients even in the absence of erythema or pus.

**E.** Serum lactate levels are more sensitive than an increase in the anion gap. An elevated anion gap is 44–67% sensitive.

**F.** Blood cultures should be obtained as soon as possible in patients evaluated for sepsis.

    **1.** If central catheters are in place and are a suspected source of infection, blood should be obtained peripherally and through the central line.

    **2.** Cultures can be negative in 10% of patients with sepsis.

## Treatment

The treatment of septic shock is complex and recommendations evolve frequently. Readers are referred to specialized texts for details.

## MAKING A DIAGNOSIS

Blood cultures and urine cultures grew *Escherichia coli*.

The positive blood cultures confirm the overwhelming clinical impression of severe sepsis. Serum lactate 8 mEq/L (nl 0.5–1.5 mEq/L) confirms lactic acidosis. Other tests are not necessary to confirm the diagnosis.

## CASE RESOLUTION

Ms. S was treated with broad-spectrum antibiotics and IV fluid resuscitation. After initial stabilization, hypotension recurred and urinary output dropped. She was transferred to the ICU. Four hours later her oxygenation deteriorated and a chest film revealed a diffuse infiltrate consistent with acute respiratory distress syndrome. She was intubated and given IV fluids, norepinephrine, antibiotics, mechanical ventilation, and activated protein C. Over the next 24 hours, her BP stabilized and her anion gap lactic acidosis resolved. Seventy-two hours later she was extubated. She eventually made a full recovery.

## CHIEF COMPLAINT

### PATIENT 3

Mr. R is a 55-year-old man with a history of COPD whose chief complaint is dyspnea. He reports that his symptoms began 5 days ago with a cough productive of green sputum. The cough worsened, and 4 days ago he had a low-grade fever of 37.2°C. He noticed increasing shortness of breath 3 days ago. He reports that previously he was able to walk about 25 feet before becoming short of breath but now he is short of breath at rest. Last night his fever reached 38.8°C, and today his dyspnea intensified. He is unable to complete a sentence without pausing to take a breath. On physical exam he appears older than his stated age. He is gaunt, sitting upright, breathing through pursed lips, and in obvious distress. Vital signs are temperature, 38.9°C; RR, 28 breaths per minute; BP, 110/70 mm Hg; pulse, 110 bpm. His pulsus paradox is 20 mm Hg. Lung exam reveals significant use of accessory muscles and markedly decreased breath sounds. Cardiac exam is notable only for diminished heart sounds.

At this point, what is the leading hypothesis, what are the active alternatives, and is there a must not miss diagnosis? Given this differential diagnosis, what tests should be ordered?

## PRIORITIZING THE DIFFERENTIAL DIAGNOSIS

### Step 1: Generate Clinical Hypotheses

Mr. R's history of very poor exercise tolerance at *baseline* suggests severe COPD. Such severe COPD could result in chronic carbon dioxide retention and chronic respiratory acidosis. A "must not miss" possibility is that his acute respiratory infection has precipitated *acute* respiratory failure (and acute respiratory acidosis). This is suggested by his worsening symptoms, respiratory distress, upright posture, pursed lip breathing, pulsus paradox, and decreased breath sounds. *It is critical to distinguish acute respiratory acidosis from chronic respiratory acidosis* because the former is more likely to progress rapidly to *complete* respiratory failure. Therefore, acute respiratory acidosis is both the leading hypothesis and the "must not miss" diagnosis. Another "must not miss" diagnosis is sepsis. His symptoms of fever and cough suggest the possibility of pneumonia, which can be complicated by sepsis resulting in an anion gap metabolic lactic acidosis. Finally, fever and lung disease may also result in *excessive* ventilation and a respiratory alkalosis. The differential diagnosis is listed in (Table 4–8).

 Patients with a history of asthma or COPD should be asked about a prior history of intubation or ICU admission. Such patients are at greater risk for respiratory failure.

## Step 2: Check the pH

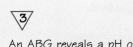

An ABG reveals a pH of 7.22, $PaCO_2$ of 70 mm Hg, and $PaO_2$ of 55 mm Hg.

The low pH on the ABG confirms the primary process is due to an acidosis.

*Table 4–8.* Diagnostic hypotheses for Mr. R.

| Diagnostic Hypothesis | Clinical Clues | Important Tests |
|---|---|---|
| **Leading Hypothesis** | | |
| Acute respiratory acidosis | Severe underlying lung disease Worsening symptoms Respiratory distress Pulsus paradox Decreased breath sounds Prior history of intubation ICU admission | Decreased pH Elevated $PaCO_2$ Near *normal* $HCO_3^-$ |
| **Active Alternatives—Most Common** | | |
| Chronic respiratory acidosis | Severe underlying lung disease Decreased breath sounds | Decreased pH Elevated $PaCO_2$ Elevated $HCO_3^-$ |
| Respiratory alkalosis | Fever Pain Anxiety | Elevated pH Decreased $PaCO_2$ Near normal $HCO_3^-$ |
| **Active Alternatives—Must Not Miss** | | |
| Sepsis: anion gap metabolic acidosis | Fever Source of infection Shaking chills Oliguria Hypotension Altered mental status | Decreased pH, $HCO_3^-$, and $PaCO_2$ Increased anion gap Positive blood cultures Increased lactate |

## Step 3: Determine Whether the Primary Disorder Is Due to a Metabolic or Respiratory Process

$Na^+$, 138 mEq/L; $K^+$, 5.1 mEq/L; $HCO_3^-$, 27 mEq/L; $Cl^-$, 102 mEq/L; BUN, 30 mg/dL; creatinine, 1.2 mg/dL.

The $PaCO_2$ and $HCO_3^-$ are elevated. Since an elevated $PaCO_2$ would lower pH and cause an acidemia (whereas an elevated $HCO_3^-$ would not), the primary process is a respiratory acidosis.

## Step 4: Calculate Whether Compensation Is Appropriate

In this case, it is critical to determine whether the $PaCO_2$ is chronically elevated or whether this represents an acute decompensation. Acute respiratory acidosis can be distinguished from chronic respiratory acidosis by evaluating the degree of metabolic compensation. Metabolic compensation takes time since it requires renal generation of $HCO_3^-$. Therefore, metabolic compensation is more complete in chronic respiratory acidosis. Formulas (see Table 4–1) allow us to calculate the $HCO_3$ levels we might expect in an acute versus chronic respiratory acidosis. In acute respiratory acidosis, the $HCO_3$ increases by only 1 mEq/L for every 10 mm Hg increase in $PaCO_2$. In Mr. R's case, the $PaCO_2$ is up by 30 mm Hg (from a normal of 40 mm Hg), so *if this were an acute respiratory acidosis* we would expect the $HCO_3^-$ to increase by only 3 mEq/L (from a normal of 24 mEq/L to 27 mEq/L).

On the other hand, in chronic respiratory acidosis we expect an increase of 3.5 mEq/L of $HCO_3^-$ per 10 mm Hg increase in $PaCO_2$. For a 30 mm Hg increase in $PaCO_2$, you would predict an increase in $HCO_3$ of $3 \times 3.5 = 10.5$ mEq *if this were a chronic respiratory acidosis.*

Mr. R's laboratory results reveal a $HCO_3$ of 27 mEq/L, an increase of only 3 mEq/L from a normal baseline of 24 mEq/L. Therefore, the tiny metabolic compensation suggests that Mr. R is suffering from an acute respiratory acidosis and you should be alert to the potential for complete respiratory failure.

 It is vital to distinguish acute from chronic respiratory acidoses.

## Step 5: Calculate the Anion Gap

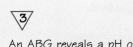

The anion gap = $138 - (102 + 27) = 9$.

Mr. R has a normal anion gap, ruling out a coexistent hidden anion gap metabolic acidosis. His laboratory test results suggest an acute respiratory acidosis.

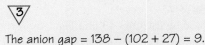

Other initial laboratory test results include WBC, 16,500/mcL with 62% granulocytes and 10% bands.

Chest radiograph reveals hyperinflated lung fields and a left lower lobe infiltrate.

**Is the clinical information sufficient to make a diagnosis? If not, what other information do you need?**

## Leading Hypothesis: Respiratory Acidosis

### Textbook Presentation

The presentation of respiratory acidosis depends primarily on the underlying cause. The most common causes are severe underlying lung or heart diseases (ie, COPD or HF). Such patients are typically in extreme respiratory distress.

### Disease Highlights

A. Insufficient ventilation results in increasing levels of $PaCO_2$. This in turn lowers arterial pH. Compensation occurs over several days, with increased renal $HCO_3^-$ regeneration.

B. Ventilation is assessed by measuring the arterial $PaCO_2$ and pH. Significant hypoventilation and acidosis may occur *without* significant hypoxia.

> Pulse oximetry should never be used to assess adequate *ventilation*. An ABG is required in patients at risk for respiratory failure.

C. Etiology: Although most commonly due to lung or heart disease, respiratory acidosis may result from any disease affecting ventilation-from the brain to the alveoli. (See differential diagnosis of acid-base disorders above.)

D. Manifestations are primarily CNS.

1. Severity depends on acuity. Patients with chronic hypercapnia have markedly fewer CNS effects than patients with acute hypercapnia.

2. Anxiety, irritability, confusion, and lethargy

3. Headache may be prominent in the morning due to the worsening hypoventilation that occurs with sleep.

4. Stupor and coma may occur when the $PaCO_2 > 70-100$ mm Hg.

5. Tremor, asterixis, slurred speech, and papilledema may be seen.

### Evidence-Based Diagnosis

A. Typically characterized by $PaCO_2 > 43$ mm Hg.

1. Occasionally, a normal $PaCO_2$ suggests respiratory failure.

   a. For example, patients with asthma typically hyperventilate and present with a $PaCO_2$ *below* normal. A *normal* $PaCO_2$ in such a patient may reflect respiratory fatigue and herald the development of frank respiratory failure.

   b. Analogously, patients with a metabolic acidosis should hyperventilate to compensate and the expected $PaCO_2$ is actually below normal. In such states, a $PaCO_2$ of 40 mm Hg would be inappropriate and represent a respiratory acidosis.

   c. Inability to compensate for a metabolic acidosis is associated with an increased risk of respiratory failure and the subsequent need for intubation.

2. The alveolar-arterial oxygen gradient ($PAO_2$-$PaO_2$) can help distinguish hypercapnia due to pulmonary disease from hypercapnia due to CNS disease (central hypoventilation).

   a. This gradient compares the *calculated alveolar* partial pressure of oxygen ($PAO_2$) with the *measured arterial* partial pressure of oxygen ($PaO_2$).

      (1) In the absence of lung disease, there is little difference between the alveolar and arterial $O_2$.

      (2) A normal A-a gradient is around 10 mm Hg.

   b. Therefore, the A-a gradient is usually normal in hypoventilation due to CNS disease but increased in pulmonary disease.

   c. The $PaO_2$ is measured in an ABG and the $PAO_2$ is calculated from the following formula:

$$PAO_2 = FIO_2 \times (pAtm - pH_2O) - PaCO_2/R.$$

   d. $FIO_2$ is the fraction of inspired oxygen: 0.21 for patients not on supplemental oxygen. pAtm = 760 at sea level, the partial pressure of $H_2O$ = 47 and $PaCO_2$ is the arterial $PCO_2$ measured in the blood gas. R refers to the respiratory quotient and is often estimated at 0.8.

B. Pulsus paradox

1. Defined as > 10 mm Hg drop in systolic BP during inspiration

2. May be seen in patients using unusually strong inspiratory effort

3. Insensitive for severe asthma

4. When pulsus paradox is marked, there is a high LR of severe disease (Table 4–9).

### Treatment

A. Treat underlying disease process (ie, bronchodilators for asthma, naloxone for narcotic overdose).

B. Supplemental oxygen should be given as necessary to prevent hypoxemia.

> Supplemental oxygen occasionally worsens hypercapnia in some patients with severe COPD, asthma, and sleep apnea but should never be withheld from hypoxic patients.

C. Avoid hypokalemia and dehydration that may worsen metabolic alkalosis, raise the serum pH and inadvertently further suppress ventilation.

**Table 4–9.** Pulsus paradox in severe asthma.

|  | Sensitivity | Specificity | LR+ | LR– |
|---|---|---|---|---|
| Pulsus > 10 mm Hg | 53–68% | 69–92% | 2.7 | 0.5 |
| Pulsus > 20 mm Hg | 19–39% | 92–100% | 8.2 | 0.8 |
| Pulsus > 25 mm Hg | 16% | 99% | 22.6 | 0.8 |

D. Mechanical ventilation with either intubation or BiPAP is life-saving in some patients.

1. Institution of mechanical ventilation is considered when pH < 7.1–7.25 or $PaCO_2$ > 80–90 mm Hg.

2. In general, patients with acute hypoventilation require mechanical ventilation with milder hypercapnia than patients with chronic hypoventilation.

## CASE RESOLUTION

Mr. R is transferred to the ICU where he is placed on ventilatory support with biphasic positive airway pressure (BiPAP) and antibiotics. Over the next 5 days, his pneumonia improves. On day 8, BiPAP is discontinued and he is sent to the medical floors.

## REVIEW OF OTHER IMPORTANT DISEASES

## General Principles of Lactic Acidosis

### Textbook Presentation

The presentation of lactic acidosis depends on the underlying etiology. The most common causes are hypoxemia, septic shock, cardiogenic shock, or hypovolemic shock.

### Disease Highlights

A. Lactic acidosis develops when oxygen delivery to the cells is inadequate. This results in anaerobic metabolism and the production of lactic acid. Therefore, the differential diagnosis can be remembered by tracing the pathway of oxygen from the environment through the blood to the cells and mitochondria. Any disease that interferes with oxygen delivery can cause lactic acidosis (Table 4–2).

1. Low oxygen carrying capacity

   a. Hypoxemia (from pulmonary or cardiac disease)

   b. Severe anemia

   c. Carbon monoxide poisoning (interferes with oxygen binding)

2. Inadequate tissue perfusion (shock)

   a. Hypovolemic shock

   b. Cardiogenic shock

   c. Septic shock

3. Regional obstruction to blood flow (eg, ischemic bowel or gangrene)

4. Inadequate cellular utilization of oxygen (cyanide poisoning)

5. Occasionally, lactic acidosis develops secondary to unusually high demand exceeding oxygen supply (eg, intense exercise, seizures).

B. As noted above, a common cause of lactic acidosis is shock, defined as inadequate tissue perfusion.

1. Manifestations of shock include hypotension, oliguria, and impaired mentation.

2. Since hypotension almost always accompanies shock, the differential of shock can be deduced by considering the components of BP:

$$BP = \text{cardiac output (CO)} \times \text{total peripheral resistance (TPR)}$$
$$CO = \text{stroke volume (SV)} \times \text{heart rate (HR)}$$
$$\text{Simple substitution: } BP = SV \times HR \times TPR$$
$$SV = \text{end-diastolic volume (EDV)} - \text{end-systolic volume (ESV)}$$
$$\text{Simple substitution: } BP = (EDV - ESV) \times HR \times TPR$$

Evaluating each constituent in turn illustrates the differential diagnosis and mechanism of hypotension and shock.

3. *Low EDV* decreases CO and if severe, results in *hypovolemic shock*. The low CO causes a compensatory increase in SVR producing cold extremities and oliguria.

   a. Common causes include massive hemorrhage and dehydration.

   b. Less common causes include massive pulmonary embolism and cardiac tamponade.

4. *Elevated ESV* occurs in left ventricular failure. When severe, this defines *cardiogenic shock*. The decreased CO causes decreased BP and a compensatory increase in SVR.

   a. Patients are usually hypotensive, oliguric, and have cold extremities.

   b. Etiologies include massive MI and severe HF of other etiologies.

5. Markedly abnormal heart rates, either tachycardias or bradycardias, can cause shock (eg, ventricular tachycardia, heart block).

6. *Low TPR* is usually caused by *septic shock*. In this case, infection and the body's response to infection triggers excessive vasodilatation.

   a. Patients are often febrile and may complain of rigors or symptoms specific to their underlying infection.

   b. Urinary tract infection, pneumonia, and bacteremia from an indwelling catheter are some of the common causes of septic shock. Extremities are often warm (due to the vasodilatation).

   c. Less common causes of low TPR include adrenal crisis and anaphylaxis.

7. Hemodynamic features of shock are summarized in Table 4–10.

C. Lactate elevation is associated with a substantially increased mortality in a variety of situations. The mortality rate of patients with shock and a lactic acidosis was 70% compared with 25–35% in patients with shock without lactic acidosis.

### Evidence-Based Diagnosis

A. Serum lactate levels are more sensitive than an increase in the anion gap.

B. An elevated anion gap is 44–67% sensitive.

C. An elevated anion gap may suggest a lactic acidosis, but a normal anion gap does not exclude a lactic acidosis.

 A serum lactate level should be ordered in critically ill patients in whom shock is suspected regardless of the anion gap.

*Table 4–10.* The hemodynamic features of shock.[1,2]

| Etiology | Clinical Clues | Mechanism | Cardiac Output | Systemic Vascular Resistance | Left Ventricular Filling Volume[3] (PcW) |
|---|---|---|---|---|---|
| Cardiogenic shock | Massive MI<br>Severe HF<br>Cold extremities<br>Arrhythmias | ↑**ESV** | ↓↓ | ↑↑ | ↑ |
| Hypovolemic shock | Hematemesis<br>Melena<br>Hematochezia<br>Vomiting Diarrhea<br>Heat stroke<br>Abdominal pain | ↓ **EDV** | ↓↓ | ↑↑ | ↓↓ |
| Septic shock | Fevers<br>Rigors<br>Dysuria<br>Flank pain<br>Cough<br>Indwelling line | ↓ **TPR** | ↑ then ↓ | ↓↓ | ↓ to normal |

[1]Principal abnormality is bolded.
[2]$BP = (EDV - ESV) \times HR \times TPR$
[3]Left ventricular (LV) filling can be estimated by using an invasive catheter and measuring the pulmonary capillary wedge pressure (PcW). This estimates LV end-diastolic pressure and thereby LV filling.
EDV, end-diastolic volume; ESV, end-systolic volume; HF, heart failure; HR, heart rate; MI, myocardial infarction; TPR, total peripheral resistance.

### Treatment

Treatment of lactic acidosis should target the underlying condition. A variety of buffering agents (ie, $NaHCO_3$) have been tried and failed to demonstrate improved hemodynamics or survival.

## Renal Tubular Acidosis (RTA)

### Textbook Presentation

Although there are a variety of RTAs, the most common type in adults is hyporenin hypoaldosterone RTA (type IV). Classically, patients have long-standing diabetes, mild renal insufficiency, a mild non-anion gap metabolic acidosis ($HCO_3^- \approx 17$ mEq/L) and hyperkalemia. Only the highlights of type IV RTA will be reviewed here.

### Disease Highlights

A. Patients with type IV RTA have hypoaldosteronism.

B. Hypoaldosteronism interferes with potassium and $H^+$ excretion resulting in hyperkalemia and acidosis.

C. The hyperkalemia also interferes with ammonia production (the major renal buffer) and further impairs acid secretion. The inability to excrete the daily acid load causes a non-anion gap acidosis.

D. In patients with diabetes mellitus, type IV RTA is associated with low renin levels.

E. The low renin, aldosterone and angiotensin levels may cause orthostatic hypotension

F. Etiologies of type IV RTA are numerous.

1. Diabetes with mild renal impairment is the most common.

2. Other causes include

a. Drugs (NSAIDs, ACE inhibitors, potassium-sparing diuretics, trimethoprim, heparin, and cyclosporine)

b. Addison disease

c. Systemic lupus erythematosus

d. AIDS nephropathy

e. Chronic interstitial renal disease

### Treatment

Dietary potassium restriction, loop diuretics, and fludrocortisone are useful.

## D-Lactic Acidosis

D-lactic acidosis is a rare disorder seen in some patients with jejunoileal bypass or short bowel. The bypass or short bowel results in carbohydrate malabsorbtion and delivery of this carbohydrate to the colon where colonic bacteria metabolize it into D-lactic acid, which is absorbed. (Endogenous lactate is L-lactic acid.) Presenting manifestations include encephalopathy and metabolic acidosis after carbohydrate ingestion. Patients may appear intoxicated and show the following symptoms and signs: altered mental status ranging from drowsiness to coma (100%), slurred speech (65%), ataxia (45%), and disorientation (21%) that may follow large carbohydrate meals. Attacks last from hours to days. It is unclear if the neurologic symptoms are secondary to the D-lactic acid or other absorbed toxins. Laboratory tests reveal an anion gap acidosis. Lactate measurements may be falsely negative since standard lactate tests measure L-lactate rather than D-lactate. Special assays must be requested to measure D-lactate. In addition, the anion gap may be smaller than expected because D-lactate is not reabsorbed by the kidney (unlike L-lactate) and is excreted.

## Starvation Ketosis

Typically, starvation ketosis occurs in patients with diminished carbohydrate intake. Ketosis is usually mild ($HCO_3^- \geq 18$ mEq/L) and serum glucose is usually normal. Serum pH is usually normal.

## Alcoholic Ketoacidosis

Alcoholic ketoacidosis usually occurs in advanced alcoholism when the majority of calories come from alcohol. It may be precipitated by decreased intake, pancreatitis, GI bleeding, or infection. The metabolic acidosis can be profound. Toxic ingestions (methanol, paraldehyde, and ethylene glycol) and lactic acidosis should also be considered.

## Metabolic Alkalosis

### Textbook Presentation

The most common clinical situations that give rise to metabolic alkalosis are recurrent vomiting or diuretic treatment. The metabolic alkalosis per se is usually asymptomatic. Muscle cramping due to coexistent hypokalemia may be seen.

### Disease Highlights

A. Metabolic alkalosis develops only when there is *both* an increased production of $HCO_3^-$ *and* a renal stimulus to reabsorb $NaHCO_3^-$. In the absence of a concomitant renal stimulus to reabsorb $NaHCO_3^-$, overproduction simply results in increased renal $HCO_3^-$ excretion.

B. The most common mechanism that promotes $NaHCO_3^-$ reabsorption is decreased renal perfusion. This occurs when the *effective circulating volume* is reduced.

   1. Examples include dehydration or other pathologic states associated with decreased renal perfusion (ie, HF, nephrotic syndrome). The decreased renal perfusion promotes avid sodium reabsorption in the proximal tubule, which in turn facilitates $HCO_3^-$ reabsorption (Figure 4–3).

   2. Hypokalemia also promotes $HCO_3^-$ reabsorption.

C. Pathologic states associated with metabolic alkalosis

   1. Vomiting or nasogastric drainage. Pathophysiology:

      a. Gastric acid production (and secretion) is matched by $HCO_3^-$ production. The $H^+$ ion enters the gastric lumen, whereas the $HCO_3^-$ enters the bloodstream.

      b. Dehydration causes increased sodium reabsorption in the nephron, which results in elevated $HCO_3^-$ reabsorption.

      c. Secondary hyperaldosteronism leads to increased sodium reabsorption in exchange for potassium and hydrogen further augmenting $HCO_3^-$ production.

      d. Chloride depletion also contributes to the metabolic alkalosis.

         (1) In health, $HCO_3^-$ excretion is facilitated by a chloride absorption.

         (2) A chloride/$HCO_3^-$ exchanger located at the luminal membrane of tubular cells secretes $HCO_3^-$ in exchange for chloride absorption.

         (3) During chloride depletion, the low intraluminal chloride levels decrease this exchange interfering with $HCO_3^-$ secretion.

         (4) In addition, the low intraluminal chloride levels facilitates chloride secretion with $H^+$ into the tubules. This also facilitates $HCO_3^-$ reabsorption.

   2. Dehydration or other causes of reduced glomerular filtration rate (GFR) (ie, HF, nephrotic syndrome)

   3. Diuretics

   4. Hypokalemia

   5. Hyperaldosteronism

      a. Adrenal adenoma

      b. Licorice ingestion (Normally, a renal enzyme converts cortisol to cortisone in order to prevent cortisol from exerting a significant mineralocorticoid effect. Licorice contains the steroid glycyrrhizic acid which blocks this enzyme resulting in a heightened mineralocorticoid effect from endogenous cortisol.)

   6. Bartter or Gitelman syndromes

   7. Respiratory acidosis also promotes a compensatory metabolic alkalosis. Occasionally, rapid resolution of the respiratory failure will correct the hypercapnia, resulting in a transient inappropriate metabolic alkalosis (posthypercapnic metabolic alkalosis).

### Treatment

A. Volume resuscitation with NaCl in patients with true volume depletion usually results in resolution.

B. Replete potassium deficiency.

C. Carbonic anhydrase inhibitors and low bicarbonate dialysis can be used in severe cases, particularly in patients with HF (and ineffective circulating volume) who cannot tolerate NaCl.

## Respiratory Alkalosis

### Textbook Presentation

The presentation of respiratory alkalosis depends on the underlying disorder. Most causes are associated with tachypnea, which can be dramatic or subtle.

### Disease Highlights

A. Hyperventilation induces hypocapnia causing respiratory alkalosis.

B. Most common causes include pulmonary disease, fever, pain, or anxiety.

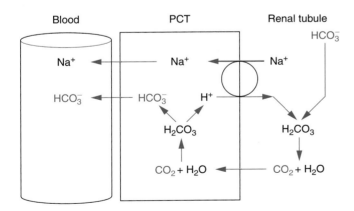

*Figure 4–3.* **Reabsorption of $HCO_3^-$ in hypovolemia.** Hypovolemia increases reabsorption of sodium in exchange for hydrogen ion at the proximal convoluted tubule (PCT). The hydrogen ion reacts with $HCO_3^-$ eventually forming $CO_2$, which crosses the cell membrane. $HCO_3^-$ is then regenerated and delivered to the bloodstream.

C. Hypocapnia acutely reduces CNS blood flow.

D. Symptoms include paresthesias (particularly perioral), vertigo, dizziness, anxiety, hallucinations, myalgias, and symptoms reflective of underlying disorder.

E. Adverse effects include decreased cerebral blood flow, hypokalemia, hypocalcemia, lung injury, seizures, angina, and arrhythmias.

## Treatment

Therapy is directed at the underlying disorder.

## Mixed Disorders and the "Delta-Delta Gap"

A. Occasionally, 2 distinct metabolic processes will be present in the same patient; for example 2 distinct acidoses, one anion gap and one non-anion gap, may develop in one patient. Another patient with vomiting and dehydration will develop a metabolic alkalosis and, if prolonged sufficiently, also develop severe dehydration, hypovolemic shock, and a lactic acidosis.

B. These multiple metabolic processes can be difficult to tease out.

C. One approach to this problem is to evaluate the delta-delta gap. Here the absolute fall in $HCO_3^-$ (the first delta) is compared with the absolute rise in the anion gap (the second delta).

   1. In simple anion gap acidoses, the deltas match.

   2. On the other hand, in a patient with both a gap and non-anion gap acidoses, the fall in $HCO_3^-$ will be greater than the rise in the anion gap.

   3. In patients with an anion gap acidosis *and* a metabolic alkalosis the fall in $HCO_3^-$ will be antagonized by the concomitant metabolic alkalosis whereas the anions will still accumulate. Therefore, the fall in $HCO_3^-$ is less than the rise in the anion gap.

D. While occasionally useful, there are several limitations to applying the delta-delta gap.

   1. The normal anion gap varies from institution to institution and with the patient's serum albumin.

   2. In anion gap acidosis both the acuity of the acidosis and the anion itself affect the magnitude of the anion gap.

## REFERENCES

Bates DW, Cook EF, Goldman L, Lee TH. Predicting bacteremia in hospitalized patients. A prospectively validated model. Ann Intern Med. 1990;113(7): 495–500.

Drage LA. Life-threatening rashes: dermatologic signs of four infectious diseases. Mayo Clin Proc. 1999;74(1):68–72.

Fall PJ, Szerlip HM. Lactic acidosis: from sour milk to septic shock. J Intensive Care Med. 2005;20(5):255–71.

Figge J, Jabor A, Kazda A, Fencl V. Anion gap and hypoalbuminemia. Crit Care Med. 1998;26(11):1807–10.

Howell MD, Donnino MW, Talmor D, Clardy P, Ngo L, Shapiro NI. Performance of severity of illness scoring systems in emergency department patients with infection. Acad Emerg Med. 2007;14(8):709–14.

Jaimes F, Arango C, Ruiz G et al. Predicting bacteremia at the bedside. Clin Infect Dis. 2004;38(3):357–62.

Kitabchi AE, Umpierrez GE, Murphy MB, Kreisberg RA. Hyperglycemic crises in adult patients with diabetes: a consensus statement from the American Diabetes Association. Diabetes Care. 2006;29(12):2739–48.

Leibovici L, Cohen O, Wysenbeek AJ. Occult bacterial infection in adults with unexplained fever. Validation of a diagnostic index. Arch Intern Med. 1990;150(6):1270–2.

Leibovici L, Greenshtain S, Cohen O, Mor F, Wysenbeek AJ. Bacteremia in febrile patients. A clinical model for diagnosis. Arch Intern Med. 1991;151(9):1801–6.

Levraut J, Bounatirou T, Ichai C et al. Reliability of anion gap as an indicator of blood lactate in critically ill patients. Intensive Care Med. 1997;23(4):417–22.

Mellors JW, Horwitz RI, Harvey MR, Horwitz SM. A simple index to identify occult bacterial infection in adults with acute unexplained fever. Arch Intern Med. 1987;147(4):666–71.

Naunheim R, Jang TJ, Banet G, Richmond A, McGill J. Point-of-care test identifies diabetic ketoacidosis at triage. Acad Emerg Med. 2006;13(6):683–5.

Rose BD PT. Clinical Physiology of Acid Base and Electrolyte Disorders. 5th edition. ed: McGraw Hill; 2001.

Safdar N, Maki DG. Inflammation at the insertion site is not predictive of catheter-related bloodstream infection with short-term, noncuffed central venous catheters. Crit Care Med. 2002;30(12):2632–5.

Slovis CM, Mork VG, Slovis RJ, Bain RP. Diabetic ketoacidosis and infection: leukocyte count and differential as early predictors of serious infection. Am J Emerg Med. 1987;5(1):1–5.

Tokuda Y, Miyasato H, Stein GH, Kishaba T. The degree of chills for risk of bacteremia in acute febrile illness. Am J Med. 2005;118(12):1417.

Umpierrez G, Freire AX. Abdominal pain in patients with hyperglycemic crises. J Crit Care. 2002;17(1):63–7.

# I have patients with AIDS-related complaints.

## I have a patient with risk factors for HIV and multiple complaints. How do I diagnose or exclude HIV infection?

## CHIEF COMPLAINT

**PATIENT** 1

Mr. O is a 29-year-old white man with a history of unprotected anal intercourse with multiple partners. He has noticed some oral lesions and weight loss. He is quite worried and wants to know if he is infected with HIV.

## PRIORITIZING THE DIFFERENTIAL DIAGNOSIS

Mr. O presents with weight loss and significant HIV risk factors. Men who have sex with men (MSM) are at very high risk for acquiring HIV infection, especially if they have multiple partners and do not use condoms consistently. Mr. O is well aware of his high-risk behavior and is rightly concerned that his weight loss and oral lesions may suggest HIV infection. He comes to your office to be tested for HIV.

This discussion will focus on his chief concern: whether he has acquired HIV infection.

1

Mr. O's past medical history is remarkable for a history of syphilis and gonorrhea. Physical exam reveals a thin white man. He is 6' tall and weighs 140 pounds. HEENT exam reveals white coating on the palate consistent with thrush. Cardiac and pulmonary exam are unremarkable.

**Is the clinical information sufficient to make a diagnosis? If not, what other information do you need?**

## Leading Hypothesis: HIV infection

### Textbook Presentation

Chronic HIV infection may present in a myriad of ways. Many patients are asymptomatic in spite of long-standing HIV infection and even advanced immune deficiency. Other patients have conditions that suggest possible HIV infection but are frequently encountered in non–HIV-infected persons (eg, tuberculosis (TB), idiopathic thrombocytopenic purpura, nephropathy, cardiomyopathy, unexplained chronic diarrhea, herpes zoster, non-Hodgkin lymphoma).

HIV infection may be diagnosed only after a patient seeks medical attention for an opportunistic infection or malignancy that is highly suggestive of severe T-cell immunodeficiency (eg, oral candidiasis, pneumocystosis, cryptococcosis, Kaposi sarcoma, primary CNS lymphoma). Nonspecific skin findings, such as severe or refractory seborrheic dermatitis, psoriasis, and prurigo nodularis (see below for skin findings in HIV infected patients), may suggest the diagnosis.

### Disease Highlights

A. Prevalence

1. In December 2007, about 33.2 [30.6–36.1] million people were reported living with HIV worldwide (Table 5–1).

2. Rates vary dramatically by gender and ethnicity (Figure 5–1).

3. The Center for Disease Control and Prevention (CDC) estimates that at the end of 2003 the total number of persons in the United States living with HIV was > 1 million (1,039,000–1,185,000). Approximately 25% are unaware that they are infected.

B. Pathogenesis

1. HIV is a retrovirus. The viral enzyme reverse transcriptase uses the viral RNA genome as a template for production of DNA that is integrated into the cell genome.

2. The HIV virus carries 3 enzymes: reverse transcriptase, integrase, and protease; all 3 enzymes are targets of highly effective inhibitors.

3. Transmission

   a. The virus is present in blood, semen, and vaginal fluid.

   b. Common modes of transmission include male to male sexual transmission (62% of cases), needle sharing among injection drug users (17% of cases), heterosexual transmission (13% of cases), and vertical transmission from mother to child.

   c. Low viral loads decrease the rate of sexual transmission. Presence of sexually transmitted diseases (STDs), especially those that cause genital ulceration, increase the risk.

   d. Transmission through blood transfusion has been greatly reduced by blood product screening, implemented in 1985. Current risk associated with blood transfusion is ≈ 1/1,800,000 units in the United States with the current use of donor screening, and blood testing for HIV 1 and 2.

   e. The highest risk of sexual transmission is among patients with unprotected receptive anal intercourse, sex-for-hire workers, sexual contacts of sex-for-hire workers, and individuals with multiple sexual partners.

***Table 5-1.*** Global summary of the AIDS epidemic.

| | | |
|---|---|---|
| **Number of people living with HIV in 2007** | Total | 33 million (30–36 million) |
| | Adults | 30.8 million (28.2–34.0 million) |
| | Women | 15.5 million (14.2–16-9 million) |
| | Children under 15 y | 2.0 million (1.9–2.3 million) |
| People newly infected with HIV in 2007 | Total | 2.7 million (2.2–3.2 million) |
| | Adults | 2.3 million (1.9–2.8 million) |
| | Children under 15 y | 370,000 (330,000–410,000) |
| AIDS deaths In 2007 | Total | 2.0 million (1.8–2.3 million) |
| | Adults | 1.8 million (1.6–2.1 million) |
| | Children under 15 y | 270,000 (250,000–290,000) |

Reproduced, with permission, from 07 AIDS Epidemic Update, Joint United Nations Programme on HIV / AIDS (UNAIDS) and World Health Organization (WHO).

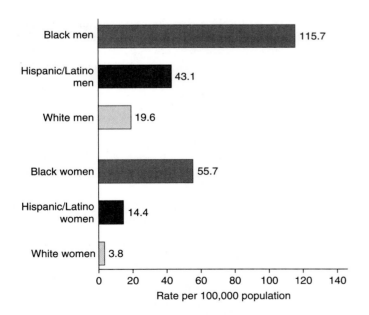

***Figure 5-1.*** Estimated rates of new HIV infections by race/ethnicity and gender, 2006. Total new infections estimated at 56,300 (95% confidence interval 48,200-64,500) new HIV infections in the United States. Source: MMWR Analysis Provides New Details on HIV Incidence in U.S. Populations. CDC HIV / AIDS Facts, September 2008.

4. Immune destruction
   a. The HIV surface protein GP 120 selectively binds first to the CD4 T receptor (main HIV receptor), then to one of two chemokine receptors (CCR5 or CXCR4) on CD4 T positive lymphocytes (helper cells).
   b. HIV replicates mostly in activated CD4 T cells.
   c. In acute HIV infection, there is a very rapid decrease in the CD4 T lymphocytes in the gut associated lymphoid tissues (GALT) but only a moderate and partially reversible decrease in the CD4 T lymphocyte count in the blood.
   d. In chronic HIV infection, there is a very slowly progressive decrease in the CD4 T lymphocyte count in the blood. This reflects about 2 billion cells destroyed and replaced every day. Both HIV-infected CD4 T lymphocytes and noninfected CD4 T lymphocytes are activated and destroyed.
   e. In most infected individuals, CD4 T cell death eventually outstrips CD4 T cell production, resulting in progressive depletion of CD4 helper lymphocytes in the blood.
      (1) When the absolute CD4 T lymphocyte count falls below 200/mcL, the patient is said to have immunologic AIDS.
      (2) A small percentage of infected individuals do not drop their CD4 counts over time (long-term nonprogressors).
   f. CD4 T cell counts below 200/mcL render patients susceptible to a wide array of opportunistic infections and malignancies.

5. Viral mutations
   a. The HIV virus mutates frequently.
   b. A high rate of mutations occurs because the reverse transcriptase enzyme is error prone and HIV replicates very rapidly (10 billion new viruses a day.)
   c. This allows for the rapid development of genetic variants.
   d. Effective therapy requires complete or near complete suppression of viral replication to prevent the production of mutations associated with drug resistance (see below).

C. Staging
   1. Stages of HIV infection include viral transmission, primary infection, seroconversion, clinically latent period, early symptomatic HIV infection, AIDS and advanced HIV infection.
      a. Primary infection
         (1) May be asymptomatic but up to 70% of patients may experience a "mononucleosis syndrome" with fever, rash, sore throat, diarrhea, lymphadenopathy, arthralgia, headache, and flu-like symptoms. Acute HIV infection should be considered when a mononucleosis syndrome fails to show evidence of infection by Epstein-Barr virus (EBV) (negative heterophile antibody, negative EBV viral capsid antibody (VCA) IgM) or cytomegalovirus (CMV) (negative CMV IgM).
         (2) Standard HIV enzyme immunoassay (EIA) and Western blot tests require an antibody response and are therefore negative during early primary infection (window period).
         (3) HIV viral load is markedly elevated (> 10,000/mcL and usually > 50,000/mcL)

**(4)** Diagnosis requires high index of suspicion and detection of HIV viral load.

**b.** Seroconversion

**(1)** Associated with a fall in HIV viral load with stabilization within 6 months to a stable level, the set point.

**(2)** In the absence of anti-HIV therapy, the set point predicts the rate of disease progression (ie, higher viral loads are associated with more rapid declines in CD4 cell counts).

**c.** Clinically latent period

**(1)** Following primary infection, viral replication continues primarily within activated CD4 T lymphocytes.

**(2)** Continued viral replication results in progressive destruction of the CD4 T lymphocyte pool.

**(3)** Persistent generalized lymphadenopathy is seen in some patients.

**(4)** Progression to an AIDS-defining illness is more common in patients with higher viral loads and lower CD4 counts (Table 5–2 and Figure 5–2).

**(5)** Progressive depletion of CD4 T lymphocytes renders patients increasingly susceptible to opportunistic infections and malignancies.

**d.** Early HIV disease before severe CD4 T cell depletion is associated with an increased risk of infections by relatively virulent pathogens (eg, bacterial pneumonia and TB).

**e.** Advanced HIV disease is accompanied by marked CD4 T cell depletion and by infection with both virulent and relatively avirulent (opportunistic) infections (eg, *Cryptococcus* and *Pneumocystis jiroveci* pneumonia (PCP)).

**(1)** Specific pathogens tend to occur only when the CD4 T cell count falls below a critical level (Figure 5–3).

**(2)** AIDS diagnostic criteria

**(a)** CD4 T count < 200/mcL and/or

**(b)** AIDS indicator condition: Common AIDS defining conditions include malignancies (primary CNS lymphoma, non-Hodgkin lymphoma, Kaposi sarcoma, and invasive cervical cancer), opportunistic infections (PCP, TB, *Mycobacterium avium* complex [MAC], recurrent bacterial pneumonia, esophageal candidiasis, cryptococcosis, progressive multifocal leukoencephalopathy [PML], toxoplasmosis,

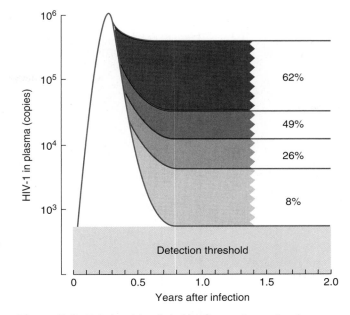

**Figure 5–2.** Relationship of viral load set point to development of AIDS. Source: http://research.bidmc.harvard.edu/VPTutorials/HIV/Tpath03a.htm

cryptosporidiosis), and other conditions (HIV-associated dementia, wasting syndrome).

**(c)** Advanced HIV infection defined as CD4 T count < 50/mcL

**Evidence-Based Diagnosis**

Similar to any other diagnosis, the positive predictive value (PPV) is determined by 3 features: the pretest probability of disease, the sensitivity of the test, and the specificity of the test. Each feature must be carefully evaluated in order to properly interpret HIV results.

**A.** Estimating pretest probability of HIV infection

**1.** Risk factors include MSM, injection drug abuse, and multiple sexual partners.

**2.** The prevalence of HIV infection varies from as low as 0.3% in the general US population to > 50% in certain high-risk groups.

**Table 5–2.** Percentage of patients not receiving HAART who progress to AIDS as a function of initial CD4 count and viral load.

| | HIV RNA ≤ 500 copies/mL | | HIV RNA 3001–10,000 copies/mL | | HIV RNA 10,001–30,000 copies/mL | | HIV RNA > 30,000 copies/mL | |
|---|---|---|---|---|---|---|---|---|
| | CD4+ > 750 cells/mcL | CD4+ ≤ 750 cells/mcL | CD4+ > 750 cells/mcL | CD4+ ≤ 750 cells/mcL | CD4+ > 750 cells/mcL | CD4+ ≤ 350 cells/mcL | CD4+ > 500 cells/mcL | CD4+ 351–500 cells/mcL |
| Percentage of patients with AIDS by 3 years | 0 | 3.7 | 3.2 | 8.1 | 9.5 | 40.1 | 32.6 | 47.9 |

HAART, highly active antiretroviral therapy.
Reproduced, with permission, from Mellors JW et al. Plasma viral load and CD4+ lymphocytes as prognostic markers of HIV-1 infection. Ann Intern Med. 1997:946–54.

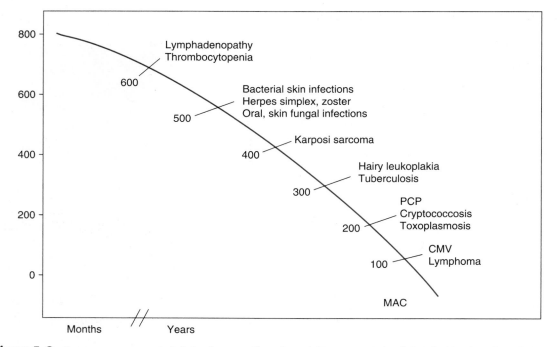

**Figure 5–3.** Common opportunistic infections as a function of CD4 count. Typical threshold values for infection (ie, *Pneumocystis jiroveci* pneumonia [PCP] is uncommon in patients with CD4 count > 200 cells/mcL). (CMV, cytomegalovirus; MAC, *Mycobacterium avium* complex.) Source: http://vhaaidsinfo.cio.med.va.gov/images/cd4.jpg

**B.** Sensitivity and specificity of tests for HIV

1. The diagnosis of chronic HIV infection involves the detection of antibody in a two-step process: initial screening with HIV-1 EIA and confirmatory HIV-1 Western blot to confirm repeatedly positive EIA.

2. HIV EIA testing

   **a.** HIV-1 EIA detects antibody to HIV-1 antigens. (Almost all HIV infections in the United States are HIV 1 of the group or type M [for main], subtype or clade B.)

   **b.** Sensitivity > 99%, specificity 98–99%

   **c.** False-positive results may be seen in a variety of circumstances, including recent influenza or hepatitis B immunization, DNA virus infections, increasing parity, positive rapid plasma reagin (RPR), improper heating, clerical error, HIV vaccine, cross reacting antibody.

   **d.** Confirmatory testing with a positive HIV-1 Western blot is required before the diagnosis of HIV infection can be made.

   **e.** False-negative EIA tests. Etiologies include

      **(1)** Recent HIV infection prior to development of antibodies (window period). With the newer tests, seroconversion occurs within 10 days to 6 weeks in most patients, and virtually all patients seroconvert within 6 months.

      **(2)** Rare causes of false-negative results include advanced AIDS with sero-*reversion* (rare), immunosuppressive therapy, malignancy, bone marrow transplant, B-lymphocyte dysfunction, replacement transfusion, hypogammaglobulinemia, and infections by rare HIV types.

 False-negative HIV-1 EIA is usually due to recent infection (window period).

3. Western blot testing

   **a.** Detects antibody to multiple HIV antigens and separates them using electrophoresis.

   **b.** Positive results require at least 2 of the following three bands: gp160/120, gp41, and p24. With such criterion, the Western blot can still very rarely be falsely positive.

   **c.** Negative results require the absence of any visible bands.

      **(1)** False-negative Western blot tests in the presence of a positive HIV EIA occur in the window period.

      **(2)** Other causes of false-negative results are rare in the United States.

   **d.** Indeterminate results

      **(1)** Occur in 10–15% of cases

      **(2)** Most patients have p24, p17, or both.

      **(3)** May represent either early HIV infection (during the window period) or lack of HIV infection (cross-reacting antibodies, HIV vaccine).

      **(4)** Infected patients in the window period will have a high viral load.

      **(5)** Patients with persistent, stable, indeterminate Western blot who have no new bands over 6 months are not infected with HIV 1.

4. Combination HIV-1 EIA and HIV-1 Western blot testing

   **a.** Combination strategy uses initial testing with HIV-1 EIA or HIV-1 and HIV-2 EIA (third-generation test).

**(1)** Patients with negative HIV EIA are not tested further; they do not have chronic HIV, although recent HIV infection is possible.

**(2)** Positive results are confirmed with the Western blot test.

**b.** Subsequent positive Western blot result confirms HIV infection.

**c.** Subsequent negative Western blot result rules out HIV infection.

**d.** This strategy further decreases the risk of false-positive results.

**e.** False-negative results may still occur in patients tested following recent infection.

**f.** Sensitivity, 99%; specificity, > 99%

 False-positive combined HIV-1 EIA and HIV-1 Western blot are very rare but need to be considered in very low prevalence populations (ie, blood donors or pregnant women) or when an undetectable viral load makes untreated HIV infection unlikely.

## Treatment

**A.** Initial work-up and vaccinations

**1.** Initial work-up should include a thorough history and physical exam, including a pelvic examination and Papanicolaou (Pap) smear in women.

**2.** Laboratory testing

**a.** Assesses current immune competence (absolute CD4 T-lymphocyte count, CD4 percentage, and HIV viral load)

**b.** Look for coinfections common in HIV-positive populations with the following tests.

**(1)** RPR

**(2)** Serology for hepatitis B and C

**(3)** Toxoplasma IgG

**(4)** PPD

**(5)** In women, test for chlamydia and gonorrhea as well as infection with the human papillomavirus (HPV), which causes an abnormal Pap smear; obtain HPV polymerase chain reaction (PCR) for high-risk HPV serotypes (type 16 and 18).

**c.** Baseline labs: CBC, comprehensive metabolic panel, lipid panel, G6PD level

**2.** Vaccinations

**a.** Pneumococcal vaccine should be given every 5 years.

**b.** Influenza vaccine should be administered each year.

**c.** Hepatitis B vaccine should be given to seronegative patients, and hepatitis A vaccine should be given to high-risk populations (ie, MSM)

**B.** Highly active antiretroviral therapy (HAART)

**1.** Has revolutionized HIV care in countries in which it is available. AIDS defining illnesses, mortality, and hospitalizations have decreased 60–80% since the introduction of HAART (Figure 5–4).

**2.** The cornerstone of therapy is the *simultaneous* and *uninterrupted* use of multiple antiretroviral drugs to which the virus is susceptible.

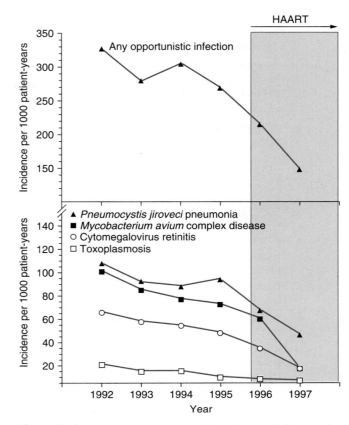

**Figure 5–4.** Reduction in opportunistic infections following the introduction of highly active antiretroviral therapy (HAART). (Reprinted, with permission, from Kovacs JA et al. Prophylaxis against opportunistic infections in patients with human immunodeficiency virus infection. N Engl J Med; 324:1416–1429.)

**3.** Complete suppression of viral replication is the goal of therapy.

**a.** The reverse transcriptase enzyme is highly error prone, resulting in a very high HIV mutation rate.

**b.** The high mutation rate of the HIV virus facilitates rapid drug resistance unless viral replication is almost completely suppressed.

**4.** Lifetime therapy is necessary to prevent viral rebound even in patients with undetectable viral loads for prolonged periods of time.

**5.** Definite indications for HAART

**a.** HIV-infected pregnant women, regardless of CD4 T cell count. (Risk of mother-to-child transmission is reduced to below 1–2% with therapy.)

**b.** Symptomatic patients with life-threatening or serious HIV-associated conditions (such as nephropathy, cardiomyopathy, idiopathic thrombocytopenic purpura, thrombotic thrombocytopenic purpura)

**c.** Asymptomatic patients with immunologic AIDS (CD4 T counts < 200/mcL)

**d.** Asymptomatic patients with CD4 T cell counts 200–350/mcL to prevent severe immunodeficiency, which is less likely to recover when HAART is started

**e.** Patients with HIV who have a coinfection with hepatitis B who require treatment of hepatitis B (because hepatitis B therapy requires 2 drugs that also have HIV activity and may select for HIV resistance)

f. Asymptomatic patients with CD4 T cell > 350/mcL may be candidates for HAART if the HIV viral load is > 100,000/mcL.

6. Controversial indications for HAART include acute HIV infections. Some experts recommend HAART therapy for individuals identified with an acute HIV infection.

7. Classifications of HAART

   a. > 20 available drugs belong to 5 classes
      (1) Protease inhibitors
      (2) Nucleoside reverse transcriptase inhibitors (NRTIs)
      (3) Non-nucleoside reverse transcriptase inhibitors (NNRTIs)
      (4) Integrase inhibitors
      (5) Entry inhibitors (CCR5 receptor inhibitors and fusion inhibitors)

   b. Protease inhibitors inhibit the HIV protease, resulting in lack of cleavage of a viral polyprotein precursor.

   c. Reverse transcriptase inhibitors block reverse transcription of viral RNA into DNA.

   d. Integrase inhibitors prevent the integration of HIV into the cellular DNA.

   e. Entry inhibitors prevent HIV entry by either inhibiting the CCR5 chemokine receptor (a co-receptor for HIV surface protein, present on all CD4 T lymphocytes), or by blocking the fusion of the HIV membrane with the cell membrane (fusion inhibitor).

8. Guidelines recommend monitoring CD4 T cell count and viral load every 3 months.

9. Patient adherence is key.

   a. Adherence of 90–95% is required to maintain viral control and prevent resistance.

   b. High adherence has been shown to decrease morbidity and mortality.

   c. Moderately poor adherence (50–90%) has some clinical benefits but promotes viral resistance, leading to eventual failure of therapy.

   d. Very poor adherence does not select for resistance but has no clinical benefits.

10. Predictors of poor adherence include substance abuse, mental illness, lack of access to medical care or medications, lack of patient education, and poor trust between patient and physician.

11. Goal of therapy: undetectable viral load (< 50/mcL) by 4–6 months.

12. Failure to achieve goal may be secondary to nonadherence, viral resistance, or rarely other factors (ie, malabsorption, interactions).

13. HIV testing for viral resistance is available (genotype and phenotype) and helps guide therapy in patients not responding to HAART. Decisions are complex and require expert guidance.

14. HAART and HIV transmission

    a. HAART has been associated with decreased risk of HIV transmission.

    b. However, HIV transmission has been documented despite undetectable viral loads.

    c. In addition to HAART, patients should be advised to use latex or polyurethane male or female condoms, use noninsertive practices avoiding mucosal exposure to genital secretions, or abstain from sexual activities to prevent acquiring or transmitting HIV sexually.

C. Primary and secondary prophylaxis of opportunistic infections

1. Primary prophylaxis prevents the *initial* infection.

2. Secondary prophylaxis prevents *subsequent symptomatic* episodes after the initial infection (may not eradicate the infection but prevent illness).

3. Primary prophylaxis

   a. The CD4 T cell count is the best predictor of susceptibility to opportunistic infections.

   b. Susceptibility is determined by the *current* CD4 T cell count rather than the nadir CD4 T cell count.

   c. HAART usually results in an increased CD4 T cell count, decreased risk of opportunistic infections and decreased need for prophylactic therapy (either primary or secondary). The current CD4 T cell count should guide decisions (Table 5–3).

4. Secondary prophylaxis may be stopped in patients in whom HAART restores the CD4 T count above the level recommended for primary prophylaxis (Table 5–4).

**Table 5–3.** Primary prophylaxis of opportunistic infections in HIV-infected patients.

| Pathogen | Indications for prophylaxis | Drug of Choice |
|---|---|---|
| PCP | CD4 count < 200 cells/mcL or oropharyngeal candidiasis | TMP-SMX double-strength once daily |
| Toxoplasmosis | Positive toxoplasma IgG *and* CD4 < 100 cells/mcL | TMP-SMX double-strength once daily |
| TB | Positive PPD (induration > 5 mm) regardless of CD4 count; recent significant exposure to active TB | INH 300 mg once daily (9 months) with pyridoxine |
| MAC | CD4 count < 50 cells/mcL | Azithromycin 1200 mg once a week |
| Varicella zoster virus | Exposure to chickenpox or shingles in patient without a history of either condition or negative antibody to varicella zoster virus | Varicella zoster immune globulin, 5 vials IM |

INH, isoniazid; MAC, *Mycobacterium avium* complex; PCP, *Pneumocystis jiroveci* pneumonia; TB, tuberculosis; TMP-SMX, trimethoprim-sulfamethoxazole.

***Table 5–4.*** Secondary prophylaxis of opportunistic infections in HIV-infected patients.

| Pathogen | Drug of choice | Indications to discontinue therapy |
|---|---|---|
| PCP | TMP-SMX double-strength once daily | CD4 count > 200 for 3 months |
| Toxoplasmosis | Sulfadiazine 500–1000 mg 4 times daily and pyrimethamine 25–50 mg once daily and leucovorin 10–25 mg once daily | CD4 count > 200/mcL for ≥ 6 months |
| TB | Not indicated | Secondary prophylaxis not indicated |
| MAC | Clarithromycin 500 mg twice daily and ethambutol 15 mg/kg once daily and rifabutin 300mg once daily | CD4 count > 100/mcL for 12 months and completed MAC therapy and asymptomatic for MAC |
| Cryptococcosis | Fluconazole 200 mg once daily | CD4 count > 100–200/mcL ≥ 6 months, completed therapy and asymptomatic for cryptococcosis |

MAC, *Mycobacterium avium* complex; PCP, *Pneumocystis jiroveci* pneumonia; TB, tuberculosis; TMP-SMX, trimethoprim-sulfamethoxazole.

## MAKING A DIAGNOSIS

HIV EIA testing is reported as positive and confirmed by a positive HIV-1 Western blot. All the bands are positive on the Western blot.

As noted above, 3 factors determine the PPV of the test: the pretest probability, the sensitivity, and the specificity. The oral lesions suggest thrush, highly suggestive of a T cell immunodeficiency (likely AIDS). Therefore, Mr. O has both clinical findings of AIDS and risk factors for HIV infection (high-risk sexual activity). His pretest probability of HIV infection is therefore very high. Combined with the excellent sensitivity and specificity of the 2-step HIV EIA and Western blot test, (99%, 99.8%) his posttest probability of HIV infection is > 99%.

Have you crossed a diagnostic threshold for the leading hypothesis, AIDS? Do other tests need to be done to exclude the alternative diagnoses?

## CASE RESOLUTION

Mr. O's CD4 T cell count is 25 cells/mcL. The viral load is 110,000/mcL. Hgb is 10 g/dL. The RPR and PPD are negative. Toxoplasma IgG is positive. Hepatitis A IgG is positive, hepatitis B surface antigen and antibody are negative. Hepatitis C antibody is negative.

At this point, HAART should be initiated because the CD4 T cell count is below 350/mcL. Fluconazole (100 mg/day) should be instituted for his thrush and continued until resolution. Primary prophylaxis is indicated for *Pneumocystis jiroveci* pneumonia (PCP), MAC, and toxoplasmosis. Trimethoprim-sulfamethoxazole (TMP-SMX) is an effective primary prophylaxis for both PCP and toxoplasmosis. Weekly azithromycin is recommended for MAC prophylaxis. Mr. O should receive hepatitis B, pneumococcal, and annual influenza vaccines.

# I have an HIV-positive patient who complains of headache. How do I determine the cause?

## CHIEF COMPLAINT

PATIENT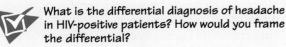

Mr. S is a 46-year-old man who is HIV- positive. He seeks medical attention for headache and vomiting.

What is the differential diagnosis of headache in HIV-positive patients? How would you frame the differential?

## CONSTRUCTING A DIFFERENTIAL DIAGNOSIS

Three pivotal considerations help frame the differential diagnosis in HIV-infected persons with neurologic complaints: the acuity of the symptoms, the degree of immunosuppression (ie, CD4 T cell count), and whether a mass lesion is seen on neuroimaging. The first pivotal step in evaluating the HIV-positive patient with headache is to determine the **acuity** of the presentation. Most opportunistic infections in HIV-infected patients are less virulent and present in a subacute fashion. However, in patients with an acute headache and fever (< 3 days), bacterial meningitis, herpes encephalitis, and West Nile virus must be considered promptly.

The next pivotal issue is to assess the **degree of immunosuppression**. HIV-positive patients with intact immunity and CD4 T cell counts > 200/mcL are at markedly diminished risk of opportunistic infections. The differential diagnosis of such headaches is similar to patients without HIV infection. These disorders are covered in Chapter 18, Headache. However, as the immunosuppression worsens and the CD4 T cell count falls below 200/mcL, the differential diagnosis broadens to include opportunistic infections and primary CNS lymphoma.

The final pivotal issue is to determine whether or not the patient has a **mass lesion**. The most common diagnoses in HIV-infected patients with low CD4 T cell counts and mass lesions are toxoplasmosis, progressive multifocal leukoencephalopathy (PML), and primary CNS lymphoma, whereas the most common diagnosis in such patients without a mass lesion is cryptococcal meningitis. CNS imaging and lumbar puncture are frequently required. In clinical practice, a CT scan is usually performed prior to lumbar puncture because it rapidly rules out a large mass lesion that may cause herniation after lumbar puncture. A platelet count, prothrombin time, and partial thromboplastin time should be checked prior to lumbar puncture to ensure the patient is not at an increased risk for developing a spinal epidural hemorrhage. An MRI is often performed subsequently due to its substantially increased sensitivity for several diagnoses. A diagnostic algorithm for the evaluation of headache in HIV-positive patients is summarized in Figure 5–5 and 5–6.

## Differential Diagnosis of Headache in Patient with HIV

A. Meningoencephalitis
1. Cryptococcal meningitis
2. HIV encephalopathy
3. CMV ventriculoencephalitis
4. TB meningoencephalitis
5. Neurosyphilis
6. Coccidioidomycosis (in southwestern United States)

B. Mass lesions
1. Toxoplasmosis
2. PML
3. Primary CNS lymphoma
4. Rare pathogens/presentations include cryptococcoma, tuberculoma, *Nocardia, Aspergillus,* bacterial abscess

Mr. S reports that his headache began 14 days previously. The headache is described as frontal, unrelenting, and pounding. He complains of subjective fevers, sweats, and chills. He admits to mild photophobia. Persistent vomiting has also developed over the last 6 days. He denies any history of confusion or seizures.

Past medical history is remarkable for a long history of injection drug use. His last reported use was 2 years ago. HIV was diagnosed 9 years ago. He has been non-compliant with HAART. He takes no medications. A CD4 count 1 year ago was 0/mcL.

 At this point, what is the leading hypothesis, what are the active alternatives, and is there a must not miss diagnosis? Given this differential diagnosis, what tests should be ordered?

## PRIORITIZING THE DIFFERENTIAL DIAGNOSIS

The first pivotal consideration is that Mr. S has had a headache for 2 weeks (subacute). This suggests a relatively less virulent opportunistic infection instead of a virulent bacterial meningitis or herpes encephalitis. Second, his prior CD4 count indicates profound immunosuppression. Therefore, he is at risk for all the serious opportunistic infections listed above. The third pivotal issue is whether there is a mass lesion. Ultimately, this will be confirmed or excluded on neuroimaging, but his headache and photophobia suggest some form of meningoencephalitis. Cryptococcal meningitis is the most common meningitis seen in patients with AIDS and is the leading hypothesis. Less common causes of meningoencephalitis include CMV, neurosyphilis, and TB. Coccidioidomycosis is uncommon but should be considered in patients in the southwestern United States. HIV meningitis may also present with headache. Should neuroimaging confirm a mass lesion, common causes include toxoplasmosis, PML, and primary CNS lymphoma. Since Mr. S has not taken TMP-SMX prophylaxis, he is at increased risk for toxoplasmosis, the most common CNS mass lesion in AIDS patients. Table 5–5 lists the differential diagnoses.

Physical exam reveals a thin man in moderate distress. Vital signs temperature, 35.9°C; BP, 154/100 mm Hg; pulse, 66 bpm; RR, 20 breaths per minute. HEENT: disks sharp, neck supple. Kernig and Brudzinski signs were negative. Cardiac, pulmonary, and abdominal exams are within normal limits. Neurologic exam: alert and oriented; cranial nerves intact; motor, sensory, and cerebellar functions were normal.

A CT scan (with contrast) is reported as normal. No mass lesions or evidence of sinusitis are seen.

The normal CT scan markedly diminishes the likelihood of the diseases associated with mass lesion and increases the likelihood of one of the remaining causes of meningitis (ie, *Cryptococcus,* CMV, neurosyphilis, etc) of which *Cryptococcus* is the most common. (An MRI is more sensitive and should be performed.)

 Is the clinical information sufficient to make a diagnosis? If not, what other information do you need?

## Leading Hypothesis: Cryptococcal Meningoencephalitis

### Textbook Presentation

Patients typically have a subacute headache, malaise, and fever that develop over days to weeks. Mental status changes may be seen. Importantly, meningismus is often absent due to the host's inability to mount an inflammatory reaction.

### Disease Highlights

A. Most common cause of meningoencephalitis in HIV-positive patients

B. Encapsulated fungus acquired via inhalation

C. Meningitis occurs due to dissemination of primary infection.

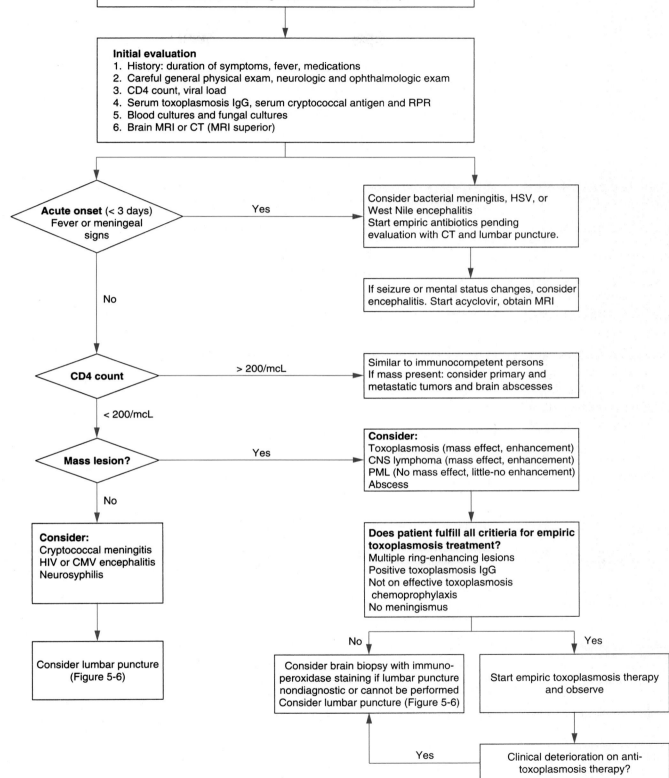

CMV, cytomegalovirus; HSV, herpes simplex virus; PML, progressive multifocal leukoencephalopathy.

***Figure 5–5.*** Diagnostic approach: headache in HIV-positive patients.

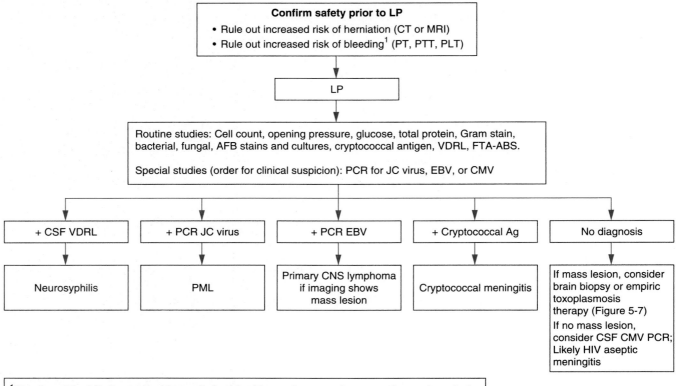

**Figure 5–6.** Evaluation of headache in HIV-positive patients: lumbar puncture.

**Table 5–5.** Diagnostic hypotheses for Mr. S.

| Diagnostic Hypotheses | Clinical Clues | Important Tests |
| --- | --- | --- |
| **Leading Hypothesis** | | |
| Cryptococcal meningitis | Headache, mental status changes | CD4 < 100/mcL<br>Serum and CSF cryptococcal antigen<br>CSF fungal culture |
| **Active Alternatives** | | |
| Mass lesions<br>Toxoplasmosis | Headache, focal findings, mental status changes<br>*Not* receiving TMP-SMX prophylaxis | Toxoplasma IgG +<br>MRI: multiple or single ring-enhancing lesions, mass effect and edema |
| Progressive multifocal leukoencephalopathy | Headache, focal findings, mental status changes | MRI single or multiple white matter nonenhancing lesions without mass effect. CSF + PCR JC virus |
| Primary CNS lymphoma | Focal findings, mental status changes | MRI single or multiple irregular enhancing lesions with mass effect<br>CSF PCR + EBV |
| Meningoencephalitis<br>CMV encephalitis | Headache, mental status changes | MRI normal or periventricular symmetric enhancement<br>CSF PCR CMV + |
| Neurosyphilis | History of chancre, rash | Serum RPR, FTA-ABS; CSF VDRL, FTA-ABS, CSF pleocytosis |

D. Usually seen in patients with CD4 T cell count < 100/mcL.

E. CNS inflammation is typically minimal and course indolent over 2–4 weeks.

F. Increased intracranial pressure common (> 20 cm $H_2O$ in lateral decubitus position)

   1. Elevated intracranial pressure associated with increased risk of death.

   2. 70% of patients with cryptococcal meningitis have significantly increased intracranial pressure.

   3. Patients with elevated intracranial pressure may have increased symptoms (headaches, clouded sensorium).

G. Mortality 6–12%

H. Pulmonary involvement has been reported in 6–23% of patients with cryptococcal meningitis.

### Evidence-Based Diagnosis

A. History

   1. Fever: 65–95%

   2. Headache: 73–100%

   3. Median duration of symptoms: 31 days (1–120 days)

B. Physical exam

   1. Stiff neck: 22–27%

   2. Photophobia: 18–22%

   3. Mental status changes: 22%

   4. Focal neurologic signs or seizures: 10%

   5. No CNS signs or symptoms: 14%

 Cryptococcal meningitis in AIDS patients is often indolent and only a small percentage of affected patients exhibit meningismus or photophobia. Some patients have only fever and malaise. A supple neck does not rule out the diagnosis, and a high index of suspicion is required.

C. Laboratory findings

   1. Blood tests

      a. Blood cultures positive in 15–35%

      b. Serum cryptococcal antigen

         (1) 95–100% sensitive, 96% specific

         (2) LR+ 24, LR– 0.05

         (3) Negative serum cryptococcal antigen makes cryptococcal meningitis highly unlikely.

         (4) Serum cryptococcal antigenemia may precede clinical cryptococcal meningitis.

   2. Lumbar puncture

      a. Neuroimaging is required prior to lumbar puncture to rule out mass effect. Mass lesions in such patients are often due to concomitant toxoplasmosis or lymphoma and only rarely due to cryptococcoma.

      b. A platelet count, prothrombin time, and partial thromboplastin time should be performed prior to lumbar puncture to rule out a bleeding diathesis, which increases the risk of a lumbar puncture–induced spinal epidural hematoma.

      c. Lumbar puncture is required in patients with suspected cryptococcal meningoencephalitis regardless of serum cryptococcal antigen results.

         (1) In patients with positive serum cryptococcal antigen, lumbar puncture is necessary to confirm cryptococcal meningitis, measure opening pressure, manage elevated intracranial pressure, and exclude other diagnoses.

         (2) In patients with negative serum cryptococcal antigen, lumbar puncture is necessary to evaluate other diagnoses.

      d. *Routine* cerebrospinal fluid (CSF) findings are often normal or minimally abnormal in many patients with cryptococcal meningitis.

         (1) Normal glucose, protein, and WBC: 19–30%

         (2) Glucose < 50 mg/dL: 64%

         (3) Protein > 40 mg/dL: 64%

         (4) CSF WBCs > 5/mcL: 35%

         (5) Increased opening pressure: 50–75%

 Routine CSF findings in patients with cryptococcal meningitis may be *normal*. Specific studies (fungal culture, cryptococcal antigen) must be obtained.

      e. Special CSF studies

         (1) CSF cryptococcal antigen: 91–100% sensitive, 93–98% specific

         (2) CSF fungal culture: 95–100% sensitive, 100% specific

### Treatment

A. Mortality is increased in patients with abnormal mental status and in patients with a marked elevated CSF cryptococcal antigen (> 1:1024). Low glycorrachia and normal CSF cell counts also predict poor outcomes.

B. Induction therapy for 2 weeks should include lipsosomal amphotericin B with or without flucytosine. Flucytosine must be dose-adjusted in patients with renal insufficiency.

C. *After* induction therapy with amphotericin and flucytosine, fluconazole (400 mg/day) can be substituted in selected patients with clinical improvement for an additional 8–10 weeks or until CSF cultures are sterile.

D. Maintenance therapy should then be continued (fluconazole 200 mg/day) for a minimum of 1 year. At this time, consideration can be given to stopping fluconazole in patients with an excellent response to HAART and a CD4 T cell count of > 100/mcL.

E. In patients with an elevated intracranial pressure, serial lumbar punctures are recommended to lower opening pressure to < 20 cm $H_2O$ or by 50%. Select patients with hydrocephalus benefit from ventricular shunts.

## MAKING A DIAGNOSIS

Blood cultures and serum cryptococcal antigen are ordered. A toxicology screen is positive for opioids and cocaine. CBC reveals a WBC of 3700/mcL (8% lymphocytes) a Hct of 36.6 and platelet count of 240,000/mcL. PT and PTT are normal. Serum RPR and

(Continued)

FTA-ABS are negative. Lumbar puncture reveals opening pressure of 30 cm H$_2$O. CSF ≥ 22 WBC/mcL; glucose, 26 mg/dL (versus serum of 127 mg/dL); and protein, 68 mg/dL (normal 15–45 mg/dL). Gram stain reveals numerous yeast forms.

 Have you crossed a diagnostic threshold for the leading hypothesis, cryptococcal meningitis? Have you ruled out the active alternatives? Do other tests need to be done to exclude the alternative diagnoses?

The CSF findings strongly suggest cryptococcal meningitis. Positive cryptococcal antigen or culture will confirm the diagnosis. A travel history to Arizona or the southwestern United States would raise the possibility of coccidioidomycosis. Neurosyphilis is unlikely with the negative RPR and fluorescent treponemal antibody absorbed (FTA-ABS). In addition, patients with AIDS may have more than one infection simultaneously. An MRI is more sensitive in the detection of CNS mass lesions than a contrast CT and is indicated to confidently exclude alternative diagnoses associated with masses. In addition, CMV encephalitis has not been excluded.

## Alternative Diagnosis: CMV Encephalitis

### Textbook Presentation

CMV encephalitis typically presents in acute or subacute fashion (< 8 weeks) with mental status changes and occasionally with focal deficits.

### Disease Highlights

**A.** Findings may include mental status changes, drowsiness, headache, and focal deficits. Cranial nerve abnormalities may be seen.

**B.** CD4 T cell counts usually < 50/mcL

**C.** Uncommon clinical cause of CNS disease in AIDS patients (< 2%): (Pathological findings frequent but clinical encephalitis rare)

**D.** Other neurologic syndromes caused by CMV include myelitis (presents with weakness and *hyperreflexia*), polyradiculopathy (presents with weakness and *hyporeflexia*), and mononeuritis multiplex.

**E.** CMV more commonly causes GI or retinal involvement than encephalitis.

**F.** CNS involvement is usually accompanied by involvement of retina, GI tract, or lung.

**G.** CMV retinitis antedates CMV ventriculoencephalitis in 50% of patients.

**H.** Disease develops secondary to reactivation of latent CMV.

**I.** Death usually occurs within 4–6 weeks.

### Evidence-Based Diagnosis

**A.** History and physical exam

1. Mental status changes common
2. Table 5–6 compares HIV and CMV encephalitis.
3. Onset of CMV encephalitis is more rapid than HIV encephalitis (3.5 vs 18 weeks).
4. Focal deficits seen in 50–70% of patients.

**Table 5–6.** Comparison of HIV and CMV encephalitis.

| | HIV encephalitis | CMV encephalitis |
|---|---|---|
| Duration of symptoms at presentation | 18 weeks | 3.5 weeks |
| Delirium | 27% | 90% |
| Apathy/withdrawal | 9% | 60% |
| Focal findings | 12% | 50–70% |
| Survival (pre-HAART) | 45 weeks | 8.5 weeks |

CMV, cytomegalovirus; HAART, highly active antiretroviral therapy.

**B.** Laboratory findings

1. CMV viremia seen in 60% but is not specific for involvement in CNS
2. MRI: A variety of nonspecific abnormalities may be seen: periventricular enhancement (45%), atrophy and ventriculomegaly (40%) and, rarely, ring-enhancing focal lesions. MRI is useful to rule out other diseases (ie, toxoplasmosis).
3. CSF
   **a.** Routine CSF findings not specific or sensitive
   **b.** CSF culture is positive in 10–25% of patients.
   **c.** CSF PCR CMV:
      **(1)** Test of choice for CMV encephalitis
      **(2)** 75% sensitive, 95% specific
      **(3)** LR+ 15; LR– 0.26

### Treatment

**A.** Ophthalmologic evaluation should be performed to rule out retinitis.

**B.** Ganciclovir, foscarnet, or both for 3–6 weeks: ganciclovir can cause neutropenia and thrombocytopenia, and foscarnet can cause hypocalcemia and renal failure.

**C.** An alternative agent is cidofovir, but it may cause serious renal toxicity.

**D.** HAART is particularly important.

## Alternative Diagnosis: Toxoplasmosis Encephalitis

### Textbook Presentation

Toxoplasmosis encephalitis in AIDS patients typically presents in a subacute fashion over 1–2 weeks, although more acute presentations with confusion or seizures may be seen. Focal neurologic manifestations are common. Confusion and mental status changes may dominate the clinical picture.

### Disease Highlights

**A.** Most common CNS mass lesion in AIDS patients

**B.** 15% of US population seropositive for toxoplasmosis

**C.** Toxoplasmosis encephalitis develops secondary to reactivation of latent toxoplasmosis; therefore, most patients have positive IgG titers (see later discussion).

D. CD4 T cell count < 100/mcL in 80% of patients

E. Probability of developing toxoplasmosis encephalitis is 30% in AIDS patients with CD4 T cell counts < 100/mcL and positive toxoplasmosis serology (if not receiving prophylaxis).

F. HAART is decreasing the incidence of toxoplasmosis encephalitis.

G. May be the initial manifestation or subsequent manifestation of HIV infection

H. 27% mortality despite treatment

I. Other concurrent CNS infections common

## Evidence-Based Diagnosis

A. History

1. Headache (often frontal and bilateral): 49–73%

2. Seizures: 15–31%

3. Hallucinations: 8%

4. Fever: 4–68%

B. Physical exam

1. Focal findings (weakness, abnormal gait, or other): 73–88%

2. Mental status changes: 50–67%

3. Mental status changes dominating clinical picture: 40%

4. Cognitive impairment (with normal arousal): 66%

5. Stiff neck: 0%

Meningismus is distinctly uncommon in cerebral toxoplasmosis and suggests an alternate or additional disease process.

C. Laboratory findings

1. Serology

a. Toxoplasma IgG: ≈ 97% sensitive

b. Toxoplasma IgM: Insensitive (15%) because disease is usually secondary to reactivation.

Cerebral toxoplasmosis is unlikely in patients with negative toxoplasma IgG.

c. Probability of toxoplasmosis encephalitis in seropositive patients with mass effect markedly reduced in patients receiving TMP-SMX prophylaxis (from 87% to 59%)

2. CSF analysis

a. Standard CSF analysis may be normal or nonspecifically elevated.

b. Percentage of patients with abnormal findings

(1) WBC > 5 cells/mcL: 50%

(2) Protein > 40 mg/dL: 81%

(3) Low glucose: 14%

(4) CSF toxoplasma IgG: 33–69%

c. CSF PCR is insensitive for toxoplasmosis but highly specific.

(1) 54% sensitive, 99% specific

(2) LR+ 54, LR– 0.46

3. Neuroimaging

a. MRI is test of choice.

(1) Superior to contrast CT and affects course in 40% of patients.

(2) Demonstrates 1 or more ring-enhancing lesions with mass effect and edema.

(3) Lesions may be located in basal ganglia, thalamus, and cortex.

(4) Single lesion in 14% of patients

(5) Single lesions make toxoplasmosis encephalitis less likely and increase likelihood of CNS lymphoma.

b. CT scan with contrast abnormal in 87–96%

(1) Single ring-enhancing lesion: 35%

(2) ≥ 2 ring-enhancing lesions: 62%

(3) Hypodense lesions: 13%

(4) Moderate to severe cerebral edema: 48%

(5) 75% of lesions located in cerebral hemispheres

(6) In patients with normal contrast CT scan or a single enhancing lesion, MRI is recommended.

c. Single photon emission CT (SPECT) thallium 201 imaging usually reveals decreased isotope activity in patients with toxoplasmosis encephalitis versus increased uptake in patients with CNS lymphoma. This distinction is less reliable in patients receiving HAART. 50% of patients with toxoplasmosis encephalitis taking HAART show increased uptake.

4. Brain biopsy

a. When positive, it is the only method that confirms cerebral toxoplasmosis with certainty.

(1) False-negative results can occur due to sampling error.

(2) Can diagnose concomitant infection

b. Sensitivity of standard hematoxylin & eosin (H & E) staining is only 50–66%. Immunoperoxidase staining adds significantly to sensitivity.

c. Brain biopsy is associated with 0.5–3.1% mortality and 10–40% morbidity.

d. Brain biopsy is not routine due to its attendant complications and imperfect sensitivity.

e. Empiric treatment for toxoplasmosis encephalitis is normally instituted in patients who fulfill all of the following criteria: multiple mass lesions, CD4 T cell count < 100/mcL, positive toxoplasma serology, and are not already receiving toxoplasmosis prophylaxis (Figure 5–7). Biopsy is reserved for atypical cases (ie, negative toxoplasmosis serology or nonresponders within 7–10 days).

## Treatment

A. Pyrimethamine plus sulfadiazine or pyrimethamine plus clindamycin

B. Folinic acid should also be administered to patients taking pyrimethamine.

C. TMP-SMX is an alternative therapy.

D. Clinical improvement occurs in > 90% of responders within first 2 weeks of drug therapy.

E. Radiologic improvement seen in most patients within 3 weeks of treatment.

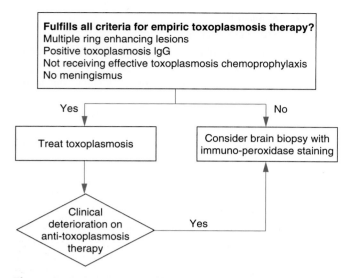

*Figure 5–7.* Empiric therapy for CNS toxoplasmosis in AIDS patients.

F. After induction therapy, suppressive therapy with lower doses should be used. Suppressive therapy can be safely discontinued in asymptomatic patients in whom HAART has restored CD4 T cell counts to > 200/mcL for ≥ 6 months. An MRI prior to discontinuation of suppressive therapy may be appropriate.

G. Corticosteroids are indicated for patients with cerebral edema *and* midline shift, or clinical deterioration within first 48 hours of therapy. Corticosteroids complicate interpretation of response to therapy since they may reduce edema and reduce the size of lesions due to primary CNS lymphoma.

H. Prevention: HIV-positive patients with a CD4 T cell count < 200/mcL and positive toxoplasma IgG should receive TMP-SMX as primary prophylaxis.

## Alternative Diagnosis: Progressive Multifocal Leukoencephalopathy

### Textbook Presentation

PML typically presents with progressive neurologic deficits, in particular weakness or gait disorders, over weeks to months. PML may also present with visual problems, headache, alterations in mental status, or dementia with focal signs.

### Disease Highlights

A. Etiologic agent is the JC virus, a polyomavirus (which should not be confused with the prion illness, Creutzfeldt-Jakob disease).

B. Primary JC virus infection is common and asymptomatic; 80–90% of population has antibodies to JC virus.

C. PML develops when profound immunosuppression allows latent virus in reticuloendothelial system and kidney to gain access to CNS and replicate.

D. Subsequent infection and lysis of the myelin-producing oligodendroglial cells results in PML. Astrocytes may also be infected.

E. Pathogenesis may involve HIV-associated immunosuppression and a direct synergistic effect of HIV and JC virus.

F. Multifocal or unifocal white matter lesions seen

G. Mean CD4 T cell count 84–104/mcL: 25% of patients have CD4 T > 200/mcL

H. PML occurs in 1–5% of AIDS patients.

### Evidence-Based Diagnosis

A. History and physical exam
   1. Limb weakness: 50–70%
   2. Gait disorder: 26–64%
   3. Speech disorder: 31–51%
   4. Visual impairment (ie, hemianopsia): 21–50%
   5. Seizures: 5–23%
   6. Headaches: 23%
   7. Cognitive abnormalities/mental status changes: 25–65%
   8. Cranial nerve palsies: 31%

B. Laboratory findings
   1. Serum antibodies to JC virus not useful due to high prevalence of JC virus infection in population.
   2. CSF
      a. Routine studies may be normal or nonspecifically elevated.
      b. CSF PCR for JCV DNA:
         (1) 80% sensitive, 98% specific
         (2) LR+ (average), 40; LR–, 0.20
         (3) Certain types of assays (repeat analysis) increase sensitivity to 90%.
         (4) Sensitivity may be diminished in patients receiving HAART.
   3. CNS imaging
      a. Typically shows extensive multifocal patchy white matter demyelination with sparing of the cortical gray matter
      b. MRI is more sensitive than CT scanning (CT 63% sensitive).
      c. Lesions are hypodense on CT scanning, low intensity on T1 weighted MRI, hyperintense on T2 weighted MRI.
      d. On imaging, lesions appear restricted to the subcortical white matter, respecting the gray-white junction of the cerebrum.
      e. There is overlap in the MRI features of toxoplasmosis, primary CNS lymphoma, and PML. However certain features *suggest* PML:
         (1) Lack of enhancement
         (2) Lack of mass effect
         (3) Less well-circumscribed lesions
      f. MRI typically shows scalloping at gray-white matter interface.
      g. CT scanning typically demonstrates white matter hypodense lesions.
      h. Brain biopsy: 100% specific but sensitivities range from 64% to 96% due to sampling error.

 MRI is markedly superior to CT for diagnosis of PML.

## Treatment

**A.** HAART associated with improvement or cure in some patients.

  **1.** Survival pre-HAART averaged 4-6 months. Survival has improved to 50% since the introduction of HAART.

  **2.** 80% of survivors have severe residual neurologic deficit.

**B.** Initiation of HAART occasionally results in PML in previously asymptomatic patients due to increased inflammation associated with immune reconstitution.

## Alternative Diagnosis: Primary CNS Lymphoma

### Textbook Presentation

Typically, patients have advanced HIV disease and profound immunosuppression. While patients may develop focal complaints (ie, weakness), many seek medical attention for altered mental status or seizures.

### Disease Highlights

**A.** Biologically distinct from primary CNS lymphoma in other immunocompromised states

**B.** Diffuse, high-grade, B cell, non-Hodgkin lymphoma arising and confined to the CNS (ie, not due to CNS involvement by *systemic* lymphoma)

**C.** CD4 T cell counts usually < 50/mcL

**D.** Consistently associated with EBV in the tumor

**E.** Pathogenesis likely involves activation of latent EBV genes due to immunodeficiency. The relative immunologic sanctuary of the CNS from immune surveillance may facilitate growth of these tumors at this location.

**F.** Rapidly progressive with a short interval from symptoms to diagnosis (1.8 months)

**G.** Median survival without treatment ≈1 month

**H.** Supratentorial location 3× more common than infratentorial

**I.** Most common cause of death in patients with primary CNS lymphoma is *other* opportunistic infection.

**J.** Marked reduction in primary CNS lymphoma incidence (≈ 90%) from 1995 to 2000 because of the introduction of HAART

### Evidence-Based Diagnosis

**A.** History and physical exam

  **1.** B symptoms (weight loss > 10%, unexplained temperatures > 38.0°C, drenching sweats): 80%

  **2.** Focal neurologic deficits: 51%

  **3.** Mental status changes: 53%

  **4.** Seizures: 27%

**B.** Laboratory findings

  **1.** CSF EBV PCR:

    **a.** 87% sensitive, 98% specific

    **b.** LR+, 43; LR−, 0.13

  **2.** Positive CSF cytology only 15–23% sensitive. Special studies are required to distinguish monoclonal proliferations from reactive T cell populations.

**C.** Radiologic studies

  **1.** CT scanning

    **a.** 90% sensitive

    **b.** Usually reveals contrast enhancement (90%)

    **c.** 48% single lesion, 52% multiple lesions

    **d.** Usually associated with mass effect (similar to toxoplasmosis but not seen in PML)

  **2.** MRI more sensitive than CT scanning

  **3.** SPECT thallium imaging

    **a.** Primary CNS lymphoma usually demonstrates early uptake and retention (compared with decreased uptake in necrotic centers of toxoplasmosis).

      **(1)** 86–100% sensitive, 77–100% specific (higher specificity was noted if retention index measured).

      **(2)** Increased uptake is noted in 15% of patients with toxoplasmosis encephalitis not receiving HAART but up to 50% of patients with toxoplasmosis encephalitis receiving HAART, making this test less useful in patients receiving HAART.

**D.** Biopsy

  **1.** Positive CSF EBV PCR may make biopsy unnecessary.

  **2.** Biopsy useful when CSF EBV PCR is negative.

  **3.** Lympholytic effect of corticosteroids may render biopsy nondiagnostic.

 Corticosteroids should not be administered before brain biopsy in patients with suspected primary CNS lymphoma unless the patient is at an increased risk for herniation.

### Treatment

**A.** Prognosis is grave with or without therapy.

**B.** Chemotherapy, whole brain radiotherapy, and corticosteroids have been used. Chemotherapy modestly prolongs survival (median survival 7 months).

**C.** Methotrexate, zidovudine, and ganciclovir have been used.

**D.** HAART therapy is beneficial in some patients. One small study noted marked increases in 2-year survival (6/7 with HAART compared with 0/18 without HAART).

**E.** Surgical resection does not improve prognosis due to multifocal nature of disease.

## CASE RESOLUTION

An MRI was performed and confirmed the absence of a CNS mass. Blood and CSF cultures grew *Cryptococcus neoformans*. Subsequent CSF AFB cultures and VDRL were negative.

Mr. S's CSF culture confirmed cryptococcal meningitis. His subacute course and lack of meningeal findings are in fact a common feature of this disease. CSF analysis did not suggest concomitant mycobacterial infection or neurosyphilis, and the MRI did not suggest toxoplasmosis, multifocal leukoencephalopathy, or primary CNS lymphoma.

Mr. S was treated and showed gradual improvement. After 2 weeks of therapy, he was discharged to follow-up with the infectious disease clinic.

## REVIEW OF OTHER IMPORTANT DISEASES

### HIV Encephalopathy (HIV-associated dementia)

#### Textbook Presentation

Patients typically have advanced HIV disease with a slowly progressive dementing process eventually accompanied by motor symptoms.

#### Disease Highlights

A. Subcortical dementia characterized by cognitive, behavioral and psychomotor slowing.

B. Prevalence 15–20% in AIDS patients prior to introduction of HAART

C. 40–50% decrease in incidence since the introduction of HAART. However, prevalence is rising due to increasing survival.

D. Severe form of encephalopathy effectively eliminated by HAART

E. Milder deficits still common

F. Principal target is perivascular CNS macrophages. Astrocytes may also become infected.

G. HIV encephalopathy develops late in infection. CD4 T cell count is typically < 200/mcL.

H. The precise pathophysiology is complex and not understood but may involve multiple inflammatory mechanisms as well as HIV proteins, which induce neuronal apoptosis.

I. Twofold increased risk in patients aged ≥ 50 years.

J. Neurotoxicity of HIV may be synergistic with that of cocaine or methamphetamine.

#### Evidence-Based Diagnosis

A. History and physical exam
   1. Memory complaints: 70%
   2. Cognitive slowing: 25–30%
   3. Gait difficulty: 45%
   4. Behavioral changes: 10–20%
   5. Seizures: 5–10%
   6. Focal findings uncommon

B. Laboratory findings
   1. MRI: T2 images may demonstrate hyperintensities in the deep white matter and basal ganglia without contrast enhancement and/or atrophy
   2. CSF
      a. Useful to rule out other infections

   b. Mild pleocytosis and protein elevations may be seen.
   c. CSF HIV RNA levels to do not correlate with HIV encephalopathy.
   d. Cannot diagnose HIV encephalopathy with certainty.
3. Neuropsychological testing is useful in evaluating the severity and response to HAART.

HIV encephalopathy is a diagnosis of exclusion. Diagnostic evaluations serve to exclude other opportunistic infections, malignancy, or substance abuse.

#### Treatment

A. HAART is recommended.

B. Most patients treated with HAART remain stable or show partial reversal of neurologic deficits. Early therapy is therefore important.

C. Elevated levels of CSF β-microglobulin (suggesting ongoing inflammation) predicted better neurologic recovery with HAART.

### Neurosyphilis in HIV-Positive Patients

#### Textbook Presentation

Patients with neurosyphilis may be asymptomatic or have meningitis, stroke-like symptoms, visual or hearing loss, or other focal deficits due to CNS gummas.

#### Disease Highlights

A. Caused by spirochete *Treponema pallidum*

B. Because infection is transmitted sexually, the group at highest risk is MSM. Other high-risk groups include injection drug users and patrons of paid sex workers.

C. Association of HIV and syphilis infection
   1. Some studies have documented a coinfection rate of HIV in patients with syphilis of 25–70%.
   2. Neurosyphilis in HIV-infected patients is less frequent (1%).

D. Syphilis commonly infects the CNS early in the course of disease in both HIV-infected and non–HIV-infected persons (25–33%).

E. The CNS infection is more often progressive in HIV-infected persons, increasing the need for detection in this group.

Coinfection with syphilis and HIV is common. Patients with either disease should be tested for the other.

F  Infections develop in characteristic stages.
   1. Primary infection
      a. Characterized by chancre: a 0.5- to 2-cm painless, indurated, well-circumscribed ulcerated papule at the site of primary inoculation approximately 2–3 weeks after contact
      b. Multiple chancres may be seen in HIV-infected patients.
      c. Lesion resolves with *or* without therapy.

**2.** Secondary stage

   **a.** Symptoms include macular or maculopapular rash involving the palms and soles in 70%, fever, myalgias and lymphadenopathy; oral mucosal patches, perineal condyloma lata (often exuberant in HIV/AIDS).

   **b.** Develops within weeks to months of primary infection

   **c.** Symptoms of secondary syphilis may or may not be seen.

   **d.** Secondary syphilis and chancres may coexist in HIV-infected patients.

**3.** Latent syphilis: Without therapy, 60–70% of patients have no disease progression.

**4.** Late or tertiary stage

   **a.** Develops in one-third of untreated patients

   **b.** Gummas (granulomas with caseating necrosis) affect involved organs and usually develop over 4–10 years but may develop within months in HIV-infected patients.

   **c.** Myriad of manifestations including cardiac (aortic root and coronary artery involvement), eyes, skin, and CNS

**5.** Neurosyphilis

   **a.** May be asymptomatic or symptomatic

   **b.** Neurosyphilis can develop early (< 1 year) or late after syphilis infection in HIV-infected patients.

     **(1)** Typical early symptoms include cranial nerve palsies, meningitis or meningovascular symptoms (strokes secondary to arteritis). One report found visual symptoms in 51%; headache in 32%; and gait difficulty, hearing loss, meningismus, or altered mental status in < 5%.

     **(2)** Early neurosyphilis develops in 1.7% of HIV-infected MSM who acquire syphilis.

     **(3)** Typical late symptoms include tabes dorsalis, general paresis (dementia associated with psychotic features) and almost any focal finding.

     **(4)** May present with visual loss secondary to ophthalmic involvement (uveitis) or hearing loss

### Evidence-Based Diagnosis

**A.** Primary syphilis

   **1.** Darkfield exam of chancre is the test of choice but availability is limited.

   **2.** Direct fluorescent antibody (DFA) may be available.

**B.** Secondary syphilis

   **1.** Nonspecific treponemal tests of serum (RPR) are highly sensitive for secondary syphilis.

   **2.** Confirmation with FTA-ABS is required to confirm diagnosis.

**C.** Tertiary syphilis

   **1.** RPR is positive in two-thirds of patients. Confirmation by FTA-ABS still required.

   **2.** FTA-ABS is 100% sensitive.

   **3.** False-negative results occur rarely.

**D.** Neurosyphilis

   **1.** Approximately half of men with neurosyphilis have no other history or evidence of syphilis.

 Consider neurosyphilis in HIV-infected patients with new visual symptoms or headache.

**2.** CD4 T cell count: 25–882/mcL. Mean CD4 T cell count: 217–312/mcL.

**3.** Estimating test accuracy is difficult due to the lack of a gold standard.

**4.** Commonly used criteria include *either* positive CSF VDRL *or* positive *serum* serology for syphilis *and* CSF pleocytosis.

   **a.** CSF VDRL is highly specific but sensitivity is ≈ 50%.

   **b.** CSF pleocytosis may be more sensitive but less specific due to other infections that increase CSF WBCs (including the HIV virus and other opportunistic infections).

   **c.** Reverse transcriptase PCR testing of CSF for *T pallidum* has been used but has limited sensitivity.

   **d.** CSF FTA-ABS is highly sensitive but less specific. A negative CSF FTA-ABS makes neurosyphilis very unlikely.

**5.** Perform lumbar puncture to look for neurosyphilis in any HIV-positive patient with syphilis and either:

   **a.** Neurologic symptoms of any type, including meningitis, stroke-like syndrome, visual loss, hearing loss, dementia, or other focal deficit

   **b.** Persistent signs of infection despite treatment (ie, failure of RPR to fall fourfold with treatment)

   **c.** Serum RPR titer ≥ 1:32

     **(1)** Increases the likelihood of neurosyphilis in HIV-infected persons with syphilis

     **(2)** 76–96% sensitive, 59% specific

   **d.** CD4 T cell count ≤ 350/mcL.

     **(1)** Increases the likelihood of neurosyphilis in HIV-infected persons with syphilis

     **(2)** 69% sensitive, 53% specific

   **e.** HIV-infected patients with late latent syphilis (> 1 year) or of unknown duration

### Treatment

**A.** Primary and secondary syphilis

   **1.** Single-dose benzathine penicillin IM

   **2.** Penicillin allergy: doxycycline

   **3.** Follow RPR every 3 months for 1 year to document 4 × fall in titer.

**B.** Latent syphilis

   **1.** If duration is unknown, lumbar puncture is recommended to rule out neurosyphilis.

   **2.** If lumbar puncture is negative, administer IM benzathine penicillin every week for 3 weeks.

   **3.** Follow RPR every 6 months for 2 years to document 4 × fall in titer.

**C.** Neurosyphilis

   **1.** IV penicillin for 10–14 days

   **2.** Penicillin allergy: high-dose ceftriaxone, oral doxycycline, or desensitization to penicillin followed by IV penicillin for 10–14 days. The latter strategy is most effective.

A summary of the clinical and radiological features, CD4 T count, and tests of choice of the common CNS disorders in AIDS patients is presented in Table 5–7.

***Table 5–7.*** Summary of findings in CNS disorders in AIDS patients.

| Disease | Common Clinical Features | Radiologic Features | Test of Choice |
|---|---|---|---|
| **Mass Lesions** | | | |
| Toxoplasmosis | Headache<br>Focal findings<br>Mental status changes<br>Onset days<br>CD4 < 100/mcL | MRI multiple ring enhancing lesions in most patients | Serum toxoplasma IgG almost always positive<br>MRI |
| PML | Headache<br>Focal findings<br>Mental status changes<br>Onset weeks-months<br>CD4 average 100/mcL (may be > 200/mcL) | MRI single or multiple, asymmetric white matter lesions<br>No mass effect or enhancement | CSF PCR JC virus<br>If negative, consider brain biopsy<br>MRI |
| Primary CNS lymphoma | Headache<br>Focal findings,<br>Mental status changes<br>Onset days-weeks<br>CD4 < 50/mcL | MRI or CT => single (50%) or multiple (50%) irregular enhancing lesions; Lesions may be large (> 4 cm) | CSF PCR EBV<br>If negative, perform brain biopsy<br>MRI |
| **Non-Mass Lesions** | | | |
| Cryptococcal meningitis | Headache<br>Mental status changes<br>CD4 < 100/mcL | Mass lesions rare | Serum or CSF cryptococcal antigen<br>CSF fungal culture |
| HIV encephalopathy | Dementia, ataxia, tremor<br>CD4 < 200/mcL | MRI may show atrophy and/or hyper-intensities in the deep white matter and basal ganglia without contrast enhancement | Diagnosis of exclusion<br>Imaging may be very suggestive |
| CMV encephalitis | Mental status changes<br>Headache<br>Focal findings CD4 < 50/mcL | MRI may show periventricular enhancement, ventricular enlargement, or be normal | CSF CMV PCR |
| TB meningitis | Mental status changes<br>Cranial nerve palsies<br>Any CD4 count | MRI demonstrates meningeal enhancement, occasional mass, or may be normal | AFB stain, large volume CSF for culture |
| Neurosyphilis | Visual symptoms, headache, cranial neuropathy, CVA, dementia<br>Any CD4 count | May demonstrate CVA, rarely mass lesion | Serum RPR,<br>Serum FTA-ABS<br>CSF RPR |

# I have an HIV-positive patient with a cough and fever. How do I determine the cause?

## CHIEF COMPLAINT

> ### PATIENT 3
>
> Mr. L is a 35-year-old man who is HIV-positive. His chief complaints are cough and fever lasting for 4 days.
>
> What is the differential diagnosis of cough and fever in HIV positive patients? How would you frame the differential?

## CONSTRUCTING A DIFFERENTIAL DIAGNOSIS

The most common pneumonias in HIV-infected patients are bacterial pneumonia, Pneumocystis jirovecii pneumonia (PCP), and TB. Taken together, they account for 91% of pulmonary infections in HIV-positive patients. Three pivotal features aid in the diagnosis of these common pneumonias in HIV-infected persons. First, the CD4 T cell count gauges the level of immunocompromise. Virulent infections, such as TB or bacterial pneumonia, may occur in patients with *any* CD4 T cell count. On the other hand, less virulent infections, such as PCP, are seen almost exclusively in patients with CD4 T cell counts < 200/mcL. Atypical mycobacteria, fungal, and CMV infections usually occur in patients with CD4 T counts < 100/mcL.

The second pivotal feature is that certain diseases present acutely (ie, bacterial pneumonia), whereas other diseases present subacutely or chronically (ie, TB or PCP).

The final pivotal feature that aids in the diagnosis of these complaints is the pattern on chest radiograph. Lobar infiltrates suggest bacterial pneumonia, whereas diffuse or interstitial infiltrates are seen in PCP, CMV, and fungal infections. Patterns that suggest TB include apical or cavitary infiltrates, hilar lymphadenopathy, or nodular infiltrates. The chest radiographic pattern in TB varies depending on the patient's degree of immunosuppression. Table 5–8 and Figure 5–8 summarize the typical CD4 T cell count, acuity, and chest radiographic pattern and approach to pulmonary infection in HIV-positive patients.

Tumors may also cause pulmonary complaints. Not surprisingly, aggressive neoplasms, such as lung cancer, may occur at any CD4 T cell count, whereas lymphoma usually develops in patients with CD4 T cell counts < 500/mcL, and Kaposi sarcoma usually develops in patients with CD4 counts < 200/mcL.

As noted above, the most common pneumonias in HIV-infected patients are bacterial pneumonia, PCP and tuberculosis. PCP is reviewed in Chapter 9 and will be mentioned here only briefly. The remainder of this section will focus on bacterial pneumonia, tuberculosis and non-tuberculous mycobacterial infection in HIV-infected patients.

## Differential Diagnosis of Pulmonary Processes in Patients with HIV

**A.** CD4 T cell count > 500/mcL
1. Bacterial pneumonia
2. TB
3. Lung cancer

**B.** CD4 T cell count 200–499/mcL: All of the above plus lymphoma

**C.** CD4 T cell count 100–199/mcL: All of the above plus PCP

**D.** CD4 T count < 100/mcL: All of the above plus the following:
1. Fungal infections uncommon (cryptococcosis, aspergillosis, histoplasmosis, blastomycosis, coccidioidomycosis)
2. CMV (commonly found, rarely pathogenic)
3. Atypical mycobacteria (MAC)
4. Kaposi sarcoma

Mr. L reports that he was feeling well until 4 days ago when sudden-onset fever of 38.8°C, cough productive of green sputum, and right-sided chest pain with inspiration developed. He feels moderately short of breath with exertion. Medical history is remarkable for sexually acquired HIV infection diagnosed 2 years ago. His last CD4 T cell count 1 month ago was 400/mcL. At that time, his viral load was undetectable. He is compliant with HAART.

At this point, what is the leading hypothesis, what are the active alternatives, and is there a must not miss diagnosis? Given this differential diagnosis, what tests should be ordered?

## PRIORITIZING THE DIFFERENTIAL DIAGNOSIS

There are 2 key features to Mr. L's presentation. The first pivotal feature is that his CD4 T cell count is only moderately reduced. This makes a variety of opportunistic infections unlikely (ie, PCP, MAC, CMV, and fungal infections). On the other hand, both TB

**Table 5–8.** Summary of findings in pulmonary infection in HIV-positive patients.

| Variable | Tuberculosis | Bacterial Pneumonia | PCP |
|---|---|---|---|
| Acuity | Subacute<br>Weeks to months | Acute<br>< 1 week | Subacute<br>Weeks to months |
| CD4 | Any count | Any count | < 200/mcL |
| Typical chest radiographic pattern | CD4 > 200 /mcL: Apical, cavitary or nodular lesions<br>CD4 < 200 /mcL: Normal, or middle or lower lobe consolidation, miliary pattern, lymphadenopathy | Lobar consolidation | Bilateral perihilar diffuse symmetric interstitial pattern |
| Risk factors | Foreign born or traveler to endemic area, recent exposure, prior positive PPD, injection drug use, prison | Injection drug use, Low CD4 count | Low CD4 count |
| Other clues | Pleural effusions may be seen | | Elevated lactate dehydrogenase, more hypoxia than expected from chest radiographic findings |
| Diagnostic tests of choice | Sputum smear and culture. BAL if no productive cough; Biopsy if miliary TB | Sputum culture, Gram stain and blood culture | Sputum obtained by BAL.[1] Silver stain, H & E, or DFA for PCP |

[1]Most institutions lack the expertise to reliably detect PCP in expectorated sputum. BAL is usually required. BAL, bronchoalveolar lavage.

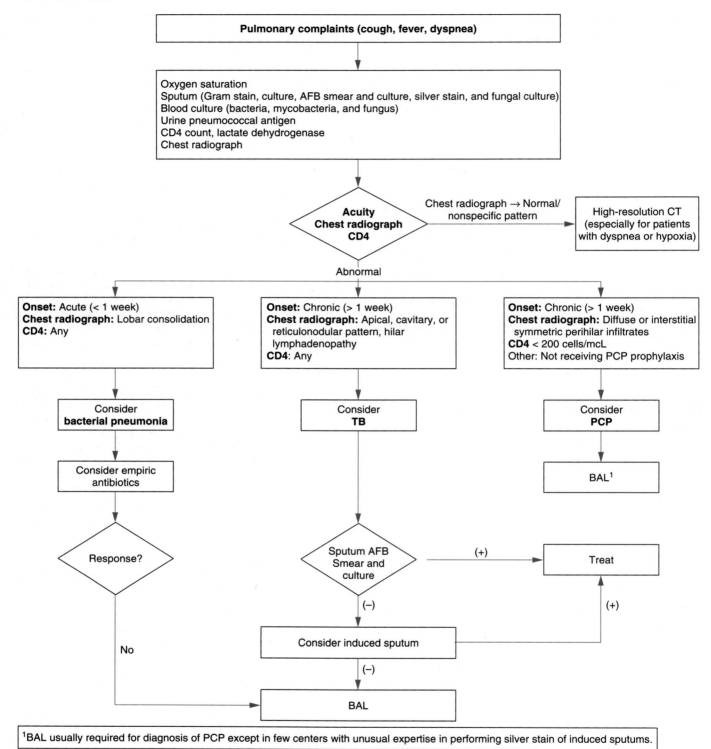

**Figure 5–8.** Evaluation of pulmonary complaints in HIV-positive patients.

AFB, acid-fast bacilli; BAL, bronchoalveolar lavage; PCP, *Pneumocystis jiroveci* pneumonia; TB, tuberculosis.

and bacterial pneumonia are sufficiently virulent to present in patients with normal or mildly impaired immune systems. The second pivotal feature is the rapid development of the pulmonary process, which strongly favors bacterial pneumonia over TB. The differential diagnosis is summarized in Table 5–9.

Physical exam reveals the following: temperature, 38.6°C; BP, 120/75 mm Hg; HR, 110 bpm; RR, 18 breaths per minute. Lung exam reveals crackles over the lower one-third of posterior right chest. Chest radiograph reveals a right lower lobe consolidation. No effusion is seen. WBC is 8000/mcL with 15% bands. Sputum

**Table 5–9.** Diagnostic hypotheses for Mr. L.

| Diagnostic Hypotheses | Clinical Clues | Important Tests |
|---|---|---|
| **Leading Hypothesis** | | |
| Bacterial pneumonia | Acute onset, any CD4 count, purulent sputum | Chest radiograph: lobar infiltrate(s) Sputum culture and Gram stain Blood culture Pneumococcal urinary antigen |
| **Active Alternative—Most Common** | | |
| Tuberculosis | Recent exposure, positive PPD, foreign born, subacute onset, any CD4 count | CD4 > 200: Chest radiograph shows apical, cavitary or nodular lesion CD4 < 200: Chest radiograph shows lower lobe consolidation, adenopathy Sputum AFB smear and culture |
| **Other Hypotheses** | | |
| PCP | Subacute/chronic process CD4 < 200/mcL, not receiving TMP-SMX prophylaxis | Chest radiograph: bilateral diffuse perihilar infiltrates |
| MAC | Systemic illness: fever, weight loss, and night sweats CD4 < 50/mcL | Chest radiograph: any pattern; AFB sputum smear and culture; blood culture |

Gram stain reveals numerous PMNs and gram-positive diplococci. The initial AFB smear is negative. Blood cultures are sent.

Is the clinical information sufficient to make a diagnosis? If not, what other information do you need?

## Leading Hypothesis: Bacterial Pneumonia

### Textbook Presentation

Typical onset is acute (< 1 week) with productive cough and fever. Patients may have purulent sputum and pleuritic chest pain. Presentation is similar to bacterial pneumonia in HIV-negative patients.

### Disease Highlights

A. Bacterial infection is the most common cause of pneumonia in HIV-positive patients.

HIV should be considered in patients with severe or recurrent community-acquired pneumonia.

B. Recurrent bacterial pneumonia (> 2 episodes within 1 year) is an AIDS-defining condition.

C. May occur at any time during course of HIV infection

D. Risk of bacterial pneumonia increases as CD4 T cell count falls. Injection drug use further increases the risk.

1. CD4 T cell count
   a. Rate of bacterial pneumonia in HIV-negative patients: 0.9%/year
   b. Rate of bacterial pneumonia all HIV-positive patients: 5.5%/year
      (1) CD4 T cell count > 500/mcL: 2.3%/year
      (2) CD4 T cell count 200–500/mcL: 6.8%/year
      (3) CD4 T cell count < 200/mcL: 10.8%/year
      (4) Two-thirds of cases in HIV-infected patients developed in those with CD4 T cell count < 200/mcL.

2. Injection drug use
   a. Pneumonia incidence in HIV-infected patients without a history of injection drug use is 4.1%/year, compared with 11.1%/year in HIV-infected persons with a history of injection drug use.
   b. Increased rate of septic emboli from infective endocarditis

3. HAART significantly reduces the risk of bacterial pneumonia (45%).

E. Etiology

1. *Streptococcus pneumoniae* is the most common cause of bacterial pneumonia. Other common causes include *Haemophilus influenzae, Mycoplasma pneumoniae, Staphylococcus aureus,* and *Pseudomonas aeruginosa.*

2. *S pneumoniae* is associated with higher WBC than *P aeruginosa* (12,400/mcL vs 5000/mcL) and higher average CD4 T count (106/mcL vs 19/mcL).

3. *M pneumoniae* was the causative agent in 21% of HIV-infected patients with pneumonia in 1 study.

4. *P aeruginosa* has been reported as causative agent in up to 38% of hospital-acquired pneumonias and 3–25% of community-acquired pneumonias. It has been associated with a 33% in-hospital mortality rate.

5. Concomitant PCP is present in 13% of patients with bacterial pneumonia.

F. Complications and prognosis

1. Bacterial pneumonia progresses more rapidly and is more often complicated in HIV-infected persons than in non-infected persons.

2. 30% of bacterial pneumonias associated with bacteremia. Bacteremia is more common in *S pneumoniae* infections than other infections.

3. Among hospitalized patients, 9.3–27% overall mortality
   a. 6–13 × higher mortality than general US population (and 1.2–2.4 × higher than population over 65 years)
   b. 5 predictors of mortality include septic shock, CD4 T count < 100/mcL, significant pleural effusion (extending beyond costophrenic angle), cavities and multilobar infiltrates. Mortality is proportional to number of risk factors (Table 5–10).
   c. Inappropriate antimicrobial therapy associated with markedly increased mortality in shock patients (85.7% compared with 25% with appropriate therapy).
   d. Mortality increases during influenza season.

***Table 5–10.*** Mortality among HIV-positive patients with bacterial pneumonia.

| No. Predictors[1] | Mortality (%) |
|---|---|
| 0 | 1.3 |
| 1 | 7.5 |
| 2 | 8.7 |
| 3 | 34.5 |
| 4 | 42.8 |

[1]Predictors: septic shock, CD4 count < 100/mcL, significant pleural effusion (extending beyond costophrenic angle), cavities and multilobar infiltrates.

G. Pyogenic bacterial bronchitis with productive cough, fever, and absence of infiltrates is more common in HIV-infected patients.

### Evidence-Based Diagnosis

A. Initial evaluation should include a chest radiograph, blood and sputum cultures, sputum Gram stain, and WBC. Urinary pneumococcal antigen is often diagnostic. Three sputum acid-fast stains should be done when TB is considered.

B. Toxic appearance is uncommon but suggests bacterial pneumonia over PCP or TB (sensitivity, 10.6%; specificity, 97.8%; LR+, 4.8)

C. Pneumococcal pneumonia
   1. A variety of symptoms are common in patients with pneumococcal pneumonia including cough (93%), subjective fever (90%), pleural pain (52–91%), and chills (74%). 51% of patients have hemoptysis and 63% have temperature > 38°C. The median duration of symptoms is 4 days.
   2. Sputum Gram stain is 58% sensitive and was more frequently positive if collected within 24 hours of antibiotics.
   3. Sputum culture was 56% sensitive.
   4. Blood cultures are positive in 31–95%.
   5. Pneumococcal urinary antigen: ≈79% sensitive and 94% specific (LR+, 13; LR–, 0.2)

D. *Legionella* pneumonia
   1. One study reported that certain findings were more common in patients with *Legionella* pneumonia than *S pneumoniae,* including extra-respiratory symptoms (57% vs 24%), hyponatremia (57% vs 13%) and elevated creatine phosphokinase (CPK) (57% vs 17%).
   2. Respiratory failure was also more common in patients with *Legionella* pneumonia than *S pneumoniae* (33% vs 2%).

E. *M pneumoniae* can be diagnosed by induced sputum culture, IgM ELISA, or cold agglutination. Their sensitivities were 90%, 67%, and 94%, respectively. Cold agglutination was 94% specific.

F. Chest radiograph
   1. Standard imaging includes posteroanterior and lateral chest radiograph.
   2. Chest radiograph typically demonstrates lobar or multifocal consolidation.
   3. Lobar consolidation is not always seen but strongly suggests bacterial pneumonia over PCP or TB (sensitivity, 54%; specificity, 90%; LR+, 5.6; LR–, 0.51).
   4. Lobar infiltrates in patients with fever for less than 1 week strongly suggests bacterial pneumonia (sensitivity, 48%; specificity, 94%; LR+, 8.0; LR–, 0.55).

5. Chest radiographic patterns did not distinguish *S pneumoniae* from *P aeruginosa,* or *Legionella* infection.
6. One report found that 82% of HIV-infected persons with pulmonary complaints had abnormalities, including pleural effusions, cavities and abscess, on high-resolution CT scans that were not detected on chest radiograph.
7. High-resolution CT scanning should be considered for patients who do not respond to therapy and for ill patients with respiratory symptoms or signs but an unexpectedly normal chest radiograph.

G. Bronchoscopy
   1. Indicated in patients who do not respond to therapy or when concomitant infection is suspected.
   2. Sensitivity of bronchoalveolar lavage (BAL) for bacterial pneumonia: 70%

### Treatment

A. Prevention
   1. TMP-SMX prophylaxis (for PCP) in patients with a CD4 T cell count < 200/mcL also decreases the incidence of bacterial pneumonia by 67%.
   2. Pneumococcal vaccine
      a. Decreases pneumococcal disease (OR 0.44)
      b. 86% of serotypes covered in 23-valent vaccine
      c. CDC recommends pneumococcal vaccine use as early as possible in HIV infection. Vaccination should be delayed 4 weeks in individuals initiating HAART to allow for immune reconstitution.
      d. A booster is recommended in 5 years. A booster may also be useful in patients whose initial CD4 T cell count is < 200/mcL after significant immune reconstitution occurs (ie, an increase of CD4 T cell count > 100/mcL).
   3. *Smoking cessation is recommended.*
   4. Therapy for typical bacterial pneumonia is usually initiated empirically.
   5. Antimicrobial therapy must cover frequent causative agents (*S pneumoniae, S aureus, H influenzae, M pneumoniae,* and *P aeruginosa*). Local resistance patterns should be considered.
   6. *P aeruginosa* is usually treated with an antipseudomonal β-lactam and an aminoglycoside.
   7. Patients with uncomplicated pneumonia have time course of clinical and radiologic response to therapy similar to non–HIV-infected persons.

## MAKING A DIAGNOSIS

Serial sputum samples are sent for AFB smear and culture. All AFB stains are negative. Induced sputum is negative for PCP.

Have you crossed a diagnostic threshold for the leading hypothesis, bacterial pneumonia? Have you ruled out the active alternatives? Do other tests need to be done to exclude the alternative diagnoses?

A critical decision at this point in the evaluation of an HIV-infected patient with pulmonary complaints is whether the patient needs bronchoscopy with BAL to establish the etiologic agent. In HIV-positive patients with infiltrates, BAL is highly sensitive (86%). Transbronchial biopsy increases the sensitivity further to 96%. Due to the large number of potential pathogens, empiric treatment is often untenable *except* in the cases in which bacterial pneumonia is strongly suspected. Acute onset and focal infiltrates suggest bacterial pneumonia whereas subacute/chronic progression, diffuse infiltrates, and cavitary lesions suggest other etiologies. Bronchoscopy is often necessary in such cases unless sputum analysis is diagnostic (positive AFB or silver stain). Figure 5–8 suggests one possible diagnostic algorithm. Mr. L' s acute illness, and focal findings on the chest radiograph strongly suggest bacterial pneumonia. You wonder if TB would present similarly in an HIV positive patient with this CD4 T cell count.

## Alternative Diagnosis: Pulmonary TB in AIDS Patients[2]

### Textbook Presentation

TB typically presents subacutely with cough and fever that have gone on for over 1 week (and often much longer) and systemic symptoms of night sweats and weight loss are common. In patients with CD4 T cell counts > 200/mcL, the chest radiographic pattern is similar to non–HIV-infected patients—that is, with apical, cavitary, or nodular infiltrates. In patients with CD4 T cell counts < 200/mcL, the pattern on chest radiograph is often atypical: lower lobe infiltrates, miliary infiltrates, and lymphadenopathy are more common. Extrapulmonary disease is also more common.

### Disease Highlights

A. More worldwide cases of TB currently than at any time in human history

B. HIV-infected persons at highest risk for TB (170× higher incidence).

   1. Risk increases further in patients from endemic areas and among patients who are injection drug users.

   2. 6000–9000 new cases in United States each year

C. TB in turn increases HIV replication and increases the risk of death.

D. Worldwide TB accounts for 30% of HIV-related deaths.

E. Epidemic in sub-Saharan Africa and parts of Asia

F. 50% of cases secondary to recent infection

G. TB may be the first manifestation of HIV infection and is an AIDS-defining illness.

TB may be the first manifestation of AIDS. All patients with TB should be tested for HIV.

H. Clinical characteristics

   1. Early HIV infection: TB is fairly typical.

   2. Advanced HIV infection

     a. Extrapulmonary TB more frequent

       (1) More common in the AIDS population (30%) than in patients without AIDS (15%)

---

**Table 5–11.** Diagnostic accuracy of radiographic findings in HIV-infected patients for tuberculosis.

| Radiographic Finding | Sensitivity | Specificity | LR+ | LR– |
|---|---|---|---|---|
| Cavitary lesions | 16.7% | 98.4% | 10.72 | 0.85 |
| Hilar lymphadenopathy | 11.1% | 98.4% | 7.15 | 0.90 |
| Nodular lesions | 25.0% | 92.7% | 3.45 | 0.81 |

       (2) Most common sites of extrapulmonary TB include blood, lymph nodes, bone marrow, genitourinary tract, CNS, and liver. 19% of patients had cervical or supraclavicular lymph node involvement.

       (3) Other syndromes seen in these patients include weight loss, fever of unknown origin, and tuberculous meningitis.

     b. Chest radiographic pattern more frequently atypical (see below).

Extrapulmonary TB is common in HIV-infected patients and can aid in the diagnosis (ie, through lymph node biopsy, bone marrow biopsy, or urine culture).

### Evidence-Based Diagnosis

A. Prolonged fever (> 7 days) is more common in HIV-infected persons with TB than in those with PCP or bacterial pneumonia (sensitivity, 56%; specificity, 78%; LR+, 2.5; LR–, 0.57).

B. Weight loss is also more common with TB infection than with PCP or bacterial pneumonia (sensitivity, 66.7%; specificity, 68%; LR+, 2.08; LR–, 0.49).

C. Standard tests in patients with suspected TB should include chest radiograph (with posteroanterior and lateral views), 3 sputum AFB stains and cultures, PPD, and blood and urine cultures.

D. Chest radiography

   1. Certain radiographic findings, including cavitary lesions, hilar lymphadenopathy, and nodular lesions, are infrequent but suggestive of TB (Table 5–11).

   2. However, the radiographic manifestations vary with degree of immunosuppression (Table 5–12).

---

**Table 5–12.** Frequency (%) of radiographic manifestations in HIV-infected patients with TB: Influence of CD4 count.

| Radiographic Finding | CD4 Count (cells/mcL) | | |
|---|---|---|---|
| | > 400 | 200–399 | < 200 |
| Cavitary lesions | 63 | 44 | 29 |
| Hilar lymphadenopathy | 0 | 14 | 20 |
| Pleural effusions | 3 | 11 | 11 |
| Miliary pattern | 0 | 6 | 9 |

---

[2]TB in the non–HIV-infected patients is covered in Chapter 9, Cough, Fever, and Respiratory Infections.

**a.** Early HIV infection (CD4 T cell count > 200/mcL): Chest radiograph usually shows the typical reactivation pattern: upper lobe disease or apical segment of lower lobe with or without cavitation

**b.** Advanced HIV infection (CD4 T cell count < 200/mcL):

(1) Middle and lower lobe consolidation, lymph node enlargement, pleural effusions, and miliary patterns are more often seen.

(2) Pleural involvement more common

(a) Often accompanied by fever (85%), cough (77%), and chest pain (36%). Weight loss is common (74%).

(b) Unilateral exudative effusion

(c) Concomitant lower lobe parenchymal infiltrate present in 44–73%

**3.** Cavitary lesions with night sweats or prolonged fever (> 7 days) was not sensitive for TB but virtually diagnostic (sensitivity, 8–11%; LR+, ∞).

**4.** Hilar lymphadenopathy with weight loss or with prolonged cough (> 7 days) was not sensitive for TB but highly suggestive (sensitivity, 8%; LR+, 8–∞).

The chest radiograph in HIV-infected patients with pulmonary TB may be typical or atypical. TB should be considered in patients with apical or cavitary disease, nodular infiltrates, or adenopathy.

**5.** Chest radiograph is normal in 10–21% of patients with pulmonary TB and advanced disease.

Pulmonary TB can be present despite a normal chest radiograph and should be considered in HIV-positive patients with CD4 T cell counts < 200/mcL and pulmonary symptoms.

**E.** PPD: Sensitivity depends on the degree of immunosuppression

**1.** CD4 T cell count > 300/mcL: 90% sensitive

**2.** CD4 T cell count < 100/mcL: 0% sensitive

A negative PPD does NOT make TB less likely in patients with low CD4 T cell counts. (A negative PPD never rules out TB.)

**F.** Sputum analysis

**1.** AFB smear results

**a.** Poor sensitivity (29–60%) is often due to the patient's inability to produce adequate sputum. Sensitivity is 67% in patients able to produce adequate sputum.

**b.** Specificity falls at lower CD4 T cell counts due to increasing incidence of MAC but remains remarkably high in this group (92%).

**2.** AFB culture

**a.** Sensitivity ranges from 43% to 100%. Sensitivity approaches 100% in patients able to produce adequate sputum.

**b.** Induced sputum is positive in 50% of patients with pleural TB without pulmonary infiltrates.

**G.** Rapid RNA or DNA testing of sputum

**1.** Helps distinguish TB from MAC or commensal organisms, which are also acid-fast positive.

**2.** Primarily used when AFB stains positive

**3.** Particularly useful if suspicion of TB is low

**a.** Positive rapid tests help confirm TB, negative tests make TB less likely

**b.** 95% sensitive and specific in this situation

**4.** May be useful when clinical suspicion is high and smear negative.

**a.** Rapid tests reported to be 53% sensitive, 93% specific.

**b.** Positive tests suggest TB

**c.** Cultures are still required to test drug susceptibility.

**5.** A diagnostic algorithm is shown in Figure 5–9.

**H.** Blood culture for mycobacteria

**1.** Blood cultures are positive in 26–42% of HIV-positive patients with TB.

**2.** Sensitivity increases to 49% in patients with CD4 T cell count < 100/mcL.

**I.** Bronchoscopy

**1.** Smear sensitivity: 50–57%; specificity: 99% in endemic area

**2.** Culture sensitivity: Nearly 100%

**3.** Some studies report similar sensitivities to *induced* sputum.

**4.** Bronchoscopy associated with increased transmission of TB to medical personnel. Risk is minimal if performed in a pressure negative room.

**5.** Induced sputum is preferred.

**6.** If bronchoscopy is performed for suspected TB, transbronchial biopsy is recommended to diagnose miliary TB.

**J.** Pleural evaluation

**1.** Pleural fluid smear is positive in 15%.

**2.** Culture of pleural fluid is positive in 33–90%.

**3.** Sputum smear or culture in patients with tuberculous pleurisy is positive in 33–50%. Sputum may be positive in patients *without* parenchymal infiltrate.

**4.** Effusion is unilateral and exudative with lymphocyte predominance.

**5.** Pleural biopsy

**a.** Positive smear: 44–69%

**b.** Positive pathology (granuloma): 88%

**Treatment**

**A.** Chemoprophylaxis

**1.** Recommended for all HIV-positive patients with positive PPD (5 mm) or those with recent close contact (eg, household) with a patient with infectious TB (regardless of PPD result)

**2.** A chest radiograph should be performed and the patient evaluated to rule out active TB (pulmonary or extra-pulmonary). In addition, even in patients with a normal chest radiograph but a CD4 T cell count < 200/mcL, sputum AFB stain and culture should be obtained if possible.

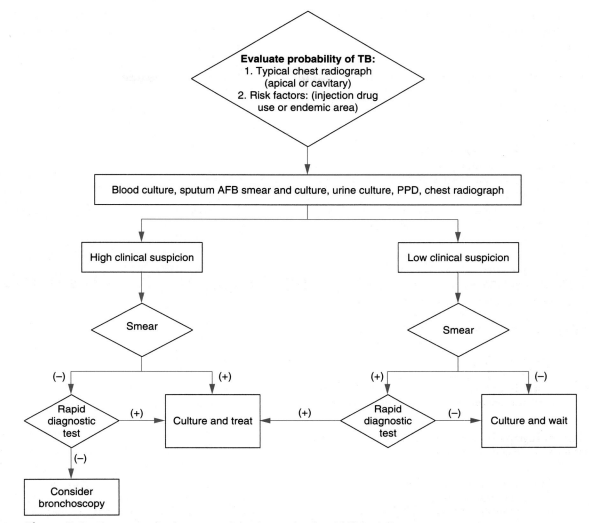

**Figure 5–9.** Diagnosis of pulmonary tuberculosis: role of rapid diagnostic tests

**3.** Isoniazid prophylaxis for 9 months (300 mg daily or 900 mg twice weekly) markedly decreases the rate of progression from latent to active TB from 7.4% to 2.6% in HIV-infected patients.

**4.** Directly observed therapy (DOT) is mandatory if twice weekly therapy is used.

5. Recent guidelines should be consulted. http://www. cdc.gov/tb/pubs/mmwr/Maj_guide/Treatment.htm

**6.** Patients should be evaluated monthly to monitor adherence and side effects of therapy.

**7.** Isoniazid liver toxicity

   **a.** Occurs in 10–20% of patients

   **b.** Isoniazid should be stopped if transaminase elevation exceeds 5× the upper limit of normal, even if the patient is asymptomatic.

   **c.** Patients with a history of alcohol abuse, liver disease, or coinfection with hepatitis B or C virus should have monthly liver function tests to rule out isoniazid-induced hepatitis. HIV-infected patients taking certain antiretroviral agents are also at higher risk for hepatotoxicity.

   **d.** Patients without risk factors for liver disease should have a baseline set of liver function tests with a single routine follow-up check at 1 month.

   **e.** Symptoms should provoke repeat transaminase evaluation.

B. Active TB

   **1.** Antituberculous regimens complicated by complex interaction with HAART

   **2.** Frequent interactions occur between rifampin, rifabutin, and HAART.

      **a.** Rifampin increases metabolism of multiple drugs, including NNRTIs and protease inhibitors.

      **b.** Rifabutin may be used but the dose has to be adjusted.

      **c.** Anti-TB therapy in patients receiving HAART requires detailed knowledge of these drug interactions. Infectious disease consultation is mandatory.

   **3.** DOT is recommended for all patients, including HIV-positive patients.

**a.** Decreases relapse rate from 20% to 5%

**b.** Decreases development of multidrug resistant TB from 6% to 1%

**4.** Monthly follow-up sputum cultures are recommended to confirm conversion to negative. If the 2-month culture remains positive, treatment is extended from the usual 6 months to 9 months.

**5.** Multidrug resistance is a major health problem.

**a.** Drug resistance is more common in HIV patients, but multidrug resistance is still uncommon in the United States (due to DOT programs).

**b.** Multidrug resistance is defined as resistance to rifampin and isoniazid.

**c.** Arises in nonadherent patients: adherence is lower in patients with psychiatric disease, illicit drug abuse, and alcoholism.

**d.** Suspect in patients with prior treatment, contact with known multidrug resistant TB or immigrants from areas of resistant TB.

**e.** Case fatality rate is very high in patients with multidrug resistant TB and HIV. In extensively drug resistant TB, almost all HIV coinfected patients died.

**f.** Multidrug resistant TB typically requires 5 to 6 drugs, including 3 drugs to which TB is susceptible. Expertise in treating multidrug resistant TB is required.

**g.** Therapy is recommended for at least 2 years.

**h.** Surgical resection of localized disease is required in some patients.

**C.** Immune reconstitution

**1.** Infiltrates worsen in 36% of patients upon institution of HAART due to immunologically mediated reactions.

**2.** Increasing fever, infiltrates, and adenopathy may be seen.

**3.** Other diagnoses must be ruled out, such as a second opportunistic infection; poor adherence, drug resistance, or low potency of TB regimen need to be excluded.

**4.** Self limited and lasts 10–40 days.

**5.** Some reactions benefit from short course of corticosteroids.

**D.** Bacille Calmette-Guérin (BCG) vaccination

**1.** BCG is a live-attenuated vaccine.

**2.** Contraindicated in HIV-positive patients due to increased incidence of active infection caused by the BCG strain.

## CASE RESOLUTION

Mr. L's acute presentation and chest radiograph suggest bacterial pneumonia. PCP and MAC are unlikely given his relatively high CD4 T cell count. Similarly, TB would be unlikely with such an acute presentation. Furthermore, at this CD4 T cell level, TB would be expected to present more typically (ie, with upper lobe or apical segment of lower lobe disease). The LR of bacterial pneumonia given the acuity of symptoms and lobar infiltrate is 8.0. Therefore, empiric therapy for bacterial pneumonia would be appropriate. There should be a low threshold for including anti-methi-cillin-resistant S aureus coverage particularly in patients

with a history of injection drug use, in MSM, and during influenza season. In addition, coverage for *Pseudomonas* should be considered when the CD4 T count is low. Bronchoscopy should be performed if Mr. L does not respond promptly to antibiotic therapy.

Mr. L is given a third-generation ceftriaxone and azithromycin. Urinary antigen is positive for S pneumoniae and blood cultures return in 36 hours positive for S pneumoniae, sensitive to penicillin. Mr. L. is treated with IV penicillin and improves over the next 3-4 days.

## REVIEW OF OTHER IMPORTANT DISEASES

### *Mycobacterium avium* complex (MAC)

**Textbook Presentation**

MAC typically presents with constitutional symptoms, including fever, drenching sweats, and weight loss.

**Disease Highlights**

**A.** MAC includes *M avium* and *Mycobacterium intracellulare*. *M avium* is by far the most common atypical mycobacterium in AIDS patients.

**B.** *M avium* is thought to be acquired through inhalation or ingestion.

**C.** No human to human transmission

**D.** Infection in immunocompetent persons is common but usually asymptomatic.

**E.** Primary infection and disease can occur in HIV-infected persons.

**1.** Usually occurs in patients with profound immunosuppression.

**a.** CD4 T cell count < 50/mcL

**b.** Mean CD4 T cell count 7/mcL

**2.** Other risk factors include African Americans, birth outside of the United States, and > 6 years of occupational exposure to soil.

**3.** Disease usually presents as a multisystemic process involving the liver, spleen, GI tract, lungs, and bone marrow.

**a.** Cultures of blood, bone marrow, and urine may all be positive.

**b.** Predominantly pulmonary disease or GI disease is also seen.

**c.** Constitutional symptoms predominate.

**4.** MAC detection in sputum and stool does not necessarily imply disease. This may indicate either colonization or disease.

**5.** Pulmonary disease occurs in < 5% of patients with disseminated disease. Nodules, infiltrates, lymphadenopathy, and cavities may be seen.

**F.** Marked decreased incidence of MAC since the introduction of HAART.

**Evidence-Based Diagnosis**

**A.** Signs and symptoms

**1.** Fever: 18–87%

**2.** Night sweats: 78%

**3.** Cough: 78%

**4.** Diarrhea: 32–47%

**5.** Weight loss: 32–100%

**6.** Hepatosplenomegaly: 24%

B. Laboratory findings
   1. Anemia: 85%
   2. Increased alkaline phosphatase: 45–53%
C. Culture
   1. Blood culture for AFB: 50–95% sensitive
   2. Bone marrow and culture: 82% sensitive
D. Sputum
   1. Smears may be positive for acid-fast bacilli.
   2. Rapid testing can distinguish MAC from TB in patients with positive smears.
E. Chest radiograph
   1. Usually normal
   2. May demonstrate patchy consolidation, nodules, or cavities
F. Table 5–13 summarizes the predictive value of clinical, radiologic, and combined findings for the diagnosis of PCP, TB, and bacterial pneumonia in HIV-infected patients.

Treatment

A. Primary prevention
   1. Recommended for patients with CD4 T cell counts < 50/mcL. Options include azithromycin weekly or clarithromycin twice daily.
   2. Therapy may be discontinued in patients responding to HAART with CD4 T counts > 100/mcL for 3 months.
B. Treatment of MAC infection
   1. Therapy usually includes clarithromycin with ethambutol and in some patients rifabutin. Drug interactions are complex and infectious disease consultation is mandatory.
   2. Susceptibility testing to macrolides should be performed if patients do not respond to the treatment regimen.
   3. Therapy may be discontinued after 1 year in patients responding to HAART with CD4 T cell counts > 100/mcL for more than 6 months.
   4. Pulmonary infiltrates, hepatosplenomegaly, lymphadenopathy, or systemic symptoms may develop anew or worsen during institution of HAART therapy (immune reconstitution inflammatory syndrome [IRIS]).

**Table 5–13.** The predictive value of clinical, radiologic, and combined findings for the diagnosis of PCP, TB, and bacterial pneumonia in HIV-infected patients.

| | Finding | LR+ |
|---|---|---|
| **Bacterial pneumonia** | | |
| Clinical findings | Toxic appearing | 4.8 |
| | Purulent sputum | 1.9 |
| Chest radiographic findings | Lobar infiltrate | 5.6 |
| Combined findings | Lobar infiltrate and cough ≤ 7 days | 11.5 |
| | Lobar infiltrate and pleuritic chest pain | 10 |
| **Pneumocystis pneumonia** | | |
| Clinical findings | Clear sputum | 2.3 |
| | Dyspneic appearing | 2.4 |
| | Dyspnea on exertion | 2.0 |
| | Oral thrush | 1.8 |
| Chest radiographic findings | Diffuse infiltrate | 2.3 |
| | Interstitial infiltrate | 4.3 |
| Combined findings | Interstitial pattern and dyspnea on exertion | 7.25 |
| | Interstitial pattern and oral thrush | 7.2 |
| **Tuberculosis** | | |
| Clinical findings | Fever > 1 week | 2.5 |
| | Weight loss | 2.1 |
| Chest radiographic findings | Cavitary lesion | 10.7 |
| | Hilar lymphadenopathy | 7.2 |
| | Nodular pattern | 3.5 |
| Combined findings | Cavitary and (night sweats or fever > 1 week) | ∞ |
| | Hilar lymphadenopathy and cough > 1 week | 8 |

# I have a patient with AIDS who complains of chronic diarrhea. How do I determine the cause?

## CHIEF COMPLAINT

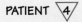

PATIENT ▽4▽

Mr. P is a 35 year-old African American man with AIDS and watery diarrhea that has persisted for at least 6 weeks.

☑ What is the differential diagnosis of chronic diarrhea in AIDS? How do you frame the differential?

## CONSTRUCTING A DIFFERENTIAL DIAGNOSIS

Chronic diarrhea is clinically defined as more than three loose bowel movements a day for > 4 weeks. Chronic diarrhea in AIDS patients is often due to infections, medications, or an array of miscellaneous causes. Three pivotal features help organize the differential diagnosis of diarrhea in AIDS patients. First, as in other AIDS-related problems, infectious etiologies can be organized based on the degree of immunosuppression (ie, CD4 T cell count). Second, opportunistic infections and GI malignancies (lymphoma and Kaposi sarcoma) are more common in patients with low CD4 T cell counts (< 100/mcL) and elevated viral loads whereas medication-induced diarrhea (protease inhibitors, antiretrovirals, antibiotics) or noninfectious etiologies (lactase deficiency) are more likely in individuals receiving HAART with high CD4 T cell counts and undetectable viral loads. The third pivotal point in the approach to AIDS patients with diarrhea recognizes that patients often have one of two clinical syndromes: an enteritis syndrome or a colitis syndrome. An enteritis syndrome ("small bowel diarrhea") is characterized by large-volume watery stools; crampy, diffuse, or epigastric abdominal pain; dehydration, and malabsorption. A colitis syndrome ("large bowel diarrhea") is characterized by frequent, small-volume stools, often containing mucus or blood and is associated with lower quadrant abdominal pain, rectal pain, and tenesmus (feeling of incomplete evacuation). The enteritis syndrome is often secondary to *Cryptosporidium, Microsporidia,* MAC, and *Giardia,* whereas the colitis syndrome is usually secondary to *Salmonella, Shigella, Clostridium difficile,* or CMV. *Salmonella* can present in either fashion. The complete differential is listed below and a diagnostic algorithm is shown in Figure 5–10.

## Differential Diagnosis of Chronic Diarrhea in Patients with AIDS

A. Infectious causes

  1. Opportunistic pathogens (CD4 T cell count usually < 100/mcL)

    a. Bacteria: *M avium* complex (10–20%)

    b. Fungus: histoplasmosis

    c. Virus

      (1) CMV (15–20%)

      (2) HIV enteropathy

    d. Protozoa

      (1) *Cryptosporidium parvum* (10–30%)

      (2) Microsporidia (15–30%)

        (a) *Enterocytozoon bieneusi*

        (b) *Encephalitozoon intestinalis*

      (3) *Isospora belli* (1–3%)

      (4) *Cyclospora cayetanensis* (< 1%)

  2. More virulent pathogens (any CD4 T count)

    a. Bacteria

      (1) *Salmonella, Shigella, Campylobacter,* enteropathogenic *Escherichia coli, Yersinia enterocolitica*

      (2) Toxin-producing *C difficile*

    b. Protozoa

      (1) *Giardia lamblia*

      (2) *Entamoeba histolytica* (1–3%)

B. Medications

  1. Protease inhibitors

  2. Reverse transcriptase inhibitors, especially didanosine

  3. Agents used in the prophylaxis or treatment of opportunistic infections: atovaquone, clarithromycin, clindamycin

  4. Ingestion of laxatives, magnesium-containing antacids, sorbitol, or lactulose

C. Miscellaneous

  1. Lactase deficiency either primary or secondary to gut infection or sprue

  2. Pancreatic insufficiency in chronic pancreatitis due to alcohol

  3. GI Lymphoma

  4. GI Kaposi sarcoma

Mr. P has 6–10 large-volume watery stools a day. The diarrhea has persisted for 6 weeks. He has not been febrile. He has no night sweats. He has lost about 15 pounds. He complains of periumbilical, crampy abdominal pain that is usually relieved by bowel movements. The stools do not appear bloody. He denies any travel history or recent antibiotic use. He denies illicit drugs, excessive alcohol intake, or smoking history. He takes no antiretrovirals or *Pneumocystis jiroveci* prophylaxis, but was advised to take both 2 years ago.

Physical exam is notable for temperature, 36.4°C; BP, 95/60 mm Hg; and HR, 90 bpm while lying down; BP, 85/55 mm Hg; and HR, 110 bpm while standing. He is cachectic: weight 45 kg, height 5'10". Oral thrush is present. No lymphadenopathy. Heart and lungs unremarkable. Abdomen scaphoid, no organomegaly.

 At this point what is the leading hypothesis, what are the active alternatives and is there a must not miss diagnosis? Given this differential diagnosis what tests should be ordered?

## PRIORITIZING THE DIFFERENTIAL DIAGNOSIS

The first pivotal point is that Mr. P has chronic diarrhea and the prior recommendation that he should be receiving TMP-SMX prophylaxis; the current finding of thrush on oral exam suggests he has advanced AIDS with a very low CD4 T cell count. This puts him at high risk for a number of opportunistic infections and GI malignancy. The second pivotal point is that the diarrheal characteristics suggest it is of small bowel origin. The most common opportunistic infections in patients like this without a travel history include *Cryptosporidium,* microsporidia, and MAC. Bacterial pathogens (*Salmonella, Shigella* and *Campylobacter*) and *Giardia* are also possible. Prior antibiotic use would increase the likelihood of *C difficile,* but recently *C difficile*–associated disease has been seen in community settings without prior antibiotic use. Lymphoma and Kaposi sarcoma are less common etiologies. *Isospora* and *Cyclospora* are more common in travelers to and immigrants from endemic areas. The differential diagnosis is found in Table 5–14.

Mr. P's CD4 T count is 25/mcL. The viral load is 110,000/mcL. Hgb is 8 g/dL. Stool fecal leukocytes are negative. Stool is sent for routine bacterial cultures

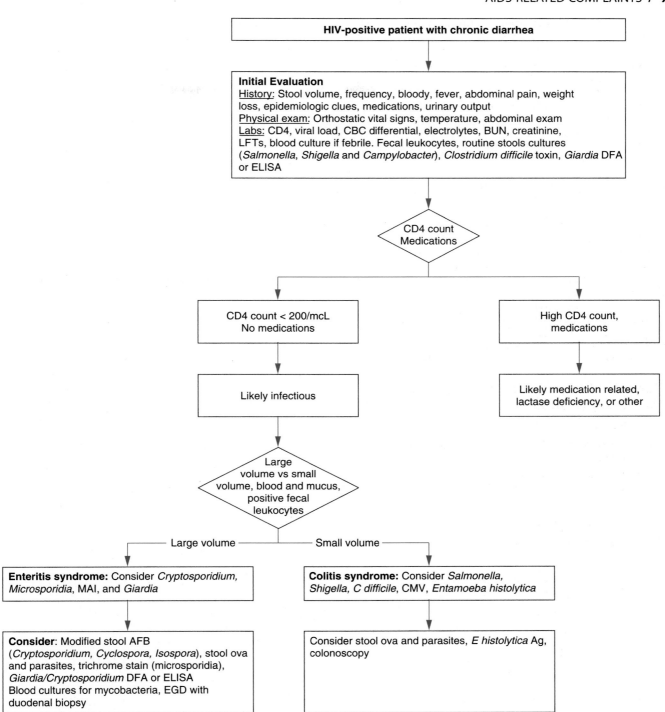

AFB, acid-fast bacilli; CMV, cytomegalovirus; DFA, direct fluorescent antibody; EGD, esophagogastroduodenoscopy; ELISA, enzyme-linked immunosorbent assay; LFTs, liver function tests; MAI, Mycobacterium avium-intracellulare.

***Figure 5–10.*** Diagnostic approach: chronic diarrhea.

(*Salmonella*, *Shigella*, and *Campylobacter*) and *C difficile* toxin. Stool is also sent for ova and parasites × 3. Blood cultures are sent for bacterial and mycobacterial cultures. Additional stools are sent for modified AFB and DFA (to evaluate for *Cryptosporidium*) and trichrome stain for microsporidia.

 **Is the clinical information sufficient to make a diagnosis of *Cryptosporidium* infection? If not what other information do you need?**

**Table 5–14.** Diagnostic hypotheses for Mr. P.

| Diagnostic Hypotheses | Clinical Clues | Important Tests |
|---|---|---|
| **Leading Hypothesis** | | |
| *Cryptosporidium parvum* | CD4 count < 150/mcL<br>Large-volume diarrhea<br>No fever<br>Dehydration<br>Weight loss | Round cysts on modified stool AFB or direct fluorescent antibody (DFA);<br>ELISA stool assay<br>Small bowel biopsy |
| **Active Alternatives—Most Common** | | |
| Microsporidia | CD4 count < 50/mcL<br>Large-volume diarrhea<br>No fever<br>Dehydration<br>Weight loss | Trichrome stool stain, calco-fluor stain;<br>Small bowel biopsy |
| Cytomegalovirus | CD4 count < 100/mcL<br>Chronic diarrhea<br>Systemic symptoms<br>Bloody stools<br>Fever, colitis<br>Severe complications | 2 fecal leukocytes<br>Colonoscopy: erythematous colitis, ulcerations, hemorrhages; colon biopsy |
| *Mycobacteriun avium* complex | CD4 count < 100/mcL<br>Chronic diarrhea<br>Fever<br>Hepatosplenomegaly | Pancytopenia<br>Positive AFB<br>Blood culture<br>Colonoscopy with biopsy and AFB stains<br>Stool AFB culture |
| **Other Alternative—Must Not Miss** | | |
| *Salmonella* | When chronic, diarrhea is moderately severe<br>Fever, bacteremia<br>Also causes colitis | Stool culture Blood culture |
| *Giardia lamblia* | Any CD4 count<br>Large-volume diarrhea, but not as severe as with other protozoa<br>Weight loss<br>Stool culture | Cysts in stools with trichrome stain or DFA<br>EGD with duodenal biopsy or aspirate |

## Leading Hypothesis: *Cryptosporidium parvum*

### Textbook Presentation

Patients typically have advanced AIDS, low CD4 T cell counts, and large-volume chronic diarrhea with weight loss.

### Disease Highlights

A. *C parvum* is an intracellular intestinal coccidian protozoa.

B. It is a common etiology of chronic diarrhea in AIDS (found in 10–30% of untreated AIDS patients with chronic diarrhea).

C. Although the small bowel is the main site of infection, the parasite may also be seen in the colon.

D. When *C parvum* infects individuals with AIDS and CD4 T counts below 150/mcL, it causes either a chronic, watery diarrhea that can be severe or, less frequently, an acute diarrhea with very large stool volumes.

E. Disseminated infection does not occur.

F. Biliary involvement occasionally occurs: acalculous cholecystitis or "AIDS cholangiopathy" with right upper quadrant pain, nausea or vomiting, and elevated alkaline phosphatases without hyperbilirubinemia.

   1. In acalculous cholecystitis, ultrasound often shows a thick-wall, dilated gallbladder without stones. HIDA scan confirms the diagnosis.

   2. In cholangiopathy, endoscopic retrograde cholangiopancreatography (ERCP) is required to show the irregular narrowing of the extrahepatic and intrahepatic bile ducts. The ampulla may be narrowed, resulting in increased diameter of the common bile duct and the pancreatic duct. Other opportunistic infections, such as CMV or MAC, may cause this presentation.

### Evidence-Based Diagnosis

A. Cryptosporidium ELISA on stools: 90–94% sensitive, > 99% specific

B. Cryptosporidium DFA on stools: 96–100% sensitive, > 99% specific

C. Modified acid-fast stain of the stools: 4–6 mcm, round, acid-fast cysts: 84% sensitive, 99% specific

D. Upper endoscopy with biopsies and brushings of the distal duodenum or proximal jejunum is 80% sensitive

### Treatment

A. Nitazoxanide is the first effective specific therapy, although only when the CD4 T count is above 200/mcL, an unusual situation in AIDS.

B. There are no other truly effective therapies: paromomycin and azithromycin are often used, to limited effect.

C. Immune reconstitution associated with effective HAART usually results in improvement or resolution of diarrhea.

## MAKING A DIAGNOSIS

Routine stool cultures for *Salmonella*, *Shigella*, and *Campylobacter* are negative. *C difficile* toxin is not detected. Stool ova and parasites with a trichrome stain are negative times three. Mycobacterial blood cultures are pending.

 Have you crossed the diagnostic threshold for the leading hypothesis, *C parvum*? Have you ruled out the active alternatives? Do other tests need to be done to exclude the alternative diagnoses?

## Alternative Diagnosis: Microsporidia

### Textbook Presentation

Microsporidia typically affect patients with low CD4 T counts who complain of large volume, chronic diarrhea, weight loss, and dehydration.

### Disease Highlights

A. Microsporidia are non-coccidian intracellular protozoa and a common (10–40%) etiology of AIDS-associated chronic diarrhea.

B. Due to either *Enterocytozoon bieneusi* (90%) or *Encephalitozoon intestinalis* (10%).

## Evidence-Based Diagnosis

A. Trichrome stain of the stools shows the small spores, some of which show a pathognomonic "belt" (> 99% sensitive, 100% specific).

B. Calco-fluor fluorescent stain is easier to read (99% sensitive, > 99% specific).

C. Upper endoscopy with small bowel biopsies may show the small intracellular parasites.

## Treatment

A. Albendazole is an effective specific therapy for *E intestinalis* but not *E bieneusi,* which is responsible for 90% of cases.

B. There is no effective specific therapy of *E bieneusi* although fumagillin may have some activity.

C. HAART is effective; symptoms resolve with immune reconstitution.

## Alternative Diagnosis: *Mycobacterium avium* complex (MAC) Infection

### Textbook Presentation

Patients typically have CD4 T counts < 50/mcL and complain of fever, night sweats, chronic diarrhea, weight loss, and abdominal pain.

### Disease Highlights

A. *M avium* is a common opportunistic infection in advanced HIV disease.

B. MAC causes 10–20% of AIDS-associated chronic diarrhea.

C. MAC involves the small bowel.

### Evidence-Based Diagnosis

A. Diagnosis may be difficult to make.

B. Physical exam
   1. Often positive for hepatosplenomegaly and anemia
   2. Intra-abdominal and thoracic lymphadenopathy is common.

C. Laboratory findings
   1. Anemia or pancytopenia is common.
   2. Blood cultures for AFB have a high sensitivity, and typically positive cultures are identified after 7–14 days.
   3. Bone marrow biopsy and culture may be useful.
   4. Stool culture for mycobacteria is of limited usefulness because a positive result does not prove the diagnosis and may simply imply colonization.
   5. Positive blood cultures or a biopsy revealing either granuloma or AFB proves the diagnosis.

### Treatment

A. Primary prophylaxis for MAC is offered when the CD4 T cell count is below 50/mcL; weekly azithromycin is often used.

B. Therapy involves a combination of at least 2 drugs, of which a macrolide is the more effective (clarithromycin, azithromycin). Other oral drugs include ethambutol, rifabutin, and rifampin.

C. Testing for susceptibility to macrolides is important.

## Alternative Diagnosis: CMV Colitis

### Textbook Presentation

Patients typically have advanced AIDS, CD4 T counts < 50/mcL, fever, myalgias, diarrhea, abdominal pain, and weight loss. Bloody stools or occult blood are commonly found.

### Disease Highlights

A. CMV causes > 20% of AIDS-associated chronic diarrhea.

B. Typically, CMV causes a colitis with erythema, ulcerations, or bleeding.

C. Complications include perforation, obstruction, ischemia, megacolon, and hemorrhage.

D. CMV can involve other parts of the gut, especially the esophagus (esophagitis, ulcers, perforation) and the small bowel (enteritis).

E. CMV colitis represents < 10% of CMV manifestations in AIDS.

F. The most common CMV disease in AIDS is sight-threatening retinitis.

### Evidence-Based Diagnosis

A. CMV colitis is best diagnosed by colonoscopy. Sigmoidoscopy may miss isolated right colonic involvement.

B. Colonoscopy shows erythema, ulcers, bleeding.

C. CMV viral inclusions are both intranuclear (the typical owl's eye inclusion) and intracytoplasmic.

### Treatment

A. Primary prophylaxis for CMV is no longer recommended.

B. 3–6 weeks of intravenous ganciclovir or foscarnet is recommended with concomitant antiretroviral therapy. Oral valganciclovir is also used when longer therapy is required.

## Alternative Diagnosis: *Giardia lamblia*

### Textbook Presentation

A patient with HIV complains of chronic diarrhea with malabsorption, flatulence, crampy abdominal pain, and weight loss.

### Disease Highlights

A. *Giardia* is an extracellular flagellate protozoa that causes acute or chronic diarrhea in individuals with advanced HIV.

B. It causes 1–3% of AIDS-associated chronic diarrhea in the United States.

C. The presentation of chronic giardiasis in AIDS is similar to what is seen in non–HIV-infected patients.

### Evidence-Based Diagnosis

A. Stool ova and parasites times three with for example a trichrome stain: 82% sensitive, > 99% specific

B. EIA: 89–99% sensitive, > 99% specific

C. DFA: 96–100% sensitive, > 99% specific

D. Esophagogastroduodenoscopy with biopsy of the distal duodenum or the jejunum is rarely required.

## Treatment

Metronidazole is effective.

## CASE RESOLUTION

RMycobacterial blood cultures are negative. Trichrome stain for microsporidia is negative. A stool modified acid-fast stain is positive for acid-fast round 4–6 mcm cysts consistent with *C parvum*.

## REVIEW OF OTHER IMPORTANT DISEASES

### Kaposi Sarcoma

#### Textbook Presentation

The rash is usually seen in HIV-positive MSM who have nodular, nontender, pink to violaceous papules and nodules (Figure 5–11).

#### Disease Highlights

A. HHV 8 (Human herpes virus 8) associated with HIV causes the angioproliferation seen in Kaposi sarcoma.

B. Most affected patients are MSM. Individual lesions are pink, red, or purple, and nontender in most cases.

C. Lesions are found on the extremities, trunk, and face.

D. With decreasing CD4 T counts, the number of lesions increases.

E. Skin involvement is almost always present in Kaposi sarcoma.

F. Extracutaneous involvement occurs: oral cavity, GI tract, lymph nodes, and lungs.

G. GI involvement is rather common (40%) but usually asymptomatic. Occasionally, bleeding and perforation occur.

H. Pleuro-pulmonary involvement is common in advanced Kaposi sarcoma.

   1. Presentations of pulmonary Kaposi sarcoma include lung nodules, infiltrates, dyspnea, pleural effusions, and respiratory failure.

   2. Patient survival is shortened.

I. The incidence of KS has decreased dramatically, only in part due to the introduction of effective antiretrovirals. A change in sexual behavior may also play a role.

#### Evidence-Based Diagnosis

A. Skin biopsy shows the typical angioproliferation with slit-like vascular spaces and spindle cells.

B. Immunohistochemistry can detect HHV 8 in the endothelial cells.

C. GI Kaposi sarcoma: endoscopy is clinically suggestive, but the submucosal location of lesions makes tissue diagnosis difficult.

D. Pulmonary Kaposi sarcoma: high-resolution chest CT suggestive; bronchoscopy; thallium scan; open-lung biopsy.

#### Treatment

Effective HAART is highly effective in early Kaposi sarcoma, but chemotherapy is required in pulmonary involvement.

## REFERENCES

Afessa B, Green B. Bacterial pneumonia in hospitalized patients with HIV infection: the Pulmonary Complications ICU Support and Prognostic Factors of Hospitalized Patients with HIV (PIP) Study. Chest. 2000;117(4): 1017–22.

Basso U, Brandes AA. Diagnostic advances and new trends for the treatment of primary central nervous system lymphoma. Eur J Can. 2002;38(10): 1298–1312.

Berenguer J, Miralles P, Arrizabalaga J et al. Clinical course and prognostic factors of progressive multifocal leukoencephalopathy in patients treated with highly active antiretroviral therapy. Clin Infect Dis. 2003;36(8): 1047–52.

Boiselle PM, Tocino I, Hooley RJ et al. Chest radiograph interpretation of *Pneumocystis carinii* pneumonia, bacterial pneumonia, and pulmonary tuberculosis in HIV-positive patients: accuracy, distinguishing features, and mimics. J Thorac Imaging. 1997;12(1):47–53.

Chuck SL, Sande MA. Infections with *Cryptococcus neoformans* in the acquired immunodeficiency syndrome. N Engl J Med. 1989;321:794–9.

de Souza MC, Nitrini R. Effects of human immunodeficiency virus infection on the manifestations of neurosyphilis. Neurology. 1997;49(3):893–4.

Eggers CH; German Neuro-AIDS Working Group. HIV-1 associated encephalopathy and myelopathy. J Neurol. 2002;249(8):1132–6.

Havlir DV, Barnes PF. Tuberculosis in patients with human immunodeficiency virus infection. N Engl J Med. 1999;340(5):367–73.

Jones D, Havlir DV. Nontuberculous mycobacteria in the HIV infected patient. Clin Chest Med. 2002;23(3):665–74.

Kovascs JA, Masur H. Prophylaxis against opportunistic infections in patients with human immunodeficiency virus infection. N Engl J Med. 2000;342(19): 1416–29.

Lin J, Nichol KL. Excess mortality due to pneumonia or influenza during influenza seasons among persons with acquired immunodeficiency syndrome. Arch Intern Med. 2001;161(3):441–6.

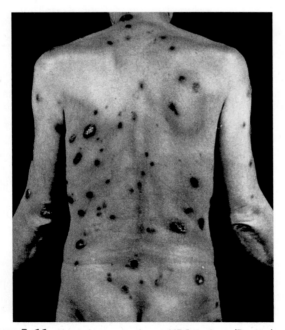

***Figure 5–11.*** Kaposi sarcoma in an AIDS patient. (Reproduced, with permission, from Wolfe K et al. Fitzpatrick's Dermatology in General Medicine, 7th edition. McGraw-Hill, 2008.)

Mamidi A, Desimone JA, Pomerantz RJ. Central nervous system infections in individuals with HIV-1 infection. J Neurovirology. 2002;8(3):158–67.

McCutchan JA. Cytomegalovirus infections of the nervous system in patients with AIDS. Clin Infect Dis. 1995;20(4):747–54.

Mellors JW, Munoz A, Giorgi JV et al. Plasma viral load and CD4+ lymphocytes as prognostic markers of HIV-1 infection. Ann Intern Med. 1997;126(12): 946–54.

Panel on Antiretroviral Guidelines for Adults and Adolescents. Guidelines for the use of antiretroviral agents in HIV-1-infected adults and adolescents. Department of Health and Human Services. November 3, 2008; 1–139. Available at http://www.aidsinfo.nih.gov/ContentFiles/AdultandAdolescentGL.pdf.

Polsky B, Gold JW, Whimbey E et al. Bacterial pneumonia in patients with the acquired immunodeficiency syndrome. Ann Intern Med. 1986;104(1):38–41.

Raoof S, Rosen MJ, Khan FA. Role of bronchoscopy in AIDS. Clin Chest Med. 1999;20(1):63–76.

Reichenberger F, Cathomas G, Weber R, Schoenenberger R, Tamm M. Recurrent fever and pulmonary infiltrates in an HIV-positive patient. Respiration. 2001;68(5):548–54.

Skiest DJ, Crosby C. Survival is prolonged by highly active antiretroviral therapy in AIDS patients with primary central nervous system lymphoma. AIDS. 2003;17(12):1787–93.

Zuger A, Louie E, Holzman RS, Simberkoff MS, Rahal JJ. Cryptococcal disease in patients with the acquired immunodeficiency syndrome. Ann Intern Med. 1986;104(2):234–40.

# I have a patient with anemia.
# How do I determine the cause?

## CHIEF COMPLAINT

**PATIENT 1**

Mrs. A is a 48-year-old white woman who has had 2 months of fatigue due to anemia.

**What is the differential diagnosis of anemia? How would you frame the differential?**

## CONSTRUCTING A DIFFERENTIAL DIAGNOSIS

The framework for organizing the differential diagnosis of anemia is a combination of pathophysiologic and morphologic. The first step in determining the cause of an anemia is to determine the general mechanism of the anemia, using a pathophysiologic framework. Anemia is caused by 1 of 3 processes:

1. **Acute or chronic blood loss** is clinically obvious. Chronic blood loss leads to iron deficiency and consequent underproduction.
2. **Underproduction** of RBCs by the bone marrow.
3. Increased **destruction** of RBCs, known as **hemolysis.**

After determining the general mechanism, the next step is to determine the cause of the underproduction or increased destruction. (This chapter will not discuss the approach to acute blood loss.) The framework for underproduction anemia is morphologic:

A. Microcytic anemias (mean corpuscular volume [MCV] < 80 mcm$^3$)
   1. Iron deficiency
   2. Thalassemia
   3. Anemia of inflammation (formerly called anemia of chronic disease)
   4. Sideroblastic anemia
   5. Lead exposure
B. Macrocytic anemias (MCV > 100 mcm$^3$)
   1. Megaloblastic anemias (due to abnormalities in DNA synthesis; hypersegmented neutrophils also occur)
      a. Vitamin B$_{12}$ deficiency
      b. Folate deficiency
      c. Antimetabolite drugs, such as methotrexate or zidovudine
   2. Nonmegaloblastic anemias (no hypersegmented neutrophils)
      a. Alcohol abuse
      b. Liver disease
      c. Hypothyroidism

C. Normocytic anemias
   1. Anemia of inflammation
   2. Early iron deficiency
   3. Infiltration of bone marrow due to malignancy or granulomas
   4. RBC aplasia
      a. Aplastic anemia
      b. Suppression by parvovirus B19 or medications

The framework for hemolytic anemias is pathophysiologic:

A. Hereditary
   1. Enzyme defects, such as pyruvate kinase or glucose-6-phosphate dehydrogenase (G6PD) deficiency
   2. Hemoglobinopathies, such as sickle cell anemia
   3. RBC membrane abnormalities, such as spherocytosis
B. Acquired
   1. Hypersplenism
   2. Immune
      a. Autoimmune: warm IgG, cold IgM, cold IgG
      b. Drug induced: autoimmune or hapten
   3. Traumatic
      a. Impact
      b. Macrovascular: shearing due to prosthetic valves
      c. Microvascular: disseminated intravascular coagulation (DIC), thrombotic thrombocytopenic purpura (TTP), and hemolytic uremic syndrome (HUS)
   4. Infections, such as malaria
   5. Toxins, such as snake venom and aniline dyes
   6. Paroxysmal nocturnal hemoglobinuria

Figure 6–1 outlines the approach to evaluating anemia caused by underproduction and increased destruction of RBCs.

**1**

Mrs. A has a past medical history of obesity, reflux, depression, asthma, and arthritis. She comes to your office complaining of feeling down with progressive fatigue for the last 2 months. She has no chest pain, cough, fever, weight loss, or edema. Her only GI symptoms are poor appetite and her usual reflux symptoms; she has had no vomiting, melena, or rectal bleeding. She still has regular menses that are occasionally heavy. She brought

(Continued)

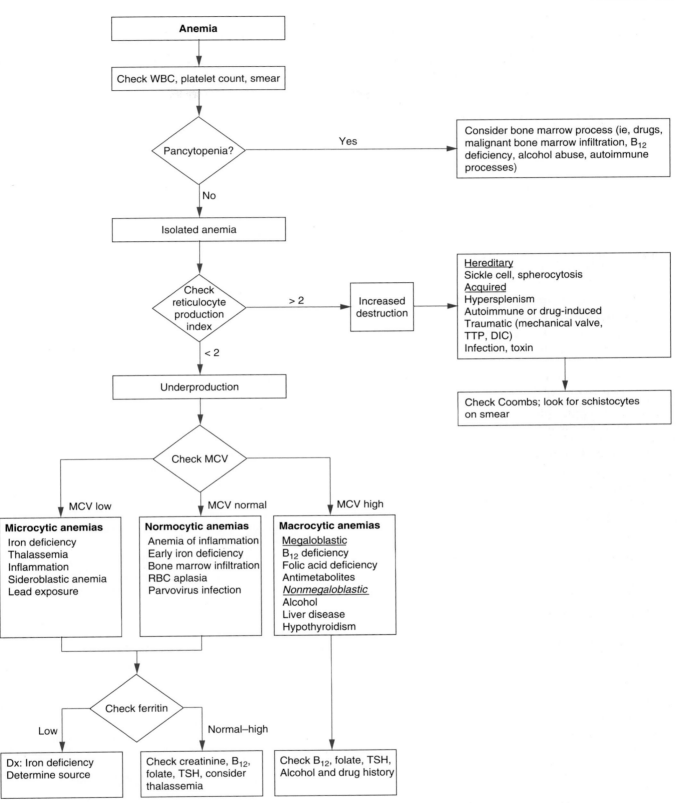

DIC, disseminated intravascular coagulation; MCV, mean corpuscular volume; TTP, thrombotic thrombocytopenic purpura.

**Figure 6–1.** Diagnostic approach: anemia.

in her medication bottles, which include ranitidine, sertraline, tramadol, cetirizine, and a fluticasone inhaler. Her physical exam shows a depressed affect, clear lungs, a normal cardiac exam, a nontender abdomen, guaiac-negative stool, no edema, and no pallor.

 **How reliable is the history and physical for detecting anemia?**

A. Symptoms in chronic anemia are due to decreased oxygen delivery to the tissues.

1. Fatigue is a common but not very specific symptom.

2. Dyspnea on exertion often occurs.

3. Exertional chest pain occurs most often in patients with underlying coronary artery disease or severe anemia or both.

4. Palpitations or tachycardia can occur.

5. Edema is sometimes seen.

   a. Due to decreased renal blood flow leading to neuro-hormonal activation and salt and water retention, similar to that seen in congestive heart failure (CHF)

   b. However, in contrast to the low cardiac output seen in patients with CHF, the cardiac output in patients with anemia is high.

6. Mild anemia is often asymptomatic

B. Symptoms of hypovolemia occur only in acute anemia due to large volume blood loss.

C. Conjunctival rim pallor

1. Present when the anterior rim of the inferior palpebral conjunctiva is the same pale pink color as the deeper posterior aspect, rather than the normal bright red color of the anterior rim.

2. The presence of conjunctival rim pallor strongly suggests the patient is anemic (LR+ 16.7).

3. However, the absence of pallor does not rule out anemia.

D. Palmar crease pallor has an LR+ of 7.9.

E. Pallor elsewhere (facial, nail bed) is not as useful, with LR+ < 5.

F. No physical sign rules out anemia.

G. The overall sensitivity and specificity of the physical exam for anemia is about 70%.

 Order a CBC if patients have suggestive symptoms, even without physical exam signs, or if you observe conjunctival rim or palmar crease pallor.

 Mrs. A's initial laboratory test results show a WBC of 7100/mcL, RBC of 3.6 million/mcL, Hgb of 6.7 g/dL, Hct of 23.3%, and MCV of 76 mcm³. A CBC 6 months ago showed an Hgb of 12 g/dL, Hct of 36%, and MCV of 82 mcm³.

 At this point, what is the leading hypothesis, what are the active alternatives, and is there a must not miss diagnosis? Given this differential diagnosis, what tests should be ordered?

## PRIORITIZING THE DIFFERENTIAL DIAGNOSIS

The first step is to determine the mechanism of Mrs. A's anemia. Mrs. A is not having any symptoms or signs of acute blood loss. She does have pivotal symptoms suggestive of diseases associated with chronic blood loss: reflux possibly causing esophagitis and occasional menorrhagia. However, it is not possible to distinguish underproduction from hemolysis based on the history. Although the change in her CBC tells you a new process is going on, it also does not distinguish between these 2 mechanisms.

 Always look at previous CBC results to see if the anemia is new, old, or progressive.

The best test to distinguish underproduction from hemolysis is the **reticulocyte count:**

A. Low or normal reticulocyte counts are seen in underproduction anemias.

B. High reticulocyte counts occur when the bone marrow is responding normally to blood loss, hemolysis, or replacement of iron, vitamin $B_{12}$, or folate.

C. Reticulocyte measures include:

1. The **reticulocyte count,** which is the percentage of circulating RBCs that are reticulocytes (normally 0.5–1.5%).

2. The **absolute reticulocyte count,** which is the number of reticulocytes actually circulating, normally 25,000–75,000/mcL (multiply the percentage of reticulocytes by the total number of RBCs).

3. The **reticulocyte production index (RPI)**

   a. Corrects the reticulocyte count for the degree of anemia and for the prolonged peripheral maturation of reticulocytes that occurs in anemia

      (1) Normally, the first 3–3.5 days of reticulocyte maturation occurs in the bone marrow and the last 24 hours in the peripheral blood.

      (2) When the bone marrow is stimulated, reticulocytes are released prematurely, leading to longer maturation times in the periphery, and larger numbers of reticulocytes present at any given time.

      (3) For a Hct of 25%, the peripheral blood maturation time is 2 days, and for a Hct of 15%, it is 2.5 days; the value of 2 is generally used in the RPI calculation.

   b. $$RPI = \frac{observed\ reticulocyte\%\ \times\ (Patient\ Hct/45)}{peripheral\ blood\ maturation\ time\ in\ days}$$

   c. The normal RPI is about 1.0, with values ≥ 2.0 indicating an adequate bone marrow response.

 The first step in evaluating anemia is checking a reticulocyte count.

Mrs. A's reticulocyte count is 1.5%, which is an absolute reticulocyte count of 54,000/mcL, and an RPI of 0.39.

Now that you have found that Mrs. A has an underproduction anemia, what is the leading hypothesis, what are the active alternatives, and is there a must not miss diagnosis? Given this differential diagnosis, what tests should be ordered?

Mrs. A's MCV is 76 mcm³, so you should consider the differential diagnosis for microcytic anemia. However, it is important to keep in mind that the **MCV is not specific and should not be used to rule in or rule out a specific cause of anemia.**

A. In one study, normal MCVs were found in 50% of patients with abnormal serum vitamin B$_{12}$, folate, or iron studies.

1. 5% of patients with iron deficiency had high MCVs

2. 12% of patients with B$_{12}$ or folate deficiency had low MCVs

B. What about the rest of the CBC? Do the other indices help?

1. Other red cell indices (mean corpuscular hemoglobin [MCH] and mean corpuscular hemoglobin concentration [MCHC]) tend to trend with the MCV and are not particularly sensitive or specific.

2. The red cell distribution width (RDW) is also not sensitive or specific in identifying the cause of an anemia.

Use the MCV to organize your thinking, not to diagnose the cause of an anemia.

Despite this caveat about the MCV, in a patient with a microcytic anemia and symptoms suggestive of possible chronic blood loss, iron deficiency is by far the most likely cause, with a pretest probability of 80%. Therefore, the leading hypothesis for Mrs. A is iron deficiency anemia. Anemia of inflammation, by virtue of being common, is the best active alternative; to make this diagnosis, keep in mind that the patient must have an inflammatory condition known to cause anemia. Sideroblastic anemia and lead exposure are other hypotheses, and isolated thalassemia is excluded by the recently normal CBC. Because the MCV lacks specificity, the causes of normocytic and macrocytic anemia also need to be kept in mind as other hypotheses. Table 6–1 lists the differential diagnosis.

## Leading Hypothesis: Iron Deficiency Anemia

### Textbook Presentation

The most classic presentation would be a young, menstruating woman who has fatigue and a craving for ice. Typical presentations include fatigue, dyspnea, and sometimes edema.

### Disease Highlights

A. The CBC varies with the degree of severity of the iron deficiency.

1. In very early iron deficiency, the CBC is normal.

2. A mild anemia then develops, with an Hgb of 9–12 g/dL, and normal or slightly hypochromic RBCs.

**Table 6–1.** Diagnostic hypotheses for Mrs. A.

| Diagnostic Hypotheses | Clinical Clues | Important Tests |
|---|---|---|
| **Leading Hypothesis** | | |
| Iron deficiency | Pica<br>Blood loss (menorrhagia, melena, hematochezia, NSAID use) | Serum ferritin |
| **Active Alternative—Most Common** | | |
| Anemia of chronic inflammation | History of renal or liver disease, inflammation, infection | Iron, TIBC, ferritin, creatinine, transaminases, ESR, CRP |
| **Other Hypotheses** | | |
| Thalassemia | Ethnic background | Hgb electrophoresis, DNA testing |
| Lead poisoning | Exposure to lead | Lead level |
| B$_{12}$ deficiency | Diet<br>Autoimmune diseases<br>Neurologic symptoms | B$_{12}$ level |
| Folate deficiency | Pregnancy<br>Sickle cell anemia<br>Alcohol abuse | Folate level |

CRP, C-reactive protein; ESR, erythrocyte sedimentation rate; NSAID, nonsteroidal antiinflammatory drug; TIBC, total iron-binding capacity.

3. As the iron deficiency progresses, the Hgb continues to decrease, and hypochromia and microcytosis develop.

B. Causes of iron deficiency

1. Blood loss, most commonly menstrual or GI

2. Inadequate intake

a. Males need 1 mg/day (need to consume 15 mg/day; absorption rate 6%).

b. Females need 1.4 mg/day (need to consume 11 mg/day; absorption rate 12%).

c. Iron is more bioavailable from meat than vegetables.

3. Malabsorption, seen in patients with gastrectomy, some bariatric surgery procedures, celiac sprue, or inflammatory bowel disease (IBD)

4. Increased demand, seen with pregnancy, infancy, adolescence, erythropoietin therapy

### Evidence-Based Diagnosis

A. Bone marrow exam for absence of iron stores is the gold standard.

B. The serum ferritin is the best serum test.

1. The LR+ for a decreased serum ferritin is very high, with reports ranging from LR+ of 51 for a ferritin < 15 ng/mL to a LR+ of 25.5 for a ferritin < 32 ng/mL.

2. Thus, a low ferritin rules in iron deficiency anemia.

3. In general populations, the LR− for a serum ferritin > 100 ng/mL is very low (0.08).

4. Thus, in general populations, a ferritin > 100 ng/mL greatly reduces the probability the patient has iron deficiency.

5. However, because ferritin is an acute phase reactant that increases in inflammatory states, interpreting it in the presence of such illnesses is difficult.

   a. There is a wide range of reported LRs, with many studies finding ferritin is *not* helpful in diagnosing iron deficiency in the presence of chronic illness.

   b. The level at which the serum ferritin suggests iron deficiency is probably much higher in patients with chronic illness, but the level may vary depending on the underlying illness.

6. Thus, the ferritin level cannot be used to absolutely rule in or rule out iron deficiency anemia in patients with chronic inflammatory diseases.

C. Other tests

1. The MCV, the transferrin saturation (serum iron/iron-binding capacity {Fe/TIBC}), red cell protoporphyrin, red cell ferritin, and RDW all are less sensitive and specific than ferritin.

2. The best of these is transferrin saturation ≤ 5%, with a LR+ of 10.46.

In patients without chronic inflammatory diseases, the serum ferritin is the best single test to diagnose iron deficiency anemia.

### Treatment

A. Iron deficiency anemia is generally treated with oral iron replacement, with IV iron therapy reserved for patients who demonstrate malabsorption or who are unable to tolerate oral iron.

B. Transfusion is necessary only if the patient is hypotensive; orthostatic; actively bleeding; or has angina, dizziness, syncope, or severe dyspnea or fatigue.

C. The best-absorbed oral iron is ferrous sulfate; the dose is 325 mg 3 times daily.

D. There are significant GI side effects including nausea, abdominal pain, and constipation; these can be reduced by taking the iron with food, and slowly titrating the dose from 1 tablet daily to 3 tablets daily over 1 to 2 weeks.

E. There should be an increase in reticulocytes 7–10 days after starting therapy, and an increase in Hgb and Hct by 30 days; if there is no response, reconsider the diagnosis.

F. It is necessary to take iron for 6 months in order to replete iron stores.

## MAKING A DIAGNOSIS

Since Mrs. A does not have any chronic, inflammatory diseases, the most useful test at this point is a serum ferritin. Serum iron and TIBC are often ordered simultaneously but are not necessary at this point.

You review the history, looking for symptoms of bleeding or chronic illness. She has no renal or liver disease and no symptoms of infection. Her ethnic background is Scandinavian, making thalassemia unlikely. You order a serum ferritin, which is 5 ng/mL.

## CASE RESOLUTION

With a pretest probability of 80% and an LR+ of 51 for this level of ferritin, Mrs. A is clearly iron deficient. It is not necessary to test for any other causes of anemia, but it is necessary to determine why she is iron deficient.

Always identify the source of blood loss in iron deficiency anemia. Be alert for occult malignancies.

Iron deficiency is almost always due to chronic blood loss and rarely due to poor iron intake or malabsorption of iron; menstrual and GI blood loss are the most common sources. Because GI blood loss can be occult, many patients need GI evaluations.

A. Who needs a GI work-up?

1. All men, all women without menorrhagia, and women over age 50 even with menorrhagia.

2. Women under age 50 with menorrhagia do not need further GI evaluation, unless they have GI symptoms or a family history of early colon cancer or adenomatous polyps.

3. Always ask carefully about minimal GI symptoms in young women, since celiac sprue often causes iron deficiency due to malabsorption, and the symptoms can easily be attributed to irritable bowel syndrome.

B. Which GI test should be done first?

1. In the absence of symptoms or in the presence of lower GI symptoms, do a colonoscopy first.

2. If there are upper GI symptoms, do an esophagogastro-duodenoscopy (EGD) first.

3. If the first test is negative, the other one must be done.

4. Small bowel imaging rarely finds important lesions in patients with normal upper and lower endoscopies and often can be omitted. However, in patients with evidence of persistent or recurrent bleeding, small bowel imaging is indicated. Imaging techniques are discussed in Chapter 17, GI Bleeding.

5. Clinicians are sometimes unsure whether a colonoscopy is necessary when the EGD shows a definitive bleeding source. Finding colonic lesions in such cases is rare, and colonoscopy can be reserved for symptomatic patients or those who need routine colorectal cancer screening.

It is unclear from Mrs. A's history whether the menorrhagia is sufficient to cause this degree of iron deficiency anemia. In addition, she has the upper GI symptoms of anorexia and reflux. Therefore, you order an EGD, which shows severe reflux esophagitis and also gastritis. Further history reveals she has been using several hundred milligrams of ibuprofen daily for several weeks because of a back strain. The severe esophagitis and gastritis are sufficient to explain her anemia, and she has no lower GI symptoms or family history of colorectal cancer. The work-up is complete.

## FOLLOW-UP OF MRS. A

Mrs. A stopped the ibuprofen, substituted a proton pump inhibitor for the H₂-blocker, and completed 6 months of iron therapy. She felt fine. A follow-up CBC showed an Hgb of 13 g/dL, an Hct of 39%, and a significantly elevated MCV of 122 mcm³.

At this point, what is the leading hypothesis, what are the active alternatives, and is there a must not miss diagnosis? Given this differential diagnosis, what tests should be ordered?

## PRIORITIZING THE DIFFERENTIAL DIAGNOSIS

Although Mrs. A is not anemic now, she has a marked macrocytosis. The approach to isolated macrocytosis is the same as the approach to macrocytic anemia. The degree of macrocytosis is not a reliable predictor of the cause, but in general, the higher the MCV, the more likely the patient has a vitamin $B_{12}$ or folate deficiency. The pretest probability of vitamin deficiency with an MCV of 115–129 mcm³ is 50%, and nearly all patients with an MCV > 130 mcm³ will have a vitamin deficiency.

Since $B_{12}$ deficiency is seen more often than folate deficiency in otherwise healthy people, that is the leading hypothesis, with folate deficiency being the active alternative. Use of antimetabolite drugs is excluded by history. Causes of nonmegaloblastic anemias need to be considered next. Hypothyroidism would be the most likely other hypothesis, with liver disease and alcohol abuse less likely based on her lack of a previous history of either. Table 6–2 lists the differential diagnosis.

**Table 6–2.** Diagnostic hypotheses for Mrs. A's follow-up.

| Diagnostic Hypotheses | Clinical Clues | Important Tests |
|---|---|---|
| **Leading Hypothesis** | | |
| $B_{12}$ deficiency | Vegan diet<br>Other autoimmune diseases<br>Elderly<br>Neurologic symptoms | $B_{12}$ level<br>Homocysteine level<br>Methylmalonic acid level (MMA) |
| **Active Alternative—Most common and Must Not Miss** | | |
| Folate deficiency | Alcohol abuse<br>Starvation<br>Pregnancy<br>Sickle cell anemia | Serum folate level<br>RBC folate level<br>Homocysteine level |
| **Other Hypothesis** | | |
| Hypothyroidism | Constipation<br>Weight gain<br>Fatigue<br>Cold intolerance | TSH<br>Free thyroxine index |

## Leading Hypothesis: B₁₂ Deficiency

### Textbook Presentation

The classic presentation is an elderly woman with marked anemia and neurologic symptoms such as paresthesias, sensory loss (especially vibration and position), ataxia, dementia, and psychiatric symptoms.

### Disease Highlights

A. It takes years to develop this deficiency because of extensive stores of vitamin $B_{12}$ in the liver.

B. Anemia and macrocytosis are not always present.

1. In 1 study, 28% of patients with neurologic symptoms due to $B_{12}$ deficiency had no anemia or macrocytosis.

2. In another study, the following clinical characteristics were found in patients with $B_{12}$ deficiency:

a. 33% white, 41% black, 25% Latino

b. 28% not anemic

c. 17% normal MCV

d. 17% leukopenia, 35% thrombocytopenia, 12.5% pancytopenia

e. 36% neuropsychiatric symptoms

The CBC can be normal in $B_{12}$ deficiency.

C. $B_{12}$ absorption requires normal gastric and intestinal function.

1. Dietary $B_{12}$ is protein bound and is released by acid peptic digestion in the stomach.

2. Although intrinsic factor is made by the parietal cells of the gastric body and fundus, it does not bind to $B_{12}$ until both reach the jejunum.

3. The $B_{12}$-intrinsic factor complex binds to receptors in the terminal ileum, where $B_{12}$ is absorbed.

D. The most common causes of $B_{12}$ deficiency are food cobalamin malabsorption, lack of intrinsic factor, and dietary deficiency.

1. Dietary deficiency is rare unless the patient follows a vegan diet.

2. Food cobalamin malabsorption occurs when $B_{12}$ is not released from food proteins due to impaired acid peptic digestion.

a. The $B_{12}$ deficiency in this condition is often subclinical.

b. It is caused by atrophic gastritis and achlorhydria, which can be seen with chronic *Helicobacter pylori* infection, gastric surgery, and long-term use of acid suppressing drugs.

3. Lack of intrinsic factor is caused by gastrectomy (all patients with total gastrectomy and 5% of patients with partial gastrectomy will become $B_{12}$ deficient) or pernicious anemia (PA).

a. PA is an immunologically mediated gastric atrophy leading to loss of parietal cells and a marked reduction in secretion of intrinsic factor.

b. It is uncommon before age 30 and most often seen in patients over age 50.

c. 25% of patients have a family history of PA and 10% have autoimmune thyroid disease.

E. B$_{12}$ deficiency can also be caused by malabsorption in the terminal ileum due to

    **1.** Ileal resection or bypass

    **2.** Tropical sprue

    **3.** Crohn disease

    **4.** Blind loop syndrome

F. Sometimes drugs interfere with B$_{12}$ absorption, most notably metformin, colchicine, ethanol, and neomycin.

G. Malabsorption may rarely be due to congenital disorders, such as transcobalamin II deficiency.

### Evidence-Based Diagnosis

A. Determining whether a patient is B$_{12}$ deficient is more complicated than it seems.

    **1.** B$_{12}$ levels can be falsely low in folate deficiency, pregnancy, and oral contraceptive use.

    **2.** B$_{12}$ levels can be falsely normal in myeloproliferative disorders, liver disease, and bacterial overgrowth syndromes.

    **3.** The sensitivity and specificity of B$_{12}$ levels for true deficiency are not well established; the sensitivity is estimated at 95%, and the specificity at 85%.

B. B$_{12}$ is a cofactor in the conversion of homocysteine to methionine, and of methmalonyl CoA (MMA) to succinyl CoA.

    **1.** Consequently, in B$_{12}$ deficiency, the levels of homocysteine and MMA increase.

    **2.** Therefore, another way to diagnosis B$_{12}$ deficiency is to measure **homocysteine and MMA levels.**

        **a.** In addition to B$_{12}$ deficiency, MMA can be elevated in renal insufficiency and hypovolemia.

        **b.** Homocysteine can be elevated in folate or pyridoxine deficiency, renal insufficiency, hypovolemia, and hypothyroidism.

        **c.** The sensitivity of MMA for the diagnosis of B$_{12}$ deficiency ranges from 86% to 98%. The sensitivity of homocysteine ranges from 85% to 96%. An elevated MMA is highly specific for B$_{12}$ deficiency in the absence of renal insufficiency; elevated homocysteine is less specific.

C. **Response to therapy** is another way to establish the presence of B$_{12}$ deficiency.

    **1.** MMA and homocysteine normalize 7–14 days after the start of replacement therapy.

    **2.** Figure 6–2 shows the response to a single IM injection of 100 mcg cobalamin on day 0 in a patient with PA.

D. An algorithm for diagnosing B$_{12}$ deficiency is the following:

    **1.** B$_{12}$ level < 100 pg/mL, deficiency present

    **2.** B$_{12}$ level 100–300 pg/mL, check MMA and homocysteine levels

        **a.** If both normal, deficiency unlikely

        **b.** If both elevated, deficiency present

        **c.** If MMA alone elevated, deficiency present

        **d.** If homocysteine alone elevated, possible deficiency

    **3.** B$_{12}$ > 300 pg/mL, deficiency unlikely

 Very low or very high B$_{12}$ levels are usually diagnostic.

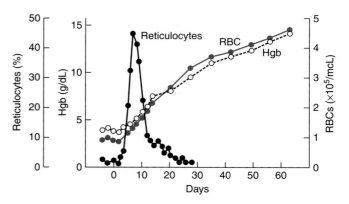

**Figure 6–2.** Response to B$_{12}$ therapy.

### Treatment

A. IM cobalamin, 1000 mcg weekly for 6–8 weeks, and then monthly for life

B. Can also use oral cobalamin, 1000–2000 mcg daily

    **1.** Oral cobalamin is absorbed by a second, nonintrinsic factor dependent mechanism that is relatively inefficient.

    **2.** Compliance can be a problem.

    **3.** Patients with dietary deficiency and food cobalamin malabsorption can be treated with lower doses of oral B$_{12}$.

C. Sublingual and intranasal formulations are available but have not been extensively studied.

## MAKING A DIAGNOSIS

Mrs. A's B$_{12}$ level is 21 pg/mL, with a serum folate of 8.0 ng/mL.

**Have you crossed a diagnostic threshold for the leading hypothesis, B$_{12}$ deficiency? Have you ruled out the active alternatives? Do other tests need to be done to exclude the alternative diagnoses?**

## Alternative Diagnosis: Folate Deficiency

### Textbook Presentation

The classic presentation is an alcoholic patient with malnutrition and anemia.

### Disease Highlights

A. Anemia and macrocytosis are the most common manifestations; neurologic symptoms are rare.

B. Most often caused by inadequate intake (especially in alcoholic patients) or increased demand due to pregnancy, chronic hemolysis, leukemia.

C. Since absorption occurs in jejunum, malabsorption is rare in the absence of short bowel syndrome or bacterial overgrowth syndromes.

D. Some drugs can cause folate deficiency, including methotrexate, phenytoin, sulfasalazine, and alcohol.

E. Along with $B_{12}$, folate is a cofactor for the conversion of homocysteine to methionine, so homocysteine levels increase in folate deficiency.

### Evidence-Based Diagnosis

A. The sensitivity and specificity of serum folate measurements for the diagnosis of folate deficiency are not clear.

B. Levels can decrease within a few days of dietary folate restriction, or with alcohol use, even though tissue stores can be normal; levels increase with feeding.

C. RBC folate, which reflects folate status over the previous 3 months, correlates more strongly with megaloblastic changes than does serum folate; however, the sensitivity and specificity of RBC folate for the diagnosis of true deficiency are both low (about 70% each).

D. Elevated homocysteine is about 80% sensitive for the diagnosis of folate deficiency; the specificity is unknown.

E. A positive response to therapy is diagnostic.
   1. Never treat folate deficiency without determining whether the patient is $B_{12}$ deficient.
   2. Folate replacement can correct hematologic abnormalities while worsening the neurologic symptoms specific to $B_{12}$ deficiency.

F. A patient with a normal serum folate, normal RBC folate, and no response to folate replacement does not have folate deficiency.

### Treatment

A. In patients with an acute deficiency, treat with 1 mg of folic acid daily for 1-4 months, or until there is complete hematologic recovery.

B. Patients with chronically increased demand, such as those with sickle cell anemia, should take 1 mg of folic acid daily indefinitely.

C. Women who are trying to conceive should take 800 mcg/day or a prenatal vitamin (contains 1 mg folic acid); pregnant women should take a prenatal vitamin.

 Always check for $B_{12}$ deficiency in a patient with folate deficiency.

## CASE RESOLUTION

1

Mrs. A's $B_{12}$ level is diagnostic of $B_{12}$ deficiency. She has no conditions associated with folate deficiency, so even though the test characteristics of the serum folate are unclear, in this case the normal level is sufficient to rule out folate deficiency.

The next step is to determine the cause of the $B_{12}$ deficiency; in most cases, this means figuring out where the malabsorption is occurring.

A. The **malabsorption is in the stomach** if:
   1. The patient has had a gastrectomy or gastric bypass
   2. The patient has detectable anti-intrinsic factor antibody
      a. Found in about 50–80% of patients with PA. The presence of anti-intrinsic factor antibody rules in PA; the absence does not rule out PA.
      b. Antiparietal cell antibodies are found in about 85% of patients with PA, but also in patients with other autoimmune endocrinopathies and up to 10% of normal patients. The presence of antiparietal cell antibodies does not rule in PA.

B. The **malabsorption is in the ileum** in patients with small bowel diseases.

It is not always possible to determine the site of malabsorption, and it is acceptable to treat such patients empirically with $B_{12}$ replacement.

1

Mrs. A's intrinsic factor antibody was positive. This is a highly specific finding and is diagnostic of $B_{12}$ deficiency due to PA. Mrs. A began receiving $B_{12}$ injections, and a follow-up CBC 4 months later was entirely normal.

## CHIEF COMPLAINT

PATIENT  2

Mrs. L is a 70-year-old woman with a history of squamous cell carcinoma of the larynx, successfully treated with surgery and radiation therapy 10 years ago. She has a tracheostomy and a jejunostomy tube. One week ago, she fell and fractured her right humeral head. On routine preoperative laboratory tests, her CBC was unexpectedly abnormal: WBC 11,100/mcL (65% polymorphonuclear leukocytes, 12% bands, 4% monocytes, 19% lymphocytes), Hgb 8.4 g/dL, Hct 26.3%, MCV 85 mcm$^3$. One month ago, her Hgb was 12.0 g/dL, with a normal WBC.

At this point, what is the leading hypothesis, what are the active alternatives, and is there a must not miss diagnosis? Given this differential diagnosis, what tests should be ordered?

## PRIORITIZING THE DIFFERENTIAL DIAGNOSIS

The relatively acute drop in Hct is a pivotal point that suggests either bleeding or hemolysis; these are also the "must not miss" diagnoses. The usual causes of normocytic anemia need to be considered next. Anemia of inflammation, previous called anemia of chronic disease, is a common cause of normocytic anemia, with bone marrow infiltration and RBC aplasia being less common. You would also include causes of macrocytic anemia in your list of other hypotheses, especially folate deficiency since it can develop fairly rapidly. Table 6–3 lists the differential diagnosis.

She has felt feverish, with a cough productive of brown sputum. She has had no nausea or vomiting, no melena, and no hematochezia. She has been postmenopausal for

**Table 6–3.** Diagnostic hypotheses for Mrs. L.

| Diagnostic Hypotheses | Clinical Clues | Important Tests |
|---|---|---|
| **Leading Hypothesis** | | |
| Acute bleeding | Melena Hematochezia Hematemesis Menorrhagia | History Rectal exam for gross blood or positive guaiac test |
| Hemolysis | Fatigue | Reticulocyte count Haptoglobin Smear for schistocytes |
| **Active Alternative—Must Not Miss** | | |
| Iron deficiency | GI bleeding Pica Menorrhagia | Ferritin |
| Hemolysis | Fatigue | Reticulocyte count Haptoglobin Smear for schistocytes |
| **Active Alternative—Most Common** | | |
| Anemia of inflammation | Acute infection Acute renal failure Chronic inflammatory diseases | Fe/TIBC Ferritin Bone marrow |
| **Other Alternatives** | | |
| Marrow infiltration | Pancytopenia Bleeding Malaise | Bone marrow |
| RBC aplasia | Drug exposure Viral symptoms | History Bone marrow |
| Folate deficiency | Diet Alcohol abuse Pregnancy Sickle cell anemia | Serum or RBC folate Bone marrow |

Fe/TIBC, serum iron/total iron-binding capacity.

a long time and has had no vaginal bleeding. The orthopedic surgeon confirms it is unlikely that she has significant bleeding at the fracture site. Her rectal exam shows brown, hemoccult-negative stool. Her chest radiograph shows a new left lower lobe pneumonia.

**Is the clinical information sufficient to make a diagnosis? If not, what other information do you need?**

## MAKING A DIAGNOSIS

Further laboratory testing shows a reticulocyte count of 1.4% (RPI = 0.8), consistent with an underproduction anemia and not hemolysis. Her serum ferritin is 200 ng/mL, substantially reducing the likelihood that she is iron deficient.

**Have you crossed a diagnostic threshold for the leading hypotheses, iron deficiency and hemolysis? Have you ruled out the active alternatives? Do other tests need to be done to exclude the alternative diagnoses?**

### Alternative Diagnosis: Anemia of Inflammation

#### Textbook Presentation

Because there is such a broad spectrum of underlying causes, there is no classic presentation of anemia of inflammation. It is most often discovered on a routine CBC that shows a normochromic, normocytic anemia, with a Hgb in the range of 8.5–9.5 g/dL.

#### Disease Highlights

A. Occurs in patients with acute or chronic immune activation

B. Cytokines (interferons, interleukins, tumor necrosis factor [TNF]) induce *changes in iron homeostasis.*

  1. Dysregulation of iron homeostasis

    a. Increased uptake and retention of iron in reticuloendothelial system cells

    b. Limited availability of iron for erythropoiesis

  2. Impaired proliferation and differentiation of erythroid progenitor cells

  3. Blunted erythropoietin response

    a. Production of erythropoietin inadequate for degree of anemia

    b. Progenitor cells do not respond normally

  4. Increased erythrophagocytosis leads to decreased RBC half-life

C. Underlying causes of anemia of inflammation include

  1. Chronic kidney disease

a. In patients with end-stage renal disease who undergo dialysis, the anemia is due to lack of erythropoietin and marked inflammation.

b. In patients with lesser degrees of chronic kidney disease, the anemia is caused primarily by lack of erythropoietin and antiproliferative effects of uremic toxins.

2. Autoimmune diseases, such as systemic lupus erythematosus (SLE), rheumatoid arthritis, vasculitis, sarcoidosis, and IBD

3. Acute infections caused by viruses, bacteria, fungi, or parasites

   a. Can occur within 24–48 hours in acute bacterial infections, with Hgb usually in the 10–12 g/dL range

   b. Occurs in as many as 90% of ICU patients, accompanied by inappropriately mild elevations of serum erythropoietin levels and blunted bone marrow response to endogenous erythropoietin

4. Chronic infections caused by viruses, bacteria, fungi, or parasites

5. Cancer, either hematologic or solid tumor

D. Noninflammatory chronic anemias also occur.

   1. Endocrinopathies, such as Addison disease, thyroid disease, panhypopituitarism can lead to mild chronic anemia.

   2. Liver disease can cause anemia.

### Evidence-Based Diagnosis

A. There is no 1 test that proves or disproves a patient's anemia is from anemia of inflammation.

B. Instead, there are several diagnostic tests that can possibly be done, sometimes simultaneously and sometimes sequentially.

A Hgb of less than 8 g/dL suggests there is a second cause for the anemia, beyond the anemia of inflammation.

1. Even in the presence of a disease known to cause anemia, it is important to rule out iron, $B_{12}$, and folate deficiencies.

2. As discussed above, it can be difficult to interpret iron studies in the presence of inflammatory diseases; however, the typical pattern in anemia of inflammation is a low serum iron, low iron-binding capacity, normal percent saturation, and elevated serum ferritin.

3. Erythropoietin levels will be low in renal insufficiency and not appropriately elevated for the degree of anemia in inflammatory conditions; interpretation is difficult and measurement of the erythropoietin level is generally not useful diagnostically.

4. Pancytopenia suggests there is bone marrow infiltration or a disease that suppresses production of all cell lines.

When you see pancytopenia, think about bone marrow infiltration, $B_{12}$ deficiency, viral infection, drug toxicity, or acute alcohol intoxication.

5. Bone marrow examination is necessary to establish the diagnosis when pancytopenia is present, serum tests are not diagnostic, the anemia progresses, or there is not an appropriate response to empiric therapy.

### Treatment

A. Treat the underlying chronic disease, if possible.

B. Indications for erythropoietin therapy and appropriate target Hgb levels are evolving; iron should be given to all patients being treated with erythropoietin.

## CASE RESOLUTION

Mrs. L has normal liver function tests and a normal creatinine. Her $B_{12}$ level is 400 pg/mL, and her serum folate is 10.0 ng/mL. Her iron studies show a serum iron of 25 mcg/dL, with a TIBC of 140 mcg/dL (% saturation = 18%).

Mrs. L has a very low RPI, ruling out hemolysis. She has no signs of bleeding, and iron studies consistent with an anemia of inflammation. In addition, she has no pancytopenia to suggest bone marrow infiltration or diffuse marrow suppression, and no evidence of vitamin deficiency. She has a disease (acute bacterial pneumonia) known to be associated with acute anemia of inflammation. Thus, the diagnosis is acute anemia of inflammation. Her pneumonia is treated with oral antibiotics, and her CBC is normal when checked 6 weeks later.

## CHIEF COMPLAINT

PATIENT

Mr. J is a 77-year-old African American man with a history of an aortic valve replacement about 2 years ago. He brought in results of tests done at another hospital: Hgb, 9.0 g/dL; Hct, 27.4%; MCV, 90 mcm³; reticulocyte count, 6%; serum ferritin, 110 ng/mL; $B_{12}$, 416 pg/mL; folate 20.0 ng/mL. The RPI is 1.8.

At this point, what is the leading hypothesis, what are the active alternatives, and is there a must not miss diagnosis? Given this differential diagnosis, what tests should be ordered?

### PRIORITIZING THE DIFFERENTIAL DIAGNOSIS

The leading hypothesis is hemolysis because of the elevated reticulocyte count. Considering the normal ferritin and vitamin levels, the pretest probability of hemolysis is high. The only potential

***Table 6–4.*** Diagnostic hypotheses for Mr. J.

| Diagnostic Hypotheses | Clinical Clues | Important Tests |
|---|---|---|
| **Leading Hypothesis** | | |
| Hemolysis | Mechanical valve<br>Known hereditary condition<br>Family history of anemia<br>Sepsis<br>Fever | Reticulocyte count<br>Haptoglobin<br>Indirect bilirubin<br>Lactate dehydrogenase<br>Examination of peripheral smear |
| **Active Alternative—Must Not Miss** | | |
| Active bleeding | Hematemesis<br>Melena<br>Hematochezia<br>Vaginal bleeding<br>Abdominal pain | |

active alternative would be active bleeding, since an elevated reticulocyte count also occurs then; however, that would be clinically obvious. All other causes of anemia are alternative diagnoses to be considered only if the diagnosis of hemolysis is not supported by further testing. Table 6–4 lists the differential diagnosis.

Mr. J has no history of hematemesis, melena, hematochezia, or abdominal pain. His abdominal exam is normal, and rectal exam shows brown, hemoccult-negative stool.

**Is the clinical information sufficient to make a diagnosis? If not, what other information do you need?**

## Leading Hypothesis: Hemolysis

### Textbook Presentation

The presentation of hemolysis depends on the cause. Patients can be asymptomatic or critically ill.

### Evidence-Based Diagnosis

A. During hemolysis, RBC products are released into the circulation, and their presence (or the absence of proteins that bind them) can be measured to support the diagnosis of hemolysis.

1. In the setting of impact, macrovascular or microvascular trauma, and some complement-induced lysis, RBCs are destroyed in the **intravascular space**.

   a. Damaged but incompletely hemolyzed cells are destroyed in the spleen.

   b. Completely destroyed cells release free Hgb into the plasma, which then binds to **haptoglobin**, reducing the plasma haptoglobin level.

   c. Some Hgb is lysed intravascularly and then is filtered by the glomerulus, causing **hemoglobinuria.**

   d. Some filtered Hgb is taken up by renal tubular cells, stored as hemosiderin, and **hemosiderinuria** occurs about a week later, when the tubular cells are sloughed into the urine.

2. Deformed RBCs and those coated with complement are usually destroyed in the **extravascular space,** in the liver, or in the spleen.

   a. Most of the Hgb is degraded into biliverdin, iron, and carbon monoxide.

   b. Biliverdin is converted to **unconjugated bilirubin** and released into the plasma, increasing the unconjugated bilirubin level.

3. Some free Hgb is released, which then binds to **haptoglobin,** again reducing the plasma haptoglobin level.

B. So, what abnormalities would you expect to see during active hemolysis?

1. The reticulocyte count should be above 4–5%; in 1 study of autoimmune hemolytic anemia, the median was 9%.

2. The serum haptoglobin should be < 25 mg/dL.

   a. Sensitivity = 83%, specificity = 96% for hemolysis; LR+ = 21, LR− = 0.18

   b. Haptoglobin is an acute phase reactant.

3. The lactate dehydrogenase (LDH) might be increased (sensitivity and specificity unknown).

   a. Finding an increased LDH *and* a decreased haptoglobin is 90% specific for the diagnosis of hemolysis.

   b. Finding a normal LDH *and* a normal serum haptoglobin (> 25 mg/dL) is 92% sensitive for the absence of hemolysis.

4. The unconjugated bilirubin may be increased (sensitivity and specificity unknown).

5. Plasma and urine Hgb should be elevated if the hemolysis is intravascular (sensitivity and specificity unknown).

### Treatment

Treatment depends on the underlying cause. In an autoimmune condition, immunosuppressive therapy, especially prednisone, is used. If hemolysis is associated with TTP and HUS, the treatment is plasmapheresis and immunosuppressives.

## MAKING A DIAGNOSIS

Mr. J's serum haptoglobin is < 20 mg/dL, his serum bilirubin is normal, and his LDH is elevated at 359 units/L.

**Have you crossed a diagnostic threshold for the leading hypothesis, hemolysis? Have you ruled out the active alternatives? Do other tests need to be done to exclude the alternative diagnoses?**

The combination of the high pretest probability and the large LR+ for this level of haptoglobin confirms the diagnosis of hemolysis.

Active bleeding has been ruled out by history and physical exam. At this point, any further testing should be aimed at determining the cause of the hemolysis. It is helpful to ask a series of questions to direct your search for the cause of a hemolytic anemia:

A. Does the patient have splenomegaly? The spleen is 1 of the major sites of extravascular hemolysis.

B. Is the direct antiglobulin (Coombs) test positive?

 1. Seen in autoimmune hemolytic anemias

 2. The Coombs test detects antibody or complement on the surface of the RBC

  a. The patient's RBCs are washed free of adherent proteins.

  b. They are reacted with antiserum containing anti-IgG and anti-C3.

  c. If IgG and/or C3 are present on the RBC, there will be agglutination.

  d. Over 99% of patients with warm antibody autoimmune hemolytic anemia will have a positive direct Coombs test.

 3. The indirect Coombs test detects antibodies to RBC antigens in the patient's serum and is sometimes positive in drug-induced hemolytic anemias.

  a. The patient's serum is incubated with normal RBCs.

  b. If the serum contains cold (IgM) antibodies, there will be agglutination.

  c. Otherwise, anti-IgG is added; if the serum contains IgG, there will be agglutination.

C. Is there concomitant thrombocytopenia and coagulopathy? This is seen in DIC.

D. Is there concomitant thrombocytopenia, renal insufficiency, or neurologic symptoms? This is seen in TTP and HUS.

E. Are there schistocytes on the peripheral smear? This is seen in traumatic hemolysis, both macrovascular and microvascular.

F. Has the patient been exposed to an infection, drug, or toxin known to cause hemolysis?

G. Does the patient have a mechanical valve or a disease known to be associated with hemolytic anemia?

## CASE RESOLUTION

▽3

His WBC and platelet count as well as his renal function are all normal; the Coombs test is negative. He does have a few schistocytes on his peripheral smear. He has hemolysis due to his mechanical valve. Since he is asymptomatic, it is not necessary to consider removal of the valve.

## REVIEW OF OTHER IMPORTANT DISEASES
## Sickle Cell Anemia

### Textbook Presentation

Sickle cell anemia is often identified at birth through screening. Adult patients generally seek medical attention for pain or some of the complications (see below). Occasionally, patients have very mild disease, and sickle cell is diagnosed late in life when evidence of a specific complication, such as sickle cell retinopathy, is identified.

### Disease Highlights

A. Epidemiology and prognosis

 1. Gene frequency for sickle cell or thalassemia is 0.17% of non-Hispanic white births.

 2. In African Americans, the gene frequency of Hgb S is 4%, of Hgb C is 1.5%, and of β-thalassemia is 4%.

 3. Median age at death is 42 for men and 48 for women.

 4. Risk factors for earlier mortality include lower Hgb F levels, episodes of acute chest syndrome, more frequent pain crises, and possibly higher WBC.

B. Clinical manifestations of sickle cell anemia

 1. Hematologic

  a. Hct usually 20–30%, with reticulocyte count of 3–15%

  b. MCV usually high normal or high

  c. Unconjugated hyperbilirubinemia, elevated LDH, and low haptoglobin are present.

  d. Hgb F level usually slightly elevated.

  e. WBC and platelet count usually elevated.

  f. Hypercoagulability: due to high levels of thrombin, low levels of protein C and S, abnormal activation of fibrinolysis and platelets

 2. Pulmonary

  a. Acute chest syndrome

   (1) Defined as a new pulmonary infiltrate accompanied by fever and a combination of respiratory symptoms, including cough, tachypnea, and chest pain

   (2) Most common cause of death in sickle cell patients

   (3) Clinical manifestations in adults (Table 6–5)

    (a) About 50% of patients in whom acute chest syndrome develops are admitted for another reason.

    (b) Over 80% have concomitant pain crises.

    (c) Up to 25% require mechanical ventilation.

   (4) Etiology

    (a) Fat embolism (from infarction of long bones), with or without infection in 12%

    (b) Infection in 27%, with 8% due to bacteria, 5% mycoplasma, and 9% chlamydia

    (c) Infarction in about 10%

    (d) Hypoventilation and atelectasis due to pain and analgesia may play a role, as might fluid overload

    (e) Unknown in about 50% of patients

   (5) General principles of management

    (a) Supplemental oxygen

    (b) Empiric treatment with a macrolide and a cephalosporin

    (c) Incentive spirometry (can be preventive)

    (d) Bronchodilators for patients with reactive airways

    (e) Transfusion

***Table 6–5.*** Clinical manifestations of acute chest syndrome in adults.

| Symptom or Sign | Frequency (%) |
| --- | --- |
| Fever | 70 |
| Cough | 54 |
| Chest pain | 55 |
| Tachypnea | 39 |
| Shortness of breath | 58 |
| Limb pain | 59 |
| Abdominal pain | 29 |
| Rib or sternal pain | 30 |
| Respiratory rate > 30 breaths per minute | 38 |
| Crackles | 81 |
| Wheezing | 16 |
| Effusion | 27 |
| Mean temperature | 38.8°C |

    **b.** Sickle cell chronic lung disease

        **(1)** 35–60% of patients with sickle cell disease have reactive airways.

        **(2)** About 20% have restrictive lung disease, and another 20% have mixed obstructive/restrictive abnormalities.

        **(3)** Up to 40% have pulmonary hypertension.

        **(4)** The relative risk of death in sickle cell patients with pulmonary hypertension, compared with those with normal pulmonary pressures, is 10.

**3.** Genitourinary

    **a.** Renal

        **(1)** Inability to concentrate urine (hyposthenuria), with maximum urinary osmolality of 400–450 mOsm/kg

        **(2)** Type 4 renal tubular acidosis

        **(3)** Hematuria

           **(a)** Usually secondary to papillary necrosis

           **(b)** Renal medullary carcinoma has been reported.

        **(4)** Proteinuria

           **(a)** Seen in 20–30% of patients with sickle cell disease; about 4% have nephrotic syndrome.

           **(b)** Progresses to chronic renal failure in about 5% of patients

           **(c)** ACE inhibitors reduce proteinuria.

    **b.** Priapism

        **(1)** 30–40% of adult males with sickle cell disease report at least 1 episode.

        **(2)** Bimodal peak incidences in ages 5–13 and 21–29.

        **(3)** 75% of episodes occur during sleep; the mean duration is 125 minutes.

        **(4)** Treatment approaches include hydration, analgesia, transfusion, and injection of α-adrenergic drugs.

**4.** Neurologic

    **a.** Highest incidence of first infarction is between the ages of 2 and 5, followed by another peak in incidence between the ages of 35 and 45.

    **b.** Hemorrhagic stroke can also occur.

    **c.** Recurrent infarction occurs in 67% of patients.

    **d.** Silent infarction is common (seen in 18–23% of patients by age 14); cognitive deficits also common.

    **e.** Patients over 2 years of age should undergo annual transcranial Doppler (TCD) screening to assess stroke risk.

        **(1)** Patients with elevated TCD velocities (> 200 cm/s) are at high risk.

        **(2)** Regular transfusions reduced the risk of stroke in such patients by 90% (10% stroke rate in control group, 1% in treatment group, number needed to treat (NNT) = 11).

**5.** Musculoskeletal

    **a.** Bones and joints often the sites of vaso-occlusive episodes.

    **b.** Avascular necrosis of hips, shoulders, ankles, and spine can cause chronic pain.

        **(1)** Often best detected by MRI

        **(2)** May require joint replacement

**6.** Other

    **a.** Retinopathy

        **(1)** More common in patients with Hgb SC disease than with sickle cell (SS) disease

        **(2)** Treated with photocoagulation

    **b.** Leg ulcers

        **(1)** Present in about 20% of patients

        **(2)** Most commonly over the medial or lateral malleoli

    **c.** Cholelithiasis: nearly universal due to chronic hemolysis

    **d.** Splenic sequestration and autosplenectomy: seen in children

    **e.** Liver disease: multifactorial, due to causes such as iron overload or viral hepatitis

### Evidence-Based Diagnosis

**A.** Newborn screening

    **1.** Universal screening identifies many more patients than screening targeted at high-risk groups.

    **2.** Homozygotes have an FS pattern on electrophoresis, which is predominantly Hgb F, with some Hgb S, and no Hgb A.

    **3.** The FS pattern in not specific for sickle cell disease, and the diagnosis should be confirmed through family studies, DNA based testing, or repeat Hgb electrophoresis at 3–4 months of age.

**B.** Testing in older children and adults

    **1.** Cellulose acetate electrophoresis separates Hgb S from other variants; however, S, G, and D all have the same electrophoretic mobility.

    **2.** Only Hgb S will precipitate in a solubility test such as the Sickledex

## Treatment

A. General principles

 1. All pediatric patients should receive prophylactic penicillin to prevent streptococcal sepsis.

 2. Transfusion indicated for acute chest syndrome, heart failure, multiorgan failure syndrome, stroke, splenic sequestration, and aplastic crisis.

   a. Do not transfuse above an Hgb of about 11 g/dL, to avoid hyperviscosity.

   b. Use simple transfusion if Hgb below 8 g/dL.

   c. Use exchange transfusion if Hgb above 8 g/dL.

 3. Hydroxyurea

   a. In patients with moderate to severe sickle cell disease, hydroxyurea therapy reduced the rate of pain crises and development of acute chest syndrome by about 50%.

   b. Hydroxyurea use is associated with a lower mortality rate.

 4. Stem cell transplant is an experimental therapy.

B. Management of vaso-occlusive crises

 1. The general approach should be similar to that used in patients with other causes of severe pain, such as cancer.

   a. Analgesics should be dosed regularly, rather than as needed.

   b. Patient-controlled analgesia can also be used.

   c. Remember that patients who use opioids long-term become tolerant and often require high doses for acute pain.

   d. Adding NSAIDs or tricyclic antidepressants to opiates is sometimes beneficial.

   e. Patients often need a long-acting opioid for baseline analgesia, combined with a short-acting opioid for breakthrough pain.

   f. A multidisciplinary approach to pain management involving nurses and social workers may help optimize pain management.

 2. Oral hydration is preferable to IV hydration.

 3. Oxygen is indicated only if the patient is hypoxemic.

## β-Thalassemia

### Textbook Presentation

β-Thalassemia major (homozygotes) presents in infancy with multiple severe abnormalities. Heterozygotes are usually asymptomatic.

### Disease Highlights

A. Impaired production of β globin chains.

B. Common in patients of Mediterranean origin.

C. β-Thalassemia minor: heterozygotes with 1 normal β globin allele and 1 β thalassemic allele

D. Anemia generally mild (Hct > 30%) and microcytosis severe (MCV < 75 mcm$^3$)

E. In pregnancy, anemia can be more severe than usual.

F. Asymptomatic splenomegaly in 15–20% of patients

### Evidence-Based Diagnosis

A. Iron studies should be normal; RDW usually normal; target cells abundant; RBCs may be normal or high.

B. On Hgb electrophoresis, the Hgb $A_2$ can be elevated, but a normal $A_2$ does not rule out β-thalassemia minor.

### Treatment of β-Thalassemia Minor

None.

## α-Thalassemia

### Textbook Presentation

Loss of 3 or 4 α globin genes causes severe disease that presents at birth or is fatal in utero. Patients with loss of 1 or 2 genes are usually asymptomatic.

### Disease Highlights

A. Impaired production of α globin chains.

B. Common in patients of African or Asian origin.

C. α-Thalassemia-2 trait: loss of 1 α globin gene; CBC normal.

D. α-Thalassemia-1 trait (α-thalassemia minor): loss of 2 α globin genes; mild microcytic anemia with target cells and normal Hgb electrophoresis.

### Evidence-Based Diagnosis

α-Thalassemia is diagnosed by polymerase chain reaction genetic analysis.

### Treatment of α Thalassemia Trait

None.

## REFERENCES

Anand IS, Chandrashekhar Y, Ferrari R, Poole-Wilson PA, Harris PC. Pathogenesis of oedema in chronic severe anaemia: studies of body water and sodium, renal function, haemodynamic variables, and plasma hormones. Br Heart J. 1993;70:357–62.

Charache S, Terrin ML, Moore RD et al. Effect of hydroxyurea on the frequency of painful crises in sickle cell anemia. N Engl J Med. 1995;332:1317–22.

Guyatt GH, Oxman AD, Ali M et al. Laboratory diagnosis of iron deficiency anemia: an overview. J Gen Intern Med. 1992;7(2):145–53.

Lindenbaum J, Healton E, Savage D et al. Neuropsychiatric disorders caused by cobalamin deficiency in the absence of anemia or macrocytosis. N Engl J Med. 1988;318:1720–28.

Marchand A, Galen R, Van Lente F. The predictive value of serum haptoglobin in hemolytic disease. JAMA. 1980;243:1909–11.

Seward SJ, Safran C, Marton KI, Robinson SH. Does the mean corpuscular volume help physicians evaluate hospitalized patients with anemia? J Gen Intern Med. 1990;5(3):187–91.

Snow C. Laboratory diagnosis of vitamin B12 and folate deficiency. Arch Intern Med. 1999;159:1289–98.

Steinberg M, Barton F, Castro O. Effect of hydroxyurea on mortality and morbidity in adult sickle cell anemia. JAMA. 2003;289:1645–51.

Vichinsky EP, Neumayr LD, Earles AN et al. Causes and outcomes of the acute chest syndrome in sickle cell disease. N Engl J Med. 2000;342:1855–65.

Weiss G, Goodnough LT. Anemia of chronic disease. N Engl J Med. 2005;352:1011–23.

Wickramasinghe SN. Diagnosis of megaloblastic anaemias. Blood Reviews. 2006;20:299–318.

# I have a patient with low back pain. How do I determine the cause?

## CHIEF COMPLAINT

> **PATIENT** ▽1
>
> Mr. Y is a 30-year-old man with low back pain that has lasted for 6 days.
>
> ☑ What is the differential diagnosis of low back pain? How would you frame the differential?

## CONSTRUCTING A DIFFERENTIAL DIAGNOSIS

Most low back pain is caused by conditions that are troublesome but not progressive or life-threatening. The primary task when evaluating a patient with low back pain is to identify those who have serious causes of back pain that require specific, and sometimes rapid, diagnosis and treatment. In practice, this means distinguishing *serious* back pain (pain due to a systemic or visceral disease or pain with neurologic symptoms or signs) from *nonspecific* back pain related to the musculoskeletal structures of the back, called mechanical back pain.

A. Back pain due to disorders of the **musculoskeletal** structures

  1. Nonspecific back pain

    a. In general, a specific anatomic diagnosis cannot be made, and there is no definite relationship between anatomic findings and symptoms.

    b. There are no neurologic signs or symptoms.

    c. It is nonprogressive.

    d. Examples include the following:

      (1) Lumbar strain and sprain

      (2) Degenerative processes of disks and facets

      (3) Spondylolisthesis (anterior displacement of a vertebra on the one beneath it)

      (4) Spondylolysis (defect in the pars interarticularis of the vertebra)

      (5) Scoliosis

  2. Specific back pain

    a. A specific anatomic diagnosis can often be made.

    b. Neurologic signs and symptoms are present.

    c. It can be progressive.

    d. Examples include the following:

      (1) Herniated disk

      (2) Spinal stenosis

      (3) Cauda equina syndrome

B. Back pain due to **systemic disease** affecting the spine

  1. Serious, requiring specific and often rapid treatment

    a. Neoplasia

      (1) Multiple myeloma, metastatic carcinoma, lymphoma, leukemia

      (2) Spinal cord tumors, primary vertebral tumors

    b. Infection

      (1) Osteomyelitis

      (2) Septic diskitis

      (3) Paraspinal abscess

      (4) Epidural abscess

  2. Serious, requiring specific treatment but not necessarily immediately

    a. Osteoporotic compression fracture

    b. Inflammatory arthritis

      (1) Ankylosing spondylitis

      (2) Psoriatic arthritis

      (3) Reiter syndrome

      (4) Inflammatory bowel disease–associated arthritis

C. Back pain due to **visceral disease** is serious and often requires specific and rapid diagnosis and treatment.

  1. Retroperitoneal

    a. Aortic aneurysm

    b. Retroperitoneal adenopathy or mass

  2. Pelvic

    a. Prostatitis

    b. Endometriosis

    c. Pelvic inflammatory disease

  3. Renal

    a. Nephrolithiasis

    b. Pyelonephritis

    c. Perinephric abscess

  4. GI

    a. Pancreatitis

    b. Cholecystitis

    c. Penetrating ulcer

It is essential to understand the clinical neuroanatomy of the lower extremity to properly examine patients with low back pain (Figures 7–1 and 7–2). Figure 7–3 outlines the diagnostic approach to low back pain.

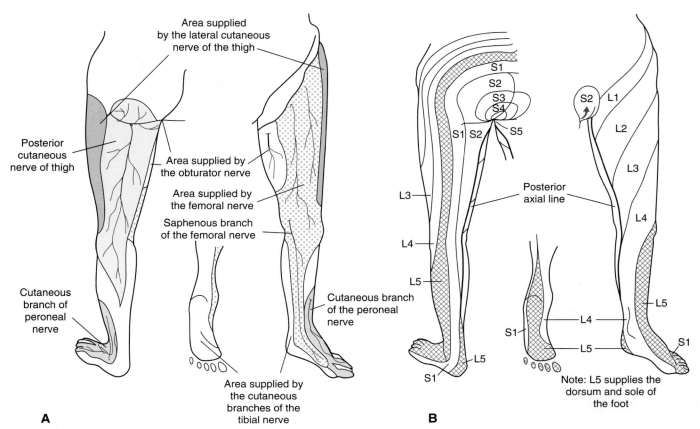

**Figure 7–1.** Distribution of cutaneous nerves (A) and nerve roots (B) in the leg. Also note that the patellar reflex reflects L4 function, and the Achilles reflex reflects S1 function. (Reproduced, with permission, from Patten J. Neurologic Differential Diagnosis, 2nd ed. Springer, 1996.)

The clinical clues for the alternative diagnoses listed in Table 7–1 have been associated with an increased likelihood of a serious etiology of back pain, and should all be considered pivotal points in refining the differential diagnosis. Likelihood ratios for these findings, when available, will be discussed later in the chapter. Table 7–1 lists the differential diagnosis.

 The clinical clues listed in Table 7–1 should be assessed in all patients with back pain.

Mr. Y felt well until 1 week ago, when he helped his girlfriend move into her third floor apartment. Although he felt fine while helping her, the next day he woke up with diffuse pain across his lower back and buttocks. He spent that day lying on the floor, with some improvement. Ibuprofen has helped somewhat. He feels better when he is in bed and had transiently worse pain after doing his usual weight lifting at the gym.

 **At this point, what is the leading hypothesis, what are the active alternatives, and is there a must not miss diagnosis? Given this differential diagnosis, what tests should be ordered?**

## PRIORITIZING THE DIFFERENTIAL

Mr. Y's history is consistent with nonspecific mechanical back pain, which is the cause of 97% of the back pain seen in a primary care practice. History and physical exam should focus on looking for **neurologic signs and symptoms** that would suggest a specific musculoskeletal cause, such as a herniated disk, and for signs and symptoms that would suggest the presence of a **systemic disease.**

Mr. Y has no history of other illnesses. He has had no trauma, weight loss, fever, chills, or recent infections. He takes no medications and does not smoke, drink, or use injection drugs. The back pain does not radiate to his legs. On physical exam, he has mild tenderness across his lower back; lower extremity strength, sensation, and reflexes are normal. Straight leg raise test is negative.

**Is the clinical information sufficient to make a diagnosis? If not, what other information do you need?**

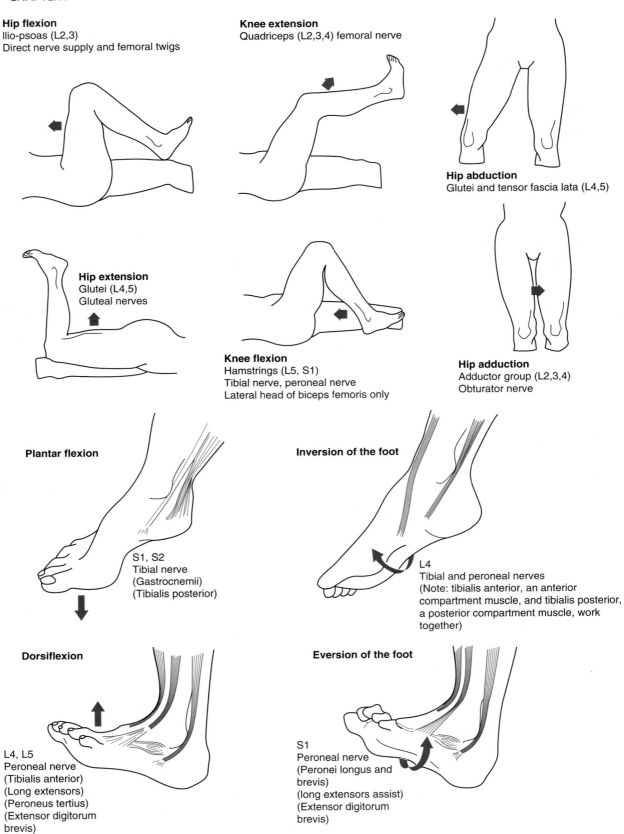

**Hip flexion**
Ilio-psoas (L2,3)
Direct nerve supply and femoral twigs

**Knee extension**
Quadriceps (L2,3,4) femoral nerve

**Hip abduction**
Glutei and tensor fascia lata (L4,5)

**Hip extension**
Glutei (L4,5)
Gluteal nerves

**Knee flexion**
Hamstrings (L5, S1)
Tibial nerve, peroneal nerve
Lateral head of biceps femoris only

**Hip adduction**
Adductor group (L2,3,4)
Obturator nerve

**Plantar flexion**
S1, S2
Tibial nerve
(Gastrocnemii)
(Tibialis posterior)

**Inversion of the foot**
L4
Tibial and peroneal nerves
(Note: tibialis anterior, an anterior
compartment muscle, and tibialis posterior,
a posterior compartment muscle, work
together)

**Dorsiflexion**
L4, L5
Peroneal nerve
(Tibialis anterior)
(Long extensors)
(Peroneus tertius)
(Extensor digitorum
brevis)

**Eversion of the foot**
S1
Peroneal nerve
(Peronei longus and
brevis)
(long extensors assist)
(Extensor digitorum
brevis)

***Figure 7–2.*** The motor exam of the leg. (Reproduced, with permission, from Patten J. Neurologic Differential Diagnosis, 2nd ed. Springer, 1996.)

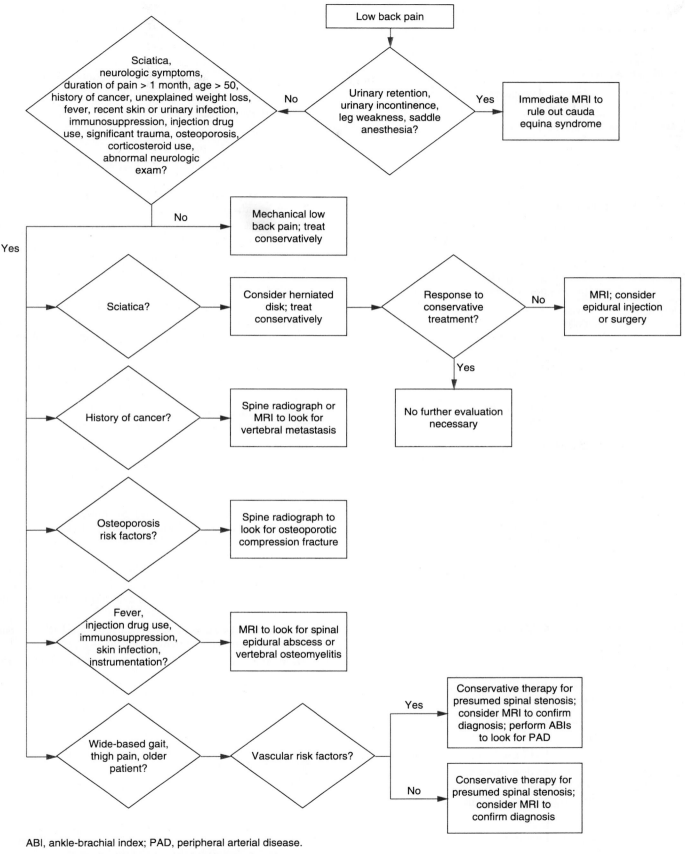

ABI, ankle-brachial index; PAD, peripheral arterial disease.

***Figure 7–3.*** Diagnostic approach: low back pain.

***Table 7–1.*** Diagnostic hypotheses for Mr. Y.

| Diagnostic Hypotheses | Clinical Clues | Important Tests |
|---|---|---|
| **Leading Hypothesis** | | |
| Mechanical back pain | Absence of symptoms listed below | Resolution within 3–4 weeks |
| **Active Alternative—Most Common** | | |
| Herniated disk | Sciatica Abnormal neurologic exam, especially in L5-S1 distribution | CT or MRI |
| **Active Alternative—Must Not Miss** | | |
| Malignancy | Duration of pain > 1 month Age > 50 Previous cancer history Unexplained weight loss (> 10 lbs over 6 months) | Spine radiograph MRI |
| Infection | Fever Chills Recent skin or urinary infection Immunosuppression Injection drug use | MRI |
| Cauda equina syndrome | Urinary retention Saddle anesthesia Bilateral sciatica Leg weakness Decreased anal sphincter tone | MRI |
| **Other Hypotheses** | | |
| Compression fracture | Age > 70 Significant trauma History of osteoporosis Corticosteroid use | Spine radiograph MRI |

## Leading Hypothesis: Mechanical Low Back Pain

### Textbook Presentation
The classic presentation is nonradiating pain and stiffness in the lower back, often precipitated by heavy lifting.

### Disease Highlights
A. Can also have pain and stiffness in the buttocks and hips
B. Generally occurs hours to days after a new or unusual exertion and improves when the patient is supine
C. Can rarely make a specific anatomic diagnosis
D. Prognosis
   1. 75–90% of patients improve within 1 month
   2. 25–50% of patients have additional episodes over the next year

3. Risk factors for persistent low back pain include
   a. A history of previous back pain
   b. Depression
   c. Substance abuse
   d. Pending or past litigation or disability compensation
   e. Low socioeconomic status
   f. Work dissatisfaction

### Evidence-Based Diagnosis
A. Many *asymptomatic* patients will have anatomic abnormalities on imaging studies.
   1. 20% of patients aged 14–25 have degenerative disks on plain radiographs.
   2. 20–75% of patients younger than 50 years have herniated disks on MRI.
   3. 40–80% of patients have bulging disks on MRI.
   4. Over 90% of patients older than age 50 have degenerative disks on MRI.
   5. Up to 20% of patients over age 50 have spinal stenosis.
B. Even in symptomatic patients, anatomic abnormalities are not necessarily causative, and identifying them does not influence initial treatment decisions.
C. A specific pathoanatomic diagnosis cannot be made in 85% of patients with isolated low back pain.

 Patients who have none of the clinical clues should not have any diagnostic testing done.

### Treatment
A. Acute low back pain
   1. Randomized controlled trials have shown that acetaminophen, nonsteroidal antiinflammatory drugs (NSAIDS), and skeletal muscle relaxants are effective in relieving acute low back pain.
   2. There is little data regarding the effects of opioids and tramadol in acute low back pain, but they are sometimes used in patients whose pain is not controlled with acetaminophen, NSAIDS, and muscle relaxants.
   3. Specific back exercises do not help acute low back pain but do help prevent recurrent back pain.
   4. Heat and spinal manipulation have been shown to reduce acute low back pain.
   5. The best approach is NSAIDs and heat during the acute phase and activity as tolerated until the pain resolves, followed by specific daily back exercises.

 Bed rest does not help acute pain and may prolong the duration of pain.

B. Subacute or chronic low back pain
   1. Tricyclic antidepressants, tramadol, opioids, gabapentin, and benzodiazepines have all been shown to be effective in treating chronic low back pain; the best evidence is for tricyclic antidepressants.

2. There is good evidence that cognitive-behavioral therapy, exercise, spinal manipulation, and interdisciplinary rehabilitation are effective for chronic low back pain.

3. There is fair evidence that acupuncture, massage, and some yoga techniques are effective.

4. Facet and epidural injection has not been shown to be beneficial; local trigger point injection might be helpful.

## MAKING A DIAGNOSIS

Considering Mr. Y's history and physical exam, there is no need to consider other diagnoses at this point. Should he not respond to conservative therapy, then the alternative diagnoses would need to be reconsidered.

## CASE RESOLUTION

You reassure Mr. Y that his pain will resolve within another 2–3 weeks. You recommend that he use ibuprofen as needed and be as active as possible within the limits of the pain. Rather than weight lifting, you suggest swimming or walking for exercise until his pain resolves. You also provide a handout on proper lifting techniques and back exercises, to be started after the pain resolves. He cancels a follow up appointment 1 month later, leaving a message that his pain is gone and he has resumed all of his usual activities.

## CHIEF COMPLAINT

PATIENT 2

Mrs. H, a 47-year-old woman, was well until 2 days ago, when she developed low back pain after working in her garden and pulling weeds for several hours. The pain is a constant, dull ache that radiates to her right buttock and hip. Yesterday, after sitting in a movie, the pain began radiating to the back of the right knee. She has taken some acetaminophen and ibuprofen without much relief. Her past medical history is unremarkable, and she takes no medicines. She has no constitutional, bowel, or bladder symptoms.

At this point, what is the leading hypothesis, what are the active alternatives, and is there a must not miss diagnosis? Given this differential diagnosis, what tests should be ordered?

## PRIORITIZING THE DIFFERENTIAL DIAGNOSIS

Similar to the patient discussed in the first case, Mrs. H developed low back pain after an unusual exertion, and has no systemic symptoms. However, her pain is worsened by sitting and radiates down the back of her leg (which suggests sciatic pain). Both of these pivotal features increase the probability that she has a herniated disk. Table 7–2 lists the differential diagnosis.

2

On physical exam, Mrs. H is clearly uncomfortable. She has no back tenderness and has full range of motion of both hips. When her right leg is raised to about 60 degrees, pain shoots down the leg. When her left leg is raised, she has pain in her lower back. Her strength and sensation are normal, but the right ankle reflex is absent.

Is the clinical information sufficient to make a diagnosis? If not, what other information do you need?

## Leading Hypothesis: Herniated Disk

### Textbook Presentation

The classic presentation is moderate to severe pain radiating from the back down the buttock and leg, usually to the foot or ankle, with associated numbness or paresthesias. This type of pain is called sciatica, and it is classically precipitated by a sudden increase in pressure on the disk, such as after coughing or lifting.

### Disease Highlights

A. Disk disease is frequently asymptomatic.

B. Numbness, paresthesias, and motor weakness are found variably; any of these can occur in the absence of pain.

**Table 7–2.** Diagnostic hypotheses for Mrs. H.

| Diagnostic Hypotheses | Clinical Clues | Important Tests |
|---|---|---|
| **Leading Hypothesis** | | |
| Herniated lumbar disk | Sciatica Neurologic signs and symptoms, especially in L5-S1 distribution Positive straight leg raise | CT or MRI |
| **Active Alternative—Most Common** | | |
| Nonspecific mechanical back pain | No neurologic or systemic symptoms | Resolution of pain |

C. Most common site of weakness is foot plantar or dorsiflexion; proximal weakness suggests a femoral neuropathy or compression of the lumbar plexus.

D. Highest prevalence is in the 45- to 64-year-old age group.

E. Risk factors include sedentary activities, especially driving, chronic cough, lack of physical exercise, and possibly pregnancy. Jobs involving lifting and pulling have not been associated with increased risk.

F. 50% of patients recover in 2 weeks and 70% in 6 weeks.

G. L4–L5 and L5–S1 cause 98% of clinically important disk herniations, so pain and paresthesias are most often seen in these distributions.

H. There are no bowel or bladder symptoms with unilateral disk herniations.

I. Coughing, sneezing, or prolonged sitting can aggravate the pain.

J. Bilateral midline herniations can cause the **cauda equina syndrome.**

1. Cauda equina syndrome is a rare condition caused by tumor or massive midline disk herniations.

2. It is characterized by the following:

   a. Urinary retention (sensitivity 90%, specificity 95%; LR+ = 18, LR− = 0.1)
   b. Urinary incontinence
   c. Decreased anal sphincter tone (80% of patients)
   d. Sensory loss in a saddle distribution (75% of patients)
   e. Bilateral sciatica
   f. Leg weakness

Suspected cauda equina syndrome is a medical emergency that requires immediate imaging and decompression.

### Evidence-Based Diagnosis

A. History and physical exam (Table 7–3)

1. Sciatica has an LR+ of 7.9 for the diagnosis of L4-5 or L5-S1 herniated disk.

2. Straight leg test is performed by holding the heel in 1 hand and slowly raising the leg, keeping the knee extended.

   a. A positive test reproduces the patient's sciatica when the leg is elevated between 30 and 60 degrees.
   b. The patient should describe the pain induced by the maneuver as shooting down the leg, not just a pulling sensation in the hamstring muscle.

3. Crossed straight leg test is performed by lifting the contralateral leg; a positive test reproduces the sciatica in the affected leg.

A straight leg raise test that elicits back pain is negative.

4. Combinations of abnormal findings (eg, positive straight leg raise and neurologic abnormalities such as absent ankle reflex, impaired plantar or dorsiflexion, impaired sensation in L5–S1 distribution) are presumably more specific than isolated findings.

**Table 7–3.** Physical exam findings for the diagnosis of disk herniation.

| Finding | Sensitivity | Specificity | LR+ | LR− |
|---|---|---|---|---|
| Sciatica | 95% | 88% | 7.9 | 0.06 |
| Positive crossed straight leg raise | 25% | 90% | 2.5 | 0.83 |
| Positive ipsilateral straight leg raise | 91% | 26% | 1.2 | 0.3 |
| Ankle dorsiflexion weakness | 35% | 70% | 1.2 | 0.93 |
| Great toe extensor weakness | 50% | 70% | 1.7 | 0.71 |
| Impaired ankle reflex | 50% | 60% | 1.3 | 0.83 |
| Ankle plantar flexion weakness | 6% | 95% | 1.2 | 0.99 |

B. Imaging

1. Plain radiographs do not image the disks and are useless for diagnosing herniations.

2. CT and MRI scans have similar test characteristics for diagnosing herniated disks.

   a. CT: sensitivity, 62–90%; specificity, 70–87%; LR+, 2.1–6.9; LR−, 0.11–0.54
   b. MRI: sensitivity, 60–100%; specificity, 43–97%; LR+, 1.1–33; LR−, 0–0.93

C. Electromyography

1. Might be useful in assessing possible nerve root dysfunction in patients with leg symptoms lasting more than 4 weeks; not useful for isolated back pain

2. Data regarding sensitivity and specificity are flawed but estimates are 71–100% sensitivity and 38–88% specificity.

### Treatment

A. In the absence of cauda equina syndrome or progressive neurologic dysfunction, conservative therapy should be tried for 1 month.

1. NSAIDs are the first choice.

2. Opioids are often necessary.

3. Bed rest does not accelerate recovery.

4. Epidural corticosteroid injections may provide temporary pain relief.

B. Surgery

1. Indications include

   a. Impairment of bowel and bladder function (cauda equina syndrome)
   b. Gross motor weakness
   c. Progressive neurologic symptoms or signs

2. Surgery should not be done for painless herniations or when the herniation is at a different level than the symptoms.

3. In the absence of progressive neurologic symptoms, surgery is elective; patients with disk herniations and radicular pain generally recover with or without surgery.

   a. Recent randomized trials of surgery versus conservative therapy for symptomatic L4-5 or L5-S1 herniated disks found short-term benefits for surgery

      1. Patients who received surgery had better pain and function scores at 12 weeks, but both groups had identical scores at 52 weeks

      2. The median time to recovery was 4 weeks for the surgery group and 12 weeks for the conservative therapy group

   b. Patient preference should drive decision making with regard to surgery.

## MAKING A DIAGNOSIS

Mrs. H has sciatica, a positive straight leg raise test, and an absent ankle reflex, a combination that strongly suggests nerve root impingement at L5–S1. However, none of these findings is so specific that nonspecific mechanical back pain has been ruled out. So, one option at this point would be to order an MRI or CT scan to positively identify a herniated disk. However, there are 2 questions to consider before ordering a scan:

1. Will the scan be diagnostic? Remember that a significant percentage of asymptomatic people have herniated disks on CT or MRI.

The abnormality on imaging studies must correlate with the findings on history and physical exam; in other words, the herniation must affect the nerve associated with the dermatome that matches the symptoms.

2. If the scan is diagnostic, will the finding change the initial management of the patient? Conservative therapy, similar to that for nonspecific back pain, is indicated initially unless the patient has cauda equina syndrome or other rapidly progressive neurologic impairment.

## CASE RESOLUTION

You decide not to order any imaging studies initially and prescribe ibuprofen (800 mg 3 times daily) and activity as tolerated. Mrs. H calls the next day, reporting that she was unable to sleep because of the pain. You then prescribe acetaminophen with codeine, which provides good pain relief. Two weeks later, she is rarely using the codeine, and is only using ibuprofen 1 to 2 times a day. Two months later, she is pain free and back to her usual activities, although her ankle reflex is still absent—a common and not significant finding. She is fine until about a year later, when she develops identical pain after a bad bronchitis. Her pain resolves with a few days of acetaminophen with codeine.

---

## CHIEF COMPLAINT

Mrs. P is a 75-year-old white woman who was well until 2 days ago when pain developed in the center of her lower back. The pain is constant and becoming more severe. There is no position or movement that changes the pain, and it is not relieved with acetaminophen or ibuprofen. It sometimes radiates in a belt like fashion across her lower back, extending around to the abdomen. She has no fever or weight loss. Her past medical history is notable for a radial fracture after falling off her bicycle 18 years ago, and breast cancer 15 years ago, treated with lumpectomy, radiation therapy, and tamoxifen. She has had annual mammograms since, all of which have been normal. She currently takes no medications.

> At this point, what is the leading hypothesis, what are the active alternatives, and is there a must not miss diagnosis? Given this differential diagnosis, what tests should be ordered?

## PRIORITIZING THE DIFFERENTIAL DIAGNOSIS

Mrs. P has several pivotal clinical findings that suggest her back pain could be due to a more serious, systemic disease rather than being nonspecific, mechanical back pain. First, she is older and has a history of previous cancer; both findings are associated with malignancy as a cause of back pain. Second, her age, race, and history of a previous fracture are established risk factors for osteoporosis. Table 7–4 lists the differential diagnosis.

On physical exam, she is in obvious pain. She is 5 ft 2 in and weighs 115 lbs. There is diffuse tenderness across her lower back, with no point tenderness of the vertebrae. There is no rash, and abdominal exam is normal. Her reflexes, strength, and sensation are all normal, and straight leg raise is negative.

> Is the clinical information sufficient to make a diagnosis? If not, what other information do you need?

**Table 7-4.** Diagnostic hypotheses for Mrs. P.

| Diagnostic Hypotheses | Clinical Clues | Important Tests |
|---|---|---|
| **Leading Hypothesis** | | |
| Metastatic breast cancer | Duration of pain > 1 month<br>Age > 50<br>Previous cancer history<br>Unexplained weight loss (> 10 lbs over 6 months) | Spine radiograph<br>MRI |
| **Active Alternative** | | |
| Osteoporotic compression fracture | Age > 70<br>Significant trauma<br>History of osteoporosis<br>Corticosteroid use | Spine radiograph<br>MRI |

**Table 7-5.** History and physical exam findings in the diagnosis of cancer as a cause of low back pain.

| Finding | Sensitivity | Specificity | LR+ | LR- |
|---|---|---|---|---|
| Previous history of cancer | 31% | 98% | 14.7 | 0.7 |
| Failure to improve after 1 month of therapy | 31% | 90% | 3.0 | 0.77 |
| Age > 50 | 77% | 71% | 2.7 | 0.32 |
| Unexplained weight loss | 15% | 94% | 2.7 | 0.9 |
| Duration of pain > 1 month | 50% | 81% | 2.6 | 0.62 |
| No relief with bed rest | 90% | 46% | 1.7 | 0.21 |
| Any of the following: age > 50, history of cancer, unexplained weight loss, or failure of conservative therapy | 100% | 60% | 2.5 | 0.0 |

## Leading Hypothesis: Back Pain Due to Metastatic Cancer

### Textbook Presentation

The classic presentation is the development of constant, dull back pain that is not relieved by rest and is worse at night in a patient with a known malignancy.

### Disease Highlights

A. Bone metastases can be limited to the vertebral body or extend into the epidural space, causing cord compression.

B. Pain can precede cord compression by weeks or even months, but compression progresses rapidly once it starts.

 Cancer + back pain + neurologic abnormalities = an emergency.

C. Malignancy causes about 1% of back pain in general but is the cause in nearly all patients with cancer who have back pain.

D. Most common sources are breast, lung, or prostate cancer.

   1. Renal and thyroid cancers also commonly metastasize to bone.

   2. Myeloma and lymphoma frequently involve the spine.

E. In most cases of cancer metastasis, the thoracic vertebrae are usually affected, while metastasis of prostate cancer most often affects the lumbar vertebrae.

F. Blastic lesions seen with prostate, small cell lung cancer, Hodgkin disease

G. Lytic lesions seen with renal cell, myeloma, non-Hodgkin lymphoma, melanoma, non–small cell lung cancer, thyroid cancer

H. Mixed blastic and lytic lesions seen with breast cancer and GI cancers

### Evidence-Based Diagnosis

A. History and physical exam

   **FP** 1. Previous history of cancer has an LR+ of 14.7 for the diagnosis of vertebral metastasis as a cause of back pain.

2. Table 7-5 lists the historical and physical exam findings associated with low back pain due to cancer.

 If the patient is younger than 50 years, has no history of cancer, has not experienced unexplained weight loss, and has not failed conservative therapy, cancer is not likely to be the cause of back pain.

B. Imaging

   1. Plain radiographs

      a. Must lose about 50% of trabecular bone before a lytic lesion is visible

      b. Blastic lesions can be seen earlier on radiographs than lytic lesions.

      c. Sensitivity, 60%; specificity, 96–99.5%

      d. LR+, 12–120; LR–, 0.4–0.42

   2. CT scan: Sensitivity and specificity for diagnosing metastatic lesions are unknown.

   3. MRI

      a. Sensitivity, 83–93%; specificity, 90–97%

      b. LR+, 8.3–31; LR–, 0.07–0.19

   4. Bone scan

      a. Sensitivity, 74–98%; specificity, 64–81%

      b. LR+, 3.9-10; LR–, 0.1–0.32

      c. Better for blastic lesions than lytic lesions; myeloma, in particular, can be missed on bone scan.

 MRI scan is the best test for diagnosing or ruling out cancer as a cause of back pain and for determining whether there is cord compression.

C. Laboratory tests: the erythrocyte sedimentation rate (ESR) is sometimes helpful

    **1.** ≥ 20 mm/h: sensitivity, 78%; specificity, 67%; LR+, 2.4

    **2.** ≥ 50 mm/h: sensitivity, 56%; specificity, 97%; LR+, 19.2

    **3.** ≥ 100 mm/h: sensitivity, 22%; specificity, 99.4%; LR+, 55.5

## Treatment

A. Surgery, radiation therapy, and chemotherapy

B. Choice of therapy depends on the type of cancer and the extent of the lesion.

## MAKING A DIAGNOSIS

Since Mrs. P has no neurologic abnormalities, and plain radiographs are relatively quick to perform, it is reasonable to start with lumbar spine films. However, because of the suboptimal LR– of about 0.4, it will be necessary to perform additional imaging if the plain radiographs are normal.

    The lumbar spine films show a vertebral compression fracture at L1, which is new when compared with films done several months ago.

 Have you crossed a diagnostic threshold for the leading hypothesis, metastatic cancer? Have you ruled out the active alternatives? Do other tests need to be done to exclude the alternative diagnoses?

## Alternative Diagnosis: Osteoporotic Compression Fracture

### Textbook Presentation

The classic presentation is acute, severe pain that develops in an older woman and radiates around the flank to the abdomen, occurring either spontaneously or brought on by trivial activity such as minor lifting, bending, or jarring.

### Disease Highlights

A. Fractures are usually in mid to lower thoracic or lumbar region.

B. Fractures at T4 or higher are more often due to malignancy than osteoporosis.

C. Pain is often increased by slight movements, such as turning over in bed.

D. Can also be asymptomatic

E. Pain usually improves within 1 week and resolves by 4–6 weeks, but some patients have more chronic pain.

F. Osteoporosis is most commonly primary, related to menopause and aging.

G. Can occur as a complication of a variety of diseases and medications.

    **1.** Most common diseases include thyrotoxicosis, primary hyperparathyroidism, vitamin D deficiency, hypogonadism, and malabsorption.

    **2.** Medications that can lead to osteoporosis include corticosteroids (most common), anticonvulsants, and long-term heparin therapy.

H. Age is the strongest risk factor for developing osteoporosis, with a RR of almost 10 for women aged 70–74 (compared with women under 65), increasing to a RR of 22.5 for women over 80.

    **1.** Other risk factors include personal history of rib, spine, wrist, or hip fracture; current smoking; white, Hispanic, or Asian ethnicity; weight < 132 lbs; family history of osteoporosis.

    **2.** Risk of developing osteoporosis is decreased in women who are obese, are of African American descent, and use estrogen postmenopausally.

I. Over 15 years, the absolute risk of vertebral fracture is about 10% for women with T scores > −1.0 and about 30% for women with T scores ≤ −2.5.

J. Women with a prevalent vertebral fracture and a T score > −1.0 have the same absolute risk of subsequent fracture, ~25%, as women without prevalent fractures and T scores ≤ −2.5.

### Evidence-Based Diagnosis

A. History and physical exam

    **1.** Not well studied

    **2.** Age > 70 has LR+ of 5.5,

     **3.** History of corticosteroid use has LR+ of 12.0 for diagnosis of osteoporotic compression fracture as a cause of back pain

B. Imaging

    **1.** MRI is thought to be more sensitive and specific than radiographs, but data are not available.

    **2.** MRI scan can distinguish between benign and malignant osteoporotic compression fractures, with sensitivity of 88.5–100% and specificity of 89.5–93% (LR+ = 8–14, LR– = 0–0.12).

    **3.** Bone scan can be useful for determining acuity.

MRI scan is the best way to distinguish malignant from benign osteoporotic compression fractures.

### Treatment

A. Osteoporosis

    **1.** Total calcium intake (dietary plus supplementation, if necessary) should be 1200–1500 mg daily; total vitamin D intake should be 700–800 international units daily.

    **2.** Bisphosphonates both increase bone density and reduce risk of subsequent spine and hip fractures.

        **a.** Alendronate and risedronate are given orally once per week

        **b.** Ibandronate is given orally once per month

        **c.** Zoledronic acid is given intravenously once per year

    **3.** Raloxifene reduces risk of spine fractures but not hip fractures.

        **a.** It also reduces the risk of estrogen receptor–positive breast cancer (RR = 0.56)

        **b.** It increases the risk of venous thromboembolism (RR about 3)

4. Parathyroid hormone (teriparatide) increases bone density and prevents fractures at the spine and the hip.

5. Estrogen can prevent fractures but is no longer recommended for long-term therapy due to adverse events such as deep venous thrombosis, pulmonary embolism, breast cancer, myocardial infarction, and cerebrovascular accidents.

6. Calcitonin does not significantly increase bone density or prevent fractures.

B. Compression fractures

1. Calcitonin may reduce the pain from an acute vertebral compression fracture.

2. Other options for treating the pain of vertebral compression fractures are vertebroplasty and kyphoplasty.

   a. Vertebroplasty consists of percutaneous injection of bone cement under fluoroscopic guidance into a collapsed vertebra.

   b. In kyphoplasty, inflatable bone tamps are also introduced into the fractured vertebral body.

   c. Neither procedure is well studied and should be reserved for patients with intractable pain.

## CASE RESOLUTION

Mrs. P undergoes an MRI scan, which confirms the diagnosis of osteoporotic compression fracture. She is treated with opioids, and her pain resolves over 3–4 weeks. Her bone density results show a spine T score of −2.1, and a hip T score of −2.6. She has no diseases or medication exposures associated with osteoporosis. She has primary osteoporosis. Treatment is started.

Regardless of Mrs. P's bone density results, the presence of a vertebral compression fracture mandates treatment for osteoporosis. Reviewing her history, she had several risk factors for osteoporosis, including her age, weight, and history of a wrist fracture.

## CHIEF COMPLAINT

PATIENT ▽ 4

Mr. F is a 65-year-old man with type 2 diabetes, hypertension, and osteoarthritis who comes into your office complaining of several months of low back pain. Sometimes the pain is limited to his back, but it sometimes radiates to his buttocks, hips, and thighs when he walks. Although generally achy in character, he sometimes feels numbness in both thighs. The pain gets better when he sits down, although he finds it also goes away while he is grocery shopping if he bends a bit to push the cart. He does not have pain while in bed, and he has more pain standing than sitting. Over-the-counter ibuprofen helps somewhat, but he feels quite limited in his activity.

 At this point, what is the leading hypothesis, what are the active alternatives, and is there a must not miss diagnosis?

## PRIORITIZING THE DIFFERENTIAL DIAGNOSIS

The differential for back pain in a man this age is broad, but 2 pivotal historical findings suggest spinal stenosis: the sensation of numbness with exertion ("pseudoclaudication"), and the improvement in the pain when he bends forward to push a grocery cart. Although he does not have the unremitting pain characteristic of metastatic cancer, that is still a possibility. Another pivotal point is that he has risk factors for vascular disease, and so peripheral arterial disease must be considered. Other possibilities include mechanical back pain, which remains common in patients over 65, although there should be no neurologic symptoms with uncomplicated mechanical back pain. Disk herniation is a final possibility, although it would have to be a central herniation to explain the bilateral symptoms. Table 7–6 lists the differential diagnosis.

**Table 7–6.** Diagnostic hypotheses for Mr. F.

| Diagnostic Hypotheses | Clinical Clues | Important Tests |
|---|---|---|
| **Leading Hypothesis** | | |
| Spinal stenosis | Wide-based gait Neurogenic claudication Age > 65 Improvement with sitting/bending forward | MRI |
| **Active Alternative—Must Not Miss** | | |
| Metastatic cancer | Duration of pain > 1 month Age > 50 Previous cancer history Unexplained weight loss (> 10 lbs over 6 months) | Spine radiograph MRI |
| Peripheral arterial disease | Vascular risk factors Leg pain with walking | ABIs |
| **Active Alternative—Most Common** | | |
| Mechanical back pain | No neurologic or systemic symptoms | Resolution of pain |
| Central disk herniation | Bilateral radicular pain | MRI |

Mr. F's past medical history is notable for hypertension, type 2 diabetes, and osteoarthritis of his knees. His medications include lisinopril, glipizide, atorvastatin, aspirin, and acetaminophen or ibuprofen. He has no history of cancer, and his prostate specific antigen (PSA) was 0.9 ng/mL 1 month ago. He has no back tenderness. Straight leg raise test is negative bilaterally; reflexes are symmetric; strength is normal; and sensation is normal, except for decreased vibratory sense in his feet. Dorsalis pedis and posterior tibialis pulses are easily palpable. His gait is normal.

**Is the clinical information sufficient to make a diagnosis? If not, what other information do you need?**

## Leading Hypothesis: Spinal Stenosis

### Textbook Presentation

The classic presentation is somewhat vague, but persistent back and leg discomfort brought on by walking or standing that is relieved by sitting or bending forward is typically seen.

### Disease Highlights

A. Leg symptoms are usually bilateral and are often described as a heaviness or numbness brought on by standing or walking ("pseudoclaudication"). Textbook descriptions of pain from spinal stenosis differ qualitatively from textbook descriptions of vascular claudication (Table 7–7).

B. Neurologic symptoms and signs are variable.

C. Stenosis is seen most often in lumbar spine, sometimes in cervical spine, and rarely in thoracic spine.

D. Spinal stenosis is due to hypertrophic degenerative processes and degenerative spondylolisthesis compressing the spinal cord, cauda equina, individual nerve roots, and the arterioles and capillaries supplying the cauda equina and nerve roots.

E. Pain is worsened by extension and relieved by flexion.

F. Patients with central stenosis generally have bilateral, non-dermatomal pain involving the buttocks and posterior thighs.

G. Patients with lateral stenosis generally have pain in a dermatomal distribution.

H. Repeating the physical exam after rapid walking might demonstrate subtle abnormalities.

I. About 50% of patients have stable symptoms; when worsening occurs, it is gradual.

   1. Lumbar spinal stenosis does not progress to paralysis and should be managed based on severity of symptoms.

   2. Progression of cervical and thoracic stenoses can cause myelopathy and paralysis and requires surgery more often than lumbar spinal stenosis.

### Evidence-Based Diagnosis

A. History and physical exam

   1. Wide-based gait has an LR+ of 14.3 for the diagnosis of spinal stenosis.

   2. Table 7–8 outlines the historical and physical exam findings associated with the diagnosis of spinal stenosis.

B. Imaging

   1. Plain radiographs can detect compromise of vertebral foramina by bone but not by soft tissue; radiography is not as sensitive as CT or MRI.

   2. CT and MRI have similar test characteristics.

      a. CT scan: sensitivity, 90%; specificity, 80–96%; LR+, 4.5–22; LR–, 0.10–0.12

      b. MRI: sensitivity, 90%; specificity, 72–99%; LR+, 3.2–90; LR–, 0.10–0.14

      c. Up to 21% of asymptomatic patients over age 65 have spinal stenosis on MRI.

CT and MRI scans can rule out spinal stenosis but cannot necessarily determine whether visualized stenosis is causing the patient's symptoms.

**Table 7–7.** Findings that differentiate vascular from neurogenic claudication.

| Vascular | Neurogenic |
|----------|-----------|
| Fixed walking distance before onset of symptoms | Variable walking distance before onset of symptoms |
| Improved by standing still | Improved by sitting or bending forward |
| Worsened by walking | Worsened by walking or standing |
| Painful to walk uphill | Can be painless to walk uphill due to tendency to bend forward |
| Absent pulses | Present pulses |
| Skin shiny with loss of hair | Skin appears normal |

**Table 7–8.** History and physical exam findings in the diagnosis of spinal stenosis.

| Finding | Sensitivity | Specificity | LR+ | LR– |
|---------|-------------|-------------|-----|-----|
| Wide-based gait | 43% | 97% | 14.3 | 0.59 |
| No pain when seated | 46% | 93% | 6.6 | 0.58 |
| Abnormal Romberg test results | 39% | 91% | 4.3 | 0.67 |
| Symptoms improve when seated | 52% | 83% | 3.1 | 0.58 |
| Vibration deficit | 53% | 81% | 2.8 | 0.58 |
| Age > 65 | 77% | 69% | 2.5 | 0.33 |
| Pseudoclaudication | 63% | 71% | 2.0 | 0.53 |

## Treatment

**A.** Evidence to guide treatment decisions is minimal.

**B.** Nonoperative treatment is successful (defined as stable or improving symptoms) in 15–70% of patients.

   **1.** Medications used for pain relief include NSAIDs, tricyclic antidepressants, gabapentin, and sometimes opioids.

   **2.** Physical therapy improves stamina and muscle strength in the legs and trunk.

   **3.** Epidural corticosteroid injection helps some patients, especially those with radicular pain.

**C.** Surgery

   **1.** Primary indication is increasing pain that is not responsive to conservative measures.

   **2.** Observational data show the following:

     **a.** More effective in reducing leg pain than back pain

     **b.** Reported improvement rates range between 64% and 91%.

     **c.** Reoperation rates range from 6% to 23%.

     **d.** Predictors of a positive response to surgery include male gender, younger age, better walking ability, better self-rated health, less comorbidity, and more pronounced canal stenosis.

   **3.** A recent trial with both a randomized and observation cohort showed the following:

     **a.** In the intention to treat analysis of the randomized cohort, patients randomized to surgery reported better scores on one measure of bodily pain at 2 years than did those randomized to conservative therapy.

     **b.** In the analysis of the observational cohort, patients who chose surgery reported better pain and function scores than those who chose conservative therapy.

## MAKING A DIAGNOSIS

Mr. F's history remains suggestive of spinal stenosis; his physical exam neither rules in nor rules out the diagnosis. You order an MRI scan.

Mr. F's lumbar MRI shows central canal stenosis at the L3-L4 level. There is also bilateral neural foraminal stenosis at L4-L5. There are no compression fractures or lytic or blastic lesions.

Have you crossed a diagnostic threshold for the leading hypothesis, spinal stenosis? Have you ruled out the active alternative, peripheral arterial disease? Do other tests need to be done to exclude the alternative diagnoses?

## Alternative Diagnosis: Peripheral Arterial Disease (PAD)

### Textbook Presentation

Classic claudication is defined as reproducible, exercise-induced calf pain that requires stopping and is relieved with less than 10 minutes of rest. Critical limb ischemia classically presents with pain in the feet at rest that may be relieved by placing the feet in a dependent position.

### Disease Highlights

**A.** In a study of outpatients over the age of 70, or aged 50–69 with a history of smoking or diabetes, the prevalence of PAD was 29%.

   **1.** Only 11% of the patients with PAD had classic claudication.

   **2.** 47% of patients had atypical symptoms (exertional leg pain that was not in the calf or was not relieved by rest), and 42% had no leg pain.

**B.** Critical limb ischemia is presenting manifestation in 1–2% of patients.

**C.** Risk factors include

   **1.** Smoking (risk of PAD increases by 1.4 for every 10 cigarettes smoked/day)

   **2.** Hypertension (risk of PAD increases by 1.5 for mild and 2.2 for moderate hypertension)

   **3.** Diabetes (risk of PAD increases by 2.6)

   **4.** Hyperlipidemia (risk of PAD increases by 1.2 for each 40 mg/dL increase in cholesterol)

**D.** Patients with PAD have a high prevalence of coronary artery disease and cerebrovascular disease with an annual rate of cardiovascular events of 5–7%.

**E.** PAD is associated with a progressive decline in walking endurance and an increased rate of depression.

**F.** Pretest probabilities of PAD in patients with a variety of risk factors are shown in Table 7–9.

### Evidence-Based Diagnosis

**A.** History

   **1.** The presence of classic claudication has an LR+ = 3.30

   **2.** The absence of claudication has an LR− = 0.89.

**Table 7–9.** Pretest probabilities of PAD.

| | Patients with leg complaints | Asymptomatic patients |
|---|---|---|
| Age 60–80 | 15% | |
| Age 60–69 | | 5% |
| Age 70–79 | | 12% |
| Stroke | 26% | 15% |
| Ischemic heart disease | 19% | 13% |
| Diabetes | 18% | 11% |
| Hypercholesterolemia | 15% | 6% |
| Hypertension | 12% | 7% |
| Male sex | 12% | 5% |
| Smoking (current or quit in last 5 years) | 11% | 7% |

PAD, peripheral arterial disease.

B. Physical exam

1. Skin changes

    **a.** In symptomatic patients, skin being cooler to the touch and the presence of a foot ulcer in the affected leg both have a LR+ = 5.9 and a LR− of about 1.0

    **b.** Skin changes (atrophic or cool skin, blue/purple skin, absence of lower limb hair) are not useful in assessing for PAD in asymptomatic patients

2. Bruits

    **a.** In symptomatic patients the presence of an iliac, femoral or popliteal bruit has a LR+ = 5.6; the absence of a bruit in ALL three locations has a LR− = 0.39

    **b.** In asymptomatic patients, the finding of a femoral bruit has a LR+ = 4.8; the absence of a femoral bruit does not change the probability of PAD

3. Pulses

    **a.** An abnormal femoral pulse has a LR+ = 7.2; an abnormal posterior tibial pulse has a LR+ = 8.10

    **b.** An abnormal dorsalis pedis pulse does not increase the probability of PAD (LR+ = 1.9); the dorsalis pedis pulse is not palpable in 8.1% of normal individuals.

    **c.** The absence of an abnormality in any pulse has a wide range of negative LRs (0.38–0.87).

4. Capillary refill time

    **a.** Apply firm pressure to the plantar aspect of the great toe for 5 seconds; after releasing the toe, normal color should return in ≤ 5 seconds

    **b.** Neither sensitive nor specific for diagnosing PAD

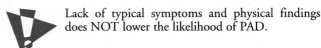 Lack of typical symptoms and physical findings does NOT lower the likelihood of PAD.

C. Ankle-brachial index (ABI)

1. Figure 7–4 shows how ABIs are done

2. Using a cutoff of 0.90 or less to define abnormal, the sensitivity is 95% and specificity 99% for the diagnosis of PAD (LR+ = 95, LR− = 0.05)

3. An ABI of 0.71–0.9 = mild PAD; 0.41–0.70 = moderate PAD; 0.00–0.40 = severe PAD

**Treatment**

A. Risk factor modification: smoking cessation, control of hypertension and diabetes, reduction of LDL to < 100 mg/dL

B. Antiplatelet therapy with aspirin or clopidogrel reduces myocardial infarction, stroke, and death from vascular causes; there is no additional benefit with combination therapy

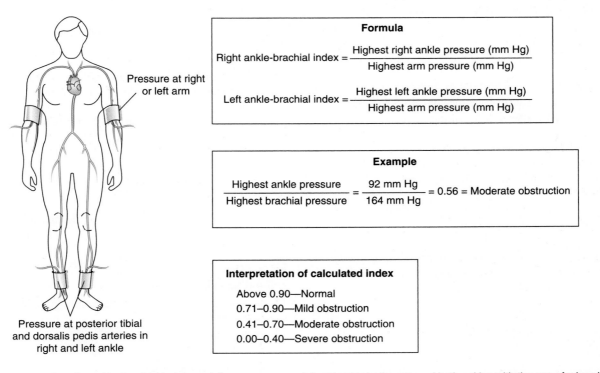

To calculate the ankle–brachial index, systolic pressures are determined in both arms and both ankles with the use of a hand-held Doppler instrument. The highest readings for the dorsalis pedis and posterior tibial arteries are used to calculate the index.

***Figure 7–4.*** Performing the ABI. (Reproduced, with permission, from White C. Intermittent claudication. N Engl J Med. 2007;356:1241–50.)

C. Cilostazol 100 mg twice daily increases walking distance by 50% after 3–6 months of use; pentoxifylline has no effect on walking distance.

D. Exercise, especially a supervised exercise program, can increase walking by up to 150% over 3–12 months.

E. Revascularization, either surgical or percutaneous transluminal angioplasty, is indicated for critical limb ischemia, and for claudication unresponsive to exercise and pharmacologic therapy that limits patients' lifestyle or ability to work.

## CASE RESOLUTION

Mr. F's pretest probability of PAD is at least 18%. You order ABIs, which show mild PAD (bilateral indices of 0.89). He begins taking 25 mg of amitriptyline at bedtime and continues using acetaminophen or ibuprofen during the day. After attending physical therapy for 8 weeks, he reports some improvement in his exercise tolerance, although he still has daily pain. An epidural corticosteroid injection provides more pain relief, and he is able to continue a walking program.

## REVIEW OF OTHER IMPORTANT DISEASES

### Spinal Epidural Abscess

#### Textbook Presentation

The classic presentation is a patient with a history of diabetes or injection drug use who has fever and back pain, followed by neurologic symptoms (eg, motor weakness, sensory changes, and bowel or bladder dysfunction).

#### Disease Highlights

A. Pathogenesis
  1. Most patients have one or more predisposing conditions.
     a. Underlying disease (diabetes mellitus, alcoholism, HIV)
     b. Spinal abnormality or intervention (degenerative joint disease, trauma, surgery, drug injection)
     c. Potential local or systemic source of infection (skin or soft tissue infection, osteomyelitis, urinary tract infection, injection drug use, epidural anesthesia, indwelling vascular access)
  2. Infection occurs by contiguous spread in 33% of cases and by hematogenous spread in 50%.
  3. *Staphylococcus aureus* is the organism in 66% of cases.
     a. Other organisms include *Staphylococcus epidermidis, Escherichia coli, Pseudomonas aeruginosa.*
     b. Anaerobes, mycobacteria, fungi, and parasites are occasionally found.
B. Clinical manifestations
  1. Back pain in 75% of patients
  2. Fever in about 50% of patients
  3. Neurologic deficits are found in about 33% of patients.
  4. More common in posterior than anterior epidural space, and more common in the thoracolumbar than cervical areas.
  5. Generally extend over 3–5 vertebrae

C. Staging
  1. Stage 1: back pain at the level of the affected spine
  2. Stage 2: nerve root pain radiating from the involved spinal area
  3. Stage 3: motor weakness, sensory deficit, bladder/bowel dysfunction
  4. Stage 4: paralysis
  5. Rate of progression from one stage to another is highly variable.
  6. The most important predictor of the final neurologic outcome is the neurologic status before surgery, with the postoperative neurologic status being as good as or better than the preoperative status.

#### Evidence-Based Diagnosis

A. ESR and C-reactive protein are usually elevated.
B. Leukocytosis is present in about 66% of patients.
C. Bacteremia is present in 60% of patients.
D. MRI is best imaging study, with a sensitivity of > 90%.

#### Treatment

A. Emergent surgical decompression and drainage
B. Antibiotics

### Vertebral Osteomyelitis

#### Textbook Presentation

The classic presentation is unremitting back pain often, but not always, with fever.

#### Disease Highlights

A. Pathogenesis
  1. Most commonly hematogenous spread; can also occur due to contiguous spread or direct infection from trauma or surgery.
  2. Generally causes bony destruction of 2 adjacent vertebral bodies and collapse of the intervertebral space.
B. Microbiology
  1. S aureus in over 50% of patients
  2. Group B and G hemolytic streptococcus, especially in diabetic patients
  3. Enteric gram-negative bacilli, especially after urinary tract instrumentation

#### Evidence-Based Diagnosis

A. History and physical exam
  1. Injection drug use, urinary tract infection, or skin infection: sensitivity, 40%
  2. Spinal tenderness
     a. Sensitivity, 86%; specificity, 60%
     b. LR+, 2.1; LR–, 0.23
  3. Fever
     a. Sensitivity, 52%; specificity, 98%
     b. LR+, 26; LR– 0.49

B. Laboratory tests

1. Leukocytosis: sensitivity, 43%; specificity, 94%; LR+, 7.2; LR– 0.6

2. ESR: sensitivity and specificity unknown, but most patients in reported case series have an elevated ESR, often over 100 mm/h

3. Blood cultures are positive in 50–70% of patients; needle aspiration is necessary to establish causative organism if blood cultures are negative.

C. Imaging

1. Radiographs: sensitivity, 82%; specificity, 57%; LR+, 1.9; LR–, 0.32

2. MRI: sensitivity, 96%; specificity, 92%; LR+, 12; LR–, 0.04

3. Bone scan: sensitivity, 90%; specificity, 78%; LR+, 4.1; LR–, 0.13

## Treatment

A. Primarily antibiotics for 6 weeks

B. Surgery is necessary only if neurologic symptoms suggest onset of vertebral collapse causing cord compression or development of spinal epidural abscess.

 Endocarditis should be considered in patients with either vertebral osteomyelitis or a spinal epidural abscess.

## REFERENCES

Cauley JA, Hochberg MC, Lui LY et al. Long-term risk of incident vertebral fractures. JAMA. 2007;298(23):2761–67.

Chou R, Qaseem A, Snow V et al; Clinical Efficacy Assessment Subcommittee of the American College of Physicians; American College of Physicians; American Pain Society Low Back Pain Guidelines Panel. Diagnosis and treatment of low back pain: a joint clinical practice guideline from the American College of Physicians, and the American Pain Society. Ann Intern Med. 2007;147:478–91.

Dauouich RO. Spinal epidural abscess. N Engl J Med. 2006;355:2012–20.

De Graaf I, Prak A, Bierma-Zeinstras S, Thomas S, Peul W, Koes B. Diagnosis of lumbar spinal stenosis. Spine. 2006;31:1168–76.

Jarvik J, Deyo R. Diagnostic evaluation of low back pain with emphasis on imaging. Ann Intern Med. 2002;137:586–97.

Khan N, Rahim S, Anad S et al. Does the clinical examination predict lower extremity peripheral arterial disease? JAMA. 2006;295:536–46.

Lurie JD. What diagnostic tests are useful for low back pain? Best Pract Res Clin Rheumatol. 2005;19:557–75.

Peul WC, van Houwelingen HC, van den Hout WB et al; Leiden–The Hague Spine Intervention Prognostic Study Group. Surgery versus prolonged conservative treatment for sciatica. N Engl J Med. 2007;356:2245–56.

Weinstein JN, Tosteson TD, Lurie JD, et al for the SPORT Investigators. Surgical versus nonsurgical therapy for lumbar spinal stenosis. N Engl J Med. 2008;358:794–810.

White C. Intermittent claudication. N Engl J Med. 2007;356:1241–50.

# I have a patient with chest pain.
# How do I determine the cause?

## CHIEF COMPLAINT

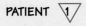

Mr. W is a 56-year-old man who comes to your office with chest pain.

> **What is the differential diagnosis of chest pain? How would you frame the differential?**

## CONSTRUCTING A DIFFERENTIAL DIAGNOSIS

A patient with chest pain poses one of the most complicated diagnostic challenges. The differential diagnosis is enormous and includes diagnoses that can be imminently life-threatening if missed. The main pivotal points when considering a history of chest pain is the acuity of onset of the pain and whether or not the pain is pleuritic (worsening with inspiration). The differential diagnosis of chest pain is the model for an anatomic approach to diagnosis. Consideration needs to be given to the structures from the skin to the internal organs. The differential below is organized anatomically.

A. Skin: Herpes zoster
B. Breast
  1. Fibroadenomas
  2. Gynecomastia
C. Musculoskeletal
  1. Costochondritis
  2. Precordial catch syndrome
  3. Pectoral muscle strain
  4. Rib fracture
  5. Cervical or thoracic spondylosis (C4-T6)
  6. Myositis
D. Esophageal
  1. Spasm
  2. Esophagitis
    a. Reflux
    b. Medication-related
  3. Neoplasm
E. GI
  1. Peptic ulcer disease
  2. Gallbladder disease
  3. Liver abscess
  4. Subdiaphragmatic abscess
  5. Pancreatitis
F. Pulmonary
  1. Pleura
    a. Pleural effusion
    b. Pneumonia
    c. Neoplasm
    d. Viral infections
    e. Pneumothorax
  2. Lung
    a. Neoplasm
    b. Pneumonia
  3. Pulmonary vasculature
    a. Pulmonary embolism (PE)
    b. Pulmonary hypertension
G. Cardiac
  1. Pericarditis
  2. Myocarditis
  3. Myocardial ischemia (stable angina, myocardial infarction [MI] or unstable angina)
H. Vascular: Thoracic aortic aneurysm or aortic dissection
I. Mediastinal structures
  1. Lymphoma
  2. Thymoma
J. Psychiatric

> Mr. W comes in regularly for management of hypertension and diabetes, both of which are under good control. He has been having symptoms since just after his last visit 4 months ago. He feels squeezing, substernal pressure while climbing stairs to the elevated train he rides to work. The pressure resolves after about 5 minutes of rest. He also occasionally feels the sensation during stressful periods at work. It is occasionally associated with mild nausea and jaw pain. Medications are metformin, aspirin, and enalapril.

>  **At this point, what is the leading hypothesis, what are the active alternatives, and is there a must not miss diagnosis? Given this differential diagnosis, what tests should be ordered?**

## PRIORITIZING THE DIFFERENTIAL DIAGNOSIS

Mr. W is a middle-aged man with risk factors for coronary artery disease (CAD), whose symptoms are consistent with stable angina. The pivotal points in this case are the chronicity, exertional nature, and substernal location of the pain. Given the seriousness and prevalence of CAD, it must lead the differential diagnosis. Gastroesophageal reflux disease (GERD) and musculoskeletal disorders are common causes of chest pain that can mimic angina (exacerbated by activity, sensation of pressure, radiation to back) and thus should be considered. The chronicity of the symptoms argues against many other worrisome diagnoses (eg, PE, pneumothorax, pericarditis, or aortic dissection). Pain from a mediastinal abnormality is possible. Table 8–1 lists the differential diagnosis.

Physical exam is entirely unremarkable except for mild, stable peripheral neuropathy presumably related to diabetes. The patient's ECG is remarkable only for evidence of left ventricular hypertrophy with strain.

**Is the clinical information sufficient to make a diagnosis? If not, what other information do you need?**

## Leading Hypothesis: Stable Angina

### Textbook Presentation

Although atypical presentations are common, stable angina usually presents with classic symptoms of substernal chest discomfort precipitated by exertion. These symptoms resolve promptly with rest or nitroglycerin and do not change over the course of weeks. Affected patients usually have risk factors for CAD.

**Table 8–1.** Diagnostic hypotheses for Mr. W.

| Diagnostic Hypotheses | Clinical Clues | Important Tests |
|---|---|---|
| **Leading Hypothesis** | | |
| Stable angina | Substernal chest pressure with exertion | Exercise tolerance test Angiogram |
| **Active Alternative—Most Common** | | |
| GERD | Symptoms of heartburn, chronic nature | EGD Esophageal pH monitoring |
| **Active Alternative** | | |
| Musculoskeletal disorders | History of injury or specific musculoskeletal chest pain syndrome | Physical exam Response to treatment |

EGD, esophagogastroduodenoscopy; GERD, gastroesophageal reflux disease.

### Disease Highlights

A. Stable angina is a chest pain syndrome caused by a mismatch between myocardial oxygen supply and demand.

   1. Usually a product of coronary artery stenosis.

   2. Can occur in the setting of normal or nearly normal coronary arteries and

      a. Anemia

      b. Tachycardia of any cause (atrial fibrillation, hyperthyroidism)

      c. Aortic stenosis

      d. Hypertrophic cardiomyopathy

      e. Heart failure (HF) (the result of high filling pressures)

 It is important to consider causes of angina other than CAD.

B. Stable angina is a common presentation for CAD.

C. Although exertional chest pain is the most common symptom of stable angina, other presentations are possible. Presentations may vary by what elicits the pain and what the symptoms are.

   1. Eliciting factors other than exercise

      a. Cold weather

      b. Extreme moods (anger, stress)

      c. Large meals

   2. Symptoms other than chest pain

      a. Dyspnea

      b. Nausea or indigestion

      c. Pain in areas other than the chest (eg, jaw, neck, teeth, back, abdomen)

      d. Palpitations

      e. Syncope

      f. Weakness and fatigue

D. The risk factors for CAD are important to elicit when the patient's history is suspicious. The traditional risk factors follow:

   1. Male sex

   2. Age > 55 years in men and > 65 years in women

   3. Tobacco use

   4. Diabetes

   5. Hypertension

   6. Family history of premature cardiovascular disease (younger than age 55 in men and younger than age 65 in women).

   7. Abnormal lipid profile

      a. Elevated low-density lipoprotein (LDL)

      b. Elevated triglycerides

      c. Elevated cholesterol/high-density lipoprotein (HDL) ratio (Ratio should be < 5:1, ideally < 3.5:1).

      d. Low HDL

E. Other risk factors

   1. Hyperhomocysteinemia

   2. Elevated levels of inflammation (C-reactive protein)

   3. Plasma fibrinogen

**4.** Microalbuminuria

**5.** Cocaine use should be asked about because although it is not a risk factor for CAD, it can cause both angina and MI.

> Asking about the traditional cardiac risk factors should be a part of the history for any patient with chest pain.

**F.** Stable angina and CAD in women

   **1.** Although the pathophysiology of stable angina is the same in men and women, it raises some unique issues in women that deserve comment.

   **2.** CAD presents differently in women than in men.

      **a.** Because CAD usually presents in women at an older age than in men, there are more comordid diseases to confuse the presentation.

      **b.** Women describe their chest pain differently, using terms like "burning" and "tender" more frequently.

   **3.** There is good evidence that the diagnostic tests used for CAD, which are discussed later in this chapter, are less accurate in women than in men.

   **4.** Because there is a lower prevalence of disease among women:

      **a.** Physicians often do not consider the diagnosis

      **b.** Lower pretest probability leads to worse positive predictive value of diagnostic tests (there are more false-positive results on noninvasive tests).

## Evidence-Based Diagnosis

**A.** History

   **1.** The first step in diagnosing CAD is taking an accurate history of the patient's chest pain.

   **2.** The vocabulary physicians use when discussing chest pain has been well validated to correlate with different risks of underlying CAD. The descriptions depend on the answers to 3 questions:

      **a.** Is your chest discomfort substernal? ("Where is your pain?")

      **b.** Are your symptoms precipitated by exertion? ("Does your pain come on or get worse when you walk, walk fast, or climb stairs?")

      **c.** Does rest provide prompt relief of your symptoms (within 10 minutes)? ("Does you pain get better with rest?")

   **3.** The number of questions to which the patient answers yes can predict the prevalence of CAD (Table 8–2).

> Use the patient's own words when taking a history (eg, pressure, burning, aching, squeezing, piercing).

   **4.** It is important to recognize that comorbidities can markedly influence the probability of disease. As an example, the rate of CAD in a 55-year-old woman with atypical angina goes from about 32% with no risk factors to 47% if the woman has diabetes, smokes, or is hypertensive.

> Almost any symptom, other than musculoskeletal ones, that reliably recurs with exertion should raise the possibility of atypical angina.

   **5.** Men over 50 and women over 60 who present with symptoms of typical angina have over a 90% likelihood of having coronary artery disease.

   **6.** The remainder of the history should be aimed at collecting evidence that makes the diagnosis of CAD more likely, such as

      **a.** Cardiac risk factors

      **b.** Past history of cardiac disease

      **c.** Symptoms classic for other causes of chest pain

   **7.** Factors that make the diagnosis of CAD less likely include

      **a.** Unremitting pain of prolonged duration

      **b.** Other explanations for the patient's symptoms

***Table 8–2.** Prevalence of coronary artery disease (%).[1]*

| Age | Asymptomatic[2] | | Nonanginal Chest Pain[3] | | Atypical Angina[4] | | Typical Angina[5] | |
|---|---|---|---|---|---|---|---|---|
| | Male | Female | Male | Female | Male | Female | Male | Female |
| 30-39 | 1.9 | 0.3 | 5.2 | 0.8 | 21.8 | 4.2 | 69.7 | 25.8 |
| 40-49 | 5.5 | 1.0 | 14.1 | 2.8 | 46.1 | 13.3 | 87.3 | 55.2 |
| 50-59 | 9.7 | 3.2 | 21.5 | 8.4 | 58.9 | 32.4 | 92 | 79.4 |
| 60-69 | 12.3 | 7.5 | 28.1 | 18.6 | 67.1 | 54.4 | 94.3 | 90.6 |

[1]See text for questions.
[2]Zero of 3 questions answered yes.
[3]One of 3 questions answered yes.
[4]Two of 3 questions answered yes.
[5]All 3 questions answered yes.
Data from Diamond GA, Forrester JS. Analysis of probability as an aid in the clinical diagnosis of coronary-artery disease. *N Engl J Med.* 1979;300:1350–1358.

**8.** Initial tests that should be done at the initial presentation include

   **a.** Glucose and lipid profile because they can identify diseases that increase the likelihood of chest pain being ischemic in origin.

   **b.** Hgb and TSH because they can identify other diseases that may cause angina.

   **c.** Resting ECG because it looks for evidence of previous infarction.

   **d.** Troponin, if the anginal symptoms had been particularly severe or long lasting.

**B.** Exercise testing

   **1.** Except in very rare cases, patients with symptoms of stable angina should have an exercise test.

   **2.** The test is used for 2 main purposes: to diagnose CAD and to determine whether patients should be treated with medication only, PCI (percutaneous intervention), or with bypass surgery.

   **3.** Decisions about treatment are based on a number factors, many coming from the results of exercise testing:

   **a.** The extent and severity of ischemia (most important)

   **b.** Other prognostic variables, such as aerobic ability, blood pressure and heart rate response to exercise, and inducible left ventricular function.

   **4.** All exercise tests attempt to induce and detect myocardial ischemia.

   **a.** Myocardial ischemia may be induced by exercise, dobutamine, adenosine, or dipyridamole.

   **b.** Myocardial ischemia may be detected by ECG, echocardiogram, or nuclear imaging.

   **5.** Exercise electrocardiography is the simplest and least expensive test. It requires a normal resting ECG.

   **a.** The sensitivity of the exercise stress test can be improved (at the cost of lower specificity) by reducing the degree of ST depression needed for a positive test.

   **b.** The sensitivity of an exercise test will fall if the patient does not reach an adequate degree of exercise, as measured by the rate-pressure product.

   **6.** The sensitivity, specificity, and LRs of some of the various tests are shown in Table 8–3. (It should be noted that the test characteristics of stress thallium and dobutamine echocardiography vary among healthcare centers.)

   **7.** The decision whether to order a routine exercise test or one with imaging is difficult. In general, definite reasons to obtain imaging are

   **a.** Abnormal resting ECG

   **b.** Previous coronary artery bypass grafting surgery (CABG) or PCI

   **c.** A more sensitive test is required to rule out CAD, such as in patients with a high likelihood of CAD.

   **8.** Means of increasing coronary demand other than exercise (pharmacologic stress tests) are indicated for patients who are unable to exercise. They may also be more accurate in patients with a left bundle-branch block.

   **9.** A patient with stable angina might not undergo an exercise test if the patient has a high likelihood of disease (a test therefore does not need to be done for diagnostic purposes) and the patient would not benefit from determining the

**Table 8–3.** Test characteristics of exercise tests.

| Test | Sensitivity | Specificity | LR+ | LR− |
|------|-------------|-------------|-----|-----|
| Exercise ECG > 1 mm depression | 65–70% | 70–75% | ≈ 2.5 | ≈ .45 |
| Exercise echocardiography | 80–85% | 80–85% | ≈ 4.8 | ≈ 0.21 |
| Dobutamine echocardiography | 80–85% | 85–90% | ≈ 6.7 | ≈ 0.23 |
| Exercise myocardial perfusion SPECT | 85–90% | 85–90% | ≈ 6.9 | ≈ 0.15 |
| Pharmacologic myocardial perfusion SPECT | 80–90% | 80–90% | ≈ 7 | ≈ 0.18 |

SPECT, single photon emission computed tomography.

distribution or severity of the disease (usually because the patient would not or could not undergo revascularization).

**C.** Angiography

   **1.** The gold standard for diagnosing CAD.

   **2.** The indications for patients with stable angina to undergo angiography include

   **a.** Abnormal stress indicating substantial ischemia

   **b.** Ischemia at a low workload on an exercise test

   **c.** Diagnostic uncertainty after an exercise test

   **3.** Patients may undergo angiography without first having an exercise test in the 2 circumstances when they will almost certainly require invasive therapy (PCI or CABG).

   **a.** When their symptoms are disabling despite therapy.

   **b.** When they have HF.

**Treatment**

**A.** The goal of treatment in patients with stable angina is to decrease symptoms and inhibit disease progression. Patients with stable angina have about a 3%/year risk of both MI and death.

**B.** Nonpharmacologic

   **1.** Smoking cessation

   **2.** Exercise (intensity guided by exercise testing)

   **3.** Low fat, low cholesterol diet

**C.** Pharmacologic

   **1.** Symptomatic treatment. It is important to recognize that patients often need a combination of medicines to control their symptoms.

   **a.** Decrease oxygen demand: β-blocker or the calcium channel blockers verapamil or diltiazem

   **b.** Increase oxygen supply: long- and short-acting nitrates

   **2.** Inhibit disease progression

   **a.** Aspirin

   **b.** Clopidogrel in patients who are intolerant of aspirin or who have had PCI

**c.** Risk factor modification

    **(1)** Lipid lowering with an HMG-CoA reductase inhibitor (statin) to a goal LDL or < 70 mg/dL.

    **(2)** ACE inhibitor or angiotensin receptor blocker (ARB) in patients at the highest risk, such as those with diabetes or HF.

    **(3)** Glycemic control in patients with diabetes

**D.** Interventional therapy (either via PCI or bypass surgery) is the mainstay of treatment for the acute coronary syndromes discussed below. For stable angina, it plays a critical role for patients with more severe disease. An overview of the data is below.

  **1.** In **low-risk patients** (such as those with single vessel disease)

    **a.** There is no difference in mortality between medical management and PCI.

    **b.** Patients who undergo a PCI tend to have better control of their symptoms but undergo more procedures.

  **2.** In **moderate-risk patients** (such as those with multivessel disease but an otherwise normal heart)

    **a.** PCI and CABG are about equal in terms of mortality and both are superior to medical therapy.

    **b.** PCI leads to more procedures.

  **3.** In **high-risk patients** (such as those with disease of the left main coronary artery, 3 vessel disease, or 2 vessel disease involving the proximal left anterior descending artery)

    **a.** Bypass surgery has a clear survival benefit compared with medical therapy.

    **b.** For selected patients, PCI can have a similar outcome to surgery.

    **c.** Bypass surgery is superior in patients with diabetes.

## MAKING A DIAGNOSIS

A tentative diagnosis of stable angina from CAD is made. Laboratory data are notable for normal blood counts and chemistries. There is hypercholesterolemia (LDL 136 mg/dL, HDL 42 mg/dL). Mr. W is referred for an exercise tolerance test. Because of his abnormal resting ECG, an exercise myocardial perfusion SPECT was performed. Although chest pain developed during the test, his results were normal without evidence of myocardial ischemia.

**Have you crossed a diagnostic threshold for the leading hypothesis, stable angina? Have you ruled out the active alternatives? Do other tests need to be done to exclude the alternative diagnoses?**

The results of the patient's exercise test are surprising. Stable angina remains high in the differential despite the normal stress test but alternative diagnoses must be considered. The intermittent nature of the pain and the lack of constitutional signs make a mediastinal lesion unlikely. The absence of a recent injury, change in activity or reproducible pain on physical exam moves musculoskeletal pain down on the differential. GERD is a common cause of chest pain and should be considered.

## Alternative Diagnosis: GERD

### Textbook Presentation

Heartburn is usually the presenting symptom in a patient with GERD. Other classic symptoms are regurgitation or dysphagia; chest pain is a common alternative presentation. Patients often report that their symptoms are worst at night and after large meals.

Although dysphagia is a common presentation of GERD, its presence raises the possibility of an obstructing lesion and thus mandates prompt evaluation, usually with upper endoscopy.

### Disease Highlights

**A.** The symptoms of GERD are so well known that most patients diagnose themselves before visiting a physician.

**B.** GERD is a common cause of chest pain that may mimic that of more sinister causes.

GERD is such a common cause of acute chest pain that it should always be considered in the differential diagnosis of chest pain.

**C.** There are GI and non-GI complications of GERD.

  **1.** GI

    **a.** Esophagitis

    **b.** Stricture formation

    **c.** Barrett esophagus

    **d.** Esophageal adenocarcinoma

  **2.** Non-GI

    **a.** Chronic cough

    **b.** Hoarseness

    **c.** Worsening of asthma

**D.** Esophageal disorders, other than GERD, might also present as chest pain.

  **1.** Esophagitis or esophageal ulcer

    **a.** Odynophagia common

    **b.** Multiple causes included infection and pill esophagitis

    **c.** Pill esophagitis is especially associated with certain medications:

      **(1)** Bisphosphonates

      **(2)** Tetracyclines

      **(3)** Antiinflammatories

      **(4)** Potassium chloride

  **2.** Esophageal cancer

    **a.** Often associated with dysphagia

    **b.** Smoking, alcohol use, and chronic reflux are risk factors.

  **3.** Esophageal rupture (Boerhaave syndrome). Often presents with acute pain after retching.

  **4.** Esophageal spasm and motility disorders. Often presents with intermittent chest pain and dysphagia.

### Evidence-Based Diagnosis

**A.** GERD should be high in the differential diagnosis of chest pain when heartburn, regurgitation, or dysphagia is present or when other commonly associated symptoms or complications (eg, chronic cough and asthma) are present.

**B.** Identifying factors that exacerbate the symptoms of GERD is helpful both in diagnosis and management.

1. Ingesting large (especially fatty) meals

2. Lying down after a meal

3. Using tobacco

4. Eating any of the delicious foods that relax the lower esophageal sphincter

   **a.** Chocolate

   **b.** Alcohol

   **c.** Coffee

   **d.** Peppermint

**C.** Historical features help differentiate esophageal from cardiac chest pain.

1. A small study analyzed the prevalence of several historical features in 100 patients in an emergency department with either esophageal or cardiac chest pain.

2. The differences that reached statistical significance are listed in Table 8–4. Although the study was small, the data are instructive.

3. From these data, it is clear that history cannot differentiate esophageal chest pain from pain due to cardiac ischemia. That said, pain that is persistent, wakes the patient from sleep, is positional, and is associated with heartburn or regurgitation is more likely to be of esophageal origin.

4. It is interesting that only 83% of patients with an esophageal cause of pain in this study had GI symptoms (ie, heartburn, regurgitation, dysphagia, or vomiting).

5. Striking were some of the features not significantly different between the 2 groups:

   **a.** Radiation to the left arm

   **b.** Exacerbation with exercise

   **c.** Relief with nitroglycerin

6. The effect of nitroglycerin in relieving chest pain has consistently been found to be useless in differentiating anginal chest pain from esophageal or other causes of chest pain.

 Response to nitroglycerin is not helpful in determining the cause of chest pain.

**D.** Esophageal pH testing, the gold standard for the diagnosis of GERD, is seldom necessary.

**E.** The combination of a suspicious history and consistent endoscopic findings has a 97% specificity for GERD.

**F.** Suggestive symptoms and response to therapy is generally considered diagnostic.

**G.** Esophagogastroduodenoscopy (EGD) should be done when

1. Patients have symptoms of complicated disease

   **a.** Dysphagia

   **b.** Extra-esophageal symptoms

   **c.** Bleeding

   **d.** Weight loss

   **e.** Chest pain of unclear etiology

2. Patients are at risk for Barrett esophagus (long-standing symptoms of reflux).

3. Patients require long-term therapy

4. Patients respond poorly to appropriate therapy

**H.** Ambulatory pH monitoring is useful in 2 settings.

1. In patients with symptoms of GERD and a normal endoscopy.

2. To monitor therapy in refractory cases.

**Treatment**

**A.** Nonpharmacologic

1. Elevate the entire head of the bed; adding extra pillows may actually worsen reflux.

2. Avoid lying down for 3 hours after meals.

3. Stop smoking.

4. Stop ingesting high-risk foods and beverages.

   **a.** Fatty foods

   **b.** Chocolate

   **c.** Alcohol

   **d.** Peppermint

   **e.** Coffee

**B.** Pharmacologic

1. Antacids

2. $H_2$-blockers

**Table 8–4.** Prevalence of symptoms in patients with cardiac and esophageal chest pain.

| Symptom | Prevalence (%) | |
| --- | --- | --- |
| | Among patients with cardiac cause | Among patients with esophageal cause |
| Lateral radiation | 69 | 11 |
| More than 1 spontaneous episode per month | 13 | 50 |
| Pain persists as ache for several hours | 25 | 78 |
| Nighttime wakening caused by pain | 25 | 61 |
| Provoked by swallowing | 6 | 39 |
| Provoked by recumbency or stooping | 19 | 61 |
| Variable exercise tolerance | 10 | 39 |
| Pain starts after exercise completed | 4 | 33 |
| Pain relieved by antacid | 10 | 44 |
| Presence of heartburn | 17 | 78 |
| Presence of regurgitation | 17 | 67 |
| Presence of GI symptoms | 46 | 83 |

Adapted from Davies HA et al. Angina-like esophageal pain: differentiation from cardiac pain by history. J Clin Gastroenterol. 1985;7:477–481.

3. Proton-pump inhibitor
   a. First-line therapy in patients with reflux severe enough to prompt physician visit.
   b. Many patients require long-term therapy.

4. Motility agents (such as metoclopramide) are useful in patients who need adjuvant therapy or who have significant symptoms of regurgitation.

5. Surgery
   a. Antireflux surgery currently has only a very small role.
   b. May be warranted in some patients with particularly severe disease.
   c. One randomized trial has suggested that patients treated with surgery had a higher mortality rate than those treated medically at a mean follow-up of about 11 years (number needed to harm [NNH] = 8.3).

 Because GERD is a common cause of chest pain, it is appropriate to prescribe an empiric course of proton-pump inhibitors after more ominous causes of chest pain have been ruled out.

## CASE RESOLUTION

 **1**

Prior to the stress test, Mr. W's probability of having CAD was at least 92%. It is important to understand why the exercise test was done in this case. The diagnosis of coronary disease was essentially made by the history and physical. The exercise test was meant to guide therapy. Considering a pretest probability of 92%, and an LR− of about 0.15 for the exercise test, the posttest probability is 60%. This is still well above the test threshold for a potentially fatal disease like CAD.

Despite the results of the stress test, stable angina was considered more likely than GERD. Mr. W was given aspirin and a β-blocker and underwent an angiogram the week after the visit. He was found to have a 90% stenosis of the mid left anterior descending artery and underwent PCI with stent placement.

 Before ordering an exercise test, ask yourself why you are doing it: Are you trying to diagnose CAD or determine how severe the disease is.

## CHIEF COMPLAINT

PATIENT  **2**

Mrs. G is a 68-year-old woman with a history of hypertension who arrives at the emergency department by ambulance complaining of chest pain that has lasted 6 hours. Two hours after eating, moderate (5/10) chest discomfort developed. She describes it as a burning sensation beginning in her mid chest and radiating to her back. She initially attributed the pain to heartburn and used antacids. Despite multiple doses over 3 hours, there was no relief. Over the last hour, the pain became very severe (10/10) with radiation to her back and arms. The pain is associated with diaphoresis and shortness of breath. The pain is not pleuritic. She called 911.

At this point, what is the leading hypothesis, what are the active alternatives, and is there a must not miss diagnosis? Given this differential diagnosis, what tests should be ordered?

## PRIORITIZING THE DIFFERENTIAL DIAGNOSIS

Mrs. G is experiencing acute, severe, nonpleuritic chest pain. This presentation is associated with multiple "must not miss" diagnoses. The acuity of the pain is a pivotal point in this history. MI with and without ST elevations and unstable angina, as a group referred to as acute coronary syndromes (ACS), are the most common life-threatening causes of acute chest pain and need to be considered first. Aortic dissection also needs to be considered given the history of hypertension and the radiation of the patient's pain to her back. PE is another possible cause even though the chest pain is not pleuritic. Other alternative, but not life-threatening, causes of this type of pain are esophageal spasm and pancreatitis. However, it would be atypical for pancreatitis to begin so acutely. Table 8–5 lists the differential diagnosis.

**2**

The patient takes enalapril for hypertension. She lives alone, is fairly sedentary, and smokes 1 pack of cigarettes each day. She has an 80 pack year smoking history.

On physical exam, the patient is in moderate distress related to the pain and is concerned that she is having a heart attack. Vital signs are temperature, 37.0°C; BP, 156/90 mm Hg in both arms; pulse, 100 bpm; RR, 22 breaths per minute. Head and neck exam, including jugular and carotid pulsations, were normal. The lung exam was clear. Heart exam was notable for a normal $S_1$ and $S_2$ and a soft, II/VI systolic ejection murmur. Abdominal exam was unremarkable with no tenderness, hepatosplenomegaly, or bruits.

Is the clinical information sufficient to make a diagnosis? If not, what other information do you need?

## Leading Hypothesis: Acute MI

### Textbook Presentation

The classic presentation of an acute MI is crushing substernal chest pressure, diaphoresis, nausea, shortness of breath, and a

**Table 8–5.** Diagnostic hypotheses for Mrs. G.

| Diagnostic Hypotheses | Clinical Clues | Important Tests |
|---|---|---|
| **Leading Hypothesis** | | |
| Acute MI | Presence of cardiac risk factors<br>Acute onset | ECG<br>Cardiac enzymes (CK and troponin)<br>Coronary angiography |
| **Active Alternative—Must Not Miss** | | |
| Unstable angina | Presence of cardiac risk factors<br>Ischemic symptoms that are new or increasing in frequency | ECG<br>Cardiac enzymes (CK and troponin)<br>Stress testing<br>Coronary angiography |
| Thoracic aortic aneurysm dissection | Presence of hypertension<br>Radiation of pain to back<br>BP differential | Transesophageal echocardiography<br>CT scan |
| **Other Alternative** | | |
| Esophageal spasm | Recurrent chest pain, often with radiation to back | Esophageal manometry and exclusion of other causes |

feeling of impending doom in a middle-aged man with risk factors for CAD. More than most other "textbook presentations," this description is often inaccurate because it does not take into account the frequency of MIs in women, younger and older patients, and the frequency of atypical presentations.

## Disease Highlights

A. MI occurs when there is a prolonged failure to perfuse an area of myocardium leading to cell death.

B. Most commonly occurs when a coronary plaque ruptures causing thrombosis and subsequent blockage of a coronary artery.

C. The universal definition of MI describes 5 subtypes of MI based on their clinical presentation:

1. Spontaneous MI related to ischemia due to a primary coronary event.

2. MI secondary to ischemia due to either increased oxygen demand or decreased supply, eg, coronary artery spasm, anemia, or arrhythmias.

3. Sudden unexpected cardiac death, including cardiac arrest, often with symptoms suggestive of myocardial ischemia.

4. MI associated with PCI or stent thrombosis.

5. MI associated with CABG.

D. Acute MIs are classified as either ST segment elevation MI (STEMI) or non–ST segment elevation MI (NSTEMI).

1. ST elevations signify transmural ischemia or infarction.

2. NSTEMI

a. Are less severe, usually injuring only subendomyocardial tissue

b. Have a higher subsequent risk for STEMI

3. These 2 types of MI are managed somewhat differently (discussed below).

## Evidence-Based Diagnosis

A. The diagnostic criteria for acute MI have been clearly established. There are 5 criteria that vary somewhat, based partly on the subtype of MI, and they are shown in Table 8–6.

B. Clinical findings suggestive of MI

1. About 15% of patients who are admitted to the emergency department with chest pain are having an MI.

2. Although historical and physical exam features are never sufficient to diagnose an MI and only rule out an MI in the lowest risk patients, a few features are fairly predictive (Table 8–7).

C. ECG findings suggestive of MI

1. All guidelines recommend an ECG be performed within 10 minutes of a patient's arrival at a healthcare facility when an MI is suspected.

 Patients with chest pain should have an ECG within 10 minutes of arriving at a healthcare facility.

2. Prevalence rates of MI among emergency department patients with chest pain and various ECG findings follow:

a. New ST elevation of 1 mm: 80%

b. New ST depression or T wave inversion: 20%

c. No new changes in a patient with known CAD: 4%

d. No new changes in a patient without known CAD: 2%

3. Table 8–8 shows the test characteristics for ECG findings in patients with acute chest pain. Because there are a range

**Table 8–6.** Criteria for diagnosing acute MI.

1. A rise and fall of cardiac biomarkers (preferably troponin) with at least one value above the 99th percentile of the URL along with one of the following:
   a. Symptoms of ischemia
   b. ECG changes consistent with new ischemia
   c. Development of pathologic Q waves
   d. Imaging evidence of new loss of viable myocardium or myocardial function.

2. Sudden cardiac death accompanied by ECG changes, angiographic findings, or autopsy findings supporting MI as the cause.

3. Elevation of cardiac biomarkers above 3 times the 99th percentile of the URL in the setting of PCI.

4. Elevation of cardiac biomarkers above 5 times the 99th percentile of the URL in the setting of CABG along with ECG changes consistent with MI, angiographic evidence of MI, or imaging evidence of new loss of viable myocardium of myocardial function.

5. Pathologic evidence of an MI.

CABG, coronary artery bypass grafting; MI, myocardial infarction; PCI, percutaneous intervention; URL, upper reference limit.

**Table 8–7.** Likelihood ratios of historical features and physical exam findings and the effect on posttest probability of acute MI.

| Feature or Finding | LR+ | Posttest Probability[1] |
|---|---|---|
| Radiation to left arm | 2.3 | 29% |
| Radiation to right shoulder | 2.9 | 34% |
| Radiation to both arms | 7.1 | 56% |
| Nausea and vomiting | 1.9 | 25% |
| Diaphoresis | 2.0 | 26% |
| Third heart sound | 3.2 | 36% |
| Hypotension | 3.1 | 35% |
| Crackles | 2.1 | 27% |

[1]Assuming 15% pretest probability.
Adapted from Panju AA et al. The rational clinical examination. Is this patient having a myocardial infarction? *JAMA.* 1998;280:1256–1263. Copyright © 1998. American Medical Association. All rights reserved.

of numbers from various studies, these numbers should be treated as estimates.

A patient with chest pain and ≥ 1-mm ST elevations in 2 contiguous leads or a new left bundle-branch block (LBBB) is having an acute MI and should receive immediate therapy.

D. Cardiac enzymes

   1. As is clear from the diagnostic criteria, the presence of cardiac enzymes define the presence of MI.

**Table 8–8.** Test characteristics for ECG findings in patients with chest pain for the diagnosis of acute MI.[1]

| ECG Finding | LR+ | LR– |
|---|---|---|
| New ST elevation > 1 mm | 5.7–53 | |
| New Q wave | 5.3–24.8 | |
| Any ST elevation | 11.2 | |
| New Q or ST elevation | 11 | 0.24 |
| New conduction defect | 6.3 | |
| Any Q wave | 3.9 | |
| T wave peaking | 3.1 | |
| Any conduction defect | 2.7 | |
| Any ECG abnormality | 1.3 | 0.04 |

[1]Data are unavailable when not given.
Adapted from Panju AA, et al. The rational clinical examination. Is this patient having a myocardial infarction? *JAMA.* 1998;280:1256–1263. Copyright © 1998. American Medical Association. All rights reserved.

2. When an MI is suspected, CK-MB and troponin should be ordered and processed immediately.

3. These tests are highly reliable in diagnosing MI. (Note that the definition of MI is based on enzyme results whenever they are available).

4. Table 8–9 lists the test characteristics for serial CK-MB and troponin I according to time after symptom onset.

5. Troponin levels in patients with renal insufficiency

   a. Patients with renal insufficiency often have elevated troponin levels raising the risk of false-positive tests for MI

   b. Patients with elevated troponin levels at baseline will still have a diagnostic rise and fall with MI

   c. In patients with renal failure, higher baseline troponin levels are predictive of poor cardiovascular outcomes.

E. MI in women

   1. Acute MIs present differently in women than in men.

      a. Women often report prodromal symptoms such as fatigue, dyspnea, and insomnia.

      b. Chest pain is only present in 57% of women at the time of MI.

Nearly half of woman having an MI present with a chief complaint other than chest pain.

      c. Dyspnea, weakness, and fatigue are the other common presenting symptoms.

   2. Women who suffer an MI are more likely to die. The cause of this disparity is multifactorial.

      a. Compared with men, women are older when they have their first MI and have more comorbid conditions.

      b. Historically, women have been less likely to undergo revascularization procedures.

   3. Women who do undergo bypass surgery and catheter-based intervention have higher complication rates than men who undergo these same procedures.

F. Unrecognized MI

   1. Although the combination of symptoms, ECG findings, and enzymes make most MIs easy to diagnose, about 2% of patients with acute MI are discharged from the emergency department.

   2. Failure to recognize an MI results in worse outcomes for patients and serious medicolegal issues.

   3. MIs most commonly go unrecognized when they present in unusual ways or in people not expected to have an MI.

   4. A patient with an MI or unstable angina who is mistakenly discharged is most likely to:

      a. Be a woman younger than age 55

      b. Be non-white

      c. Have a chief complaint of shortness of breath

      d. Have a nondiagnostic ECG

   5. MI may present without chest pain; patients tend to be older women or have diabetes mellitus or a history of HF.

   6. The most common alternative presentations of MI are listed below. MI should at least be considered in patients

***Table 8–9.*** Test characteristics for the diagnosis of acute MI by time after symptom onset.

| Test | Time Frame | Sensitivity (%) | Specificity (%) | LR+ | LR– |
|---|---|---|---|---|---|
| Serial CK-MB | < 24 h | 99 | 98 | 50 | 0.01 |
| | > 24 h | 55 | 97 | 18 | 0.46 |
| Troponin I | 9 h | 95 | 98 | 47 | 0.03 |
| | > 24 h | 95 | 98 | 47 | 0.03 |

Adapted from Black ER. Diagnostic strategies for common medical problems. P. 64. Philadelphia: American College of Physicians, 1999.

being discharged from the emergency department with one of these diagnoses.

**a.** HF

**b.** Stable angina

**c.** Arrhythmia

**d.** Atypical location of pain

**e.** CNS manifestations (symptoms of cerebrovascular accident)

**f.** Nervousness, mania, or psychosis

**g.** Syncope

**h.** Weakness

**i.** Indigestion

 MI can present in many different ways. A high index of suspicion should always be present. Certain groups of patients (elderly, women, minorities, diabetics) are most likely to be misdiagnosed.

## Treatment

**A.** A patient with an acute MI needs to receive immediate treatment with antianginals and pain medications. The initial treatment is outlined below, ranked by the level of evidence supporting their use:

**1.** Aspirin, β-blocker

**2.** Oxygen

**3.** Nitroglycerin

**4.** Although frequently used in NSTEMI and occasionally in STEMI, there is only weak evidence that unfractionated or low-molecular-weight heparin is beneficial around the time of thrombolysis or primary PCI.

**5.** Other therapy based on presentation

**a.** Opioids for patients in pain

**b.** Atropine for patients with pathologic bradycardia

**c.** Antiarrhythmic agents

**B.** The next and most important step is opening the culprit vessel. The 2 options are systemic thrombolysis or primary PCI.

**1.** Although less widely available, primary PCI is the preferred option.

**2.** Primary PCI is associated with

**a.** Lower mortality (even in patients who must be transferred—albeit quickly—to a hospital with the capability)

**b.** Significantly lower risk of serious bleeding complication. Hemorrhagic stroke is not a potential complication as it is with systemic thrombolysis.

**3.** The ability to do primary PCI depends on the presence of a skilled team of interventional cardiologists who can rapidly (within 90 minutes) bring the patient to the catheterization laboratory.

**4.** Primary PCI with stent placement is probably the most efficacious treatment.

**5.** Both primary angioplasty and thrombolysis are most effective when completed within 12 hours of symptom onset.

**C.** Once the culprit vessel has been opened, various medications have been shown to improve survival after acute MI.

**1.** β-Blockers

**2.** ACE inhibitors

**3.** Aspirin

**4.** Clopidogrel (duration based on intervention and risk of bleeding)

**5.** HMG-CoA reductase inhibitors, dosed to achieve an LDL < 70 mg/dL.

**6.** Glycoprotein IIB/IIIA inhibitors are recommended for patients with STEMIs and most patients with NSTEMIs.

**D.** An exercise test is also recommended within 3 weeks of an MI in patients not undergoing PCI or angiography for information on prognosis, functional capacity, and risk stratification.

## MAKING A DIAGNOSIS

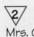 Mrs. G's ECG shows ST depression in leads II, III, AVL, and V3–V6. The chest radiograph is normal.

**Have you crossed a diagnostic threshold for the leading hypothesis, acute MI? Have you ruled out the active alternatives? Do other tests need to be done to exclude the alternative diagnoses?**

The ECG is consistent with cardiac ischemia but does not make the diagnosis of an acute MI; the diagnosis will be confirmed when the laboratory results for the enzymes are available. The abnormal ECG certainly makes the alternative diagnosis, unstable angina, quite likely if an MI is excluded. Aortic dissections can cause cardiac ischemia, so this too must remain in the differential.

## Alternative Diagnosis: Unstable Angina

### Textbook Presentation

Classically, new or worsening symptoms of CAD are the presenting manifestations of unstable angina. Unstable angina and an acute MI without ST elevation may be identical in their presentation, only differentiated by the presence or absence of myocardial enzyme elevation.

### Disease Highlights

A. Unstable angina is defined as angina that is new, worsening in severity or frequency, or occurs at rest.

B. Pathophysiology
   1. Primarily caused by acute plaque rupture followed by platelet aggregation.
      a. 67% of episodes occur in arteries with < 50% stenosis.
      b. 97% occur in arteries with < 75% stenosis.
   2. Caused less commonly by changes in oxygen demand or supply (eg, hyperthyroidism, anemia, high altitude).

C. The diagnosis of unstable angina can be difficult, often depending on a careful history to differentiate stable from unstable angina.

D. The clinician seeing a patient with unstable angina or a NSTEMI must
   1. Recognize that the patient has an ACS
   2. Institute care
   3. Determine the patient's risk of progressing to an MI or death
   4. Treat accordingly

E. Vasospastic angina
   1. Vasospastic angina (also called Prinzmetal or variant angina) is a phenomenon that is related to unstable angina in presentation.
   2. Patients with vasospastic angina periodically have episodes of cardiac ischemia with ST elevation.
   3. The attacks
      a. Are often associated with chest pain or other ischemic symptoms
      b. Resolve spontaneously or with nitroglycerin
      c. May occur in normal or diseased coronary arteries
      d. Can result in MI or death (often secondary to arrhythmia)
      e. Often occur at the same time each day
   4. Vasospastic angina is usually diagnosed clinically but can also be diagnosed by inducing it with ergonovine infusion in the catheterization laboratory.
   5. Vasospastic angina is treated effectively with calcium channel blockers and nitrates.

 Vasospastic angina should be considered in patients whose symptoms are consistent with cardiac ischemia and occur at about the same time each day. The diagnosis should also be considered when transient ST elevations develop.

### Evidence-Based Diagnosis

The diagnostic considerations for a patient in whom unstable angina is suspected are 2-fold: diagnose unstable angina or NSTEMI and risk stratify the patient.

A. Diagnosis
   1. There are 3 presentations of unstable angina.
      a. Rest angina
      b. New onset (< 2 months) angina
      c. Increasing angina
   2. The American College of Cardiology (ACC) and American Heart Association (AHA) have endorsed a number of findings that increase the likelihood that a patient's symptoms represent an ACS. These include
      a. Chest or left arm pain that reproduces prior angina
      b. Known history of CAD
      c. Transient mitral regurgitation murmur
      d. Hypotension
      e. Diaphoresis
      f. Pulmonary edema
      g. Crackles

B. Risk stratification
   1. Appropriate risk stratification ensures that the patient is triaged to the proper location for care (ICU, inpatient ward, home) and eventually receives the most beneficial therapy.
   2. Patients can be stratified by various validated scores. The TIMI score is probably most commonly used and is shown in Table 8–10.
   3. Other characteristics that portend high risk are
      a. Recurrent angina or ischemia at rest or with low-level activities despite intensive medical therapy
      b. Elevated cardiac biomarkers (TnT or TnI)
      c. Signs or symptoms of heart failure or new or worsening mitral regurgitation
      d. High-risk findings from noninvasive testing

***Table 8–10.*** TIMI risk score for unstable angina/NSTEMI.

| TIMI Score[1] | All cause mortality, new or recurrent MI, or severe or recurrent ischemia requiring urgent revascularization within 14 days |
|---|---|
| 0–1 | 4.7 |
| 2 | 8.3 |
| 3 | 13.2 |
| 4 | 19.9 |
| 5 | 26.2 |
| 6–7 | 40.9 |

[1]Patients receive one point for each of the following variables: age ≥ 65, ≥ cardiac risk factors, prior coronary stenosis of ≥ 50%, ST segment deviation on admission ECG, ≥ 2 anginal events in preceding 24 hours, use of aspirin in previous 7 days, elevated cardiac biomarkers.
MI, myocardial infarction; NSTEMI, non-ST segment elevation MI.

  e. Hemodynamic instability

  f. Sustained ventricular tachycardia

  g. PCI within 6 months

  h. Prior CABG

  i. Reduced left ventricular function

## Treatment

A. The following treatments should be started as soon as unstable angina is suspected:

1. Aspirin

2. β-Blockers

3. Nitrates

B. Patients whose risk stratification identifies them as having a low risk of death or complications should undergo conservative management strategy.

1. Enoxaparin or unfractionated heparin

2. Clopidogrel

3. If the patient is stable (no ongoing ischemia, arrhythmias or decreased ejection fraction on echocardiogram), a stress test should be done to determine if angiography is indicated.

4. If the stress test finds the patient to be at low risk, the patient can be discharged with prescriptions for aspirin, clopidogrel, β-blockers, and an HMG-CoA reductase inhibitor.

C. Patients found to be at higher risk benefit from an early invasive strategy:

1. Enoxaparin or unfractionated heparin

2. Clopidogrel or glycoprotein IIb/IIIA inhibitor, or both

3. Angiography

4. Further management is dictated by the findings on angiography: PCI, CABG, or medical therapy for coronary disease.

## Alternative Diagnosis: Aortic Dissection

### Textbook Presentation

The textbook presentation of an aortic dissection is an older man with a history of hypertension and possibly atherosclerotic disease who complains of "tearing" chest or back pain. The pain might be associated with vascular complications such as syncope, stroke, cardiac ischemia, or HF secondary to acute aortic regurgitation. On physical exam, there is asymmetry in the upper extremity BPs, and the chest radiograph shows a widened mediastinum.

### Disease Highlights

A. Dissection begins with a tear in the aortic intima allowing blood to dissect the aorta between the intima and media.

B. The primary risk factors for aortic dissection are hypertension and atherosclerosis, present in 72% and 31% of patients, respectively. Other risk factors include

1. Known aortic aneurysm (present in 16% of patients)

   a. Aortic aneurysms are usually detected while they are asymptomatic on a chest radiograph.

   b. They may also present with aortic regurgitation, pain, or through impingement on other structures such as the trachea, esophagus, or recurrent laryngeal nerve.

2. Prior aortic dissection (6%)

3. Diabetes (5%)

4. Marfan syndrome (5%)

C. An additional risk factor for aortic dissection is cocaine use. This is associated with dissections in younger patients (mean age 41).

In addition to MI, thoracic aortic dissection should be considered in the differential of a young hypertensive patient who has chest pain after using cocaine.

D. The symptoms of dissection include pain as well as symptoms of vascular complications of the dissection. The type of complication depends on what type of dissection occurs.

E. Type A dissections involve the ascending aorta with or without the descending aorta.

1. Account for about 60% of dissections

2. Carry a mortality of about 35%

3. May be associated with

   a. Acute aortic insufficiency

   b. Myocardial ischemia due to coronary occlusion

   c. Neurologic deficits

   d. Cardiac tamponade due to hemopericardium

F. Type B dissections involve only the descending aorta and are associated with a mortality of about 15%.

### Evidence-Based Diagnosis

A. The diagnosis of aortic dissection is reliably difficult. There are no signs or symptoms that are consistently associated with very high or very low LRs.

B. A study of 464 patients with aortic dissection helps describe the common presenting signs and symptoms of people with this diagnosis.

1. The demographic findings were not surprising:

   a. Mean age ≈ 63 years

   b. 73% of patients had hypertension

2. The presenting signs and symptoms were notable for the infrequency of some classic findings.

   a. Pulse deficit was noted in only 15% of patients, syncope in 9%, cerebrovascular accident in 5%, and HF in 7%.

   b. Some of the more common symptoms are shown in Table 8–11.

   c. Chest radiograph and ECG were found to be very insensitive diagnostic tools.

The aorta is normal on the chest film in about 40% of patients with a dissection of the thoracic aorta.

C. Another study stratified patients by 3 independent predictors of aortic dissection: aortic type pain (pain of acute onset or tearing or ripping character), aortic or mediastinal widening on chest radiograph, and pulse or BP differentials.

1. Low-risk patients had none of the characteristics.

   a. Only 7% of these patients had a dissection

   b. The test characteristics of these findings for excluding dissection were sensitivity, 96%; specificity, 48%; LR+, 1.85; LR−, 0.08.

**Table 8–11.** Prevalence of various findings and symptoms in patients with thoracic aortic aneurysm dissection (type A).

| Finding or Symptom | Prevalence |
|---|---|
| Abrupt onset pain | 85% |
| Chest pain | 79% |
| Back pain | 47% |
| Severe or worst ever pain | 90% |
| Sharp pain | 62% |
| Tearing pain | 51% |
| Normal chest film | 11% |
| Widened mediastinum | 63% |
| Normal mediastinum and aortic contour | 17% |
| Nonspecific ST-segment or T-wave changes | 43% |

Adapted from Hagan PG et al. The International Registry of Acute Aortic Dissection (IRAD): new insights into an old disease. JAMA. 2000;283:897–903. Copyright © 2000. American Medical Association. All rights reserved.

2. Intermediate-risk patients had only consistent pain or a consistent chest radiograph. Between 30% and 40% of these patients had a dissection.

3. High-risk patients had pulse or BP differentials or any combination of the 3 of the variables.

 a. > 84% of these patients had a dissection.

 b. The test characteristics of these findings for predicting dissection were sensitivity, 76%; specificity, 91%; LR+, 8.4; LR−, 0.26.

FP 4. The test characteristics for pulse or blood pressure differentials in a patient in whom aortic dissection is suspected were sensitivity, 37%; specificity, 99%; LR+, 37; LR−, 0.64.

D. Summarizing the clinical diagnosis of aortic dissection

1. Patients with dissections are likely to have a history of hypertension and experience severe, acute pain.

2. Patients with chest pain are unlikely to have a dissection if they do not have any of the following:

 a. Acute or tearing or ripping pain

 b. Aortic or mediastinal widening

 c. Asymmetric pulse or BPs

E. The gold standard for diagnosis is angiography but most patients undergo only noninvasive tests.

F. All the commonly used noninvasive tests have sensitivities and specificities above 95%.

G. The most commonly used tests are CT scans and transesophageal echocardiography.

H. Angiography is recommended to help guide therapy if there is evidence of organ ischemia.

## Treatment

A. Because dissection is associated with extremely high mortality, the ideal is to identify and repair the aneurysm prior to rupture.

B. Thoracic aortic aneurysms

1. When aneurysms are detected prior to rupture, the goal of therapy is to slow their growth and operate when the aneurysm reaches a certain size.

2. Patients with aneurysms should have tight BP control.

3. Patients should be closely monitored for increasing aneurysm size.

4. Indications for surgery are based on the size of the aneurysm

 a. 5.5 cm for ascending aneurysms

 b. 6.5 cm for descending aneurysms

 c. Rapid growth

5. There is growing enthusiasm for using intravascular stents to repair some aneurysms.

C. Thoracic aortic dissection

1. Dissection of the thoracic aorta is a medical emergency.

2. Type A dissections are generally operated on immediately.

3. Type B dissections usually are managed medically.

## CASE RESOLUTION

Mrs. G's initial troponin was elevated at 3.5 ng/mL with a CK of 750 units/L and positive MB fraction. The final diagnosis is NSTEMI. Following treatment in the emergency department with oxygen, β-blockers, nitrates, and enoxaparin, she was taken directly to the cardiac catheterization laboratory. There she was found to have a left dominant system and an acute thrombosis of a branch of the left circumflex artery. This was opened with intracoronary thrombolysis and a stent was placed.

The patient's troponin and CK make the diagnosis of an acute MI. It should be realized that the presence of an MI does not rule out dissection of the thoracic aorta. Between 3% and 5% of patients with dissections have associated MIs. Even before the catheterization results, the subacute onset of the pain, the normal chest film, the lack of "tearing pain," and symmetric pulses made aortic dissection unlikely.

Four days after her MI, Mrs. G was discharged with prescriptions for the following medications:

1. Atorvastatin 80 mg
2. Enalapril 20 mg
3. Atenolol 100 mg
4. Aspirin 81 mg
4. Clopidogrel 75 mg

# CHIEF COMPLAINT

PATIENT 3

Mr. H is a 31-year-old man, previously in excellent health who arrives at the emergency department complaining of chest pain. He reports that the pain began 10 days earlier. It was initially mild but has become more severe. The pain is accompanied by mild cough and shortness of breath. Five days earlier, he had come to the emergency department and musculoskeletal chest pain was diagnosed; he was given nonsteroidal antiinflammatory drugs (NSAIDs) and discharged.

Since the pain has become more severe, it has become pleuritic. He says it is located over the right lateral lower chest wall. His dyspnea is still only mild. He also has noted low-grade fevers with temperatures running about 38°C.

> ☑ At this point, what is the leading hypothesis, what are the active alternatives, and is there a must not miss diagnosis? Given this differential diagnosis, what tests should be ordered?

## PRIORITIZING THE DIFFERENTIAL DIAGNOSIS

This is a healthy young man with an acute illness. He reports pleuritic chest pain, cough, dyspnea, and fevers. The acuity of the symptoms as well as the pleuritic nature of the pain are pivotal points in this case. The first diagnoses to consider are infectious diseases that could cause pleuritic chest pain. Pneumonia or pleural effusion could cause these symptoms, either individually or as part of the same process. (Pleural effusions will be discussed below while pneumonia will be diagnosed in Chapter 9). Pericarditis can also cause pleuritic chest pain and can be associated with fevers. PE is a classic cause of pleuritic chest pain and shortness of breath and may be associated with fever (see Chapter 14, Dyspnea). Intra-abdominal processes, such as subdiaphragmatic abscess should be kept in mind as causes of pleuritic chest pain. The combination of fever, dyspnea, and chest pain places pneumonia or pleural effusion at the top of the list. Table 8–12 lists the differential diagnosis.

3

During further history taking, Mr. H reports no radiation of the pain. He denies abdominal pain, nausea, vomiting, or change in appetite. Deep breathing and sudden movements tend to worsen the pain. There are no other palliative or provocative features.

On physical exam, Mr. H is a healthy appearing man who appears in mild distress. He moves somewhat gingerly because of the pain and is dyspneic. He coughs occasionally during the history. This causes great pain. Vital signs are temperature, 38.9°C; BP, 130/84 mm Hg; pulse, 110 bpm; RR, 26 breaths per minute. Head and neck exam is normal; there is no jugular venous distention. Lung exam is notable for dullness to percussion and decreased breath sounds at the right base. There is an

**Table 8–12.** Diagnostic hypotheses for Mr. H.

| Diagnostic Hypotheses | Clinical Clues | Important Tests |
|---|---|---|
| **Leading Hypothesis** | | |
| Pleural effusion or pneumonia associated physical exam findings | Cough and shortness of breath with pleural effusion | Chest radiograph Thoracentesis for |
| **Active Alternative** | | |
| Pericarditis | Pain relieved by leaning forward Friction rub ECG changes | ECG Echocardiogram |
| **Active Alternative—Must Not Miss** | | |
| Pulmonary embolism | Risk factors Tachycardia | Ventilation-perfusion scan Helical CT Pulmonary angiogram |
| **Other Alternative** | | |
| Subdiaghragmatic abscess | Intra-abdominal process Fevers | Abdominal ultrasound CT |

area of egophony just superior to the decreased breath sounds and normal breath sounds superior to this. The left chest is clear. Heart exam is normal as are the abdomen and extremities.

> ☑ Is the clinical information sufficient to make a diagnosis? If not, what other information do you need?

## Leading Hypothesis: Pleural Effusion

### Textbook Presentation

Small effusions are usually asymptomatic while large effusions reliably cause dyspnea with or without pleuritic chest pain. Presentation depends on the cause of the effusion. Parapneumonic effusions will be accompanied by the signs and symptoms of pneumonia while neoplastic effusions will usually present with dyspnea alone and symptoms of the underlying cancer. Pleural effusions related to rheumatologic disease are usually accompanied by signs of the specific illness. Physical exam reveals dullness to percussion and decreased breath sounds over the area of effusion.

### Disease Highlights

A. Pathophysiology of pleural effusions vary by etiology but may be due to 1 or any combination of the following:

  1. Increased capillary permeability

  2. Increased hydrostatic pressure

  3. Decreased oncotic pressure

**Table 8–13.** The incidences of several causes of pleural effusion.

| Etiology | Incidence |
|---|---|
| HF | 500,000 |
| Pneumonia | 300,000 |
| Malignancy | 200,000 |
| Pulmonary embolism | 150,000 |
| Viral disease | 100,000 |
| Coronary artery bypass surgery | 60,000 |
| Cirrhosis with ascites | 50,000 |
| Less common but prevalent causes, including uremia, tuberculosis, chylothorax, and rheumatologic disease (RA and SLE) | |

HF, heart failure; RA, rheumatoid arthritis; SLE, systemic lupus erythematosus. Data from Light RW. Clinical practice. Pleural effusion. N Engl J Med. 2002;346:1971–1977. Copyright © 2002 Massachusetts Medical Society. All Rights Reserved.

4. Increased negative intrapleural pressure
5. Disruption of pulmonary lymphatics

B. The differential diagnosis of a pleural effusion is enormous. The most common causes with their approximate yearly incidence are listed in Table 8–13.

C. The most useful way of organizing the differential diagnosis is by whether the effusion is exudative or transudative.

1. Exudative effusions are caused by increased capillary permeability or disruption of pulmonary lymphatics.

2. Transudative effusions are caused by increased hydrostatic pressure, decreased oncotic pressure, or increased negative intrapleural pressure.

D. Table 8-14 lists some common transudative and exudative effusions.

**Table 8–14.** Common transudative and exudative effusions.

| Transudative Effusions | Exudative Effusions |
|---|---|
| Heart failure | Parapneumonic effusions |
| Cirrhosis with ascites | Malignancy |
| Pulmonary embolism (1/4) | Pulmonary embolism (3/4) |
| Nephrotic syndrome | Viral infections |
| Severe hypoalbuminemia | Post CABG |
| | Subdiaghragmatic infections and inflammatory states |
| | Chylothorax, uremia, connective tissue diseases |

CABG, coronary artery bypass grafting.

E. Exudative effusions commonly complicate the following diagnoses:

1. Pneumonia

   a. Any effusion associated with pneumonia, lung abscess, or bronchiectasis is considered a parapneumonic effusion.

   b. Empyemas are parapneumonic effusions that have become infected.

   c. Empyemas, and certain parapneumonic effusions called complicated parapneumonic effusions, are more likely to form fibrotic, pleural peels. The diagnostic criteria for these types of effusions are given below.

   d. Parapneumonic effusions accompany 40% of all pneumonias while empyemas occur 2% of the time, at most.

   e. Effusions are more likely to form and more likely to become infected if the treatment of the underlying pneumonia is delayed.

   f. The bacteriology of parapneumonic effusions is shown in Table 8–15.

2. Malignancy

   a. Most common cancers leading to effusions are

      (1) Lung

      (2) Breast

      (3) Lymphoma

      (4) Leukemia

      (5) Adenocarcinoma of unknown primary

   b. The effusion may occur as the presenting symptom of the cancer or occur in patients with a previously diagnosed malignancy.

   c. The presence of a malignant effusion is generally a very poor prognostic sign.

3. PE

   a. Effusions are present in 26–56% of patients with PE.

   b. Effusions accompany PE most commonly in patients with pleuritic pain or hemoptysis.

4. Viral infections

   a. Considered to be a common cause of effusions

   b. Difficult to diagnose; definitive diagnosis is rarely made

   c. Usually diagnosed in patients with febrile or nonfebrile illness with transient effusion and negative work-up.

   d. Other clues such as atypical lymphocytes, monocytosis, and leukopenia are helpful in diagnosing viral infection.

**Table 8–15.** Bacteriology of parapneumonic effusions.

| Bacteria | Percentage of pneumonias with effusion | Percentage of effusions that are empyemas |
|---|---|---|
| *Streptococcus pneumoniae* | 40–60 | < 5 |
| Anaerobes | 35 | 90 |
| *Staphylococcus aureus* | 40 | 20 |
| *Haemophilus influenzae* | 50 | 20 |
| *Escherichia coli* | ~50 | ~99 |

A pleural effusion should only be diagnosed as viral in an appropriate clinical setting when more serious causes of effusion have been ruled out.

5. CABG surgery
   a. Pleural effusions develop in up to 90% of patients immediately following CABG.
   b. Can be left sided or bilateral
   c. Usually resolve spontaneously
6. Other diseases that are not uncommon causes of pleural effusions include
   1. Uremia
   2. Tuberculosis (TB)
   3. Chylothorax
   4. Rheumatologic disease (eg, rheumatoid arthritis and systemic lupus erythematosus)

F. The most common causes of transudative effusions are
   1. HF
      a. Most common cause of transudative effusions in the United States
      b. Effusions are accompanied by other findings of left heart failure.
      c. Effusions are usually small and resolve with diuresis alone.
      d. Effusions are usually bilateral; unilateral effusions can occur, but they are less common.
   2. Cirrhosis with ascites
      a. About 6% of patients with ascites have pleural effusions.
      b. Effusion is thought to be secondary to ascites moving into the thorax via defects in the diaphragm.
      c. Extremely rare to have pleural effusions on the basis of cirrhosis without ascites.

## Evidence-Based Diagnosis

A. The diagnosis of a pleural effusion itself is based on the recognition of fluid in the pleural space on physical exam.
   1. The sensitivity and specificity of dullness to chest percussion for detecting pleural effusions is very good.
      a. Sensitivity, 96%; specificity, 95%
      b. LR+, 18.6; LR–, 0.04
   2. There is often an area of egophony just superior to the effusion.
   3. Once detected, a pleural effusion is confirmed on chest radiograph, ultrasound, or other form of chest imaging.

B. After diagnosing a pleural effusion, the next step is to determine the cause. If the effusion is clinically significant (usually considered > 1 cm on a chest film), it should be sampled.
   1. A cause should be determined for any new pleural effusion.
   2. The only exception to this is in the case of HF. If the clinical suspicion for HF as the sole cause of the effusion is high, the effusion can be observed while the patient is treated. If the effusion persists or the diagnosis becomes unclear, the effusion should then be sampled.

 Pleural effusions are abnormal; any new pleural effusion should be evaluated.

C. The first step in determining the cause of an effusion is to differentiate transudative from exudative effusions.
D. Light's criteria are the most widely used criteria for differentiating transudative from exudative effusions.
   1. An effusion is considered to be an exudate if any of the following 3 criteria are met:
      a. Pleural fluid protein/serum protein > 0.5
      b. Pleural fluid LDH/serum LDH > 0.6
      c. Pleural fluid LDH > 2/3 upper limit of normal for serum LDH
   2. The test characteristics for these are
      a. Sensitivity, 98%; specificity, 83%
      b. LR+, 5.76; LR–, 0.02
   3. The most specific test for an exudative effusion is a difference between the serum albumin and pleural fluid albumin of < 1.2 g/dL (LR+ 10.88).
E. Once the diagnosis of a transudate or exudate is made, various other tests will help determine the exact diagnosis. Besides lactate dehydrogenase (LDH) and protein, certain tests are routinely sent when pleural fluid is sampled.
   1. Positive Gram stain or culture makes the diagnosis of an empyema.
   2. Fluid pH. A low pH (< 7.2) is commonly seen with
      a. Empyemas
      b. Malignant effusions
      c. Esophageal rupture
   3. Cell count
      a. Neutrophil count over 50% argues for an acute process
         (1) Parapneumonic effusion (sensitivity = 91%)
         (2) PE
      b. High neutrophil count is rarely seen in other diseases, such as TB and malignancy.
      c. Lymphocyte predominant exudative effusions are almost always caused by TB or malignancy (positive predictive value = 97%).
      d. Pleural fluid eosinophilia is a nonspecific finding. It is seen frequently with inflammatory diseases, pneumococcal pneumonia, viral pleuritis, TB, and even repeated thoracentesis.
      e. A low mesothelial cell count (< 5%) count is highly suggestive of TB.
   4. Cytology
      a. Highly specific for the diagnosis of cancer
      b. Sensitivity is 70% at best, with significantly lower values for some cancers.
F. Other tests are done if the clinical suspicion for certain diseases is high.
   1. Tuberculous effusions
      a. Usually suspected based on clinical presentation and pleural fluid lymphocytosis
      b. The sensitivity of commonly used tests for the diagnosis of tuberculous pleurisy are
         (1) Pleural fluid culture, 42%
         (2) Pleural biopsy culture, 64%
         (3) Pleural biopsy histology (caseating granulomas), 70–80%

(4) Histology and pleural tissue culture > 90%

(5) Sputum culture, 20–50%

c. A recent meta-analysis has shown that interferon-γ levels in the pleural fluid are very useful for diagnosing tuberculous pleurisy with the following test characteristics:

(1) Sensitivity, 89%; specificity, 95%

(2) LR+, 23.45; LR–, 0.11

2. Glucose levels < 60 mg/dL are helpful and are seen in

a. Empyema

b. TB

c. Rheumatoid arthritis and systemic lupus erythematosus

3. Triglycerides are greater than 110 mg/dL in patients with chylothorax. The fluid is also a milky white.

4. Thoracoscopy with pleural biopsy often used when suspicion for malignancy is high and cytology is negative.

 Pleural fluid testing should always include LDH, protein, albumin, pH, and cell count. Other tests, such as cytology, are often sent.

## Treatment

A. Pleural effusions are treated by treating the underlying disease (eg, pneumonia, uremia, and HF). Specific treatment of the effusion is called for in certain circumstances.

B. Complicated parapneumonic effusions

1. Evacuation by chest tube drainage prevents pleural scarring and the development of restrictive pleural disease.

2. Indications for chest tube placement are

a. Purulent fluid or positive Gram stain

b. pH < 7.2

c. LDH > 1000 units/L

d. Glucose < 40 mg/dL

e. Small effusions that are close to the above 3 cutoffs can sometimes be carefully monitored.

C. Malignant pleural effusions

1. Usually managed by treating the underlying disease and periodic therapeutic thoracentesis.

2. If thoracentesis is required frequently and the patient's life expectancy is long, there are a number of options among which are

a. Pleurodesis, obliteration of the pleural space by the installation of a chemical irritant

b. Catheter drainage, in which a semi-permanent catheter is placed to allow constant drainage of the effusion.

3. Pleurodesis is usually done with talc.

D. Chylothorax

1. Caused by nontraumatic (primarily lymphoma) or traumatic (usually surgical) disruption of the thoracic duct.

2. In nontraumatic cases, the underlying disease is treated.

3. In both nontraumatic and traumatic disease, the pleural space is evacuated with chest tube drainage.

4. A diet of medium chain fatty acids or a trial of total parenteral nutrition is used to decrease flow through the thoracic duct.

5. Pleurodesis and surgical management reserved for refractory cases.

## MAKING A DIAGNOSIS

The patient's physical exam findings are consistent with a pleural effusion. A posteroanterior, lateral, and decubitus chest film were done that revealed an effusion. The effusion was tapped and yielded pale, turbid fluid. The initial results are glucose, < 20 mg/dL; LDH = 38,400 units/L; protein = 4.4 g/dL; fluid pH, 6.2; RBC, 3200/mcL; WBC, 144,000/mcL; Gram stain positive for gram-positive cocci in pairs and chains. Serum values at the time included total protein of 7.8 g/dL and LDH 141 units/L.

 Have you crossed a diagnostic threshold for the leading hypothesis, pleural effusion? Have you ruled out the active alternatives? Do other tests need to be done to exclude the alternative diagnoses?

Mr. H has a pleural effusion. Given the size of the effusion on the chest film, a thoracentesis was clearly indicated. The results of the tap are diagnostic. The fluid is an exudate and the low glucose, low pH, high WBC, and positive Gram stain make the diagnosis of an empyema.

It is worth noting that Mr. H's previous diagnosis of musculoskeletal chest pain was incorrect. A chest radiograph done on his previous visit to the emergency department may have made the correct diagnosis and treatment could, potentially, have prevented the development of an empyema. There are many indications for chest films, one is to diagnose a cause for chest pain.

 A chest film should be performed in any patient with chest pain and no clear diagnosis.

## Alternative Diagnoses: Acute Pericarditis

### Textbook Presentation

Acute pericarditis typically presents in young adults, with 1 week of viral symptoms and chest pain that improves with leaning forward. Physical exam reveals a 3-part friction rub. ECG reveals ST elevations and PR depressions in all leads.

### Disease Highlights

A. Although the causes of pericarditis are extremely varied, most (85–90%) are considered idiopathic or due to an undiagnosed virus. The common causes are listed below:

1. Viral pericarditis is primarily caused by coxsackie, echo, and adeno viruses.

2. Other infectious causes of pericarditis include TB (historically the most common) and HIV and related diseases.

3. Pericarditis may occur after myocardial injury (post MI and postcardiac surgery).

4. Rheumatologic causes include systemic lupus erythematosus and rheumatoid arthritis.

**5.** Procainamide and hydralazine are among the drugs that can cause it.

**6.** Neoplastic causes

  **a.** Malignancy metastatic to the pericardium

  **b.** Pericarditis can also be caused by exposure of the chest to radiation.

**7.** Uremia

**B.** About 50% of patients with uremia have pericardial effusions.

## Evidence-Based Diagnosis

**A.** The diagnosis of pericarditis is made based on a pericardial friction rub or in a patient with chest pain and characteristic ECG findings.

  **1.** History

   **a.** Chest pain is almost always present.

   **b.** The pain is usually pleuritic.

   **c.** It classically radiates to the trapezius ridge.

   **d.** Pain improves with sitting and worsens with reclining.

  **2.** Physical exam

   **a.** The pericardial friction rub is insensitive but nearly 100% specific; it is diagnostic of pericarditis.

   **b.** The rub is usually triphasic.

     **(1)** Triphasic in 58% of cases

     **(2)** Biphasic in 24% of cases

     **(3)** Monophasic in 18% of cases

   **c.** Although the physical exam is insensitive for effusions, it is good for detecting tamponade.

     **(1)** Sensitivity of jugular venous distention to detect tamponade is 100%.

     **(2)** Sensitivity of tachycardia to detect tamponade is 100%.

     **(3)** Pulsus paradoxus > 12

       **(a)** Sensitivity, 98%; specificity, 83%

       **(b)** LR+, 5.9; LR−, 0.03

  **3.** ECG

   **a.** The ECG most commonly shows widespread ST elevations and PR depressions. This finding is highly specific but the sensitivity is only about 60%.

   **b.** The differentiation of pericarditis from acute MI on ECG can be difficult. Some of the key differentiating factors are

     **(1)** ST elevation in pericarditis is usually diffuse while in MI it is usually localized.

     **(2)** ST elevations in MI are often associated with reciprocal changes.

     **(3)** PR depression is very uncommon in acute MI.

     **(4)** Q waves are not present with pericarditis.

 Pericarditis can mimic MI. The presence of a rub and careful analysis of the ECG should enable their distinction.

  **4.** Other diagnostic tests

   **a.** An echocardiogram is always done when pericarditis has been diagnosed to evaluate the presence of a significant pericardial effusion and exclude the presence of tamponade.

   **b.** Cardiac enzymes are frequently positive and are therefore not helpful for distinguishing the chest pain of pericarditis from that of cardiac ischemia.

**B.** Once the diagnosis of pericarditis is made, the cause needs to be determined.

  **1.** Because most pericarditis is either idiopathic or viral, requiring only supportive care, extensive work-up is generally not indicated.

  **2.** After a thorough history, most experts recommend only a few diagnostic tests.

   **a.** Chest radiograph

   **b.** BUN and creatinine

   **c.** PPD

   **d.** Antinuclear antibodies

   **e.** Blood cultures

  **3.** More extensive evaluation is appropriate for patients with refractory or recurrent disease. Even the most invasive diagnostic studies, pericardiocentesis and pericardial biopsy, are generally not helpful. Their diagnostic yield is only about 20%.

## Treatment

**A.** Because most patients have viral or idiopathic disease, the treatment of acute pericarditis is supportive.

  **1.** NSAIDs are the treatment of choice, usually providing good pain relief.

  **2.** The addition of colchicine may improve response to therapy and decrease rates of recurrent disease.

**B.** Prednisone is effective in patients with refractory disease but only after excluding the presence of diseases (such as TB) that are potentially exacerbated by corticosteroids.

**C.** Pericardiocentesis is required in patients with tamponade.

## CASE RESOLUTION

Mr. H underwent chest tube drainage of the effusion. Three tubes were placed with thoracoscopic guidance because the effusion was loculated. He was given a third-generation cephalosporin while sensitivities of his presumed pneumococcus were pending. He became afebrile after 2 days of antibiotics and chest tube drainage. The tube output declined over 5 days and the tubes were removed on day 6. Total output was about 3 L.

He was discharged and given oral antibiotics for 6 weeks for treatment of an empyema.

 Empyemas are a medical emergency. They are closed space infections that need to be drained in order to cure them and preserve future lung function. As soon as one is detected, steps should be taken to drain it.

# REFERENCES

Abrams J. Clinical practice. Chronic stable angina. N Engl J Med. 2005;352(24): 2524–33.

Anderson JL, Adams CD, Antman EM, et al. ACC/AHA 2007 Guidelines for the Management of Patients With Unstable Angina/Non ST-Elevation Myocardial Infarction. J Am Coll Cardiol. 2007;50(7):e1–157.

Antman EM, Anbe DT, Armstrong PW, et al. ACC/AHA guidelines for the management of patients with ST-elevation myocardial infarction. J Am Coll Cardiol. 2004;44(3):E1–E211.

Jiang J, Shi HZ, Liang QL, Qin SM, Qin XJ. Diagnostic value of interferon-gamma in tuberculous pleurisy: a metaanalysis. Chest. 2007;131(4):1133–41.

Kimble LP, McGuire DB, Dunbar SB, et al. Gender differences in pain characteristics of chronic stable angina and perceived physical limitation in patients with coronary artery disease. Pain. 2003;101:45–53.

Klompas M. Does this patient have an acute thoracic aortic dissection? JAMA. 2002;287(17):2262–72.

Light RW. Parapneumonic effusions and empyema. Clin Chest Med. 1985;6(1):55–62.

McGee SR. Evidence-based physical diagnosis. Philadelphia, PA: Saunders; 2001.

Permanyer-Miralda G, Sagrista-Sauleda J, Soler-Soler J. Primary acute pericardial disease: a prospective series of 231 consecutive patients. Am J Cardiol. 1985;56(10):623–30.

Spodick DH. Pericardial friction. Characteristics of pericardial rubs in fifty consecutive, prospectively studied patients. N Engl J Med. 1968;278(22):1204-7.

Thygesen K, Alpert JS, White HD. Universal definition of myocardial infarction. Circulation. 2007;116(22):2634–53.

von Kodolitsch Y, Schwartz AG, Nienaber CA. Clinical prediction of acute aortic dissection. Arch Intern Med. 2000;160(19):2977–82.

Williams SV, Fihn SD, Gibbons RJ. Guidelines for the management of patients with chronic stable angina: diagnosis and risk stratification. Ann Intern Med. 2001;135(7):530–47.

Yeghiazarians Y, Braunstein JB, Askari A, Stone PH. Unstable angina pectoris. N Engl J Med. 2000;342(2):101–14.

# I have a patient with acute respiratory complaints of cough and congestion. How do I determine the cause?

## CHIEF COMPLAINT

PATIENT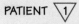

Ms. L is a 22-year-old woman who comes to your office in August complaining of cough and fever. She reports that she was in her usual state of health until 3 days ago when a cough developed. Two days ago, a low-grade fever (37.2°C) developed, which increased to 38.8°C yesterday. She reports that her sputum is yellow and that she has no chest pain or shortness of breath.

## CONSTRUCTING A DIFFERENTIAL DIAGNOSIS

The framework for the differential diagnosis of acute respiratory complaints is anatomic and microbiologic. Although there are a myriad of viral and bacterial (and occasional mycobacterial) infections that infect the respiratory tree, a practical approach addresses 3 issues:

1. Where is the infection (sinuses, tracheobronchial tree, alveoli)?
2. Will the patient benefit from antibiotics?
3. Among patients with pneumonia, clinicians must separate the common community-acquired pneumonias (CAPs) from the less common but important pneumonias due to aspiration, tuberculosis (TB), and opportunistic infections. Diagnostic and treatment algorithms that summarize the approach to patients with acute respiratory infections appear at the end of the chapter. (see Figures 9–3 and 9–4)

### Differential Diagnosis of Acute Cough and Congestion

A. Common cold
B. Sinusitis
C. Bronchitis
D. Influenza
E. Pneumonia
  1. CAP
  2. Aspiration pneumonia
  3. TB
  4. Opportunistic (eg, *Pneumocystis jiroveci* pneumonia [PCP])

On physical exam, Ms. L is in no acute distress. Vital signs are RR, 18 breaths per minute; BP, 110/72 mm Hg; pulse, 92 bpm; temperature, 38.6°C. Pharynx is unremarkable; lung exam reveals normal breath sounds without crackles, dullness, bronchophony, or egophony.

 At this point, what is the leading hypothesis, what are the active alternatives, and is there a must not miss diagnosis? Given this differential diagnosis, what tests should be ordered?

## PRIORITIZING THE DIFFERENTIAL DIAGNOSIS

The differential diagnosis for Ms. L includes acute bronchitis, influenza, aspiration pneumonia, and CAP. Ms. L's high fever is a pivotal feature of this case. Acute bronchitis is *not* usually associated with significant fever (unless caused by influenza). Influenza can cause high fevers and chest symptoms but almost always occurs between December and May. Therefore, despite Ms. L's normal lung exam, the high fever raises the possibility of CAP and makes this the leading diagnosis. Table 9–1 lists the differential diagnosis.

 A high fever should raise the suspicion of pneumonia.

Influenza occurs from December to May in the northern hemisphere; it is highly unlikely at other times.

Ms. L reports drinking only an occasional glass of wine and denies recent intoxication, loss of consciousness, or substance abuse. She reports no travel history and no sick contacts.

 Is the clinical information sufficient to make a diagnosis of CAP? If not, what other information do you need?

**Table 9-1.** Diagnostic hypotheses for Ms. L.

| Diagnostic Hypothesis | Clinical Clues | Important Tests |
|---|---|---|
| **Leading Hypothesis** | | |
| CAP | Cough<br>Shortness of breath<br>High fever<br>Crackles or dullness on lung exam | Chest radiograph<br>Blood culture<br>Sputum Gram stain and culture (occasionally) |
| **Active Alternatives-Most Common** | | |
| Acute bronchitis | Cough<br>Absence of high fever<br>Normal lung exam | Chest radiograph (if abnormal lung exam, dyspnea or high fever) |
| Influenza | Sudden onset<br>High fever<br>Severe myalgias<br>December to May | Diagnosis is usually clinical;<br>Direct immunofluorescence or ELISA can be used |
| Aspiration pneumonia | Impaired mentation (dementia, prior stroke, substance abuse) | Chest radiograph |

ELISA, enzyme-linked immunosorbent assay.

# Leading Hypothesis: CAP

## Textbook Presentation

Productive cough and fever are often the presenting symptoms in patients with pneumonia. Symptoms may worsen over days or develop abruptly. Pleuritic chest pain, shortness of breath, chills, and rigors may also develop.

## Disease Highlights

A. Most common cause of infectious death in the United States

B. Most common identified pathogens

1. *Streptococcus pneumoniae*

2. *Mycoplasma pneumoniae*

   a. More common in younger patients

   b. Cannot be distinguished from other pyogenic infections based on clinical presentation or chest radiograph

3. *Haemophilus influenzae*

4. *Chlamydia*

5. Influenza (and other viruses)

6. Polymicrobial infection

7. *Legionella*

8. *Staphylococcus aureus* infection may develop post influenza.

C. 3.4% of pneumonias are associated with underlying malignancy

D. Complications

1. Respiratory failure

2. Death

3. Empyema (See Chapter 8, Chest Pain)

E. Prognosis is good overall.

1. 8% hospitalization rate

2. 95% radiographic cure in 1 month

3. Mortality 1.2%

## Evidence-Based Diagnosis

A. Diagnosis of pneumonia

1. Diagnosis is usually clinical, based on constellation of cough, fever, and infiltrate on chest film

2. Prevalence of symptoms in patients with pneumonia

   a. Cough, 96%

   b. Fever, 81% but 53% in the elderly

 Elderly patients with pneumonia often *do not* have a fever. Clinicians should have a low threshold for obtaining a chest radiograph in elderly patients or in patients with COPD with cough or with mental status changes.

   c. Dyspnea, 46–66%

   d. Pleuritic chest pain, 37–50%

   e. Chills, 59%

   f. Headache, 58%

3. Physical exam

   a. No single finding is very sensitive. Therefore, the absence of any single finding does not rule out pneumonia (Table 9–2).

      (1) Neither a normal lung exam nor the absence of fever rule out pneumonia (LR–, 0.6 and 0.8, respectively).

 A normal lung exam *does not* rule out pneumonia.

      (2) Normal vital signs make pneumonia less likely (LR 0.18).

      (3) Combination of normal vital signs and normal chest exam make pneumonia highly unlikely (95% sensitive, LR 0.09).

**Table 9-2.** Likelihood ratios for physical findings in pneumonia.

| Finding | LR+ | LR– |
|---|---|---|
| Fever > 37.8°C | 4.4 | 0.8 |
| Any chest finding | 1.3–3.0[1] | 0.6 |
| Normal vital signs HR < 100 bpm, temperature ≤ 37.8°C, RR ≤ 20 breaths per minute | 1.2 | 0.18 |
| Normal vital signs and lung exam | 2.2 | 0.09 |
| Egophony | 8.6 | 1.0 |
| Crackles | 2.7 | 0.9 |

**b.** Egophony is fairly specific and significantly increases the likelihood of pneumonia when present (LR+ 8.6).

**4.** WBC > 10,400 cells/mcL: LR+, 3.7; LR−, 0.6

**5.** Chest film

   **a.** Sensitivity is lower in dehydrated patients.

   **b.** Compared with high-resolution chest CT scan, chest film sensitivity is 69%.

A normal chest radiograph does *not* rule out pneumonia when the pretest probability is high (ie, a patient with cough, fever and crackles), and antibiotics should still be administered.

   **c.** 94% of infiltrates are in the lower and middle regions.

CAP rarely affects the upper lobes; consider TB or aspiration pneumonia when upper lobe involvement is seen.

**6.** Determining the etiologic agent

   **a.** A variety of tests, including sputum culture, sputum Gram stain, blood culture and urinary antigen tests for pneumococcus and *Legionella,* can help determine the pathogen in CAP.

   **b.** The yield of these tests in outpatients with CAP is low and routine testing is optional in outpatients.

   **c.** Sputum cultures are often unreliable due to contamination by oral flora.

   **(1)** Normal flora should not be misinterpreted to mean no infection.

   **(2)** When positive, sputum cultures can help determine the resistance pattern.

   **d.** Sputum Gram stains are also often unreliable due to poor quality, preparation, and interpretation.

   **(1)** One study reported that only 14% of hospitalized patients had an adequate specimen with a dominant organism.

   **(2)** One study reported positive sputum Gram stains in 63–80% of patients with pneumococcal bacteremia.

   **e.** Blood cultures are positive in 5–14% of patients.

   **f.** Pneumococcal urinary antigen

   **(1)** Sensitivity for pneumococcal pneumonia, 50–80%

   **(2)** Specificity, 90% (false-positives may occur secondary to colonization)

   **g.** *Legionella* urinary antigen 70–90% sensitive, 99% specific

**Treatment**

**A.** Prevention: Indications for polyvalent pneumococcal vaccine

   **1.** Persons ≥ 65 years old and adults of any age with:

   **2.** Diabetes

   **3.** Chronic heart, lung, renal, or liver disease

   **4.** Alcoholism

   **5.** Immunosuppression (including asplenia)

   **6.** Native Americans, Alaskans, or residents of long-term care facilities

**B.** One time revaccination is recommended after 5 years in immunocompromised adults and those who received their first dose before age 65.

**C.** Determine need for hospitalization

   **1.** Prospective validated clinical tools can help determine the need for admission (see Figure 9–4).

   **2.** Indications for admission

   **a.** Hypoxia

   **b.** Shock

   **c.** Pleural effusion

   **d.** Multilobar infiltrates on CXR

   **e.** Failure of prior outpatient therapy

   **f.** Confusion

   **g.** Unable to tolerate oral intake

   **h.** Unreliable social situation

   **i.** Certain underlying diseases (sickle cell disease, immunocompromise, severe chronic obstructive pulmonary disease [COPD] or heart failure [HF])

   **3.** The CURB-65 score is a validated model that predicts mortality.

   **a.** Criteria are **c**onfusion (to person, place or time), **u**remia (BUN > 20 mg/dL), **R**R ≥ 30 breaths per minute, systolic **B**P < 90 mm Hg or diastolic BP ≤ 60 mm Hg, age ≥ **65.**

   **b.** A score of > 1 is associated with an increased mortality and the need for hospital admission.

**D.** Evaluation

   **1.** Chest film is recommended in the evaluation of all patients with CAP.

   **2.** Evaluate oxygenation in all patients (ABG or $SaO_2$)

   **3.** An ABG is required in patients with respiratory distress, particularly those with preexistent COPD.

A normal $SaO_2$ on pulse oximetry does not exclude *hypercarbia* and respiratory failure. A blood gas to check *$PaCO_2$* is required for patients with respiratory distress.

   **4.** Determining the causative agent

   **a.** Most patients are treated empirically, to cover the most common organisms responsible for CAP

   **b.** The Infectious Diseases Society of America (IDSA) has published guidelines for more extensive testing on select inpatients (Table 9–3).

   **c.** Patients with severe pneumonia should have blood and sputum cultures, sputum Gram stain, and urinary tests for pneumococcal and *Legionella* antigen.

   **d.** CAP is the most common pneumonia among outpatients with an infiltrate and fever.

   **e.** Nonetheless, clinicians should always consider other less common pneumonias including aspiration, TB, and pneumocystis.

   **(1)** A history of neurologic impairment or drug abuse should suggest aspiration.

   **(2)** Chronic symptoms, upper lobe disease, or cavitary lesions should suggest TB.

**Table 9–3.** IDSA guidelines for more extensive testing in persons with CAP.

| Indication | Blood culture | Sputum culture | *Legionella* UAT | Pneumococcal UAT | Other |
|---|---|---|---|---|---|
| Intensive care unit admission | X | X | X | X | X[a] |
| Failure of outpatient antibiotic therapy | | X | X | X | |
| Cavitary infiltrates | X | X | | | X[b] |
| Leukopenia | X | | | X | |
| Active alcohol abuse | X | X | X | X | |
| Chronic severe liver disease | X | | | X | |
| Severe obstructive/structural lung disease | | X | | | |
| Asplenia (anatomic or functional) | X | | | X | |
| Recent travel (within past 2 weeks) | | | X | | X[c] |
| Positive *Legionella* UAT result | | X[d] | NA | | |
| Positive pneumococcal UAT result | X | X | | NA | |
| Pleural effusion | X | X | X | X | X[e] |

NOTE. NA, not applicable; UAT, urinary antigen test.
[a]Endotracheal aspirate if intubated, possibly bronchoscopy or nonbronchoscopic bronchoalveolar lavage.
[b]Fungal and tuberculosis cultures.
[c]See table 8 for details.
[d]Special media for *Legionella*.
[e]Thoracentesis and pleural fluid cultures.
CAP, community-acquired pneumonia; IDSA, Infectious Diseases Society of America; NA, not applicable; UAT, urinary antigen test.
(Reproduced, with permission, from Mandell LA, Wunderink RG, Anzueto A et al. Infectious Diseases Society of America/American Thoracic Society consensus guidelines on the management of community-acquired pneumonia in adults. Clin Infect Dis. 2007;44 Suppl 2:S27–72.)

**(3)** HIV risk factors or bilateral fluffy infiltrates should suggest PCP (see Figure 9–4).

**5.** Patients with pleural effusions require diagnostic thoracentesis to rule out empyema or complicated parapneumonic effusions, which require chest tube drainage in addition to antibiotics.

**6.** HIV testing is recommended for all adults aged 15–54 years who have CAP.

E. Antibiotics

**1.** Treatment must cover pyogenic and atypical (*Mycoplasma* and *Chlamydia*) organisms.

**2.** Penicillin-resistant *S pneumoniae* (PRSP)

**a.** Increasing resistance in United States

**b.** Marked geographic variability in frequency of resistance but up to 65% in some areas

**c.** PRSP often resistant to cephalosporins and macrolides but not quinolones with extended activity against *S pneumoniae*.

**3.** Empiric therapy (recommendations from the IDSA 2007)

**a.** Outpatients

**(1)** Previously healthy outpatients without recent use of antibiotics (3 months) are usually treated with an advanced macrolide (azithromycin or clarithromycin). In areas with a high rate of macrolide resistance, a respiratory quinolone (moxifloxacin, levofloxacin, or gemifloxacin) should be substituted.

**(2)** Outpatients recently treated with antibiotics or with comorbidities (heart, lung, liver, or kidney disease; diabetes mellitus; alcoholism; cancer; asplenia; immunosuppression) are treated with a respiratory fluoroquinolone or an advanced macrolide plus a β-lactam (high-dose amoxicillin or amoxicillin-clavulanate).

**b.** Inpatients

**(1)** Inpatients should be treated with respiratory fluoroquinolone or advanced macrolide with β-lactam.

**(2)** Drotrecogin alpha (activated protein C) should be considered in patients with pneumonia and septic shock that persists despite fluid resuscitation and in those with pneumonia, sepsis, and leucopenia.

**(3)** Hypotensive patients with severe CAP should be screened for adrenal insufficiency and treated if their cortisol response to stimulation is inadequate.

## MAKING A DIAGNOSIS

Ms. L does not have risk factors for aspiration pneumonia. Influenza is highly unlikely in August. The differential diagnosis is narrowed to CAP and acute bronchitis.

Have you crossed a diagnostic threshold for the leading hypothesis, CAP? Have you ruled out the active alternatives? Do other tests need to be done to exclude the alternative diagnosis?

## Alternative Diagnosis: Acute Bronchitis

### Textbook Presentation

Acute bronchitis presents in the healthy adult primarily as a cough of 1–3 weeks duration. Myalgias and low-grade fevers may be seen. This is distinct from an acute exacerbation of COPD (see Chapter 28, Wheezing and Stridor).

### Disease Highlights

A. Etiology

   1. Viruses

      a. Influenza

      b. Parainfluenza

      c. Respiratory syncytial virus

      d. Adenovirus

      e. Rhinovirus

      f. Coronavirus

   2. Bacterial

      a. < 10% of cases are caused by bacteria

      b. Organisms include *Bordetella pertussis, Mycoplasma,* and *Chlamydia*

   3. Noninfectious

      a. Asthma

      b. Pollution

      c. Tobacco

      d. Cannabis

B. Symptoms

   1. Initial phase: Cough and systemic symptoms secondary to infection are seen.

   2. Fever may be low grade. Consider pneumonia in patients whose fever is high-grade or persistent.

   3. Protracted phase

      a. In 26% of patients, cough persists secondary to bronchial hyperresponsiveness and lasts 2–4 weeks or more.

      b. 40–65% of patients without prior pulmonary disease show evidence of reactive airway disease during acute bronchitis.

### Evidence-Based Diagnosis

A. Sputum may be clear or discolored. Discoloration arises from tracheobronchial epithelium cells and WBCs and is *not* diagnostic of bacterial infection.

*Purulent* sputum is not an indication for antibiotic therapy in patients with acute bronchitis.

B. Chest film is not routine but is indicated when pneumonia is being considered; (See Figure 9–3) indications include

   1. Abnormal vital signs including high fever (temperature > 38°C), tachypnea (RR > 24 breaths per minute), tachycardia (HR > 100 bpm)

   2. Dyspnea

   3. Focal findings on lung exam

   4. Elderly patients

   5. Presence of COPD, HF, cancer, or immunocompromised state

C. Testing for influenza can be considered in febrile patients who present during influenza season within 48 hours of symptoms onset in whom antiviral therapy is being considered (see below).

### Treatment

A. Antibiotics

   1. Antibiotics do not provide major clinical benefit and are *not* recommended in the treatment of acute bronchitis.

   2. Influenza treatment shortens the course of illness in patients with influenza treated within 48 hours of symptoms (see below) and can be considered in patients with bronchitis due to this pathogen.

B. Bronchodilators significantly reduce cough in patients with bronchial hyperreactivity, wheezing, or airflow obstruction at baseline.

C. Antitussives are useful symptomatic measures.

## CASE RESOLUTION

At this point, obtaining a chest radiograph is critical. WBCs and sputum and blood cultures can be obtained but are too insensitive to rule out pneumonia.

    A chest film reveals a left lower-lobe infiltrate, confirming the diagnosis of pneumonia.

25–50% of patients with pneumonia do not have crackles on auscultation. Chest film is required when pneumonia is suspected.

WBC is 10,200 cells/mcL with 67% neutrophils and 5% bands. Her SaO₂ is 96% on room air. An HIV test should be ordered, antibiotics must be chosen, and a decision must be made to admit or discharge Ms. L.

Ms. L's CURB-65 score is 0 and she has no indications for admission (see Figure 9–4). She has no risk factors for aspiration, and her chest radiograph does not suggest TB or PCP. Her HIV test is negative. She is treated for CAP with azithromycin and instructed to call immediately if her fever increases or increasing shortness of breath or chest pain develop.

    One week later, she reports feeling much better. A follow-up chest film 6 weeks later shows resolution of the pneumonia.

A follow-up chest radiograph is indicated in patients with pneumonia to exclude an underlying obstructing mass.

## CHIEF COMPLAINT

PATIENT 2

Mr. P is a 32-year-old man with cough and progressive shortness of breath over the last 4 weeks. He complains of a persistent cough productive of purulent sputum and low-grade fever. His past medical history is unremarkable. Social history: Mr. P reports that he is homeless. He admits to drinking 1 pint of gin per day. He reports no history of recreational or injection drug use. He reports that he has rarely used paid sex workers. He has no history of sex with men. He denies using condoms.

On physical exam he appears disheveled and smells of alcohol and urine. Vital signs are pulse, 95 bpm; temperature, 37.0°C; RR, 20 breaths per minute; BP, 140/90 mm Hg. There is temporal wasting. Lung exam reveals diffuse fine crackles in the lower lung fields bilaterally. Cardiac exam is normal. His chest radiograph demonstrates bilateral lower lobe infiltrates. No cardiomegaly is seen. A CBC is normal. SaO$_2$ is 88%. His BUN is 18 mg/dL.

> At this point, what is the leading hypothesis, what are the active alternatives, and is there a must not miss diagnosis? Given this differential diagnosis, what tests should be ordered?

## PRIORITIZING THE DIFFERENTIAL DIAGNOSIS

The clinical findings of cough, shortness of breath, crackles on pulmonary exam, and infiltrates on chest film all suggest pneumonia. One pivotal feature of this case is the long duration of symptoms. CAP is possible but less likely with such protracted symptoms. More chronic processes such as aspiration pneumonia or TB should be considered. Another pivotal feature of Mr. P's case is his alcoholism. Alcoholism, substance abuse, and neurologic disorders are leading risk factors for aspiration, and his alcoholism makes aspiration pneumonia the leading diagnosis. The duration of his complaints and temporal wasting also raise the possibility of more chronic pneumonias caused by TB, fungi, or PCP. TB is more common in alcoholic patients and malnourished patients. Given the public health risks, TB is a must not miss possibility. A third pivotal feature in this patient is his high-risk sexual behavior increasing his risk for HIV infection and PCP. PCP primarily affects HIV-infected patients. It is important to consider PCP even in patients without a history of *known* HIV infection because PCP can be the first sign of HIV infection. The sexual history makes PCP (or another HIV-related pneumonia) an active alternative diagnosis. Finally, uncomplicated influenza does not persist for 4 weeks, although a postinfluenza pneumonia could be considered in the proper season. Table 9–4 lists the differential diagnosis.

> Is the clinical information sufficient to make a diagnosis? If not what other information do you need?

**Table 9–4.** Diagnostic hypotheses for Mr. P.

| Diagnostic Hypothesis | Clinical Clues | Important Tests |
|---|---|---|
| **Leading Hypothesis** | | |
| Aspiration pneumonia | Impaired mentation (dementia, prior stroke, substance abuse) | Chest radiograph |
| **Active Alternatives-Most Common** | | |
| CAP | Cough<br>Shortness of breath<br>High fever<br>Crackles or dullness on lung exam | Chest radiograph<br>Blood culture<br>Sputum culture and Gram stain (occasionally) |
| PCP | Injection drug use, men who have sex with men, engaging in sex with paid sex workers | HIV<br>CD4 count<br>Chest radiograph demonstrating diffuse bilateral infiltrates |
| **Active Alternatives-Must Not Miss** | | |
| TB | Long duration of symptoms<br>Risk factors for TB (alcoholism, HIV infection, foreign-born persons, cancer, diabetes, homeless persons, end-stage renal disease, use of corticosteroids, incarceration) | Chest radiograph shows upper lobe, cavitary or reticulonodular disease<br>Sputum for acid-fast stain and culture |

CAP, community-acquired pneumonia; PCP, *Pneumocystis jiroveci* pneumonia; TB, tuberculosis.

## Leading Hypothesis: Aspiration Pneumonia

### Textbook Presentation

Aspiration pneumonia typically develops in patients with impaired mentation (ie, the demented elderly patient or alcoholic). Classic symptoms include fever, cough, chest pain, and putrid sputum. The syndrome most commonly evolves over days to weeks rather than acutely.

### Disease Highlights

A. Patients can aspirate oropharyngeal secretions or gastric contents.

   1. Gastric acid aspiration may result in chemical damage (aspiration *pneumonitis*) and may be accompanied by subsequent infection (aspiration *pneumonia*).

   2. Factors that contribute to the development of aspiration pneumonia include aspiration, colonization, impaired immunity, and decreased pulmonary clearance.

B. Risk factors for aspiration

   1. Neurologic disease (dementia, cerebrovascular accident, seizures)

2. Sedation (illicit drug or alcohol overdose, general anesthesia)

3. Impaired oral pharyngeal clearance (status post head and neck surgery)

4. Gastroesophageal reflux disease, vomiting

5. Endoscopy, tracheostomy, bronchoscopy, nasogastric feeding

C. Aspiration *pneumonitis*

1. Aspirated contents with lower pHs and larger volumes leads to more damage

2. Clinical syndrome

   a. Usually follows large volume aspiration (ie, during anesthesia)

   b. Cyanosis and shortness of breath develop within 2 hours

   c. Fever is usually low grade

   d. Outcome varies

      (1) Rapid recovery within 24–36 hours (62%), bacterial superinfection (26%), acute respiratory distress syndrome (12%)

      (2) Bacterial superinfection may lead to pneumonia, lung abscess, or empyema.

D. Aspiration *pneumonia* refers to infection due to aspirated organisms.

1. Accounts for 5–15% of pneumonias

2. Poor dentition increases the risk of aspiration pneumonia.

3. Aspiration is usually not witnessed.

4. Clinical features include cough, fever, sputum production, and shortness of breath, which may progress over days to weeks.

5. Organisms

   a. Community-acquired aspiration pneumonia may be caused by anaerobes, *S pneumoniae, S aureus,* and *H influenzae.*

   b. Hospital-acquired aspiration pneumonias may be caused by anaerobes, gram-negative organisms (including *Pseudomonas*), and *S aureus.*

### Evidence-Based Diagnosis

A. Often presumptive based on aspiration risk factors, putrid sputum and typical chest film. Many patients have periodontal disease.

B. Oropharyngeal motility studies can identify certain patients at risk, particularly those with neurologic impairment.

C. Rigors and acute onset suggest more virulent organisms (ie, *S pneumoniae* and *S aureus*).

D. Chest film

1. The classic location of infection is in the basal segment of lower lobes, but it can involve upper lobes if aspiration occurred while the patient was recumbent.

2. Cavitation is more common in aspiration pneumonia than in CAP.

### Treatment

A. Prevention

1. Soft diets and feeding strategies can reduce subsequent aspiration.

2. Tube feedings decrease the incidence of aspiration pneumonia in patients with dysphagia (54% vs 13% with oral feeding). However, despite tube feedings, patients can still aspirate from gastroesophageal reflux, vomiting, and aspiration of oropharyngeal contents.

3. Several studies suggest that ACE inhibitors increase the cough reflex and decrease the rate of pneumonia in persons at-risk (NNT 9-19).

4. Amantadine promotes dopamine release (which facilitates cough and decreases dysphagia). It also has been shown to decrease the rate of pneumonia in elderly patients with prior stroke (NNT 4.3).

5. Oral hygiene decreases colonization and subsequent pneumonia.

6. Postprandial semi-recumbent positions decrease the rate of aspiration pneumonia compared with supine positions.

B. Supportive treatment

1. Suction any material in airway.

2. Intubation if necessary for ventilation, oxygenation, or to protect airway in patients with altered level of consciousness.

C. Aspiration *pneumonitis*

1. Antibiotics are recommended if the infiltrates do not resolve within 48 hours or if the patient likely has gastric colonization (resulting from a $H_2$-blocker, proton pump inhibitor, or from bowel obstruction).

2. Corticosteroids are controversial.

D. Aspiration *pneumonia*: antibiotics are indicated.

1. Community-acquired aspiration

   a. First-line options include clindamycin or amoxicillin/clavulanate or amoxicillin with metronidazole.

   b. Other options include piperacillin-tazobactam, moxifloxacin, ceftriaxone, cefotaxime.

2. Hospital-acquired aspiration: Coverage requires addition of an antibiotic that is effective against gram-negative organisms and *S aureus.*

## MAKING A DIAGNOSIS

At this point, it is appropriate to order blood cultures, sputum cultures, and Gram stain. The patient's chest radiograph does not have any features that suggest TB (see below), which makes TB less likely. Nonetheless, PPD placement and obtaining sputum for acid-fast bacillus (AFB) stain and culture would be reasonable. Finally, given the diffuse symmetric infiltrate on chest radiography and his sexual history, PCP must be considered and testing for HIV is mandatory. Although the patient's CURB-65 score is 0, his hypoxia and lack of a reliable social structure make admission mandatory. Antibiotics that cover both CAP and aspiration pneumonia should be started.

Mr. P is admitted to an isolation bed on the general medical floor. He is empirically treated with clindamycin (for presumed aspiration pneumonia), azithromycin, and ceftriaxone. The PPD test is done and is negative. Blood cultures are negative and sputum cultures reveal normal flora.

**Have you crossed a diagnostic threshold for the leading hypothesis, aspiration pneumonia? Have you ruled out the active alternatives TB and PCP? Do other tests need to be done to exclude the alternative diagnosis?**

# Alternative Diagnosis: PCP

## Textbook Presentation

Patients with PCP may have diagnosed or *undiagnosed* advanced HIV disease. Patients commonly complain of progressive shortness of breath and dry cough of 1 to 3 week duration.

 PCP is often the presenting manifestation of AIDS. Suspect PCP in patients with diffuse bilateral pneumonia, particularly of subacute onset.

## Disease Highlights

A. PCP presents as diffuse bilateral pneumonia.

B. PCP occurs most commonly in patients with HIV disease and CD4 counts < 200 cells/mcL.

C. PCP is the most common cause of acute *diffuse* lung disease in immunocompromised patients and is the leading cause of AIDS-related death in HIV-infected patients.

D. PCP may also develop in patients undergoing organ transplantation or chemotherapy and in patients with idiopathic CD4 lymphocytopenia.

E. The exact classification of the organism is unclear.

## Evidence-Based Diagnosis

A. History

    1. Patients may *or may not* already carry diagnosis of HIV or AIDS.

    2. Fever is present in 79–100% of cases.

    3. Cough is present in 95% of cases. It is usually (but not always) nonproductive.

    4. Progressive dyspnea is present in 95% of cases.

B. Physical exam

    1. Fever is present in 84%.

    2. Tachypnea is present in 62%.

    3. Chest auscultation is normal in 50% of cases.

C. Chest film

    1. Usually shows diffuse symmetric bilateral alveolar or interstitial infiltrates (81–93% of cases)

    2. In HIV-infected patients, interstitial infiltrates are present in 69% of patients and increase the likelihood of PCP (versus TB or bacterial pneumonia) (LR+ 4.25).

    3. Dyspnea or oral thrush combined with a diffuse interstitial pattern on chest radiograph strongly suggest PCP in HIV-infected persons (sensitivity 58% and 36%, respectively; LR+ ≈7.25).

    4. Isolated upper lobe disease may be seen in patients taking inhaled pentamidine as PCP prophylaxis.

    5. Occasionally shows pneumothorax

    6. Normal in 10–25% of cases

 PCP should be considered in dyspneic patients with HIV and CD4 counts < 200 cells/mcL even when the chest exam and chest radiograph are normal.

D. Specific diagnostic tests

    1. Although the chest radiograph and lactate dehydrogenase (LDH) (see below) can suggest PCP or make the diagnosis less likely, patients require specific tests to confirm or exclude PCP.

    2. Clinical diagnosis (without confirmational staining of sputum or bronchoalveolar lavage [BAL]) is incorrect in 43% of patients.

    3. Induced sputums are typically the first test used to diagnose PCP.

        a. 55–92% sensitive, 100% specific

        b. The addition of immunofluorescent staining increases sensitivity.

    4. BAL is used to diagnose PCP when sputum stains are negative.

        a. Diagnosis is based on staining the fluid obtained during BAL.

        b. Silver or Giemsa staining and monoclonal antibodies have been used.

        c. Sensitivity is 86–97%.

        d. Sensitivity of BAL is lower (62%) after inhaled pentamidine prophylaxis.

    5. The most common diagnostic strategy is sputum analysis with silver stain and immunofluorescence. Positive results confirm PCP. Negative results should prompt BAL.

    6. Other diagnostic tools being investigated include the study of sputum, blood and nasal pharyngeal specimens with polymerase chain reaction (PCR) and the measurement of serum s-adenosylmethionine (which falls in patients infected with PCP).

E. Nonspecific diagnostic tests

    1. Lactate dehydrogenase (LDH) is a nonspecific test; it is elevated in 90% of cases, but specificity is low. Although LDH can be helpful, some patients with PCP have normal LDH levels.

    2. High-resolution chest CT scan

        a. Patchy or nodular ground-glass appearance; ground glass most marked in perihilar regions. Cystic lesions may be seen.

        b. 100% sensitive, 83–89% specific

        c. LR+, 5.9; LR–, 0

    3. Pulmonary function tests

        a. Carbon monoxide diffusing capacity of the lungs (DLCO) is usually low in PCP and highly sensitive.

        b. Likelihood of PCP is < 2% if DLCO is > 75% predicted.

## Treatment

A. Antimicrobial therapy

    1. Trimethoprim-sulfamethoxazole (TMP-SMX) is initial treatment of choice.

    2. Antibiotic therapy may markedly *worsen* preexistent hypoxia. Many patients require concomitant glucocorticoids to prevent acute respiratory distress syndrome (see below).

    3. IV pentamidine and TMP-SMX have similar efficacy.

    4. Occasional resistance to TMP-SMX has been reported.

    5. Both TMP and pentamidine may cause hyperkalemia.

    6. Patients allergic to TMP-SMX may be desensitized.

**7.** Other options reserved for patients with mild to moderate PCP infections include clindamycin plus primaquine, dapsone plus TMP or atovaquone.

**B.** Glucocorticoids

    **1.** Reduce mortality and respiratory failure in patients with severe PCP treated with TMP-SMX.

    **2.** Initiate at time of PCP therapy if room air $PaO_2 < 70$ mm Hg or the A-a gradient $\geq 35$ mm Hg.

    **3.** Prednisone 40 mg twice daily for 5 days, then 40 mg daily for 5 days, then 20 mg daily for 11 days.

 Concomitant glucocorticoid therapy is lifesaving in patients with PCP whose $PaO_2 < 70$ mm Hg.

**C.** Prophylaxis

    **1.** Indications

        **a.** Prior PCP

        **b.** CD4 counts < 200 cells/mcL

        **c.** HIV-infected patients with unexplained persistent fevers or oral candidiasis for more than 2 weeks

    **2.** TMP-SMX is superior to pentamidine and the drug of choice. In addition, it is effective prophylaxis against toxoplasmosis and some bacterial infections.

    **3.** Significant adverse reactions are common with TMP-SMX. Rash, fever, neutropenia, and hypotension may necessitate discontinuation of TMP-SMX. Consultation with an infectious disease specialist is recommended.

    **4.** Dapsone, pentamidine, and atovaquone are alternative therapies in patients intolerant of TMP-SMX. Some authorities recommend screening patients for glucose 6-phosphate dehydrogenase (G6PD) deficiency prior to instituting dapsone.

    **5.** HAART can restore the CD4 count and allow for discontinuation of prophylaxis when CD4 count > 200 cells/mcL for approximately 3 months.

## Alternative Diagnosis: TB

### Textbook Presentation

TB pneumonia usually develops due to reactivation of latent mycobacteria residing in the upper lobes. Symptoms are chronic and include cough, fever, weight loss, and night sweats. By the time patients seek medical attention, they have often had these symptoms for weeks or months. The weight loss and duration of symptoms often suggest cancer.

### Disease Highlights

**A.** Obligate aerobe has predilection for lung apices.

**B.** The organism is slow growing; the generation time is 12–18 hours, resulting in slow progression.

**C.** Common and serious

    **1.** Infects 33% of the world's population

    **2.** 9 million new cases per year and 2 million deaths (worldwide)

**D.** Epidemiology

    **1.** 7% of US population is PPD positive.

    **2.** Foreign-born persons have the highest rate of TB (9.7 times higher than US-born persons) and account for 85% of multidrug resistant TB (MDR-TB) in the United States.

    **3.** Asians, blacks, and Hispanics have higher rates of TB than whites (22.9, 8.3 and 7.4 times, respectively). Foreign-born persons account for a majority of TB cases in Asians and Hispanics but not blacks.

    **4.** 67% of cases occur in the nonwhite population.

    **5.** In the nonwhite population, the median age is 39. In whites, the median age is 62.

    **6.** Reactivation TB accounts for 90% of TB in older patients and 67% of TB in younger patients.

    **7.** High risk groups

        **a.** HIV

            **(1)** HIV-infected patients are at highest risk for TB (200 times increased incidence).

            **(2)** TB may be the first manifestation of HIV.

 Patients with active or latent TB should be tested for HIV.

            **(3)** Extrapulmonary TB without pulmonary disease is more common in patients with AIDS (30%) than in those without AIDS (15%).

            **(4)** In early HIV infection, TB is fairly typical. However, in advanced HIV infection, pulmonary TB is much more often atypical.

        **b.** Alcoholics

        **c.** Other high-risk groups

            **(1)** Foreign-born persons

            **(2)** Immunosuppressed patients (including patients taking corticosteroids)

            **(3)** Patients with cancer, diabetes mellitus, end-stage renal disease, transplants, or malnutrition

            **(4)** PPD-positive patients

            **(5)** Patients with evidence of prior TB on chest film

            **(6)** Economically disadvantaged, inner city residents

            **(7)** Nursing home residents

            **(8)** Hispanics and African Americans

            **(9)** Drug-dependent persons, homeless persons, prison inmates

**E.** Pathophysiology

    **1.** Inhaled organism lands in the middle and lower lobes (due to increased ventilation).

    **2.** Multiplies over next 3 weeks, spreads to hilar nodes and often bloodstream.

    **3.** Organism lodges preferentially in areas of high $PaO_2$ (lung apices, renal cortex, vertebrae).

    **4.** In 90% of patients, the immune system then contains the organism resulting in typical scarring (Ghon complex). However, the chest film can be normal.

    **5.** Above sequence usually asymptomatic.

    **6.** In some patients a few viable organisms remain. This is referred to as **latent TB infection** (LTBI). Latent TB can reactivate later (**reactivation TB**).

    **7.** The PPD is positive 6–8 weeks after the initial infection. These patients are resistant to subsequent *exogenous* infection.

8. Primary TB
   a. In approximately 10% of patients (higher in immuno-compromised patients and children), the initial infection is not controlled and causes primary TB.
   b. Primary TB accounts for 23–34% of adult cases.
   c. Chest radiograph shows patchy lower lobe pneumonia.
      (1) Disease is usually unilateral.
      (2) Lymphadenopathy is seen in 10–65% of adults.
      (3) Often occurs in those unable to mount a sensitized macrophage response.
      (4) PPD may be negative in these patients.
      (5) Most cases of primary TB resolve spontaneously without treatment.
      (6) Pneumonia progresses without treatment in 15% of patients.
9. Reactivation TB
   a. 3–5% of patients with LTBI experience reactivation due to declining immune function
   b. Reactivation TB results in 90% of adult non–AIDS-related TB.
   c. 71% of cases occur in foreign-born patients
   d. Symptoms are usually insidious and include chronic cough, weight loss, night sweats, anorexia, and low or high-grade fevers.
   e. Reactivation TB progresses unless patient is treated.
10. Pleural TB takes 2 forms: tuberculous empyema and tuberculous pleural effusions.
    a. Tuberculous empyema
       (1) Secondary to direct infection of pleural space (often from rupture of neighboring tuberculous cavity)
       (2) Rare
       (3) Pleural fluid characterized by pus and numerous TB organisms
    b. Tuberculous effusions
       (1) Tuberculous effusions result from a delayed hypersensitivity reaction to mycobacterial antigens in the pleural space.
       (2) Usually due to reactivation in adults (75%)
       (3) Typical features include acute high fever, cough (94%), and pleuritic chest pain (78%).
       (4) Chest radiograph shows unilateral effusion in 95% of cases. Parenchymal infiltrate is seen in 50% of cases.
       (5) Effusion usually exudative (see below)
       (6) PPD is usually positive (69–93%).
11. Extrapulmonary TB may involve the spine, kidney, pericardium, and CNS.

### Evidence-Based Diagnosis

A. History
   1. Only 31–62% of patients with TB have fever.
   2. 50% of patients with TB have fever and night sweats or night sweats alone.
   3. Cough was present for more than 1 month in 70% of patients and may be mild, nonproductive, purulent, or bloody.

4. Hemoptysis develops in 24% of patients with tuberculous pneumonia compared with 15% of those with CAP (LR+ 1.6).
5. 33% of TB cases are diagnosed after admission for an unrelated complaint.

 Patients with TB may complain primarily of night sweats and weight loss and have a normal lung exam. Pulmonary TB still needs to be considered in such patients.

6. Symptoms and risk factors for disease tend to vary between older patients who often have reactivation TB and younger patients in whom primary TB is more common. Compared with older patients, younger patients have a higher incidence of alcoholism (66% vs 37%). In addition, younger patients more frequently have fever (62% vs 31%), night sweats (48% vs 6%), and hemoptysis (40% vs 17%).

B. PPD
   1. Immune response to 0.1 mL intradermal PPD
   2. Turns positive 4–7 weeks after primary infection
   3. Test results are determined by measuring the maximal diameter of *induration* (not redness).
   4. Maximal induration occurs 48–72 hours after injection.
   5. Table 9–5 lists the criteria for a positive reaction.
   6. *Significant* reaction suggests prior infection, not necessarily active disease. Patients with positive tests who do not have active TB are classified as having LTBI.
   7. Sensitivity (for active TB) 70–80%
      a. Primary TB: PPD is often negative
      b. Reactivation TB: PPD is positive in 80% of cases
      c. Tuberculous pleurisy: PPD usually positive
      d. AIDS patients with TB: PPD is positive in 50% of cases

 A negative PPD does *not* rule out active TB.

   8. Specificity 98–99% but lower in patients who received bacillus Calmette-Guérin (BCG) vaccination after infancy
   9. Interferon γ assays can also suggest LTBI or active TB infection and are more accurate in previously vaccinated patients (see below).
   10. Annual PPD
       a. Useful to determine whether patient has recently converted
       b. Recent converters are at higher risk for developing active TB
       c. Conversion defined as *increase* in induration of ≥ 10 mm
       d. Therapy is indicated for patients who have recently converted due to high risk of developing active TB.
       e. Indications for annual PPD
          (1) HIV infection
          (2) Health care workers

**Table 9–5.** Criteria for a positive PPD test.

| Diameter of Induration | Population |
|---|---|
| ≥ 5 mm | Patients with marked impaired immune response or high pretest probability<br>  HIV infection<br>  Immunosuppressed patients[1]<br>  Close contacts with persons with infectious TB<br>  Chest radiograph consistent with prior TB[2] |
| ≥ 10 mm | Patients with modest impaired immunity of moderate pretest probability<br>  Medical condition that carry an increased risk of active TB in patients with latent TB infection[3]<br>  Foreign born persons arriving from high prevalence area within 5 years<br>  Injection drug abuse<br>  Homeless persons<br>  Residents and staff of long-term care facilities (including prisons, shelters, nursing homes)<br>  Health care workers<br>  Children younger than 4 years<br>  Recent PPD converters (within 2 year period) |
| ≥ 15 mm | Patients with normal immunity and low pretest probability<br>  All others[4] |

[1]Equivalent to ≥ 15 mg of prednisone per day ≥ 1 month, recipient of tumor necrosis factor (TNF)-α inhibitors, organ transplant recipients.
[2]Chest radiographic findings suggestive of tuberculosis (TB) include fibrotic opacities occupying more than 2 cm of upper lobe; pleural thickening or isolated granuloma suggestive of TB.
[3]End-stage renal disease, malnutrition (or > 10% loss of ideal body weight), diabetes mellitus, lymphoma, leukemia, carcinoma of head, neck or lung, silicosis, gastrectomy or jejunoileal bypass.
[4]These patients should not be screened.
Adapted, with permission, from Jasmer RM et al. Latent tuberculosis infection. N Engl J Med. 2002;347:1860–66. Copyright © 2002. Massachusetts Medical Society. All rights reserved.

     (3) Correctional facility workers
     (4) Residents in long-term care facilities
     (5) Medical conditions that carry an increased risk of active TB (see above)
     (6) Homeless persons
  11. Indications for single PPD test
    a. Clinical suspicion of active TB
    b. Immigrants from high-incidence areas (eg, Africa, Asia, Latin America)
    c. Status post exposure to TB
    d. Fibrotic lung lesion
  12. Effect of BCG on PPD
    a. Vaccine used in some countries to prevent TB
    b. BCG has some similarities to PPD and may cause false-positive PPD reactions
     (1) False-positive PPD reactions (≥ 10 mm) are rare in adults who received BCG in infancy (≈1%)
     (2) However, false-positives are more common in BCG recipients who were vaccinated ≥ 2 years of

age (40%). False-positive PPDs remained common in this group even more than 10 years later (20%).
  13. Booster phenomenon
    a. In patients with latent TB, the PPD may revert to negative many years after infection.
    b. In such patients, the *initial* PPD may be negative but stimulate immune memory cells such that *subsequent* PPD tests may be positive.
    c. Subsequent positive tests may be *misinterpreted* as recent conversion.
    d. Misinterpretation can be avoided by performing the 2-step skin tests in patients scheduled for annual PPD.
    e. Patients with initial negative PPD are retested 1 week later.
     (1) Patient in whom the second PPD test is positive should be treated as though the first test was positive.
     (2) Patients in whom the second PPD test is negative are truly negative. Any future positive reactions in these patients should be considered recent conversions.
C. Interferon γ assays
  1. Lymphocytes from patients with LTBI or active TB produce interferon γ when exposed to TB antigens.
  2. Blood tests have been recently developed that expose the patient's lymphocytes to *highly* specific TB antigens (not shared with BCG or most non-tuberculous mycobacteria) and measure the production of interferon γ by the patient's lymphocytes.
  3. These tests are highly specific for *active* or *latent* TB infection.
    a. Prior BCG vaccination and infection with non-tuberculous mycobacteria do not cause false-positive reactions that might be seen with PPD.
    b. A recent meta-analysis summarized the sensitivity and specificity of these tests (and PPD) in patients with and without prior BCG vaccination and is shown in Table 9–6.
    c. Interferon γ assays are markedly superior to the PPD in patients with prior BCG vaccination LR+ > 10 versus 1.9, respectively.
  4. Positive results confirm either active or latent TB.
  5. Positive results do not distinguish active TB from LTBI. In patients with pneumonia, a positive result could be due to active TB, or non-tuberculous pneumonia (ie, streptococcal) in a patient with latent TB.
  6. Negative tests decrease the likelihood of TB infection but are not sufficiently sensitive to rule out active TB when the clinical suspicion is high (LR– 0.13–0.25).
  7. One paper suggested the likelihood of TB was very low in patients with both a negative PPD and a negative interferon γ assay (LR– 0.02–0.04). If confirmed in other studies, this could be used to rule out TB.
  8. Interferon assays are more sensitive to TB infections in immunocompromised patients (ie, HIV infection) and in patients with active TB.
  9. When used for the evaluation of latent TB, patients with positive results on interferon γ assays are more likely to develop active TB (if left untreated) than patients with a positive PPD (14.6% vs 2.3%).

**Table 9–6.** Characteristics of various TB tests in patients with and without prior BCG vaccination.

| Test | Sensitivity | Specificity | LR+ | LR– |
|---|---|---|---|---|
| **Patients without prior BCG vaccination** | | | | |
| QuantiFERON-TB | 78% | 99% | 78 | 0.22 |
| QuantiFERON-TB Gold In-Tube | 70% | 99% | 70 | 0.3 |
| T-SPOT.TB | 90% | 93% | 12.9 | 0.11 |
| PPD | ≥ 15mm: 70%<br>≥ 10mm: 73%<br>≥ 5mm: 80% | 97% | 25.6[1] | 0.24 |
| **Patients with prior BCG Vaccination** | | | | |
| QuantiFERON-TB | 78% | 96% | 19.5 | 0.23 |
| QuantiFERON-TB Gold In-Tube | 70% | 96% | 17.5 | 0.31 |
| T-SPOT.TB | 90% | 93% | 12.9 | 0.11 |
| PPD | ≥15 mm: 70%<br>≥10 m: 73%<br>≥5 mm: 80% | 59% | 1.9[2] | 0.39 |

[1]Calculated using an average sensitivity of PPD of 77%.
[2]Calculated using an average sensitivity of PPD of 77%.

**Table 9–7.** Sensitivity of test according to the number of sputum specimens sent to the laboratory.

| Number of Specimen | Sensitivity | | |
|---|---|---|---|
| | Culture Alone | Sputum Stain Alone | Either |
| 1 | 79% | 58% | 81% |
| 2 | 96% | 82% | 97% |
| 3 | 99% | 93% | 99% |

Reprinted, with permission, from Scott B. Early identification and isolation of inpatients at high risk for tuberculosis. Arch Intern Med. 1994;154:326–30.

10. In addition to the higher specificity and sensitivity of these assays over PPD, they have the added advantage of not requiring a return visit by the patient to have the test read, and do not require the expertise of an intradermal injection or reading. The CDC has recommended that interferon assays replace PPD for the diagnosis of active and latent TB infections.

D. Diagnosis of active TB

  1. Chest x-ray and clinical features on admission

    a. The chest radiograph in TB usually presents in 1 of 3 patterns: apical disease, cavitary disease, or reticular nodular pattern. Such patterns are *consistent* with TB.

      (1) Sensitivity, 86%; specificity, 83%

      (2) LR+, 5.0; LR–, 0.16

 TB should be considered in patients with apical, cavitary, or reticulonodular patterns on chest radiograph. TB is unlikely if none of these features are present.

    b. Cavitation is seen in 19–50% of cases (OR for TB 3.9). The walls are usually thick and irregular. Air-fluid levels are rare and may indicate anaerobic abscess or superinfection.

    c. Endobronchial spread may result in nodular disease that clusters in the dependent portion of the lung.

    d. Calcification can be seen in active lesions. Demonstrating stability requires comparison of prior films.

    e. 5% of patients with reactivation pulmonary TB have normal chest radiographs.

    f. The chest radiograph in HIV-positive patients is often atypical (see Chapter 5, HIV/AIDS).

  2. AFB stain and culture

    a. Culture is the gold standard and is specific.

    b. Sensitivity depends on the number of specimens (Table 9–7).

    c. Patients with positive smears are more infectious that patients who are culture positive but have negative smears; 35% of family members of persons with positive smears are PPD positive compared with 9% of family members when patients are smear negative.

    d. Other mycobacteria may lead to false-positive smears.

    e. Specific nucleic amplification tests of sputum for TB RNA or DNA are specific for TB and can help distinguish TB from other mycobacteria.

      (1) Helps distinguish TB from *Mycobacterium avium* complex (MAC) or commensual organisms that are also acid-fast positive.

      (2) Primarily used when AFB stains positive

      (3) Particularly useful if suspicion of TB is low

        (a) Positive rapid tests help confirm TB, negative tests make TB less likely

        (b) 95% sensitive and specific in this situation

      (4) May also be useful when clinical suspicion is high and smear is negative

        (a) Rapid tests reported to be 53% sensitive, 93% specific.

        (b) Positive tests suggest TB.

        (c) Cultures still required to test drug susceptibility

      (5) A diagnostic algorithm for TB is shown in Figure 9–1.

  3. BAL

    a. Smears: 38% sensitive, 100% specific

    b. Culture or smear: 74% sensitive, 75% specific

    c. Comparable to data for a single induced sputum

    d. Not routine or superior to induced sputums

    e. Use when induced sputums are unavailable.

E. Tuberculous pleurisy with effusion

  1. Typical pleural fluid findings

    a. Exudative effusion

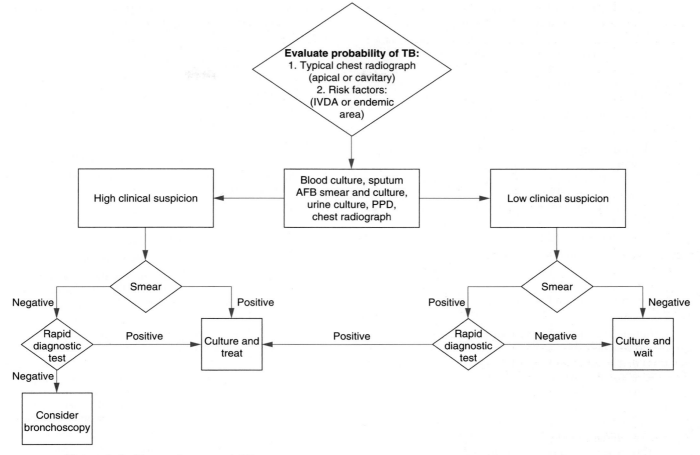

**Figure 9–1.** Diagnostic approach: TB.

b. Pleural fluid glucose variable

c. Pleural fluid pH always < 7.4

d. WBC 1000–6000 cells/mcL with neutrophilic predominance early and lymphocytic predominance later. Pleural fluid eosinophils > 10% suggests alternative diagnosis (unless prior thoracentesis).

2. Sensitivity of tests for diagnosis of tuberculous pleurisy

a. Pleural fluid culture, < 30%

b. Pleural biopsy culture, 40–80%

c. Pleural biopsy histology (caseating granulomas), 50–97%

d. Histology and pleural tissue culture > 60–95%

e. Sputum culture, 20–50%

3. Adenosine deaminase: Utility unclear due to different cut points and different isoenzymes.

4. Pleural fluid interferon γ 89% sensitive, 97% specific

**Treatment**

A. Isolation

1. Only 1% of all patients tested for TB are proven to have TB. Consider isolation of hospitalized patients with upper lobe, cavitary, or reticulonodular disease.

2. Highest risk of contagion among household contacts, schoolmates, or other close contacts.

3. Patients with cavitary disease, HIV, or watery sputum have the highest infectivity.

B. Principles of therapy

1. Multi-drug resistance is a significant problem.

2. Precise drug recommendations evolve due to resistance.

3. Susceptibility testing is critical to ensure an appropriate regimen is used.

4. Premature discontinuation and nonadherence promotes drug resistance and must be avoided. Direct observed therapy (DOT) refers to treatment protocols where public health officials directly observe patients swallow *each* dose of medication (administered 2–3 times/week). DOT is strongly recommended.

5. Due to the public health risks of MDR-TB, the responsibility for prescribing appropriate therapy and ensuring adherence rests on the public health program and clinician.

6. Effective regimens require at least 2 drugs to which the organism is susceptible.

7. Effective therapy takes many months.

8. TB therapy in HIV-infected patients is complex due to innumerable drug interactions with highly active antiretroviral

therapy (HAART) and the need for differing regimens depending on the degree of immunosuppression.

9. To determine the duration of therapy, all patients should have monthly sputums smears analyzed for AFB stain and culture until 2 consecutive sputum cultures are negative.

10. All patients should be seen monthly to assess symptoms, side effects, and adherence to therapy.

11. Infectious disease consultation is advised.

C. Multidrug resistant TB (MDR-TB)

1. Defined as organisms that are resistant to isoniazid and rifampin

2. Suspect MDR-TB in patients previously treated for TB, in patients who are HIV positive, in close contacts of patients with MDR-TB, and in patients who have not responded to therapy.

3. DOT should be used for patients with MDR-TB.

4. Surgery is occasionally used for patients with localized disease and persistently positive sputums. Antituberculous therapy is continued.

5. Expert consultation is mandatory.

D. Treatment in patients at low risk for MDR-TB

1. Initiate therapy with isoniazid, rifampin, pyrazinamide, and ethambutol.

2. After 2 months, the regimen is simplified to isoniazid and rifampin, if the organism is fully susceptible, for an additional 4 months.

3. Patients with cavitary TB who have positive sputum culture at 2 months should receive isoniazid and rifampin for an additional 3 months (9 months of therapy altogether).

4. The median duration of fever after the institution of antituberculous drugs was 10 days but ranged from 1 to 109 days. For patients with tuberculous effusion, resorption can take 4 months.

E. Pleural fluid drainage does not improve outcome in patients with tuberculous effusions (nonempyema).

F. Latent TB

1. Definition of positive PPD test depends on the population (see Table 9–5).

2. The patients with the highest priority for treatment of latent TB include recent contacts of infectious TB, patients with HIV infection, and recent immigrants from high TB prevalence areas.

3. Prior to treatment for LTBI, active infection must be ruled out with a careful history, physical exam, and chest radiograph.

4. Expert consultation is recommended if exposure to drug-resistant TB is likely.

5. Isoniazid

   a. Drug most commonly used for latent TB

   b. Dose is 300 mg/d for 9 months or 900 mg twice a week with DOT.

   c. Side effects

      (1) Hepatitis

         (a) Reported incidence is 0.1–2.3%

         (b) Incidence may be higher in older patients.

         (c) Alcohol consumption is the most important risk factor for isoniazid hepatitis. Patients who are taking isoniazid should avoid drinking alcohol.

         (d) Monitoring monthly for *clinical* symptoms of hepatitis

         (e) Obtain baseline and monthly liver function tests in patients with risk factors for hepatitis (alcohol consumption, pregnant and postpartum patients, HIV-infected patients, patients with chronic liver disease or other hepatotoxic medications).

         (f) Repeat liver function tests in symptomatic patients (right upper quadrant pain, anorexia, or nausea)

      (2) Peripheral neuropathy develops in 2% of patients taking isoniazid and can be prevented with pyridoxine (10–25 mg/d).

6. Other options are available in patients with isoniazid-resistant TB and in those intolerant of isoniazid.

## CASE RESOLUTION

Fortunately, Mr. P's HIV result was negative. His PPD and AFB smears were negative. On day 3 of his hospitalization, he became agitated, tachycardic, and complained of visual hallucinations. He was treated for delirium tremens with high doses of IV benzodiazepines. By day 5, he was improving. He was afebrile and his appetite improved. He was given a prescription for oral antibiotics and discharged to an outpatient alcohol treatment center.

Patients with a history of alcohol abuse must be monitored for withdrawal during any hospitalization.

## REVIEW OF OTHER IMPORTANT DISEASES

### Influenza

**Textbook Presentation**

Although there is a wide range of severity of influenza symptoms, patients typically complain of a severe, febrile, respiratory illness that began abruptly. Complaints include an abrupt onset ("like being hit by a train"), severe myalgias (even their eyes hurt when they look around), diffuse pain (they may complain that their hair or skin hurts), respiratory symptoms (cough, rhinitis, pharyngitis), and fever that is often pronounced and peaks within 12 hours (occasionally as high as 40–41°C). Influenza typically occurs between December and May. Patients may have rigors (frankly shaking chills) and headache (Figure 9–2).

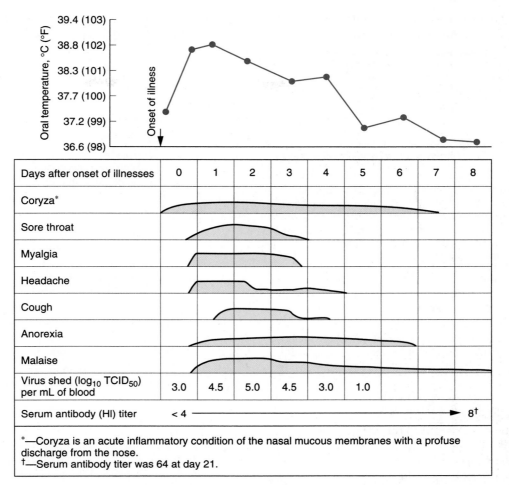

**Figure 9–2.** The typical clinical course of influenza. (Reproduced with permission from Montalto NJ. An office-based approach to influenza: Clinical diagnoses and laboratory testing. Am Fam Physician. 2003;67:111–18. Copyright © 2003. American Academy of Family Physicians.)

 Influenza is an unlikely diagnosis in the late spring, summer, or early fall.

## Disease Highlights

A. Pathogenesis
  1. Influenza virus A or B infects respiratory epithelium.
  2. Antigenic change in the virus surface glycoprotein (hemagglutinin or neuraminidase) renders populations susceptible to the virus. Antigenic shifts are most common with influenza virus A and are associated with epidemics. The pandemic of 1918 is believed responsible for 40 million deaths.
  3. Adults are infectious from the day prior to the onset of symptoms until about 5 days later (10 days in children).
  4. The incubation period is 1–4 days.

B. Manifestations
  1. History
     a. Onset is sudden in 75% of cases.

  b. Fever present in 51% of cases.
     (1) Peaks within 12–24 hours of onset of illness
     (2) Typically 38.0-40.0°C, occasionally 41.0°C
     (3) Typical duration is 3 days but may last 1–5 days

 High fever within 12–24 hours of symptom onset is typical of influenza but not other viral respiratory pathogens.

 Fever that increases over several days is not typical of influenza. When accompanied by cough, such a fever suggests bacterial pneumonia.

  c. Prevalence of other symptoms in influenza
     (1) Headache, 58–81%
     (2) Cough, 48–94%
     (3) Sore throat, 46–70%
     (4) GI symptoms are not characteristic of influenza.

***Table 9–8.*** Comparison of features in influenza, community-acquired pneumonia, and acute bronchitis.

| Infection | High Fever[1] | Localized Lung Findings[2] | Shortness of Breath[3] | Season |
|---|---|---|---|---|
| Community acquired pneumonia | Common | Common | Variable | Anytime |
| Influenza | Common | Uncommon | Uncommon[4] | December–May |
| Acute bronchitis | Uncommon | Uncommon | Uncommon | Anytime |

[1]Indication for chest film (unless flu season *and* patient has normal lung exam).
[2]Findings include crackles, dullness, bronchophony or egophony. All such findings indication for chest film.
[3]Indication for chest film.
[4]Unless influenza pneumonia.

 Patients with significant diarrhea or vomiting should be evaluated for an alternative diagnosis.

    **d.** Symptoms help distinguish influenza from acute bronchitis or pneumonia (Table 9–8).

  **2.** Crackles are seen in < 25% of patients.

**C.** Complications

  **1.** Pneumonia

    **a.** High-risk groups for pneumonia and death include

      **(1)** Elderly. Influenza mortality rates are 200 times greater in patients over age 65 than in patients aged 0–49 years.

      **(2)** HIV-infected patients also suffer a 100 times increase in mortality.

      **(3)** Other high-risk groups include patients with HF and COPD; immunocompromised patients; pregnant patients; and patients with renal disease, diabetes mellitus, or hemoglobinopathies.

    **b.** Two types of pneumonia are seen in influenza patients.

      **(1)** Influenza pneumonia per se

      **(2)** *Post*-influenza bacterial pneumonia

    **c.** Influenza pneumonia

      **(1)** Often develops within 1 day of onset of influenza

      **(2)** Most frequent in patients with underlying cardiopulmonary disease, diabetes, immunodeficiency states, and pregnancy.

      **(3)** Patients with influenza pneumonia complain of shortness of breath more often than patients with uncomplicated influenza (82% vs 17%).

 Obtain a chest film in patients with influenza and shortness of breath to rule out pneumonia.

      **(4)** Associated with tachycardia, tachypnea, cyanosis, and crackles on pulmonary exam

      **(5)** Hypoxemia and leukocytosis may be seen

      **(6)** Chest film shows bilateral or lobar pulmonary infiltrates.

      **(7)** 29% mortality

      **(8)** Treatment

        **(a)** Antiviral therapy

        **(b)** Empiric antibacterial agents pending culture

        **(c)** Oxygen

        **(d)** Intubation, with positive end-expiratory pressure as necessary

        **(e)** Antibiotics should cover methicillin-resistant *S aureus* in endemic regions.

    **d.** Postinfluenza (secondary) bacterial pneumonia

      **(1)** Suspect when initial improvement is followed by worsening cough, purulent sputum, and increasing fever.

      **(2)** Among patients hospitalized for influenza pneumonia, 30% have concomitant bacterial pneumonia caused by *S aureus* or *S pneumoniae*

      **(3)** Chest film may show either bilateral or lobar infiltrates.

      **(4)** *S pneumoniae* is most common (29–48%).

      **(5)** *S aureus* is next most common (7–40%), highly destructive, and associated with significant incidence of empyema and death.

      **(6)** *Haemophilus* and *Moraxella* may also cause secondary pneumonia.

  **2.** Exacerbation of asthma or COPD

  **3.** Less common complications include HF, myositis, myocarditis, pericarditis, meningoencephalitis, Guillain-Barré syndrome

### Evidence-Based Diagnosis

**A.** History, physical exam, and vaccination status

  **1.** Current prevalence of influenza helps determine risk

    **a.** www.cdc.gov/flu/weekly/fluactivity.htm

    **b.** 888/232-3228

  **2.** Summary of findings and likelihood ratios is presented in Table 9–9.

    **a.** The negative likelihood ratios are modest, suggesting it is difficult to rule out influenza clinically. The absence of fever and cough helps decrease the likelihood of flu in patients of all ages, but less so in patients ≥ 60.

    **b.** Fever and cough, particularly in older patients, increases the likelihood of influenza.

    **c.** A clinical prediction rule helps rule in influenza (fever ≥ 37.8°C with at least 2 of the following: headache, myalgia, cough, or sore throat and symptom onset within 48 hours. In addition, the rule requires at least 2 cases of confirmed influenza in the community).

**B.** Laboratory results

  **1.** Confirmation is usually not required.

  **2.** During influenza outbreaks, empiric therapy without laboratory confirmation is appropriate in patients with typical symptoms, clear lung fields, and no history of vaccination who present within 48 hours of symptom onset.

**Table 9–9.** Likelihood ratios for signs and symptoms in influenza.

| Finding | Patients: all ages | | Patients ≥ 60 y | |
|---|---|---|---|---|
| | LR+ | LR– | LR+ | LR– |
| Fever | 1.8 | 0.40 | 3.8 | 0.72 |
| Cough | 1.1 | 0.42 | 2.0 | 0.57 |
| Chills | 1.1 | 0.68 | 2.6 | 0.66 |
| Fever and cough | 1.9 | 0.54 | 5.0 | 0.75 |
| Fever and cough and acute onset | 2 | 0.54 | 5.4 | 0.77 |
| Decision rule[1] | 6.5 | 0.3 | | |
| Vaccine history | 0.63 | 1.1 | | |

[1]See text.

3. Rapid testing is most appropriate in *non*influenza periods.
   a. Various methods are available including fluorescent antibody, reverse transcriptase PCR, enzyme immunoassays, and others.
   b. Sensitivity and specificity vary from test to test, source of sample, duration of illness, and patient age.
      (1) In general, the tests are highly specific (90–95%) and help rule in influenza when positive (LR+ 28.2).
      (2) However, the tests are not terribly sensitive (70–75%) and cannot rule out influenza (LR– 0.7).
   c. Nasopharyngeal swabs are more effective than throat swab specimens.
4. Institutionalized patients are at higher risk for respiratory syncytial virus, which can mimic influenza. Testing may be useful in such patients.

**Treatment**

A. Prevention
   1. Options include vaccination or chemoprophylaxis with neuraminidase inhibitors.
   2. Trivalent inactivated influenza vaccine (TIV)
      a. Prophylactic strategy of choice
      b. IM vaccine uses inactivated (killed) viruses that are currently prevalent.
      c. Updated and administered annually.
      d. 50% fewer cases of influenza, associated pneumonia, and hospitalizations
      e. 68% decrease in all cause mortality
      f. Contraindications
         (1) Egg allergy
         (2) Significant febrile illness at time of vaccination (Patients may be vaccinated during mild nonfebrile upper respiratory tract infections.)
         (3) History of Guillain-Barré syndrome following prior vaccination

   g. Adverse effects
      (1) Soreness at injection site occurs in 10–64% of patients
      (2) No increase in systemic symptoms (compared with placebo)
      (3) Guillain-Barré may increase by 1 case per million recipients.
      (4) Upper respiratory tract infection symptoms are *not* more common than placebo.
      (5) TIV cannot *cause* influenza.
   h. Indications
      (1) Patients older than 50 years
      (2) Patients with diabetes; cardiopulmonary disease (including asthma, smokers); renal, hepatic or hematologic disease (ie, sickle cell disease)
      (3) Any individual wishing to reduce their chance of influenza
      (4) Residents of long-term care facilities
      (5) Immunosuppression (including corticosteroid use, HIV disease)
      (6) Women who will be pregnant during flu season
      (7) Health care personnel
      (8) Employees or household members having contact with high-risk groups (including vaccinating contacts of children < 6 months)
      (9) Neurologic disease that impairs handling of respiratory secretions
      (10) Travelers to the Southern Hemisphere during April to December can consider vaccination or revaccination (if already vaccinated). Persons traveling with organized groups from many parts of the world can also consider vaccination.

3. Live-attenuated intranasal vaccine (LAIV)
   a. Uses live-attenuated strains administered intranasally that replicate poorly in the warmer lower respiratory tract.
   b. Increases upper respiratory symptoms due to intranasal viral replication. Compared with placebo, LAIV increases nasal congestion (45% vs 27%) and sore throat (28% vs 17%).
   c. Persons vaccinated with LAIV can transmit the attenuated infection to other persons.
   d. Should not be given to contacts of severely immunosuppressed individuals (ie, hematopoietic stem cell recipients).
   e. Approved for *healthy* nonpregnant persons 5–49 years
   f. Updated and administered annually
   g. Should not be given to patients with significant nasal congestion that may impair delivery
   h. Still under study in older adults
   i. Contraindications include egg allergy, pregnancy, a prior history of Guillain-Barré syndrome, or underlying medical conditions that serve as an indication for TIV.

4. Chemoprophylaxis
   a. Significantly more costly than vaccination

b. Oseltamivir and zanamivir are neuraminidase inhibitors active against influenza viruses A and B and are usually highly effective as chemoprophylaxis.

c. Amantadine and rimantadine are not effective against influenza B (and often not to influenza A) and should not be used for chemoprophylaxis or treatment.

d. Indications for chemoprophylaxis:

(1) Persons at high risk (or those who come in contact with such persons) who were vaccinated after exposure to influenza (treat for 2 weeks after vaccination).

(2) Persons with immune deficiencies who are unlikely to mount a response to vaccination (ie, those with advanced HIV disease) could also receive prophylaxis.

(3) Persons with contraindications to vaccination.

(4) Persons living in institutions during outbreaks (ie, nursing homes) regardless of vaccination status.

B. Treatment of influenza

1. Zanamivir and oseltamivir

a. When given within 48 hours of symptom onset, they reduce the symptom severity and the duration of symptoms approximately 1–2 days. Oseltamivir has also been demonstrated to reduce the incidence of pneumonia.

b. Minimal to no benefit is seen when started > 2 days after symptom onset.

c. Safety during pregnancy is unknown.

d. Studies suggest that empiric therapy is cost effective for several groups.

e. Rapid influenza testing is recommended if prevalence of influenza is low.

2. Oseltamivir

a. Route of administration is oral. Taking the drug with food decreases nausea and vomiting, which occurs in 10% of patients.

b. Transient neuropsychiatric events have been recorded.

c. Reduce the dose by 50% if creatinine clearance < 30 mL/min.

d. Drug resistance

(1) A strain of influenza A (H1N1) was discovered to be resistant to oseltamivir in the 2008–2009 season.

(2) The CDC has recommended combining oseltamivir with rimantadine or using zanamivir alone for this strain or if the influenza strain is unknown.

(3) Oseltamivir alone is recommended for other strains of influenza (influenza B or influenza A, H3N2).

3. Zanamivir

a. Route of administration is inhalation; can cause bronchospasm.

b. Not recommended in patients with asthma or COPD.

4. Indications for treatment

a. All people at high risk for complications in whom influenza develops, regardless of their vaccination status

b. Persons with severe influenza

c. Consider for persons with influenza who wish to shorten the duration of illness.

## REFERENCES

Call SA, Vollenweider MA, Hornung CA, Simel DL, McKinney WP. Does this patient have influenza? JAMA. 2005;293(8):987–97.

Dosanjh DP, Hinks TS, Innes JA et al. Improved diagnostic evaluation of suspected tuberculosis. Ann Intern Med. 2008;148(5):325–36.

Kikawada M, Iwamoto T, Takasaki M. Aspiration and infection in the elderly: epidemiology, diagnosis and management. Drugs Aging. 2005;22(2):115–30.

Kunimoto D, Long R. Tuberculosis: still overlooked as a cause of community-acquired pneumonia—how not to miss it. Respir Care Clin N Am. 2005;11(1): 25–34.

Metlay JP, Fine MJ. Testing strategies in the initial management of patients with community-acquired pneumonia. Ann Intern Med. 2003;138(2):109–18.

Metlay JP, Kapoor WN, Fine MJ. Does this patient have community-acquired pneumonia? Diagnosing pneumonia by history and physical examination. JAMA. 1997;278(17):1440–5.

Metlay JP, Schulz R, Li YH et al. Influence of age on symptoms at presentation in patients with community-acquired pneumonia. Arch Intern Med. 1997;157(13):1453–9.

Montalto NJ. An office-based approach to influenza: clinical diagnosis and laboratory testing. Am Fam Physician. 2003;67(1):111–8.

O'Brien WT Sr, Rohweder DA, Lattin GE Jr et al. Clinical indicators of radiographic findings in patients with suspected community-acquired pneumonia: who needs a chest x-ray? J Am Coll Radiol. 2006;3(9):703–6.

Pai M, Zwerling A, Menzies D. Systematic review: T-cell-based assays for the diagnosis of latent tuberculosis infection: an update. Ann Intern Med. 2008;149(3):177–84.

Rapid Diagnostic Testing for Influenza: Information for Health Care Professionals. (Accessed at http://www.cdc.gov/flu/professionals/diagnosis/rapidclin.htm.)

Role of Laboratory Diagnosis of Influenza. (Accessed at http://www.cdc.gov/flu/professionals/diagnosis/labrole.htm.)

Selwyn PA, Pumerantz AS, Durante A et al. Clinical predictors of *Pneumocystis carinii* pneumonia, bacterial pneumonia and tuberculosis in HIV-infected patients. AIDS. 1998;12(8):885–93.

Stein J, Louie J, Flanders S et al. Performance characteristics of clinical diagnosis, a clinical decision rule, and a rapid influenza test in the detection of influenza infection in a community sample of adults. Ann Emerg Med. 2005;46(5):412–9.

Tietjen PA. Clinical presentation and diagnosis of *Pneumocystis carinii* (*P. jiroveci*) infection in HIV-infected patients. In: UpToDate; 2008.

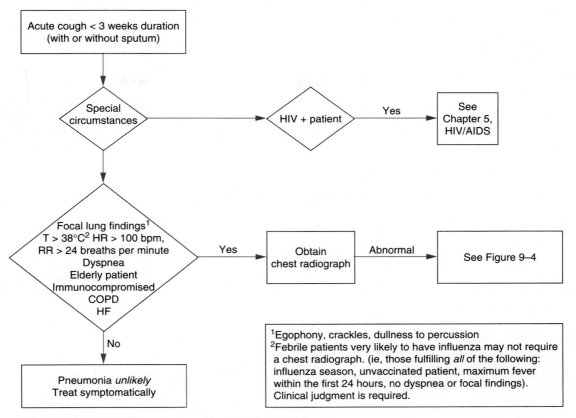

COPD, chronic obstructive pulmonary disease; HF, heart failure.

***Figure 9–3.*** Diagnostic approach: acute cough and fever.

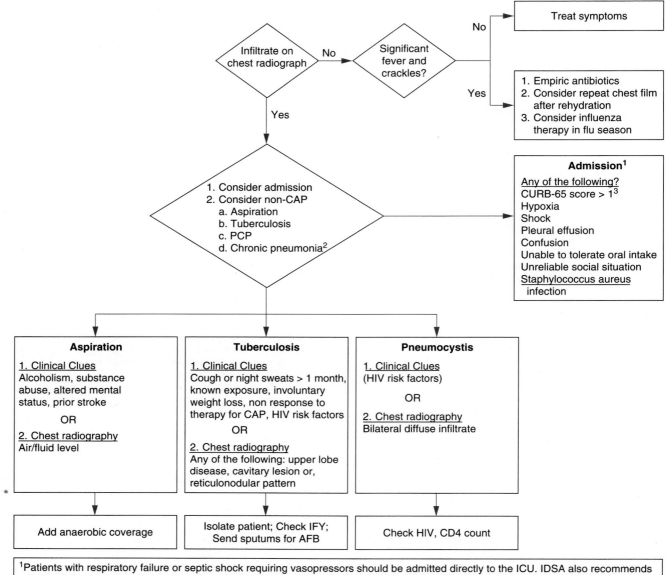

Treat symptoms

Infiltrate on chest radiograph — No → Significant fever and crackles? — No →

Yes ↓

Significant fever and crackles? — Yes →

1. Empiric antibiotics
2. Consider repeat chest film after rehydration
3. Consider influenza therapy in flu season

1. Consider admission
2. Consider non-CAP
   a. Aspiration
   b. Tuberculosis
   c. PCP
   d. Chronic pneumonia[2]

**Admission[1]**

Any of the following?
CURB-65 score > 1[3]
Hypoxia
Shock
Pleural effusion
Confusion
Unable to tolerate oral intake
Unreliable social situation
Staphylococcus aureus
  infection

**Aspiration**

1. Clinical Clues
Alcoholism, substance abuse, altered mental status, prior stroke

OR

2. Chest radiography
Air/fluid level

**Tuberculosis**

1. Clinical Clues
Cough or night sweats > 1 month, known exposure, involuntary weight loss, non response to therapy for CAP, HIV risk factors

OR

2. Chest radiography
Any of the following: upper lobe disease, cavitary lesion or, reticulonodular pattern

**Pneumocystis**

1. Clinical Clues
(HIV risk factors)

OR

2. Chest radiography
Bilateral diffuse infiltrate

Add anaerobic coverage

Isolate patient; Check IFY; Send sputums for AFB

Check HIV, CD4 count

[1]Patients with respiratory failure or septic shock requiring vasopressors should be admitted directly to the ICU. IDSA also recommends ICU admission for patients with 3 or more of the following: RR > 30, $PaO_2/FIO_2$ < 250 mm Hg, multilobar infiltrates, confusion, BUN > 20 mg/dL, leukopenia resulting from infection, thrombocytopenia, hypothermia or hypotension requiring aggressive fluid resuscitation.
[2]Chronic: Consider fungal pneumonia and tuberculosis. Consider bronchoscopy.
[3]Curb-65 criteria: Confusion (to person, place or time), Uremia (BUN > 20 mg/dL), RR ≥ 30 breaths per minute, Systolic BP < 90 mm Hg or diastolic BP ≤ 60 mm Hg, age ≥ 65.

AFB, acid-fast bacilli; CAP, community-acquired pneumonia; IDSA, infectious diseases society of America; PCP, pneumocystis pneumonia; TX algorithm-expansion of abbrev.

***Figure 9–4.*** Response to the results of the CXR in patients with cough and fever.

# I have a patient with delirium or dementia. How do I determine the cause?

## CHIEF COMPLAINT

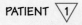

PATIENT 1

Mr. B is a previously healthy 70-year-old man who underwent right upper lobectomy for localized squamous cell lung cancer 5 days ago. On morning rounds, he comments that he is in a military barracks and that he is ready to go home.

> What is the differential diagnosis of delirium and dementia? How would you frame the differential?

## CONSTRUCTING A DIFFERENTIAL DIAGNOSIS

Delirium and dementia are both syndromes of neurologic dysfunction. Both present as a "change in mental status." Their similarities end here. Whereas delirium is acute, usually reversible and nearly always has an underlying, non-neurologic etiology, dementia is chronic and seldom reversible. The definitions of these syndromes, as included in the DSM-IV-TR follow:

A. Delirium
   1. Disturbance of consciousness with reduced ability to focus, sustain, or shift attention.
   2. Cognitive change that is not better explained by dementia.
   3. Symptoms develop rapidly (hours to days) and tend to vary during the day.
   4. History, physical exam, or laboratory data suggest that a general medical condition has directly caused the condition.

B. Dementia
   1. Impaired memory plus at least 1 of the following:
      a. Aphasia (inability to produce or comprehend language)
      b. Apraxia (inability to execute purposeful movements)
      c. Agnosia (inability to recognize objects by feel)
      d. Impaired executive functioning (eg, abstracting and organizing)
   2. Symptoms must also impair work, social, or personal functioning.

Because any illness can cause delirium in a susceptible patient, the differential diagnosis of delirium is long and needs to consider a broad range of illnesses, comorbidities, and medication effects. The differential diagnosis of dementia is more finite; disorders have been listed in order of their approximate prevalence as etiologic factors.

A. Delirium
   1. Metabolic
      a. Dehydration
      b. Electrolyte abnormalities
      c. Hyperglycemia or hypoglycemia
      d. Acidosis or alkalosis
      e. Liver disease
      f. Hypoxia or hypercarbia
      g. Uncontrolled thyroid disease
      h. Azotemia
      i. Thiamine deficiency (Wernicke encephalopathy)
   2. Infectious disease
      a. CNS infection
      b. Systemic infection of any kind
      c. HIV
   3. Cerebrovascular event
      a. Ischemic stroke
      b. Hemorrhagic stroke
      c. Vasculitis
   4. CNS mass
      a. Tumor
      b. Subdural hematoma
   5. Cardiovascular
      a. Myocardial infarction
      b. Heart failure
      c. Arrhythmia
   6. Drugs
      a. Alcohol withdrawal
      b. Diuretics
      c. Anticholinergics
      d. Nonsteroidal antiinflammatory drugs
      e. Corticosteroids
      f. Digoxin
      g. Opioids
      h. Antidepressants
      i. Anxiolytics
   7. Miscellaneous
      a. Fecal impaction
      b. Urinary retention
      c. Sensory deprivation
      c. Severe illness

B. Dementia

   1. Alzheimer dementia

   2. Dementia with Lewy bodies

   3. Vascular dementia

   4. Frontotemporal dementia

   5. Alcohol-related

   6. Uncommon dementias

     a. Subdural hematoma

     b. Hypothyroid

     c. Vitamin $B_{12}$ deficient

     d. Infectious

       (1) Syphilis

       (2) Prion disease

     e. Normal-pressure hydrocephalus

Almost any illness can cause delirium in a susceptible patient.

Mr. B was previously healthy with only mild chronic
obstructive pulmonary disease. His surgery went well but
was complicated by transient hypotension and excessive
blood loss. He was extubated on postoperative day 3. On
postoperative day 4, his wife noted some confusion. The
medical team did not detect any abnormalities when
they evaluated him.

Today, postoperative day 5, he is more confused. He is
oriented only to person. He is unable to answer any minimally complicated questions.

At this point, what is the leading hypothesis,
what are the active alternatives, and is there
a must not miss diagnosis? Given this differential diagnosis, what tests should be
ordered?

## PRIORITIZING THE DIFFERENTIAL DIAGNOSIS

Based on his history, Mr. B's subacute mental status change
appears to fulfill the definition of delirium. The pivotal points are
that his symptoms seem to vary, he is disoriented, and he is inat-
tentive. He certainly has many potential causes of delirium.
Although Mr. B does not have a history of alcohol abuse, alcohol
withdrawal is always a possible diagnosis for acute mental status
changes in the hospital and should not be missed. Stroke and
seizure, although commonly considered in the differential diagnosis of mental status change, are rare causes of delirium. Table 10–1
lists the differential diagnosis.

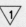

On physical exam, Mr. B is lying in bed. He is irritable and
somewhat hypervigilant, becoming frustrated during

**Table 10–1.** Diagnostic hypotheses for Mr. B.

| Diagnostic Hypotheses | Clinical Clues | Important Tests |
|---|---|---|
| **Leading Hypothesis** | | |
| Delirium caused by postsurgical state, fluid and electrolyte abnormalities, hypoxia or hypercarbia, medications, or cardiac ischemia | Subacute onset and fluctuating course | Confusion Assessment Method Basic metabolic panel Pulse oximetry/ABG Urinalysis ECG Review of medications |
| **Active Alternative—Must Not Miss** | | |
| Delirium caused by alcohol withdrawal | History of alcohol use Predictable syndrome with systemic and neurologic symptoms | Clinical diagnosis |
| **Other Alternative** | | |
| Delirium caused by stroke, seizure, or meningitis | Focal neurologic exam Seizure activity Fever or meningismus | Rarely needed (see text) CNS imaging EEG Lumbar puncture |

questioning. His vital signs are temperature, 37.0°C; BP,
146/90 mm Hg; pulse, 80 bpm; RR, 18 breaths per
minute. General physical exam reveals a healing surgical
scar, normal lung, heart, and abdominal exam. On neurologic exam, he scores a 3 out of 4 on the confusion
assessment method. The remainder of the neurologic
exam is normal.

Initial laboratory data, including basic metabolic panel,
liver function tests (LFTs), and urinalysis, are normal.

Is the clinical information sufficient to make
a diagnosis? If not, what other information
do you need?

## Leading Hypothesis: Delirium

### Textbook Presentation

Delirium commonly manifests as inattention and confusion (often
referred to as mental status change). It is usually seen in older
patients with severe illness. Clouding of consciousness has classically been used to describe a patient's symptoms.

### Disease Highlights

A. Almost any illness can present as delirium in a susceptible
patient.

B. Delirium often complicates medical or surgical hospitalizations.

C. The most important clue to delirium is the acuity of onset and fluctuation in course.

D. It is most common in older persons and in patients with underlying neurologic disease.

 There is always a cause of delirium. Clinicians must recognize delirium and identify the cause.

E. Several diseases are more likely to cause delirium than others.
1. Severe illness
2. Drug toxicity
3. Fluid and electrolyte disturbances (hyponatremia and azotemia)
4. Infections
5. Hypothermia or hyperthermia

F. Delirium is very common in sick, hospitalized patients over the age of 65.
1. 10% of emergency department patients
2. 12–25% of medical patients
3. 20–50% of surgical patients (highest in patients after hip replacement)

 Assume that a sick, older patient, with an acute deterioration in mental status is delirious until proved otherwise.

G. The prognosis of delirium is poor.
1. Although studies provided mixed data as to whether there are mortality differences when patients with delirium are compared with matched controls, patients in whom delirium develops will have worse functional status and less independence at discharge.
2. Patients with dementia and delirium have the worst prognosis.
3. Delirium can also persist. Many studies show that most patients in whom delirium develops have at least some persistent symptoms at discharge that may continue to be present months later.

 Only in a small percentage of patients will delirium resolve completely with cure of the underlying disease or returning home.

H. Delirium can occasionally "unmask" an underlying dementia. This occurs when a patient with a mild, undiagnosed dementia becomes delirious in the hospital and is evaluated more fully for cognitive impairment after recovery.

## Evidence-Based Diagnosis

A. Pretest probability
1. Predictors of delirium have been identified in various studies. These help provide pretest probabilities.
2. One study developed a model to determine a patient's risk of delirium developing while in the hospital. Predictors included:
   a. Vision impairment
   b. Severe illness
   c. Cognitive impairment
   d. High BUN/creatinine ratio
3. In a patient population with a mean age of 78, the number of risk factors present correlated with the risk of developing delirium.
   a. No risk factors: 3% chance of delirium developing.
   b. 1 or 2 risk factors: 14% chance of delirium developing.
   c. 3 or 4 risk factors: 26% chance of delirium developing.
4. Several predictors from another study, with ORs for association with delirium, are listed in Table 10–2.

 Consider a patient's risk for delirium upon hospital admission; a prior identification potentially lessens the likelihood of delirium and promotes a more appropriate response if it does.

B. Diagnosis
1. Doctors are generally not very good at recognizing delirium.
2. A routine exam is very specific but not very sensitive for the diagnosis of delirium.
3. The confusion assessment method (CAM) is one of the best-validated and most widely used tools for diagnosing delirium.
4. The CAM is considered positive when a patient fulfills criteria a and b and either c or d:
   a. Acute onset and fluctuating course
      (1) Is there evidence of an acute change in mental status from the patient's baseline?
      (2) Does the behavior fluctuate during the day?
   b. Inattention: Does the patient have difficulty focusing his or her attention (is the patient easily distracted or have trouble following the conversation)?
   c. Disorganized thinking: Is the patient's thinking disorganized or incoherent (such as rambling or irrelevant conversation, unclear or illogical flow of ideas, or unpredictable switching from subject to subject)?
   d. Altered level of consciousness: Anything other than alert (vigilant, lethargic, stupor)

**Table 10–2.** Predictors for delirium.

| Predictor | Odds Ratio |
| --- | --- |
| Abnormal sodium level | 6.2 |
| Severe illness | 5.9 |
| Chronic cognitive impairment | 5.3 |
| Hypothermia or hyperthermia | 5.0 |
| Moderate illness | 4.0 |
| Psychoactive drug use | 3.9 |
| Azotemia | 2.9 |

Modified from Francis J, Martin D, Kapoor WN. A prospective study of delirium in hospitalized elderly. JAMA. 1990;263:1097–1101. Copyright © 1990, American Medical Association. All rights reserved.

***Table 10–3.*** Test characteristics for the CAM and emergency department evaluation in the diagnosis of delirium.

| Criteria | Sensitivity | Specificity | LR+ | LR– |
|---|---|---|---|---|
| Evaluation in emergency department | 17–35 | 98–100 | 8.5–∞ | 0.65–0.85 |
| CAM | 94–100 | 90–95 | 9.4–20 | 0.00–0.07 |

CAM, Confusion Assessment Method.

 When using the CAM, make use of information from family members and medical staff; do not rely on a single mental status exam.

5. Table 10–3 compares the test characteristics of the CAM with those from a routine evaluation in the emergency department.

6. A positive CAM is essentially diagnostic of delirium.

C. Etiology

  1. Common causes

    a. The search for a cause of delirium involves a review of the most common causes of delirium.

    b. Repeat a full physical exam, focusing on sources of infection.

    c. Review medications in detail, including reconciling home and hospital medication to ensure that psychoactive medications have not been inadvertently discontinued (eg, benzodiazepines, opioids).

 Medication toxicity, even at therapeutic doses, is a common cause of delirium and is particularly common in older patients. Review all medications, especially psychoactive ones.

    d. Always order basic laboratory tests, such as a CBC, basic metabolic panel, LFTs, and urinalysis.

    e. Consider other tests (based on the clinical situation) such as ECG, chest radiograph, pulse oximetry (with ABG if the patient is at risk for $CO_2$ retention), and blood and urine cultures.

  2. Uncommon causes

    a. A common question when evaluating a patient with delirium is: If the initial work-up is negative, is it reasonable to assume the delirium is related to the acute illness or should the patient be assessed for diseases that directly affect the CNS (eg, stroke, seizure, and meningitis or encephalitis)?

      (1) Stroke

        (a) Very rare cause of delirium

        (b) A very good study has only about 7% of cases of delirium caused by stroke.

        (c) 97% of these patients had focal abnormalities on a careful neurologic exam.

      (2) Seizure

        (a) Nonconvulsive seizures, such as temporal lobe epilepsy, are usually recognized by their intermittent nature.

        (b) Nonconvulsive status epilepticus is very rare but is a potential cause of mental status consistent with severe delirium. Patients with nonconvulsive status epilepticus almost always have risk factors for seizures or abnormal eye movements, defined as eye jerking, hippus (unprovoked changes in pupil size), repeated blinking, and persistent eye deviation.

      (3) Meningitis: Fever and mental status change may be the only presenting symptoms.

    b. In the work-up of delirium, consider neuroimaging, EEG, and lumbar puncture only in certain conditions.

      (1) **Neuroimaging** is only necessary if delirium is associated with a focal neurologic exam or if there is a very high suspicion of a cerebrovascular event.

      (2) **EEG** is only necessary if there is no other explanation for delirium and the patient has either risk factors for, or signs of, seizures.

      (3) **Lumbar puncture** is only necessary if there is fever with no other source or a suspicion for a CNS infection.

**Treatment**

A. Prevention

  1. Because of the poor prognosis of delirium, prevention is the goal.

  2. Multidisciplinary interventions have been shown to prevent delirium. One study demonstrated a decrease in the rate of delirium from 15% to 9.9% (number needed to treat ≅ 20).

  3. The intervention addressed the risk factors in the following ways:

    a. Cognitive impairment: Repeated orientation of the patient and performance of cognitively stimulating activity (eg, discussion of current events).

    b. Sleep deprivation: Noise reduction and minimizing of nighttime activities.

    c. Immobility: Early mobilization.

    d. Visual and hearing impairment: Visual and hearing aids as well as adaptive devices.

    e. Dehydration: Aggressive volume repletion.

B. Treatment

  1. Once delirium occurs, the causes must be addressed and then supportive measures must be instituted.

    a. Administer fluids to prevent dehydration.

    b. Avoid sleep deprivation.

    c. Provide quiet environment.

    d. Keep nighttime awakenings to a minimum.

    e. Protect from falls or self-inflicted injury.

      (1) "Sitters" are preferable to restraints as the latter can increase the risk of physical injury.

      (2) Sitters can also provide constant reorientation and reassurance.

**(3)** Occasionally, medications such as low doses of neuroleptics can be used for sedation. Long-term use should be avoided whenever possible.

## MAKING A DIAGNOSIS

Review of Mr. B's medication list revealed that 0.5 mg doses of lorazepam ordered to be given as needed, were being given every 8 hours. Laboratory data was normal with the exception of an ABG: 7.36/46/70.

Have you crossed a diagnostic threshold for the leading hypothesis, delirium? Have you ruled out the active alternatives? Do other tests need to be done to exclude the alternative diagnoses?

By CAM criteria, Mr. B is clearly delirious. He has recently undergone a major surgery, he is taking medications known to cause delirium, and he is found to be hypoxic. Despite his intraoperative blood loss and hypotension there are no signs of a stroke, cardiac ischemia, heart failure, or anemia.

## Alternative Diagnosis: Alcohol Withdrawal

### Textbook Presentation

A typical presentation of inpatient alcohol withdrawal is the development of agitation, hypertension, and tachycardia in a patient during the first 2 days after hospital admission. Seizures may soon follow with delusions and delirium occurring during the first 3–5 days.

### Disease Highlights

**A.** Symptoms of alcohol withdrawal are stereotypical, occurring on a predictable time line as outlined in Figure 10–1.

**B.** The predominant symptoms of minor withdrawal are irritability, hypertension, and tachycardia.

**C.** Alcoholic hallucinosis is a syndrome of hallucinations, usually visual, with a clear sensorium that makes this easily distinguishable from delirium.

**D.** Major withdrawal is synonymous with delirium tremens.

   **1.** Occurs in patients with history of severe alcohol abuse.

   **2.** Confusion, disorientation, and autonomic hyperactivity are the hallmarks of this disorder.

**3.** Delirium tremens can be fatal if the patient does not receive appropriate supportive care.

**E.** Wernicke encephalopathy

   **1.** Wernicke encephalopathy is not an alcohol withdrawal syndrome but is caused by thiamine deficiency.

   **2.** Alcohol abuse is the most common cause of thiamine deficiency.

   **3.** Symptoms include the triad of confusion, disorders of ocular movement, and ataxia. The confusion commonly manifests as disorientation and indifference.

   **4.** Korsakoff syndrome is the chronic form of Wernicke encephalopathy. Korsakoff syndrome presents with memory problems and resulting confabulation.

### Evidence-Based Diagnosis

**A.** Delirium tremens and Wernicke encephalopathy are the alcohol-related syndromes most likely to be confused with nonalcohol-related delirium. Various features clearly differentiate these syndromes.

**B.** Wernicke encephalopathy

   **1.** Generally requires long-term alcohol abuse. (Rare cases of Wernicke encephalopathy with hyperemesis gravidarum or after bariatric surgery do occur.)

   **2.** It is important to recognize that Wernicke encephalopathy usually presents with only one or two of the features of the classic triad.

   **3.** Fluctuation that characterizes nonalcohol-related delirium is absent.

**C.** Delirium tremens

   **1.** Always preceded by minor withdrawal.

   **2.** Minor withdrawal is sometimes overlooked in the hospital if a patient is critically ill, sedated, or anesthetized.

   **3.** History of heavy alcohol use required.

   **4.** Adrenergic overactivity always present unless masked by medications.

     **a.** Hypertension

     **b.** Tachycardia

     **c.** Fever

**D.** The diagnoses of delirium tremens and Wernicke encephalopathy are clinical. They are based on suggestive clinical signs in the setting of a history of alcohol use. An appropriate response to treatment is helpful. There are specific MRI findings that are seen in Wernicke encephalopathy.

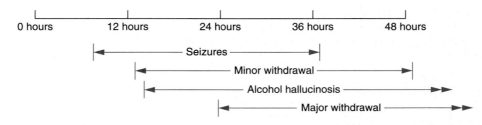

***Figure 10–1.*** Symptoms of alcohol withdrawal. (Reproduced from Virtual Naval Hospital. A Digital Library of Naval Medicine and Military Medicine. http://www.vnh.org/)

Every patient should have an alcohol history taken on admission. If a clinical syndrome suggestive of alcohol withdrawal occurs in a patient who denied alcohol use, information about alcohol use should be sought from other sources.

## Treatment

**A.** Both Wernicke encephalopathy and delirium tremens are preventable.

**B.** Wernicke encephalopathy

    **1.** Any patient in whom thiamine deficiency is suspected should receive 100 mg of IV thiamine prior to receiving glucose-containing fluids.

    **2.** Patients in whom Wernicke encephalopathy is suspected should receive thiamine until symptoms resolve.

**C.** Alcohol withdrawal and delirium tremens

    **1.** Supportive care

    **2.** Benzodiazepines

        **a.** Benzodiazepines decrease the symptoms of withdrawal and can prevent delirium tremens, seizures, and death.

        **b.** Some patients can be treated with benzodiazepines as outpatients.

        **c.** Indications for inpatient therapy

            **(1)** Moderate to severe withdrawal

            **(2)** Prior history of seizures or delirium tremens

            **(3)** Patient unable to cooperate with outpatient therapy

            **(4)** Comorbid psychiatric or medical conditions

            **(5)** Unsuccessful outpatient detoxification

        **d.** Inpatient management

            **(1)** The optimal dose of benzodiazepines cannot be determined in advance and must be titrated to the particular needs of the patient.

            **(2)** Benzodiazepines may either be given on a fixed-scheduled or be given to treat symptoms. Both strategies require careful patient monitoring and medication adjustment.

            **(3)** The Addiction Research Foundation Clinical Institute Withdrawal Assessment for Alcohol (CIWA-Ar) developed a tool to predict the level of alcohol withdrawal.

                **(a)** The tool scores the severity of symptoms in various categories such as tremor, anxiety, and sensory disturbances.

                **(b)** A higher score (> 8–12) generally calls for active pharmacologic management, whether using a fixed-dose or symptom-triggered protocol.

                **(c)** Printable version of the tool is available online at http://images2.clinicaltools.com/images/pdf/ciwa-ar.pdf

            **(4)** Fixed-schedule therapy

                **(a)** Delivers regular fixed doses of benzodiazepines to the patients.

                **(b)** Careful monitoring is still required to avoid undertreatment or oversedation.

                **(c)** Fixed-schedule therapy may provide a slight margin of safety if careful monitoring cannot be performed adequately.

            **(5)** Symptom-triggered therapy

                **(a)** Avoids unnecessary medications in the group of patients who will not need them.

                **(b)** Careful monitoring is required to avoid withdrawal and delirium tremens.

Careful monitoring and prompt patient-specific adjustment of the benzodiazepine dose is the key to successful management of the alcoholic patient.

    **3.** β-Blockers

        **a.** Can decrease sympathetic overactivity in patients during withdrawal

        **b.** Are useful adjuncts but because they can mask sympathetic signs that alert the clinician to increasingly severe withdrawal, they increase the risk of inadequate use of benzodiazepines.

## CASE RESOLUTION

On the afternoon of the fifth postoperative day, Mr. B pulled out his IV and attempted to climb out of bed while his chest tube was still attached. Around the clock observation was ordered.

Further history revealed no history of alcohol use. Mr. B was placed on oxygen with near normalization of his blood gas. The benzodiazepines were discontinued.

By postoperative day 8 (3 days after the onset of his delirium) Mr. B's mental status had returned nearly to baseline. He was still occasionally disoriented to time.

He was discharged on postoperative day 14. His wife noted him to still be occasionally "spacey" at the time of discharge. The patient was completely back to normal at a postoperative visit 14 days later.

The patient's delirium was severe for 3–4 days and persisted for at least 1 week. The delirium was assumed to be a symptom of hypoxia, the postsurgical state, and medication complication. No specific therapy was given. The patient's safety was ensured with a "sitter" and the reversible factors (hypoxia, medication dosing mistakes) were addressed.

## CHIEF COMPLAINT

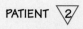

PATIENT 2

Mr. R is a 75-year-old man who comes to see you in clinic accompanied by his wife because she is concerned that his memory is getting worse. She states that, for the last few months, he has been getting lost driving 20 miles from his home to his local VA hospital where he volunteers. He has done this job twice weekly for 25 years.

At this point, what is the leading hypothesis, what are the active alternatives, and is there a must not miss diagnosis? Given this differential diagnosis, what tests should be ordered?

## PRIORITIZING THE DIFFERENTIAL DIAGNOSIS

Mr. R has had a decline in cognitive status. He is unable to do a higher-level task that he used to do. Given that this patient is exhibiting cognitive decline, dementia—most commonly Alzheimer disease (AD)—has to be included in the differential diagnosis. The subacute onset of this patient's symptoms, with loss of recall, makes AD likely. Another common cause of dementia in older persons is vascular dementia (VaD). It will be important to determine whether this patient has risk factors for cerebrovascular disease. In an older person, clinicians have to consider the normal cognitive decline that comes with aging, but normal cognitive aging never causes functional compromise. An alternative diagnosis is mild cognitive impairment (MCI), a syndrome of memory loss more severe than the memory loss that occurs with normal aging. MCI, however, also does not cause functional decline. Delirium and depression should always be considered in an older patient with cognitive decline because they are highly treatable. Table 10–4 lists the differential diagnosis.

A patient who is unable to successfully live independently because of cognitive issues always has an abnormality.

2

Mr. R's past medical history is notable for chronic leg pain resulting from a war injury. He also has a history of ischemic bowel, which has been asymptomatic since a hemicolectomy 3 years ago, and gout.

His medications are

1. Paroxetine, 20 mg daily
2. Methadone, 20 mg 3 times a day
3. Meloxicam, 7.5 mg daily, orally
4. Acetaminophen with codeine (300/60), 2 tablets 3 times a day
5. Allopurinol 300 mg daily, orally

Mr. R is a retired accountant. He completed 4 years of college on the GI bill after his service in Korea.

His physical exam reveals an alert, pleasant man. His vital signs are normal. He answers about half the history questions himself but turns to his wife for assistance with details about doctors he

**Table 10–4.** Diagnostic hypotheses for Mr. R.

| Diagnostic Hypotheses | Clinical Clues | Important Tests |
|---|---|---|
| **Leading Hypothesis** | | |
| Dementia, most commonly Alzheimer type | Memory loss with impairments in instrumental activities of daily living | MMSE Neuropsychiatric testing |
| **Active Alternative** | | |
| Vascular dementia | Risk factors for vascular disease | Evidence of vascular disease Positive ischemia score |
| **Active Alternative---Must Not Miss** | | |
| Delirium | Altered level of consciousness with variation during the day | Confusion Assessment Method |
| Depression | May present as patient-reported memory loss | Fulfillment of DSM-IV-TR criteria |

has seen, medications he takes, and the timing of his surgery. He and his wife deny any symptoms of depression, although they note this has been a problem in the past and he has taken paroxetine for years. His physical exam is normal except for evidence of bilateral knee osteoarthritis. His initial neurologic exam, including motor, sensory, and reflex examination, is normal.

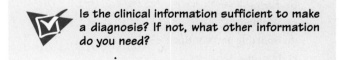

Is the clinical information sufficient to make a diagnosis? If not, what other information do you need?

## Leading Hypothesis: AD

### Textbook Presentation

Typically, a family member brings in an older patient because of confusion, memory loss, or personality change. The patient may deny that a problem exists and detection of dementia during casual conversation may be difficult. Dementia, especially early in its course, is sometimes difficult to detect on casual questioning; more formal assessment is frequently necessary.

### Disease Highlights

A. AD most commonly occurs after the age of 65.

B. Earlier presentations are possible.

C. AD may present with memory loss, behavioral or personality change, functional impairments, or social withdrawal.

D. Language disturbances are usually present early in the course of disease and often become severe with time.

E. Eventually, global cognitive impairment develops and patients become unable to independently accomplish the most basic activities of daily living.

Although present, memory loss may not be the presenting symptom in patients with AD; rather, behavioral or personality changes, functional impairments, social withdrawal, and language disturbances may be the initial symptoms.

F. AD accounts for about 67% of cases of dementia.

G. Early symptoms of AD include memory loss, social withdrawal, and language disturbances.

1. Language disturbances are often the most obvious finding.

2. As the disease progresses, fluent aphasia, paraphasias, and word substitutions may develop.

H. Strictly speaking, the diagnosis of AD can only be made pathologically. That said, the diagnosis of AD is always made clinically.

I. All definitions of AD include the deterioration in a person's ability to function independently. A patient's level of functioning can be evaluated by assessing his ability to do the instrumental activities of daily living (IADLs):

1. The IADLs include

   a. Cooking

   b. House cleaning

   c. Laundry

   d. Management of medications

   e. Management of the telephone

   f. Management of personal accounts

   g. Shopping

   h. Use of transportation

2. Late in the disease, a patient's ability to perform the activities of daily living (ADLs) often becomes compromised. These ADLs are:

   a. Bathing

   b. Eating

   c. Walking

   d. Toileting and continence

   e. Dressing

   f. Grooming

J. The prognosis of AD is poor.

1. Estimates of median survival have traditionally ranged from 5 to 9 years with more recent data suggesting median survival close to 3 years with a range of 2.7 to 4 years.

2. Patients with AD also have a much worse prognosis after an acute illness. Mortality after an episode of pneumonia or a hip fracture is about 4 times that of matched controlled (~50% vs ~15%).

**Evidence-Based Diagnosis**

A. Diagnosing AD can be challenging because patients often have subtle symptoms early in the disease course.

1. AD presents with self-reported memory loss in only a minority of patients.

   a. Memory loss reported by a spouse, relative, or close friend is more predictive of dementia.

   b. Memory loss reported by a patient is more predictive of depression.

2. Behavioral changes and mood changes are commonly recognized by family members.

**Table 10–5.** Prevalence of dementia by age

| Age | Prevalence | |
| --- | --- | --- |
| | Outpatient | Inpatient |
| 65–75 | 2.1% | 6.4% |
| > 75 | 11.7% | 13% |
| > 85 | — | 31.2% |

3. Physicians sometimes recognize behavioral changes such as increased anxiety, increased somatic complaints, or delusional thinking regarding illness as early symptoms of the disease.

B. The most efficient way to diagnose AD is to follow these 3 steps:

1. Consider the probability that a patient has dementia.

2. Diagnose dementia.

3. Diagnose AD by ruling out other causes and ensuring that the presentation fits.

C. Diagnosing dementia

1. The prevalence of dementia in the older population is very high. The prevalence at different ages is given in Table 10–5.

2. The Mini-Mental Status Exam (MMSE) is the most commonly used test to screen for dementia. The test characteristics for this test, some of its components, and some other common tests, are listed in Table 10–6.

   a. An important point about the MMSE is that its performance is influenced by the patient's level of education.

   b. The exam tends to underestimate the level of dementia in highly educated people and overestimate it in the poorly educated.

3. The Memory Impairment Screen (MIS) is another test for dementia that seems to be less affected by the level of education and may perform better than the 3-item recall.

   a. In this test, patients are given 4 words.

**Table 10–6.** Test characteristics for the MMSE, some of its components, and other tests in the diagnosis of dementia.

| Test | Sensitivity | Specificity | LR+ | LR− |
| --- | --- | --- | --- | --- |
| MMSE score < 24 | 87% | 82% | 4.83 | 0.16 |
| Unable to name month | | | 16 | 0.4 |
| Unable to name year | | | 37 | 0.5 |
| Unable to do serial 7s to 79 | | | 1.9 | .06 |
| 3-item recall < 2 | 65% | 85% | 4.33 | 0.41 |
| Clock drawing | | | | |
| Normal | | | | 0.2 |
| Almost normal | | | | 0.8 |
| Abnormal | | | 24 | |

MMSE, Mini-Mental Status Exam.

**b.** They are then asked to match them to a category (for example apple and fruit) and then asked to recall the words 2–3 minutes later.

**c.** Patients receive 2 points for words remembered without prompting and 1 point for those remembered after prompting with the category.

**d.** A positive test is a score of less than 5/8 points. The test characteristics are given below:

    **(1)** Sensitivity, 86%; specificity, 97%

    **(2)** LR+, 28.67; LR−, 0.14

**e.** The MIS is a very specific test for dementia.

**4.** Neuropsychiatric testing

  **a.** When the diagnosis of dementia is especially difficult, neuropsychiatric testing can be very helpful.

  **b.** Some of the situations in which neuropsychiatric testing is commonly used are:

    **(1)** When there is disagreement between the clinical suspicion and in-office tests.

    **(2)** To specifically gauge deficits in order to recommend ways of compensating.

    **(3)** When present or suspected psychiatric disease (usually depression) complicates the diagnosis.

    **(4)** When a more definitive diagnosis would be helpful for the patient or family members.

**D.** The diagnosis of AD is a clinical one based on the diagnosis of dementia and the presence of features consistent with AD.

**1.** Various office-based tests are useful in making this diagnosis. The National Institute of Neurological and Communicative Disorders and Stroke and the Alzheimer's Disease and Related Disorders Association (NINCDS-ADRDA) criteria for probable AD are currently the most commonly used by specialists.

**2.** Criteria for the clinical diagnosis of probable AD

  **a.** Dementia

  **b.** Deficits in 2 or more areas of cognition

    **(1)** Orientation

    **(2)** Registration

    **(3)** Visuospatial and executive functioning

    **(4)** Language

    **(5)** Attention and working memory

    **(6)** Memory

  **c.** Progressive worsening of memory and other cognitive functions

  **d.** No disturbance of consciousness

  **e.** Onset between ages 40 and 90, most often after age 65

  **f.** Absence of other disorders that could account for the symptoms

**3.** The test characteristics for these criteria follow:

  **a.** Sensitivity, 83%; specificity, 84%

  **b.** LR+, 5.19; LR−, 0.2

**4.** The NINCDS-ADRDA also gives factors that support the diagnosis. These are very helpful clinically although none are necessary to make the diagnosis. Some of these are included below:

  **a.** Progressive deterioration of specific cognitive functions

    **(1)** Aphasia

    **(2)** Apraxia

    **(3)** Agnosia

  **b.** Impaired ADLs and altered patterns of behavior

  **c.** Family history of dementia

  **d.** Normal lumbar puncture, normal or nonspecific EEG findings, and cerebral atrophy on neuroimaging

**5.** Because these criteria are not perfect in the diagnosis of AD, patients in whom dementia or AD is suspected but who do not meet the criteria should be monitored closely or referred for more detailed neuropsychiatric testing.

**E.** Reversible dementias

**1.** An important issue when diagnosing AD is how much more of a work-up should be done? The concern is that when making a clinical diagnosis, potentially reversible dementias might be missed. These reversible dementias include:

  **a.** CNS infections

  **b.** Hypothyroidism

  **c.** $B_{12}$ deficiency

  **d.** CNS masses

    **(1)** Neoplasms

    **(2)** Subdural hematomas

  **e.** Normal-pressure hydrocephalus

  **f.** Medications

**2.** Current practice is to order the following tests:

  **a.** CBC

  **b.** TSH

  **c.** Basic metabolic panel and LFTs

  **d.** Vitamin $B_{12}$ level

  **e.** Rapid plasma reagin

  **f.** Consider neuroimaging (MRI or CT)

    **(1)** Imaging is not required in most patients with dementia.

    **(2)** In practice, most patients will undergo imaging both to assess for diagnoses other than AD and to detect brain atrophy that may support the diagnosis of AD.

## Treatment

**A.** Counseling

**1.** When the diagnosis of AD is made, patients and families should be educated on course, complications, and prognosis of the disease.

**2.** Decisions need to be made regarding health care proxies, financial and estate planning, and end-of-life care.

**3.** It is crucial to make these decisions while the patient is still a competent decision maker and referral to support services, such as the Alzheimer's Association, my be helpful.

**B.** Safety

**1.** At some point in the disease, patient safety often becomes an issue.

**2.** Driving, wandering, and cooking are often early concerns.

  **a.** Driving is usually the most difficult to address because patients lack insight into the dangers they pose and resist the loss of independence that not driving brings.

    **b.** Physicians should raise this issue since it is often difficult for caregivers to bring up.

    **c.** Patients with even mild dementia should be told not to drive, or they should undergo frequent performance evaluations.

    **d.** Home safety checklists are available online that can help family members protect patients with dementia.

**C.** Behavioral

    **1.** Caregivers should be told to expect behavioral and personality changes, and be instructed on how to respond.

    **2.** Maintenance of routines is important.

    **3.** Situations likely to be stressful to patients, such as those in which a patient's deficits interfere with his functioning, should be avoided.

 The fact that medications are only moderately effective in treating AD does not mean that the physician's role is limited.

**D.** Pharmacotherapy

    **1.** Cholinesterase inhibitors

        **a.** 4 cholinesterase inhibitors are approved for treatment

            **(1)** Donepezil

            **(2)** Tacrine

            **(3)** Rivastigmine

            **(4)** Galantamine

        **b.** These medications have been shown to have modest effects on objective measures of dementia and functional status.

    **2.** Memantine is an NMDA receptor antagonist also approved for the treatment of AD. It has similar efficacy to the drugs above.

    **3.** Associated neuropsychiatric symptoms

        **a.** May include agitation (60–70%) or either delusions or hallucinations (30–60%)

        **b.** Atypical neuroleptics, such as olanzapine and risperidone, are frequently used but the evidence base for their efficacy is poor and they have been associated with higher mortality. Neither of these drugs are approved for this indication.

    **4.** Depression

        **a.** Very common in patients with AD

        **b.** Present in up to 50% of patients

        **c.** All patients with AD should be screened for depression and treated if it is found.

    **5.** Caregiver care

        **a.** Taking care of a friend or relative with AD can be extremely challenging.

        **b.** Caregivers should be counseled on the importance of taking time off and the availability of respite care.

        **c.** They should be counseled that behavioral difficulties are a result of the disease and not the patient's anger or heartlessness.

        **d.** Caregiver support groups can be extremely helpful.

## MAKING A DIAGNOSIS

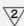

Mr. R's exam thus far reveals some difficulty with recalling recent events. Given his age, his baseline risk of dementia is at least 10%. The first step in his work-up would be to screen for dementia with the MMSE or MIS. If this is positive, an effort should be made to see if he fulfills the NINCDS-ADRDA criteria for probable AD.

Further history revealed that the patient's wife had taken over bookkeeping because a few bills had gone unpaid during the last 3 months.

    The patient was given the MMSE and scored a 20 out of 30. He was not able to give the day of the month, could only register 2 of 3 items and recalled 0 of 3. He only got 1 of the serial 7s and could not draw pentagons.

    Consideration of the NINCDS-ADRDA criteria showed him to have dementia with deficits in 2 or more areas of cognition (orientation, visuospatial and executive functioning, attention and working memory, and memory). At the time of the visit, it was not clear whether his cognitive functioning was worsening and there were no disturbances in consciousness.

    The plan was made for initial laboratory work to be done and for a 3-month follow-up visit. Given that he was taking multiple psychoactive medications, his regimen was scaled back to the minimum doses necessary to control his pain.

 **Have you crossed a diagnostic threshold for the leading hypothesis, AD? Have you ruled out the active alternatives? Do other tests need to be done to exclude the alternative diagnoses?**

## Alternative Diagnosis: Multi-infarct Dementia (Vascular Dementia, VaD)

### Textbook Presentation

A patient with VaD may have dementia that has an abrupt onset or is slowly worsening. The patient usually has risk factors for vascular disease or has previously diagnosed vascular disease. The patient often has difficulty walking or a focal neurologic exam.

### Disease Highlights

**A.** Generally considered to be the most common cause of dementia after AD.

**B.** Disease seen most commonly in patients with risk factors for vascular disease or embolic stroke.

**C.** Patients have dementia and evidence that cerebrovascular disease has caused the dementia.

    **1.** A classic, but insensitive, clue is a "step-like deterioration" related to intermittent cerebrovascular accidents.

    **2.** Other clues may be a focal neurologic exam or evidence of strokes, white matter changes, or atrophy on neuroimaging.

**D.** Clues to the diagnosis of VaD are gait disturbance, urinary symptoms, and personality changes.

## Evidence-Based Diagnosis

A. The DSM-IV-TR criteria for the clinical diagnosis of VaD include:

   1. The development of cognitive deficits including memory deficits

   2. A resulting significant impairment in social or occupational functioning

   3. Focal neurologic signs, symptoms, or diagnostic studies indicative of cerebrovascular disease judged to be etiologically related to the cognitive change

B. Features consistent with the diagnosis of VaD are

   1. Exaggeration of deep tendon reflexes

   2. Extensor plantar response

   3. Gait abnormalities (consider history of unsteadiness and frequent, unprovoked falls)

   4. Pseudobulbar palsy (pathologic laughing, crying, grimacing; and weakness of the muscles associated with cranial nerves V, VII, IX, X, XI, and XII)

   5. Focal neurologic signs

C. The actual diagnosis of VaD is complicated by the presence of multiple different criteria.

D. The Hachinski Ischemic Score seems to be a clinically useful test for determining whether ischemic disease is playing a role in a patient's dementia.

   1. In the score, 2 points are given for each of the following features:

      a. Abrupt onset

      b. Fluctuating course

      c. History of stroke

      d. Focal neurologic signs

      e. Focal neurologic symptoms

   2. 1 point is given for each of the following features:

      a. Stepwise deterioration

      b. Nocturnal confusion

      c. Preservation of personality

      d. Depression

      e. Somatic complaints

      f. Emotional lability

      g. Hypertension

      h. Atherosclerosis

   3. A score of greater than 7 carries a LR+ of 8.3 for differentiating VaD from AD. The score performs less well for differentiating AD or VaD from a mixed dementia.

## Treatment

A. Behavioral, pharmacologic, and surgical means of modifying risk factors for cerebrovascular disease and preventing recurrent vascular events should be used.

B. Behavioral interventions include smoking cessation and dietary intervention to decrease vascular risk.

C. Pharmacologic interventions include treatment of hypertension and diabetes mellitus, treatment of hypercholesterolemia (to an LDL < 100 mg/dL), aspirin therapy, and anticoagulation when indicated.

D. Surgical therapy includes carotid endarterectomy when indicated.

## CASE RESOLUTION

Initial laboratory evaluation, including CBC, TSH, basic metabolic panel and LFTs, vitamin $B_{12}$ level, and rapid plasma reagin was normal. He was able to wean his medications and felt like he had a little more energy. On a follow-up visit 3 months later, the patient's wife reported that he was no longer driving to his job as it had become too difficult. On physical exam, his language skills had worsened, and he frequently answered questions with short affirmative phrases and nods that were often contradicted by his wife. (He would subsequently agree with her.) A CT scan with contrast was ordered and showed only cerebral atrophy.

AD can be confidently diagnosed in this patient. His only risk factor for VaD is a history of ischemic bowel. His ischemia score is only 2. Dementia was diagnosed at his previous visit; since his symptoms have progressed, he now fulfills the criteria for AD. Reversible causes of dementia are unlikely given the normal evaluation. The patient's functional limitations exclude MCI as a cause. The patient has no symptoms of delirium or depression.

## REVIEW OF OTHER IMPORTANT DISEASES

## Mild Cognitive Impairment (MCI)

### Textbook Presentation

Usually presents in an older patient complaining of memory loss. Common complaints are difficulty remembering names and appointments or solving complex problems. Detailed testing shows abnormal memory, but patients have no functional impairment.

### Disease Highlights

A. Memory complaints are very common in older people.

B. Concern for AD is also very common.

C. The definition of MCI includes the lack of any functional impairment and

   1. Memory complaint

   2. Normal ADLs

   3. Normal general cognitive function

   4. Abnormal memory for age

   5. No dementia

D. Patients with this disorder are not neurologically normal.

   1. Their memory is worse than age-matched controls.

   2. They have a higher rate of progression to dementia than those without memory impairments (12% per year vs 1–2% per year).

### Evidence-Based Diagnosis

The diagnosis of this disease is made by the above criteria. The memory deficits are sometimes difficult to detect and distinguish from normal, age-related changes. If it is desirable to obtain a definite diagnosis, neuropsychiatric testing is helpful.

### Treatment

Presently, there is no proven treatment for MCI. Patients should be monitored closely for development of more severe cognitive or functional decline.

## Dementia with Lewy Bodies (DLB)

### Textbook Presentation

DLB is typically seen in a patient with Parkinson disease who has dementia. The predominant symptoms of the dementia are a fluctuating course and the presence of hallucinations. In patients without a previous diagnosis of Parkinson disease, motor symptoms similar to those seen in Parkinson disease are often present.

### Disease Highlights

A. Lewy bodies are seen in the cortex of about 20% of patients with dementia.

   1. Includes some patients with a clinical diagnosis of AD

   2. Probably among the most common types of dementia after AD. It may coexist with AD.

B. The most important features of DLB are included in the Evidence-Based Diagnosis section below.

C. The fluctuating course can mean that early in the disease patients may seem nearly normal at times and demented at other times. Because of the fluctuation in symptoms, delirium needs to be included in the differential diagnosis.

D. Visual hallucinations are common in DLB, unlike in most other types of dementia.

E. Mild extrapyramidal motor symptoms (rigidity and bradykinesis) are often seen. These may occur late in the course of other dementias but occur early with DLB and worsen over time.

### Evidence-Based Diagnosis

The diagnostic criteria for DLB are presented below.

A. There is dementia that might be mild at the onset of disease.

B. Two of the following are essential for a diagnosis of probable DLB:

   1. Fluctuating cognition with pronounced variations in attention and alertness

   2. Recurrent visual hallucinations that are typically well formed and detailed

   3. Spontaneous motor features of parkinsonism

C. The following features are supportive of the diagnosis of DLB

   1. Repeated falls

   2. Syncope

   3. Transient loss of consciousness

   4. Neuroleptic sensitivity

   5. Systematized delusions and hallucinations

### Treatment

A. Supportive treatment of patients with DLB is the same as for patients with AD.

B. Cholinesterase inhibitors have also been shown to be effective.

C. Neuroleptics can be dangerous, potentially worsening symptoms.

 Patients with dementia with parkinsonian features, a fluctuating course, and visual hallucinations should be evaluated for DLB before they are treated with neuroleptics.

## REFERENCES

Benbadis SR, Sila CA, Cristea RL. Mental status changes and stroke. J Gen Intern Med. 1994;9:485–7.

Black ER. Diagnostic strategies for common medical problems. Philadelphia: American College of Physicians; 1999:674.

Elie M, Rousseau F, Cole M, Primeau F, McCusker J, Bellavance F. Prevalence and detection of delirium in elderly emergency department patients. CMAJ. 2000;163:977–81.

Francis J, Martin D, Kapoor WN. A prospective study of delirium in hospitalized elderly. JAMA. 1990;263:1097–101.

Husain AM, Horn GJ, Jacobson MP. Non-convulsive status epilepticus: usefulness of clinical features in selecting patients for urgent EEG. J Neurol Neurosurg Psychiatry. 2003; 74:189–91.

Inouye SK. The dilemma of delirium: clinical and research controversies regarding diagnosis and evaluation of delirium in hospitalized elderly medical patients. Am J Med. 1994;97:278–88.

Inouye SK, Bogardus ST Jr, Charpentier PA et al. A multicomponent intervention to prevent delirium in hospitalized older patients. N Engl J Med. 1999;340:669–76.

Inouye SK, Viscoli CM, Horwitz RI, Hurst LD, Tinetti ME. A predictive model for delirium in hospitalized elderly medical patients based on admission characteristics. Ann Intern Med. 1993;119:474–81.

Lewis LM, Miller DK, Morley JE, Nork MJ, Lasater LC. Unrecognized delirium in ED geriatric patients. Am J Emerg Med. 1995;13:142–5.

Moroney JT, Bagiella E, Desmond DW et al. Meta-analysis of the Hachinski Ischemic Score in pathologically verified dementias. Neurology. 1997;49(4):1096–105.

Rockwood K. The occurrence and duration of symptoms in elderly patients with delirium. J Gerontol. 1993;48:M162–6.

Siu AL. Screening for dementia and investigating its causes. Ann Intern Med. 1991;115:122–32.

Wiederkehr S, Simard M, Fortin C, van Reekum R. Comparability of the clinical diagnostic criteria for vascular dementia: a critical review. Part I. J Neuropsychiatry Clin Neurosci. 2008;20(2):150–61.

# I have a patient who is concerned that she has diabetes. How do I confirm the diagnosis and treat patients with diabetes?

## CHIEF COMPLAINT

PATIENT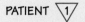

Mrs. D is a 50-year-old African American woman who is worried she has diabetes.

 What is the differential diagnosis of diabetes? How would you frame the differential?

## CONSTRUCTING A DIFFERENTIAL DIAGNOSIS

The differential diagnosis of diabetes mellitus (DM) is actually a classification of the different causes of diabetes:

A. Type 1 DM

1. Of the persons with DM in Canada, the United States, and Europe, 5–10% have type 1.

2. Caused by cellular-mediated autoimmune destruction of the pancreatic beta cells in genetically susceptible individuals, triggered by an undefined environmental agent

   a. Some combination of antibodies against islet cells, insulin, glutamic acid decarboxylase ($GAD_{65}$), or tyrosine phosphatases IA-2 and IA-2$\beta$ are found in 85–90% of patients.

   b. Strong HLA association

   c. Risk is 0.4% in patients without family history, 5–6% in siblings and children, and 30% in monozygotic twins

   d. Patients are also prone to autoimmune thyroid disease, Addison disease, vitiligo, celiac sprue, autoimmune hepatitis, myasthenia gravis, and pernicious anemia.

3. Occasionally idiopathic

   a. Usually seen in patients of African or Asian ancestry

   b. Strongly inherited but no HLA link or autoimmunity

4. Insulin therapy is always necessary.

5. Patients are at high risk for diabetic ketoacidosis (DKA).

B. Type 2 DM

C. Other causes of diabetes

1. Genetic defects of beta cell function or insulin action

2. Exocrine pancreatic diseases (pancreatitis, trauma, infection, pancreatectomy, pancreatic carcinoma)

3. Endocrinopathies (acromegaly, Cushing syndrome, glucagonoma, pheochromocytoma)

4. Medications (especially corticosteroids)

5. Infections

D. Gestational diabetes

Type 1 DM generally occurs in children, although approximately 7.5–10% of adults assumed to have type 2 DM actually have type 1, as defined by the presence of circulating antibodies. Type 2 DM is becoming more prevalent in teenagers and young adults, presumably related to the increased prevalence of obesity.

In most patients, the distinction between type 1 and type 2 DM is clear. Thus, the primary tasks of the clinician are to determine who should be tested for diabetes, who has diabetes, which complications to monitor, and how to treat the patient.

Mrs. D has worried about having diabetes since her father died of complications from the disease. Over the last couple of weeks, she has been urinating more than usual. She is aware that excess urination can be a symptom of diabetes, so she scheduled an appointment.

 At this point, what is the leading hypothesis, what are the active alternatives, and is there a must not miss diagnosis? Given this differential diagnosis, what tests should be ordered?

## PRIORITIZING THE DIFFERENTIAL DIAGNOSIS

Mrs. D's pretest probability of diabetes is high because of 2 pivotal points in her history, the urinary frequency and the positive family history. The rest of the differential diagnosis consists of other entities that can cause urinary frequency, such as urinary tract infection, excess fluid intake, and bladder dysfunction. Other diseases that cause true polyuria, defined as urinary output of > 3 L/day, should also be considered. Table 11–1 lists the differential diagnosis.

Mrs. D has no dysuria or hematuria. She takes no medications, drinks 1 cup of coffee per day, and uses alcohol rarely. She has been trying to lose weight and has been drinking more water in an attempt to reduce her appetite.

On physical exam, she looks a bit tired. Vital signs are as follows: BP, 138/82 mm Hg; pulse, 96 bpm; RR, 16 breaths per minute. The remainder of the physical exam is normal. A random plasma glucose is 152 mg/dL.

 Is the clinical information sufficient to make a diagnosis? If not, what other information do you need?

**Table 11–1.** Diagnostic hypotheses for Mrs. D.

| Diagnostic Hypotheses | Clinical Clues | Important Tests |
|---|---|---|
| **Leading Hypothesis** | | |
| Type 2 diabetes mellitus | Family history Obesity Hypertension Ethnic group Polyuria Polydipsia | Fasting plasma glucose |
| **Active Alternatives—Most Common** | | |
| Urinary tract infection | Urgency Frequency Hematuria | Urinalysis Culture |
| Excess fluid intake | Polyuria Frequency | History |
| Bladder dysfunction | Urgency Frequency Incontinence | Postvoid residual Urodynamic testing |
| **Other Hypotheses** | | |
| Diabetes insipidus | Polyuria > 3 L/day | Water restriction test |
| Primary polydipsia | Polyuria > 3 L/day Excess water intake | Water restriction test |

## Leading Hypothesis: Type 2 DM

### Textbook Presentation

Patients with type 2 DM can have the classic symptoms of polyuria, polydipsia, and weight loss. The presentation can also be more subtle, with patients complaining that they feel tired or "just not right." Many patients are asymptomatic; the diagnosis is made after plasma glucose testing. The complications of diabetes may already be present by the time patients seek medical attention.

### Disease Highlights

A. Caused by a combination of impaired insulin secretion and insulin resistance with no evidence of autoimmunity

B. Accounts for 90–95% of cases of DM, with prevalence in the United States of about 13–14%; up to 50% of patients are unaware that they have DM.

C. The lifetime risk of diabetes developing in individuals born in 2000 is estimated to be 32.8% for males and 38.5% for females; rates are as high as 50% for African American and Hispanic women.

D. Strong genetic component

  1. In the United States, type 2 DM is 2–6 times more prevalent among African Americans, Native Americans, Pima Indians, and Latinos than among whites.

  2. 39% of patients have at least 1 parent with diabetes

  3. 60–90% concordance in monozygotic twins

  4. The lifetime risk of a first-degree relative of a patient with type 2 DM is 5–10 times higher than that of age- and weight-matched individuals without a family history.

E. The most important risk factor is obesity, which induces insulin resistance.

  1. The RR of diabetes developing in a woman who has a body mass index (BMI) > 35 kg/m² is 93, compared with a woman who has a BMI < 22 kg/m².

  2. The RR of diabetes developing in a man who has a BMI > 35 kg/m² is 42, compared with a man who has a BMI < 23 kg/m².

F. DKA develops less often in patients with type 2 DM than those with type 1; however, DKA can occur in persons with type 2 DM.

 Do not assume all patients with DKA have type 1 DM; DKA can develop in persons with type 2 DM.

G. Risk factors for type 2 DM include

  1. Age ≥ 45

  2. BMI ≥ 25 kg/m²

  3. A first-degree relative with diabetes

  4. Physical inactivity

  5. Being a member of a high-risk ethnic group (African American, Latino, Native American, Asian American, Pacific Islander)

  6. Having delivered a baby weighing > 9 pounds or having had gestational DM

  7. Hypertension

  8. Metabolic syndrome (high-density lipoprotein [HDL] cholesterol < 35 mg/dL or triglycerides > 250 mg/dL, or both)

  9. Polycystic ovary syndrome

  10. Vascular disease

  11. History of impaired glucose tolerance (IGT) or impaired fasting glucose (IFG)

H. IFG and IGT: Metabolic stage between normal glucose homeostasis and diabetes, sometimes called **prediabetes**

  1. Patients with IFG or IGT have normal HgbA$_{1c}$ levels.

  2. Both IFG and IGT are risk factors for the development of diabetes and cardiovascular disease.

  3. Both are associated with the metabolic syndrome (insulin resistance, compensatory hyperinsulinemia, obesity, hypertension, and dyslipidemia consisting of high triglycerides and low HDL).

  4. Table 11–2 lists the defining criteria for IFG and IGT.

**Table 11–2.** American Diabetes Association diagnostic criteria for diabetes.

| | Fasting Plasma Glucose | 2-Hour Plasma Glucose (After 75-g Oral Glucose Load) |
|---|---|---|
| Normal | < 100 mg/dL | ≤ 140 mg/dL |
| Impaired fasting glucose | 100–125 mg/dL | |
| Impaired glucose tolerance | | 140–199 mg/dL |
| Diabetes | ≥ 126 mg/dL | ≥ 200 mg/dL |

I. Screening for diabetes

1. American Diabetes Association (ADA) recommends screening patients every 3 years beginning at age 45, especially those with a BMI ≥ 25 kg/m²; those with ≥ 2 risk factors should be screened earlier and more often.

2. In 2008, the US Preventive Services Task Force recommended screening asymptomatic adults with sustained BP > 135/80 mm Hg. The Task Force concluded that evidence is insufficient to assess the benefits and harms of routine screening in asymptomatic patients with BP of 135/80 mm Hg or lower.

## Evidence-Based Diagnosis

A. Table 11–2 lists the diagnostic criteria established by the ADA; in addition, a random plasma glucose > 200 mg/dL in a symptomatic patient is diagnostic.

B. The ADA recommends that all abnormal results be confirmed with a second test.

C. The criteria for diagnosing diabetes were chosen based on the observation that the risk for retinopathy increases substantially at a fasting plasma glucose (FPG) of 126 mg/dL.

D. FPG measurements are more reproducible and easier to obtain than oral glucose tolerance test (OGTT) measurements.

1. Either test is acceptable for screening.

2. The OGTT, consisting of an FPG and a second glucose measurement 2 hours after a 75-g oral glucose load, does identify more prediabetic people than the FPG.

3. The 2 tests do not necessarily detect the same individuals; some patients will have normal results on 1 test but abnormal results on the other.

E. The HgbA$_{1c}$ should not be used to screen for diabetes because of a variable correlation with FPG.

1. The LR– is unacceptably high for A$_{1c}$ levels of 6.1–6.5% (Table 11–3).

2. However, the HgbA$_{1c}$ should always be ordered in patients with hyperglycemia on a random sample, or a fasting glucose > 100 mg/dL.

## Treatment of IFG/IGT

A. The goals are to prevent or delay the onset of diabetes and to modify other cardiac risk factors.

B. Large randomized trials have shown that lifestyle modification or medication can prevent or delay diabetes.

**Table 11–3.** Test characteristics of the HgbA$_{1c}$ in the diagnosis of diabetes.

| HgbA1$_c$ Cutoff (%) | Sensitivity (%) | Specificity (%) | LR+ | LR– |
|---|---|---|---|---|
| 5.6 | 83.4 | 84.4 | 5.35 | 0.2 |
| 6.1 | 63.2 | 97.4 | 24.3 | 0.38 |
| 6.5 | 42.8 | 99.6 | 107 | 0.57 |
| 7.1 | 28.3 | 99.9 | 283 | 0.72 |

1. Finnish patients with IGT were randomized to brief diet/exercise counseling or intensive individualized instruction.

a. There was a 58% relative reduction in the development of diabetes in the intensive group, (NNT = 22 to prevent 1 case of DM over 1 year; NNT = 5 to prevent 1 case of DM over 5 years).

b. The study cohort was monitored for 3 years after the intervention; the group of patients initially assigned to the lifestyle intervention tended to continue their lifestyle changes after the trial ended, and continued to have a reduced risk of developing diabetes.

2. Patients in the United States (45% African American or Hispanic) were randomized to intensive diet/exercise program, metformin, or placebo.

a. There was a 58% relative reduction in the development of DM in the intensive diet/exercise group and a 31% relative reduction in metformin group.

b. NNT = 7 over 3 years to prevent 1 case of diabetes for the intensive diet/exercise group, and NNT = 14 for the metformin group.

3. Acarbose, orlistat, and rosiglitazone have also been studied, but the ADA does not recommend their use in diabetes prevention.

 Lifestyle modification is the best way to prevent or delay the onset of diabetes.

C. Recommended lifestyle modification goals are 30 minutes of modest physical activity daily and loss of 5–10% of body weight.

D. The ADA recommends considering the addition of metformin in patients who have a BMI > 35, are under 60 years old, and have combined IFG and IGT plus at least 1 other risk factor.

E. The goal of hypertension therapy in patients with IFG or IGT is to achieve a BP < 140/90 mm Hg.

F. Lipids should be treated according to National Cholesterol Education Program (NCEP) guidelines for nondiabetic patients (see Chapter 20, Hypertension).

## MAKING A DIAGNOSIS

Mrs. D's random glucose is elevated but is not diagnostic of diabetes. She reports that even though she is urinating often, the urine volumes are small. You ask her to return for more testing:

FPG, 120 mg/dL

HgbA$_{1c}$, 5.8%

Urinalysis: negative for protein, glucose, and blood; no WBCs or bacteria; specific gravity, 1.015.

 **Have you crossed a diagnostic threshold for the leading hypothesis, type 2 DM? Have you ruled out the active alternatives? Do other tests need to be done to exclude the alternative diagnoses?**

Mrs. D does not have diabetes, but she does have IFG. This does not cause glycosuria of a degree sufficient to cause urinary frequency. A urinary tract infection is ruled out by the normal urinalysis. She has increased her water consumption, so excess fluid intake is a likely cause of her symptoms. Bladder dysfunction should be considered if her symptoms do not resolve with reduction in fluid intake. Diabetes insipidus and primary polydipsia are rare diseases that do not need to be considered unless she has a documented urinary output of more than 3 L/day. The next diagnostic test should be reducing her fluid intake.

## CASE RESOLUTION

Mrs. D stops forcing herself to drink extra water, and her urination pattern returns to normal. She is very concerned about her elevated FPG and wants to know how to prevent progression to diabetes. Her BMI is 30 kg/m², and her fasting lipid panel shows total cholesterol of 220 mg/dL; HDL, 38 mg/dL; triglycerides, 250 mg/dL; and low-density lipoprotein (LDL), 132 mg/dL. You refer her to a nutritionist for dietary counseling and recommend that she walk 30 minutes a day 5 days a week. When she returns to see you 4 months later, she has lost 8 pounds. Her FPG is 112 mg/dL; total cholesterol 197 mg/dL, HDL, 42 mg/dL; triglycerides, 150 mg/dL; and LDL, 125 mg/dL.

## FOLLOW-UP OF MRS. D

Mrs. D returns 5 years later, having lived in another city in the meantime. She reports that she did quite well with her diet and exercise program for several years, maintaining a 10% weight loss. However, over the last couple of years, she has not been able to continue her exercise program or be as careful about her diet because of the stresses of caring for her chronically ill mother as well as working and caring for her own family. Her mother died recently, so Mrs. D has moved back. She knows that she has gained weight and is especially worried about her blood sugar level because she did not have time to see a doctor herself during her mother's illness.

On physical exam, her BMI is 34 kg/m², and her BP is 155/88 mm Hg. Her lungs are clear, and on cardiac exam you hear an $S_4$ but no $S_3$ or murmurs. Abdominal exam is normal, and there is no peripheral edema. Her peripheral pulses are normal, and there are no ulcerations on her feet. She does have tinea pedis. Her fingerstick glucose measurement is 335 mg/dL.

**At this point, what is the leading hypothesis, what are the active alternatives, and is there a must not miss diagnosis? Given this differential diagnosis, what tests should be ordered?**

## PRIORITIZING THE DIFFERENTIAL DIAGNOSIS

Clearly, Mrs. D now has type 2 DM. At this point, in addition to starting treatment, the clinician should focus on identifying and managing diabetic complications and associated cardiovascular risk factors rather than ruling out other diagnoses (Table 11–4).

Mrs. D does not report any vision loss, numbness, edema, dyspnea, or chest pain.

**Is the clinical information sufficient to make a diagnosis? If not, what other information do you need?**

## Leading Hypothesis: Diabetic Complications

### 1. Retinopathy

**Textbook Presentation**

Most patients with retinopathy are asymptomatic. Other patients experience either gradual or sudden vision loss.

**Table 11–4.** Diagnostic hypotheses for Mrs. D's follow-up.

| Diagnostic Hypotheses | Clinical Clues | Important Tests |
|---|---|---|
| **Leading Hypothesis: Diabetic Complications** | | |
| Retinopathy | Asymptomatic Decreased vision | Ophthalmologic exam |
| Nephropathy | Long duration diabetes mellitus Poor glycemic control Hypertension | Albumin/creatinine ratio |
| Peripheral neuropathy | Paresthesias | Monofilament test |
| Diabetic foot ulcers | Neuropathy Peripheral arterial disease | Physical exam |
| Vascular disease | Coronary artery disease Heart failure Peripheral arterial disease Transient ischemic attack/cerebrovascular accident symptoms | Stress test Ankle-brachial index Carotid duplex ultrasound |
| **Active Alternatives that Increase Cardiovascular Risk— Must Not Miss:** | | |
| Hypertension | | Physical exam |
| Hyperlipidemia | | Fasting lipid panel |
| Smoking | | History |
| Obesity | | Body mass index |

## Disease Highlights

A. Most common cause of new cases of blindness in adults aged 20–74 years

B. Occurs in nearly all patients with type 1 and > 60% of patients with type 2 DM after 20 years.

C. Stages of diabetic retinopathy (DR)

    1. Nonproliferative (NPDR)

        a. Earlier stage of DR

        b. Earliest signs are microaneurysms and retinal hemorrhages

        c. Progressive capillary nonperfusion leads to ischemia, manifested by increasing cotton wool spots, venous beading, and intraretinal vascular abnormalities.

    2. Proliferative diabetic retinopathy (PDR)

        a. Most advanced form of DR

        b. Progressive retinal ischemia causes formation of new blood vessels on the retina or optic disk

        c. The new vessels bleed, leading to vision loss because of vitreous hemorrhage, fibrosis, or retinal detachment.

        d. Present in 50% of persons with type 1 and 15% of those with type 2 who have had DM for 15 years

    3. Diabetic macular edema (DME)

        a. Can develop at any stage of retinopathy

        b. Now the leading cause of vision loss in persons with diabetes

        c. Increased vascular permeability causes plasma leaks from the macular vessels, leading to swelling and formation of hard exudates at the central retina.

        d. Incidence over 10 years

            (1) 20% in persons with type 1 DM

            (2) 25% in persons with type 2 DM who require insulin

            (3) 14% in persons with type 2 DM who do not require insulin

D. Risk factors

    1. Most consistently identified risk factors are duration of DM, elevated $HgbA_{1c}$ level, hypertension, hyperlipidemia, pregnancy, nephropathy

    2. Less consistently identified risk factors include obesity, smoking, moderate alcohol consumption, physical inactivity

## Evidence-Based Diagnosis

A. Evaluation should include dilated indirect ophthalmoscopy or fundus photography, or both, by an ophthalmologist

B. Patients with type 1 diabetes should have an exam within 3–5 years of disease onset, followed by at least annual exams.

C. Patients with type 2 diabetes should have an exam at the time of diagnosis, followed by at least annual exams.

 All patients with type 2 DM need eye exams by an ophthalmologist at least annually.

## Treatment

A. Glycemic control

    1. In persons with type 1 DM *without* retinopathy, the risk of developing DR is reduced 76% by tight control ($HgbA_{1c}$ 7.2 vs 9.1% in the Diabetes Control and Complications Trial [DCCT]).

    2. In persons with type 1 DM *with* retinopathy, the risk of progression is reduced by 54% by tight control.

    3. In persons with type 2 DM, better control reduces the risk of microvascular complications (retinopathy and nephropathy) by 16–25%. ($HgbA_{1c}$ 7% vs 7.9% in the United Kingdom Prospective Diabetes Study [UKPDS] [1998]; $HgbA_{1c}$ 6.5 vs 7.2% in the ADVANCE trial [2008].)

    4. In persons with type 2 DM, there is a 35% reduction in the risk of microvascular complications for every percentage point decrease in $HgbA_{1c}$.

B. Better BP control reduces the risk of progression of retinopathy.

C. Aspirin neither improves nor worsens retinopathy.

D. Pan-retinal photocoagulation is indicated for PDR and selected cases of severe NPDR; focal laser photocoagulation is indicated for DME.

E. Vitrectomy (removal of the vitreous, the gel-like substance in the eye) is indicated for selected patients who do not respond to photocoagulation and for patients who have type 1 DM with DR and vitreous hemorrhage.

F. Intravitreal steroids may have a role in diffuse DME not responsive to laser treatment.

## 2. Neuropathy

### Textbook Presentation

Diabetic peripheral neuropathy (DPN) classically presents as paresthesias or burning pain in a "glove-stocking" distribution. Diabetic autonomic neuropathy can manifest in a variety of ways, including orthostatic dizziness, diarrhea, urinary incontinence, and gastroparesis.

### Disease Highlights

A. Types of DPN

    1. Symmetric distal polyneuropathy (most common)

    2. Focal neuropathies

        a. Cranial (0.05% of mononeuropathies)

            (1) Usually cranial nerve III or VI

            (2) Usually acute and transient

            (3) Caused by ischemia

        b. Thoracolumbar

        c. Limb

            (1) Median nerve most common site (5.8% of mononeuropathies)

            (2) Ulnar (2.1%), femoral, and peroneal also affected

    3. Diabetic amyotrophy (pain, severe asymmetric muscle weakness, and wasting of the iliopsoas and quadriceps)

B. Epidemiology of symmetric distal polyneuropathy

    1. Affects up to 50% of persons with diabetes, with chronic neuropathic pain in 20% of patients with diabetes for over 10 years

2. Severity is related to duration of disease, degree of glycemic control, and presence of hypertension and hyperlipidemia.

3. DPN is an independent risk factor for foot ulceration and amputation; patients with neuropathy have a 15% lifetime risk of amputation.

C. Clinical manifestations of symmetric distal polyneuropathy

1. History

   a. Up to 50% of patients asymptomatic

   b. Burning, shooting, or lancinating pain

   c. Paresthesias, hyperesthesias

   d. Often worse at night

   e. When symptoms ascend to the knees, upper extremity symptoms start

2. Physical exam

   a. Loss of vibration, pain, pressure, and temperature sensation

   b. Loss of ankle reflexes

   c. Distal muscle atrophy late in the course

3. Charcot joints develop, usually in the tarsometatarsal region, in 10% of patients.

D. Differential diagnosis symmetric distal polyneuropathy

1. Consider other causes of neuropathy if

   a. Neuropathy develops before the onset of or early in the course of the diabetes

   b. Patient has a history of excellent glycemic control

   c. Neuropathy is asymmetric

   d. There is proximal or upper extremity involvement disproportionate to distal lower extremity involvement

2. Be sure to check for other treatable causes (eg, hypothyroidism and vitamin $B_{12}$ deficiency), even in patients with long-standing diabetes.

 Think about other causes of neuropathy in diabetic patients.

E. Diabetic autonomic neuropathy can affect any organ innervated by the autonomic nervous system.

1. Cardiovascular autonomic neuropathy: many possible manifestations

   a. Reduced heart rate variability; associated with increased risk of silent ischemia and cardiac death

   b. Fixed heart rate

   c. Resting sinus tachycardia

   d. Inadequate increase in heart rate/BP with exercise

   e. Postural hypotension with systolic BP drop of > 30 mm Hg, without an appropriate heart rate response

   f. Intraoperative cardiac instability

2. Gustatory sweating

   a. Facial sweating, often accompanied by flushing, that occurs after eating

   b. Generally occurs in patients with nephropathy or peripheral neuropathy

   c. Cause unknown

3. GI dysfunction

   a. Reduced esophageal motility

   b. Gastroparesis

      (1) Abnormality of gastric motility leading to delayed gastric emptying

      (2) Symptoms include nausea, vomiting, anorexia, postprandial fullness, early satiety.

      (3) Poor correlation between demonstrated motility abnormalities and symptoms

   c. Diabetic diarrhea

      (1) Characterized by intermittent, brown watery, voluminous stools, occasionally accompanied by tenesmus

      (2) Can be episodic, separated by periods of normal bowel movements or constipation

      (3) Rare in the absence of other manifestations of neuropathy, either peripheral or autonomic

   d. Constipation

      (1) Constipation specifically resulting from autonomic neuropathy occurs in 20% of patients with type 2 DM

      (2) Caused by abnormality in autonomic neural control of colonic motility

   e. Anorectal dysfunction

      (1) Results in fecal incontinence, even in the absence of diarrhea

      (2) Patients can generally sense the presence of stool, but cannot prevent passage

4. Genitourinary dysfunction

   a. Bladder dysfunction

      (1) Initially motor function normal, but sensation of bladder distention impaired

      (2) Then, detrusor muscle hypocontractility occurs, leading to urinary retention and overflow incontinence.

   b. Erectile dysfunction

      (1) Present in 28–45% of diabetic men

      (2) Most common organic cause of erectile dysfunction

      (3) Risk factors include duration of DM, glycemic control, smoking, other diabetic complications.

## Evidence-Based Diagnosis

A. Symmetric distal polyneuropathy

1. Nerve conduction studies are the gold standard.

2. Several physical exam maneuvers have been compared with nerve conduction studies.

   a. Semmes-Weinstein monofilament examination

      (1) Apply a 5.07/10-g monofilament to a noncallused site on the dorsum of the first toe just proximal to the nail bed.

      (2) Repeat 4 times on both feet in an arrhythmic manner.

      (3) Add up the total number of times the monofilament is perceived by the patient (score range = 0–8).

   b. On–off vibration testing

      (1) Apply a vibrating 128-Hz tuning fork to the bony prominence at the dorsum of the first toe just proximal to the nail bed.

**(2)** Repeat twice on each foot.

**(3)** Add up the total number of times the patient perceives the application of the vibrating tuning fork and the cessation of the vibration (score range = 0–8).

**c.** Timed vibration testing

**(1)** Apply a vibrating 128-Hz tuning fork to the same location used for the on–off vibration test.

**(2)** Ask the patient to report the time at which vibration diminished beyond perception, and compare with the number of seconds perceived by the examiner when the tuning fork is applied to the examiner's thumb.

**(3)** Record number of times patient's perception time less than examiner's (score range = 0–8).

**d.** Superficial pain sensation

**(1)** Apply a sterile sharp to the same sites used for the monofilament.

**(2)** Repeat 4 times on each foot.

**(3)** Add up the total number of times the patient did not perceive the painful stimulus (score range = 0–8).

**e.** All tests have high LR+; monofilament and timed vibration have best LR– (Table 11–5).

**f.** Monofilament more reproducible than timed vibration.

 The monofilament is the preferred physical exam method for detecting diabetic peripheral neuropathy.

**3.** The absence of ankle reflexes has a sensitivity of 60% and specificity of 90% in 1 study, compared with a clinical gold standard (LR+ = 6; LR– = 0.44).

**4.** Another study compared 3 criteria (symptoms, abnormal temperature sensation, and absent ankle reflexes) to a clinical gold standard; if 2 of the 3 criteria were present, the sensitivity was 87% and specificity 91% (LR+ = 10.8; LR– = 0.14).

**5.** The ADA recommends screening for neuropathy at least annually by checking ankle reflexes and assessing sensation by testing pinprick, temperature, vibration, and pressure sensation with a monofilament.

**Table 11–5.** Physical exam findings in diabetic peripheral neuropathy.

| Test | Able to perceive stimulus ≥ 4 times (normal test) | | Able to perceive stimulus ≤ 3 times (abnormal test) | |
| --- | --- | --- | --- | --- |
| | Sensitivity (%) | LR– | Specificity (%) | LR+ |
| Monofilament | 77 | 0.34 | 96 | 10.2 |
| Timed vibration | 80 | 0.33 | 98 | 18.5 |
| Superficial pain | 59 | 0.5 | 97 | 9.2 |
| On-off vibration | 53 | 0.51 | 99 | 26.6 |

**B.** Diabetic autonomic neuropathy

**1.** Cardiovascular autonomic neuropathy

**a.** There are standardized ways to measure heart rate variability.

**b.** Postural change in systolic BP is used to diagnose orthostatic hypotension caused by diabetic autonomic neuropathy; the systolic BP is measured with the patient supine and again after 2 minutes of standing.

**(1)** A drop of < 10 mm Hg is normal.

**(2)** A drop of 10–29 mm Hg is borderline.

**(3)** A drop of > 30 mm Hg is definitely abnormal.

**2.** Gustatory sweating is diagnosed by history.

**3.** GI dysfunction

**a.** Esophageal dysmotility: Esophagogastroduodenoscopy and manometry

**b.** Gastroparesis: Diagnosed clinically or by a "gastric emptying" study, consisting of double-isotope scintigraphy of either solids or liquids

**c.** Diabetic diarrhea: Rule out other causes of chronic diarrhea.

**d.** Anorectal dysfunction: Anorectal manometry and defecography can be done to document abnormalities.

**4.** Genitourinary dysfunction

**a.** Urinary bladder dysfunction: Ultrasound and urodynamic testing

**b.** Erectile dysfunction: History

**Treatment**

**A.** Tight glycemic control

**1.** Definitely prevents and improves neuropathy in persons with type 1 DM (RR reduction of 60%, NNT of 15 to prevent 1 case of neuropathy in tightly controlled patients)

**2.** Possibly prevents and improves neuropathy in persons with type 2 DM

**B.** Otherwise, treatment is symptomatic.

**1.** Peripheral neuropathy

**a.** Tricyclic antidepressants, gabapentin, and pregabalin all shown to effectively reduce neuropathic pain

**b.** Tramadol and opioids also effective

**c.** Capsaicin possibly effective

**d.** Nonsteroidal antiinflammatory drugs generally not effective

**2.** Autonomic neuropathy

**a.** Cardiovascular

**(1)** Orthostatic hypotension is usually the most disabling symptom.

**(a)** Patients should raise head of bed, and rise slowly.

**(b)** Patients can try an elasticized garment that extends from the feet to the costal margins.

**(c)** Fludrocortisone is sometimes used, but must beware of supine hypertension, excessive salt, and water retention

**(2)** Cardioselective β-blockers sometimes helpful

**b.** Sweating: no specific treatment available; clonidine may be effective.

**c.** Esophageal dysmotility: can try prokinetic agents such as metoclopramide

**d.** Gastroparesis

    **(1)** Severe gastroparesis is very difficult to manage.

    **(2)** Small meals sometimes help.

    **(3)** Prokinetic agents, such as metoclopramide or erythromycin, sometimes are effective.

    **(4)** Gastric electrical stimulation is being studied for refractory cases.

**e.** Constipation

    **(1)** Increase fiber

    **(2)** Drug choices include lactulose, polyethylene glycol, stool softeners.

    **(3)** Avoid senna, cascara due to stimulant activity

**f.** Urinary bladder dysfunction

    **(1)** Bethanecol

    **(2)** Intermittent self-catheterization

**g.** Erectile dysfunction: sildenafil and other similar agents

## 3. Nephropathy

### Textbook Presentation

Diabetic nephropathy is asymptomatic until it is so advanced that the patient has symptoms of renal failure.

### Disease Highlights

**A.** Occurs in 20–40% of patients with diabetes

**B.** The most common cause of end-stage renal disease (ESRD) in the United States and Europe, accounting for about 40% of new cases of ESRD.

**C.** Definitions (based on spot collection and calculation of the albumin/creatinine ratio in mcg/mg)

    **1.** Normal < 30

    **2.** Microalbuminuria = 30–299

    **3.** Macroalbuminuria (overt nephropathy) ≥ 300

**D.** Natural history: much better defined for type 1 than for type 2 DM

    **1.** Type 1 DM

        **a.** Renal enlargement and hyperfunction at onset of diabetes; continues for 5–15 years

        **b.** Microalbuminuria appears 10–15 years after onset of DM; glomerular filtration rate (GFR) and BP initially normal.

        **c.** Over the ensuing 10–15 years, 80% of patients progress to macroalbuminuria; GFR declines and hypertension develops.

        **d.** ESRD develops in 50% of patients with overt nephropathy within 10 years and in 75% by 20 years.

    **2.** Type 2 DM

        **a.** Natural history is less well defined because onset of type 2 DM is usually not well defined, and other causes of renal insufficiency (such as hypertension and vascular disease) are more common.

        **b.** 20–40% of patients with microalbuminuria progress to overt nephropathy.

        **c.** 20% have ESRD within 20 years of the onset of overt nephropathy.

**E.** Risk factors for development of nephropathy

    **1.** Poor glycemic control

    **2.** Hypertension

    **3.** Long duration of diabetes

    **4.** Male sex

    **5.** Ethnic predisposition (Native American, African American, Hispanic [especially Mexican American])

**F.** Patients with microalbuminuria have an increased risk of cardiovascular events.

### Evidence-Based Diagnosis

**A.** ADA recommends annual screening for microalbuminuria beginning at the time of diagnosis for patients with type 2 DM and at year 5 for patients with type 1 DM.

**B.** The recommended screening is a spot urinary albumin/creatinine ratio

    **1.** There is diurnal variation, so first-void or early-morning specimens are best; otherwise, try to obtain confirmatory specimen at same time of day as initial specimen.

    **2.** Short-term hyperglycemia, exercise, urinary tract infection, marked hypertension, heart failure, and acute febrile illness can cause transient elevations in albumin excretion.

    **3.** All abnormal tests should be confirmed by a second test.

    **4.** For morning specimens, sensitivity ranges from 70% to 100% and specificity ranges from 91% to 98%.

    **5.** For random specimens, sensitivity ranges from 56% to 97% and specificity ranges from 81% to 92%.

**C.** It is not clear whether it is necessary to measure the albumin/creatinine ratio annually in patients being treated with an ACE inhibitor or angiotensin receptor blocker (ARB).

**D.** All patients should have a serum creatinine checked at least annually.

### Treatment

**A.** Tight glycemic control reduces nephropathy.

    **1.** Type 1 DM

        **a.** Incidence of microalbuminuria reduced by 34% (NNT = 83) in patients without retinopathy and by 43% (NNT = 47) in patients with retinopathy

        **b.** Incidence of macroalbuminuria reduced by 56% (NNT = 125) in patients with retinopathy

    **2.** Type 2 DM

        **a.** Better control reduces the risk of microvascular complications (retinopathy and nephropathy) by 16–25%. ($HgbA_{1c}$ 7% vs 7.9% in the UKPDS [1998]; $HgbA_{1c}$ 6.5% vs 7.2% in the ADVANCE trial [2008].)

        **b.** NNT = 36 over 10 years in the UKPDS; NNT = 66 over 5 years in the ADVANCE trial

        **c.** The microvascular complication rate was 58% for patients with an $HgbA_{1c}$ ≥ 10% and 6.1% for patients with an $HgbA_{1c}$ < 6.0% (UKPDS).

        **d.** Microvascular complication rate decreases by 37% for every 1% reduction in $HgbA_{1c}$.

**B.** BP control and choice of agents

1. BP should be < 130/80 mm Hg.

2. Either ACE inhibitors or ARBs should be used

 **a.** ACE inhibitors have been shown to reduce

 **(1)** Progression to nephropathy in type 1 and type 2 diabetics with hypertension and albuminuria

 **(2)** Progression to microalbuminuria in type 2 diabetics with hypertension and normoalbuminuria

 **(3)** Cardiovascular events in patients with type 2 diabetes

 **b.** ARBs have been shown to reduce progression to nephropathy in type 2 diabetics with hypertension and albuminuria.

**C.** Protein restriction to about 10% of daily calories may reduce progression of overt nephropathy.

**D.** Refer to a nephrologist if the creatinine clearance is < 60 mL/min or hypertension cannot be controlled.

# 4. Diabetic Foot Ulcers

## Textbook Presentation

A patient with peripheral neuropathy is unaware of minor trauma and the beginning of plantar ulceration. By the time the ulcer is discovered incidentally, it is often advanced, sometimes with associated osteomyelitis.

## Disease Highlights

**A.** Lifetime risk of developing an ulcer is about 15%.

**B.** 90% of patients with ulcers have neuropathy, and 15–20% have peripheral vascular disease.

**C.** Tend to occur at pressure points, so plantar surface and sites of calluses are common locations

1. Venous ulcers generally occur above the medial or lateral malleolus

2. Arterial ulcers generally occur on the toes or shins

**D.** Risk factors

1. Duration of diabetes > 10 years

2. Male sex

3. Poor glycemic control

4. Coexisting cardiovascular, renal, or retinal complication

5. Peripheral neuropathy

6. Altered biomechanics

7. Evidence of increased pressure on the foot

8. Bony deformity of the foot or ankle

9. Peripheral vascular disease

10. A history of ulcers or amputation

11. Severe nail pathology

**E.** Pathophysiology

1. Repetitive mechanical stress occurs as a result of altered biomechanics, foot deformities, ill-fitting shoes.

2. Peripheral neuropathy causes loss of protective sensation, so the patient is unaware of the incipient ulceration.

3. Ischemia, resulting from macrovascular peripheral arterial disease (commonly in the tibioperoneal vessels) or microvascular dysfunction from autonomic neuropathy, inhibits healing and promotes progression.

**F.** Classification

1. Non–limb-threatening

 **a.** Superficial infection, purulent discharge, and minimal (< 2 cm extension from the ulcer) or absent cellulitis

 **b.** No systemic toxicity (fever, leukocytosis, severe hyperglycemia, or osteomyelitis)

2. Limb-threatening

 **a.** Ulceration to deep tissues, extensive purulent drainage, cellulitis extending more than 2 cm from the ulcer, and lymphangitis

 **b.** Systemic toxicity and significant ischemia, with or without gangrene, present

3. Life-threatening

 **a.** Ulceration to deep tissues, extensive purulent drainage, cellulitis, necrosis, gangrene, osteomyelitis

 **b.** Marked systemic toxicity, including septic shock

**G.** Microbiology

1. Non–limb-threatening infections average 2 species/ulcer, but are often monomicrobial.

2. Limb-threatening and life-threatening infections are generally polymicrobial.

3. *Staphylococcus aureus* is most common organism and is present in 50% of infections.

4. Streptococci present in one-third of cases.

5. Gram-negative organisms, especially *Proteus, Klebsiella, Escherichia coli,* and *Pseudomonas,* present in polymicrobial infections.

6. Anaerobic gram-positive cocci and *Bacteroides* present in up to 80% of polymicrobial infections.

**H.** Osteomyelitis develops in 15% of patients with foot ulcers.

## Evidence-Based Diagnosis

**A.** ADA recommendations include at least annual foot examinations that should include screening for neuropathy and assessing foot structure, biomechanics, vascular status, and skin integrity.

1. Patients with neuropathy should have a foot exam at every visit.

2. ADA recommends screening for peripheral arterial disease with ankle-brachial index measurements in patients over age 50 and those under age 50 with other vascular risk factors in addition to diabetes.

 You cannot examine the feet of your diabetic patients too often!

**B.** Culturing ulcers

1. Can be difficult to distinguish between colonizing organisms and true pathogens

2. Deep cultures of the ulcer or the bone are more reliable but are more invasive to perform

3. Swab cultures identify the same pathogens as bone culture in only 19–36% of patients.

4. If the patient is responding to empiric therapy, it is not necessary to culture.

C. Diagnosing complications

1. Cellulitis: clinical diagnosis (see Chapter 15, Edema)

2. Osteomyelitis (Table 11–6)

   a. Open bone biopsy with culture is the gold standard.

   b. Needle bone biopsy subject to sampling error (sensitivity, 87%; specificity, 93%; LR+, 12.4; LR–, 0.14)

   c. Being able to see bone or to probe the ulcer down to bone increases the probability the patient has osteomyelitis

   d. C-reactive protein (CRP), erythrocyte sedimentation rate (ESR), CBC, blood cultures not sufficiently sensitive or specific to diagnose osteomyelitis.

   e. MRI is the imaging procedure with the best test characteristics; bone scan and WBC scans are less specific.

 MRI scan is the best imaging procedure to diagnose osteomyelitis in a patient with a diabetic foot ulcer.

 A normal CBC, CRP, or ESR does not rule out osteomyelitis.

## Treatment

A. Preventive foot care

1. Improve glycemic control to reduce risk of neuropathy.

2. Reduce vascular risk factors (smoking cessation, BP control, lipid management, glycemic control).

3. Examine the feet of high-risk patients at every visit (patients with peripheral neuropathy, evidence of increased pressure, limited joint mobility, bony deformity, severe nail pathology, peripheral vascular disease, or a history of ulcers or amputation).

4. Examine the feet of low-risk patients at least annually.

5. Ensure patients wear well-fitted shoes.

**Table 11–6.** Test characteristics for the diagnosis of osteomyelitis in patients with diabetic foot ulcers.

|  | LR+ | LR– |
|---|---|---|
| **Physical Exam Findings** | | |
| Bone exposure | 9.2 | 0.7 |
| Ulcer area > 2 cm² | 7.2 | 0.48 |
| Positive probe to bone | 6.4 | 0.39 |
| Ulcer inflammation (erythema, swelling, purulence) | 1.5 | 0.84 |
| **Laboratory Tests** | | |
| ESR > 70 mm/h | 11 | 0.34 |
| **Imaging Studies** | | |
| MRI | 5.1 | 0.12 |
| Radiographs | 2.3 | 0.63 |

6. Educate patients regarding need for daily visual inspection of feet.

7. Refer to podiatrist for débridement of calluses, assessment of bony deformities.

B. Treatment of ulcers

1. Treat any infection.

   a. Patients with non–limb-threatening infections

      (1) Can generally be treated with oral antibiotics in the outpatient setting

      (2) Oral antibiotic choices include clindamycin, amoxicillin–clavulanate, and fluoroquinolones; the increasing prevalence of community-acquired methicillin-resistant *S aureus* (MRSA) should be considered when choosing empiric therapy.

      (3) Patients should be reassessed after 24–48 hours and switched to IV therapy if there is no response.

   b. All other patients should be hospitalized and given IV antibiotics.

      (1) IV antibiotic choices include ampicillin–sulbactam, ticarcillin–clavulanate, levofloxacin, imipenem– cilastin, with vancomycin often added to cover MRSA.

      (2) 10–14 days of therapy are generally adequate for patients without osteomyelitis; those with osteomyelitis need 3–10 weeks.

      (3) Can often switch from IV to oral therapy if patients are improving

2. Determine need for revascularization, and revascularize as early as possible in patients with treatable peripheral vascular disease.

3. Heal the ulcer.

   a. Off loading: use orthotics or fiberglass casts to remove pressure from the wound while allowing the patient to remain active.

   b. Débride ulcers (surgically or with débriding agents such as hydrogels).

   c. Control edema.

   d. Growth factors are being studied.

4. Institute preventive measures once the ulcer has healed.

 A multidisciplinary approach, including internal medicine, vascular surgery, and podiatry is necessary for the optimal treatment of diabetic foot ulcers.

## MAKING A DIAGNOSIS

The ophthalmologist reports that Mrs. D has no retinopathy. Her neurologic exam, including monofilament testing, is normal. She does not complain of orthostatic dizziness or any GI or genitourinary symptoms. She has bilateral bunions but no calluses or ulcers. Her albumin–creatinine ratio is 50 mcg/mg, confirmed on repeat testing. Her HgbA$_{1c}$ is 9.1%.

Have you crossed a diagnostic threshold for the leading hypothesis, diabetic complications? Have you ruled out the active alternatives? Do other tests need to be done to exclude the alternative diagnoses?

The evaluation for diabetic complications is complete. Mrs. D has no evidence of retinopathy, neuropathy, or diabetic foot disease. She does have microalbuminuria. However, before formulating a treatment plan for Mrs. D, it is necessary to assess for the presence or absence of other cardiovascular risk factors and cardiovascular disease:

1. Dyslipidemia
2. Hypertension
3. Obesity
4. Smoking
5. Coronary artery disease (CAD)
6. Cerebrovascular disease
7. Peripheral vascular disease

Table 11–7 outlines a summary of testing that must be performed on all patients with diabetes.

**Table 11–7.** Summary of testing and monitoring recommended for patients with diabetes.

| Condition | Required Test/Action |
|---|---|
| Retinopathy | Ophthalmologic exam[1] |
| Peripheral neuropathy | Monofilament testing, ankle reflexes, vibration sense[1] |
| Nephropathy | Albumin/creatinine ratio, serum creatinine[1] |
| Diabetic foot ulcers | Foot exam[1] |
| Dyslipidemia | Fasting total cholesterol, HDL, triglycerides, LDL[1] |
| Hypertension | BP measurement[1] |
| Smoking | Obtain history and counsel cessation[1] |
| Obesity | Measure weight and calculate BMI[1] |
| Coronary artery disease | Assess for symptoms; screening asymptomatic patients controversial |
| Cerebrovascular disease | Carotid duplex ultrasound in patients with symptoms |
| Peripheral vascular disease | ABIs in patients over 50 and those under 50 with other vascular risk factors in addition to diabetes |

[1]Should be performed at least annually and may need to be done more often in patients with abnormalities.
ABI, ankle-brachial index; BMI, body mass index; HDL, high-density lipoprotein; LDL, low-density lipoprotein.

## CASE RESOLUTION

Mrs. D has no symptoms of vascular disease on careful questioning, and her exercise tolerance is more than 1 mile. Her fasting lipid panel shows total cholesterol of 230 mg/dL, HDL of 45 mg/dL, triglycerides of 200 mg/dL, and LDL of 145 mg/dL. You refer Mrs. D to a diabetes educator and a nutritionist for instruction about diet and exercise. You also prescribe metformin for the diabetes and atorvastatin for the hyperlipidemia. Because she has hypertension and microalbuminuria, you elect to start an ACE inhibitor, lisinopril, to treat her hypertension. You also recommend that she start taking aspirin, 81 mg daily. Over the next 12–18 months, Mrs. D loses 5 pounds. You increase the dose of metformin, add glipizide, and her $HgbA_{1c}$ decreases to 6.7%. After increasing the dose of lisinopril and adding hydrochlorothiazide, her BP is 128/80 mm Hg. Her LDL is now 85 mg/dL.

### Treatment of Type 2 Diabetes

The treatment of type 2 diabetes involves not only the treatment of the hyperglycemia but the management of associated complications and cardiovascular risk factors as well. According to survey data, only 37% of participants reach $HgbA_{1c}$ goals, 35.8% reach BP goals, and 48% reach cholesterol goals; only 7.3% reach all 3 goals.

It is common for patients to require 6–7 medications to meet accepted treatment goals.

### Treatment of Hyperglycemia

A. Treatment goals

   1. The ADA recommends treating to a $HgbA_{1c}$ < 7.0%

      a. $HgbA_{1c}$ levels < 7% have been clearly shown to reduce microvascular events in patients with type 2 DM (see data above).

      b. Intensive control has not been consistently shown to reduce macrovascular events; intensive control may be harmful in *older* diabetics *with* cardiovascular disease, and may be beneficial in younger persons in whom diabetes was recently diagnosed.

      (1) UKPDS (1998)

        (a) About 4200 persons with *newly* diagnosed type 2 DM without CV disease, mean age 53, randomized to conventional therapy ($HgbA_{1c}$ 7.9%) vs intensive therapy with sulfonylureas with or without insulin ($HgbA_{1c}$ 7.0%) and monitored for 10 years

        (b) RR of myocardial infarction (MI) in the intensive group = 0.84 (95% CI, 0.71–1.00)

        (c) A separate study arm randomized obese patients to receive metformin or conventional therapy; there was a significant reduction in MI with metformin (RR = 0.61, 0.41–0.89)

(2) UKPDS 10-year follow up (2008)

    (a) About 3200 of the original 4200 patients were monitored for an additional 10 years after the intervention trial ended, with patients returning to their personal physicians for diabetes care

    (b) Endpoints included death from any cause, diabetes-related death, MI, stroke, peripheral arterial disease, microvascular disease, any diabetes-related endpoint.

    (c) The mean $HgbA_{1c}$ was about 8% in all groups (conventional, sulfonylurea/insulin, metformin) 1 year after the intervention trial ended

    (d) Patients originally assigned to sulfonylurea/insulin had significant reductions in all endpoints measured (RR for MI 0.85, 95% CI 0.74–0.97; RR for death from any cause = 0.87, 0.79–0.96)

    (e) Patients originally assigned to metformin had significant reductions in any diabetes-related endpoint, death from any cause (RR = 0.73, 0.59–0.89), diabetes-related death, and MI (RR = 0.67, 0.51–0.89)

    (f) These results suggest a "legacy" effect from initial intensive therapy in type 2 diabetes, similar to that seen in long-term follow-up of type 1 diabetics.

(3) ADVANCE trial (2008)

    (a) About 11,000 type 2 diabetics with cardiovascular disease or multiple risk factors, mean age 66, randomized to intensive control with a sulfonylurea-based regimen ($HgbA_{1c}$ 6.5%) vs conventional control ($HgbA_{1c}$ 7.2%) and monitored for 5 years

    (b) No difference in macrovascular events (RR = 0.94, 0.84–1.06)

(4) ACCORD trial (2008)

    (a) About 10,000 type 2 diabetics with cardiovascular disease or multiple risk factors, mean age 62, randomized to intensive control ($HgbA_{1c}$ 6.4%) vs conventional control (7.5%) and monitored for 3.5 years

    (b) No difference in primary endpoint (nonfatal MI, nonfatal stroke, or cardiovascular death)

    (c) Increase in any cause death with intensive treatment (RR = 1.22 (1.01–1.46), NNH = 100)

    (d) Increase in cardiovascular death with intensive treatment (RR = 1.35 (1.04–1.76), NNH = 125)

    (e) Most patients in the intensive group received rosiglitazone, which is associated with increased risk of MI.

2. Goals should be modified for frail elderly, in whom avoidance of hypoglycemia and optimization of functional status may be more important than tight glycemic control.

**Table 11–8.** Correlation between plasma glucose and $HgbA_{1c}$.

| $HgbA1_c$ (%) | Mean Plasma Glucose (mg/dL) |
|---|---|
| 6 | 135 |
| 7 | 170 |
| 8 | 205 |
| 9 | 240 |
| 10 | 275 |
| 11 | 310 |
| 12 | 345 |

B. Monitoring

  1. $HgbA_{1c}$ levels every 3–6 months (Table 11–8 shows correlation between plasma glucose and $HgbA_{1c}$.)

    a. The $HgbA_{1c}$ is altered unpredictably by Hgb variants.

    b. Processes that shorten RBC life span, such as kidney disease, liver disease, hemolytic anemia, hemoglobinopathies, and recovery from blood loss, will decrease the $HgbA_{1c}$.

    c. Processes that slow erythropoiesis, such as iron deficiency anemia, increase the $HgbA_{1c}$.

    d. 50% of $HgbA_{1c}$ is determined by glycemia during the month before the measurement, 25% from the 30–60 days before, and 25% from 60–90 days before.

  2. Home glucose monitoring

    a. Patients taking insulin should test blood levels several times a day (fasting, before lunch, before dinner, and before bed) if not well controlled and perhaps less often if well controlled.

    b. Optimal frequency for patients taking oral agents is unclear; recent studies suggest home glucose monitoring does not improve $HgbA_{1c}$ levels in patients with type 2 diabetes taking oral agents but does increase anxiety.

C. Lifestyle modification

  1. Weight loss (goal of at least 10% of body weight), diet modification, and exercise (goal of at least 150 minutes/week) are the foundations of all treatment for diabetes.

  2. Best instituted in conjunction with a certified diabetes educator or nutritionist

D. Oral hypoglycemics

  1. Sulfonylureas

    a. Examples: glyburide, glipizide, glimepiride

    b. Increase insulin secretion.

    c. Average decrease in $HgbA_{1c}$ about 1–2%

    d. Side effects include weight gain (2–5 kg) and hypoglycemia, especially in the elderly, patients with reduced renal function, and those with erratic eating habits.

**e.** Shown to reduce microvascular outcomes; no change in cardiovascular events.

**f.** Can be used as monotherapy or in combination with insulin or other oral agents (except non-sulfonylurea secretagogues)

**g.** May become less effective with time, as beta cell function decreases

2. Biguanides

**a.** Example: metformin

**b.** Reduce hepatic glucose production.

**c.** Average decrease in HgbA$_{1c}$ about 1–2%

**d.** Associated with weight loss (or at least no weight gain); hypoglycemia rare

**e.** Most common side effects are GI (abdominal pain, nausea, diarrhea).

**f.** Because of risk of lactic acidosis, contraindicated in patients with creatinine ≥ 1.5 mg/dL, decompensated heart failure (HF), significant hepatic dysfunction, metabolic acidosis, and alcoholism.

 Metformin should be withheld in patients with acute illness and those undergoing surgery or procedures using radiocontrast.

**g.** Has been shown to decrease microvascular and macrovascular outcomes, and total mortality in obese type 2 diabetics (UKPDS, 1998)

**h.** Can be used as monotherapy or in combination with all other oral agents and insulin

3. α-Glucosidase inhibitors

**a.** Example: acarbose

**b.** Delay and decrease intestinal carbohydrate absorption, decreasing postprandial glucose swings

**c.** About 50% less efficacious than sulfonylureas and metformin in reducing HgbA$_{1c}$

**d.** Side effects include flatulence, abdominal discomfort, and diarrhea.

**e.** No studies of effects on macrovascular or microvascular outcomes

**f.** Can be used as monotherapy, but this is rarely done because of relatively poor efficacy; can also be used in combination with sulfonylureas

4. Thiazolidinediones (TZDs)

**a.** Examples: rosiglitazone, pioglitazone

**b.** Increase insulin-stimulated glucose uptake by skeletal muscle cells.

**c.** Average decrease in HgbA$_{1c}$ about 1–2%

**d.** Tend to increase HDL and decrease triglycerides

**e.** Can take weeks or months to obtain maximum effect

**f.** Side effects include weight gain (as great as or more so than that seen with sulfonylureas) and edema.

**g.** Increased risk of HF with both agents (RR ~ 3)

**h.** Increased risk of cardiovascular events with rosiglitazone; current data suggest pioglitazone either does not affect or reduces cardiovascular events

 Do not use TZDs in patients with HF or edema.

**i.** Can be used as monotherapy or in combination with sulfonylureas, metformin, and insulin.

5. Non-sulfonylurea secretagogues

**a.** Examples: repaglinide, nateglinide

**b.** Because of short half-life, cause brief, episodic increases in insulin secretion

**c.** Primarily reduce postprandial glucose, with less risk of hypoglycemia than with sulfonylureas

**d.** Efficacy of repaglinide similar to that of sulfonylureas and metformin; nateglinide less efficacious

**e.** No long-term studies of effects on macrovascular or microvascular outcomes

**f.** Must be dosed with every meal

**g.** Should be used cautiously in patients with hepatic or renal dysfunction

**h.** Can be used as monotherapy or in combination with metformin

6. DPP4 inhibitors

**a.** Incretins (glucose-dependent insulinotropic polypeptide [GIP] and glucagonlike peptide 1 [GLP-1]) are intestinal peptides that augment insulin secretion in the presence of glucose or nutrients in the gut; they are inactivated by the enzyme dipeptidyl peptidase 4 (DPP4).

**b.** Sitagliptin and vildagliptin are selective DPP4 inhibitors.

**c.** Decrease HgbA$_{1c}$ by ~0.75%

**d.** No GI side effects; average weight gain < 1 kg

**e.** Less effective than metformin in a direct comparison

**f.** No data on macrovascular or microvascular outcomes

E. GLP-1 receptor analogues

1. Example: exenatide

2. Given subcutaneously twice daily

3. Decrease HgbA$_{1c}$ by about 1%, similar in efficacy to insulin

4. Most common side effects are nausea and vomiting.

5. Average weight loss of ~1.5 kg when compared with placebo and of ~4.75 kg when compared with insulin

6. No data on macrovascular or microvascular outcomes

F. Insulin

1. Types of insulin (Table 11–9)

2. Adverse effects of insulin

**a.** Hypoglycemia, especially with short-acting forms

**b.** Weight gain of 2–4 kg

G. Choosing a medication to treat type 2 DM

1. Most studies compare an agent to placebo, so direct comparison data are limited

***Table 11–9.*** Types of insulin.

| | Onset of Action | Peak | Duration of Action |
|---|---|---|---|
| **Rapid Acting** | | | |
| Lispro (Humalog) Aspart (Novolog) | 5–15 min | 45–75 min | 2–4 h |
| **Short Acting** | | | |
| Regular U100 | ~30 min | 2–4 h | 5–8 h |
| **Intermediate Acting** | | | |
| Isophane (NPH, Humulin N, Novolin N) | ~2 h | 4-10 h | 10–16 h |
| Insulin zinc (Lente, Humulin L, Novolin L) | ~2 h | 4-12 h | 12–18 h |
| **Long Acting** | | | |
| Glargine (Lantus) | ~2 h | No peak | 20 to > 24 h |
| Detemir (Levemir) | ~2 h | No peak | 6–24 h |
| **Premixed** | | | |
| Humulin 70/30 (70% NPH/ 30% regular) | | | |
| Humalog Mix 75/25 (75% NPL [neutral protamine lispro, similar to NPH]/25% lispro) | | | |
| Novalog Mix 70/30 (70% NPH/30% aspart) | | | |

2. Sulfonylureas, metformin, and insulin have the best long-term outcome data.

3. 75% of patients require more than 1 drug by 9 years; there is no evidence that any specific combination is better than another.

4. There is not a standard, evidence-based approach to treatment; the algorithm in Figure 11–1 is consistent with ADA consensus recommendations.

5. Using insulin to manage type 2 diabetes
   a. Beta cell function declines over time in type 2 DM, so many patients will eventually need insulin.
   b. The first step is to add long-acting basal insulin to oral agents, titrating the insulin dose to the fasting blood sugar.
      (1) There are fewer nocturnal hypoglycemic episodes with bedtime glargine than with bedtime NPH.
      (2) There is less weight gain with metformin and insulin than with sulfonylureas or TZDs and insulin.
   c. If the HgbA$_{1c}$ target is not achieved, options include adding a short-acting insulin, such as lispro, with meals, or switching to twice daily biphasic insulin.
   d. Sulfonylureas should be stopped when short-acting insulins are used because of increased hypoglycemia.

## Treatment of Hypertension

The treatment goal is to achieve a BP < 130/80 mm Hg. See Nephropathy section and Hypertension chapter for details.

## Treatment of Hypercholesterolemia

A. Statin therapy should be used, *regardless of baseline lipid levels*, in diabetic patients with cardiovascular disease, and those without cardiovascular disease who are over age 40 and have at least 1 other cardiovascular risk factor.

B. Low-risk patients (those under age 40 or those over age 40 without cardiovascular disease or additional risk factors) do not require statin therapy if their LDL is < 100 mg/dL.

C. The LDL goal is < 100 mg/dL for patients without known cardiovascular disease.

D. The LDL goal is < 70 mg/dL for patients with known cardiovascular disease.

E. Reduction of LDL by 40% is an alternative therapeutic goal in patients who cannot achieve targets on maximal tolerated doses of statins.

F. There are no data regarding whether the addition of ezetimibe to statins reduces cardiovascular outcomes.

G. Although ideally triglycerides are < 150 mg/dL, and HDL is > 50 mg/dL in women and 40 mg/dL in men, there are no data regarding whether the addition of a fibrate or niacin to a statin further reduces cardiovascular outcomes.

## Antiplatelet Therapy

A. Low-dose aspirin (75–162 mg/day) prevents vascular events in diabetics with or without preexisting vascular disease.

B. ADA guidelines recommend low-dose aspirin for the following groups:
   1. All patients with preexisting vascular disease
   2. All type 2 diabetics older than 40 years
   3. Type 2 diabetics younger than 40 years who have additional risk factors such as family history, hypertension, smoking, dyslipidemia, microalbuminuria

 The optimally treated patient with type 2 diabetes does not smoke, exercises regularly, takes low-dose aspirin, an ACE inhibitor, and a statin, and has an HgbA$_{1c}$ < 7.0%, BP < 130/80 mm Hg, and LDL < 100 mg/dL.

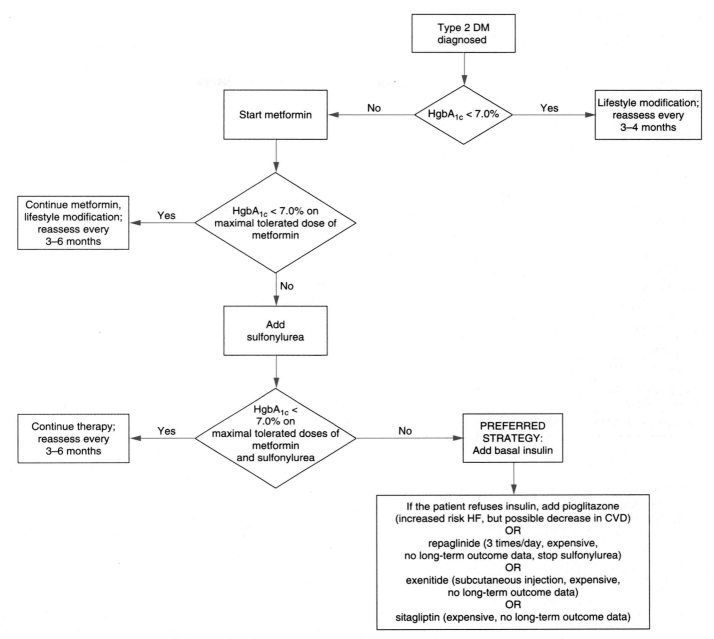

CVD, cardiovascular disease; DM, diabetes mellitus; HF, heart failure.

*Figure 11–1.* Approach to treatment of type 2 DM.

## CHIEF COMPLAINT

PATIENT  2

Mr. G is a 56-year-old African American man with diabetes, chronic hepatitis B, CAD status post MI 2 months ago, hypertension, and a history of stroke 1 year ago. He is taking many medications, including Humulin 70/30 20 units twice daily, metoprolol, aspirin, atorvastatin, lisinopril, furosemide, and ribavirin. Despite all of these problems, he has been slowly improving and reported at his last visit 3 weeks ago that he had recently given up his walker for a cane. Today you are paged by his sister, who reports that Mr. G is very weak and cannot get up; his home glucose monitor reading is "critical high." Mr. G's voice is barely recognizable over the phone, and he is unable to respond to your questions. You advise his sister to call 911.

**At this point, what is the leading hypothesis, what are the active alternatives, and is there a must not miss diagnosis? Given this differential diagnosis, what tests should be ordered?**

## PRIORITIZING THE DIFFERENTIAL DIAGNOSIS

The differential diagnosis at this point is very broad and difficult to organize. It is helpful to recognize that Mr. G appears to be suffering from the syndrome of delirium and to use the framework for delirium to organize your thinking (see Chapter 10, Delirium and Dementia). It is also reasonable to consider Mr. G's underlying chronic medical problems as pivotal points and initially focus on the serious complications of these conditions; in other words, initially focus on diseases for which he has a high pretest probability:

1. Diabetes: DKA, hyperosmolar hyperglycemic state (HHS), infection with or without sepsis.
2. CAD: recurrent MI, possibly with HF or cardiogenic shock
3. Cerebrovascular disease: recurrent stroke
4. Chronic hepatitis B: hepatic encephalopathy

Mr. G could have any of these conditions or more than 1 of them. His critical high blood sugar makes a complication of diabetes the leading hypothesis; all of the other diagnoses are "must not miss" hypotheses (Table 11–10).

When Mr. G arrives in the emergency department, he is barely responsive but able to move all 4 extremities. His BP is 85/50 mm Hg; pulse, 120 bpm; RR, 24 breaths per minute; temperature, 37.2°C. His lungs are clear, and cardiac exam shows an $S_4$ with no $S_3$ or murmurs. His abdomen is nontender, and there is no peripheral edema. Initial laboratory tests include the following:

Sodium, 138 mEq/L; K, 4.9 mEq/L; Cl, 88 mEq/L; $HCO_3$, 37 mEq/L; BUN, 99 mg/dL; creatinine, 4.3 mg/dL; glucose, 1246 mg/dL

Arterial blood gases: pH 7.40; $PO_2$, 88 mm Hg; $PCO_2$, 35 mm Hg

WBC is 8400/mcL, with 75% polymorphonuclear neutrophils, 3% bands, 18% lymphocytes, and 4% monocytes.

Albumin, 4.4 g/dL; total bilirubin, 0.3 mg/dL; alkaline phosphatase, 175 units/L; AST (SGOT), 40 units/L; ALT (SGPT), 56 units/L; INR, 1.1.

Serum ketones, negative

$$\text{Corrected Na (sodium)} = \frac{\text{measured Na} + (2.4 \times \text{glucose} - 100)}{100}$$

$$= 138 + 2.4(11) = 164$$

Urinalysis: 2+ protein, 4+ glucose, no ketones, 3–5 WBC/high-power field, occasional bacteria

 Is the clinical information sufficient to make a diagnosis? If not, what other information do you need?

## Leading Hypothesis: Hyperosmolar Hyperglycemic State

### Textbook Presentation

Patients with HHS are usually older type 2 diabetics who present with the gradual onset of polydipsia, polyuria, and lethargy. They are extremely dehydrated and have very high serum glucose levels.

**Table 11–10.** Diagnostic hypotheses for Mr. G.

| Diagnostic Hypotheses | Clinical Clues | Important Tests |
|---|---|---|
| **Leading Hypothesis** | | |
| Hyperosmolar hyperglycemic state (HHS) | Delirium/coma Polyuria Polydipsia Dehydration | Plasma glucose Serum/urine ketones |
| **Active Alternatives—Must Not Miss** | | |
| Diabetic ketoacidosis | Delirium/coma Polyuria Polydipsia Dehydration | Blood glucose/ bicarbonate Serum/urine ketones pH |
| Sepsis | Hypotension Fever | Blood cultures Urinalysis Chest radiograph |
| Myocardial infarction | Chest pain Dyspnea | ECG Cardiac enzymes |
| Cerebrovascular accident | Hemiparesis Aphasia | Physical exam Head CT or MRI |
| Hepatic encephalopathy | Delirium Liver disease | Clinical diagnosis |

### Disease Highlights

A. Epidemiology

1. Incidence is 1/1000 person-years (DKA incidence is 4.6–8.0/1000 person years).

2. Mortality rate about 15%

3. Risk factors include older age, nursing home residence, inability to recognize thirst, and lack of access to fluids.

**Table 11–11.** Laboratory findings in HHS and DKA.

| Laboratory Parameter | HHS | DKA |
|---|---|---|
| Plasma glucose (mg/dL) | > 600 | > 300 |
| Arterial pH | > 7.30 | < 7.3 (< 7.0 in severe DKA) |
| Serum bicarbonate (mEq/L) | > 15 | < 15 (< 10 in severe DKA) |
| Urine ketones | Negative or small | > 3+ |
| Serum ketones | Negative or small | Positive |
| Anion gap | Variable | > 12 |
| Effective serum osmolality (mOsm/L)[1] | > 320 | Variable |

[1]Effective serum osmolality = 2 × Na (mEq/L)+ glucose (mg/dL)/18
HHS, hyperosmolar hyperglycemic state; DKA, diabetic ketoacidosis.

**B.** Pathogenesis

**1.** A reduction in the effective action of circulating insulin and a concomitant increase in counterregulatory hormones leads to increased hepatic and renal glucose production and impaired glucose utilization in peripheral tissues.

**2.** Glycosuria leads to an osmotic diuresis with loss of free water in excess of electrolytes, leading to hyperosmolality.

**3.** As volume depletion occurs, urinary output drops, and hyperglycemia worsens.

**4.** The absence of ketoacidosis in HHS is not completely understood; possible explanations are as follows:

**a.** There are higher intraportal insulin levels than seen in DKA, sufficient to prevent lipolysis.

**b.** The levels of counterregulatory hormones are lower than in DKA.

**c.** The hyperosmolar state inhibits lipolysis.

**C.** Precipitating factors

**1.** The 3 most common precipitants are infection, lack of compliance with insulin, and first presentation of diabetes.

**2.** Other precipitants include postoperative state, cerebrovascular accident (CVA), MI, pancreatitis, alcohol abuse, trauma, thyrotoxicosis, and medications (eg, corticosteroids, total parenteral nutrition).

**D.** Clinical manifestations

**1.** History

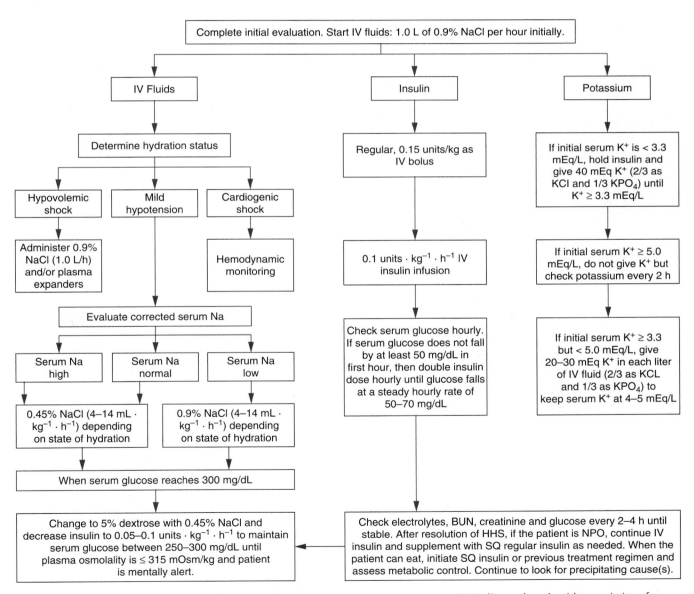

***Figure 11–2.*** Management of adult patients with hyperosmolar hyperglycemic state (HHS). (Reproduced, with permission, from American Diabetes Association, Diabetes Care. 2004;27:S94–S102.)

a. Symptoms and signs usually evolve over several days or even weeks.

b. Common findings include polyuria, polydipsia, fatigue, and weight loss.

c. Abdominal pain generally does not occur in HHS, as it does in DKA, but there are reports of a hypertonicity-induced gastroparesis leading to abdominal pain, distention, nausea, and vomiting.

d. Neurologic manifestations

   (1) Lethargy and disorientation common

   (2) Focal neurologic findings, including seizures, can occur with hyperglycemia and resolve with normalization of serum glucose.

   (3) Changes in mental status correlate with the degree of hyperosmolarity.

     (a) 20–25% present with coma.

     (b) Coma present in half of patients with effective serum osmolality of > 350 mOsm/L

     (c) Must search for another cause of coma if osmolality < 345–350 mOsm/L

2. Physical exam

a. Hypothermia often seen resulting from peripheral vasodilation

b. Signs of dehydration (see Chapter 25, Acute Renal Failure) often seen

c. Tachycardia and hypotension suggest severe dehydration or underlying sepsis.

### Evidence-Based Diagnosis

A. Typical total body water deficit is 20–25% (about 9 L).

B. See Table 11–11 for laboratory findings in HHS compared with DKA.

### Treatment

A. Patients with HHS generally need more fluid and less insulin than those with DKA

B. Figure 11–2 outlines the treatment approach.

## MAKING A DIAGNOSIS

Mr. G's glucose is > 600 mg/dL, ketones are negative, and calculated serum osmolality is 345 mOsm/L (effective serum osmolality = 2 × measured Na + glucose/18 = (2 × 138) + 1246/18 = 345).

**Have you crossed a diagnostic threshold for the leading hypothesis, HHS? Have you ruled out the active alternatives? Do other tests need to be done to exclude the alternative diagnoses?**

Mr. G fulfills the diagnostic criteria for HHS. It is not necessary to consider other diagnoses, but it is essential to determine the precipitant for this event. Considering Mr. G's complicated

history, he is at risk for many of the precipitants of HHS, especially infection, MI, and CVA.

 Always look for the precipitant when patients present with either HHS or DKA.

## CASE RESOLUTION

Mr. G's chest radiograph is clear, his urine and blood cultures are negative, his ECG shows no acute changes, and his cardiac enzymes are normal. He responds well to IV hydration and insulin therapy. When he becomes more alert, he reports that he had become depressed and had stopped taking his insulin.

## REFERENCES

American Diabetes Association. Diagnosis and classification of diabetes mellitus. Diabetes Care. 2008;31:s55–s60.

American Diabetes Association. Hyperglycemic crises in patients with diabetes mellitus. Diabetes Care. 2004;27:S94–S102.

American Diabetes Association. Standard of medical care in diabetes—2008. Diabetes Care. 2008;31:S12–s54.

Bax JJ, Young LH, Frye RL et al. Screening for coronary artery disease in patients with diabetes. Diabetes Care. 2007;30:2729–36.

Bolen S, Feldman L, Vassy J et al. Systematic review: comparative effectiveness and safety of oral medications for type 2 diabetes mellitus. Ann Intern Med. 2007;147:386–99.

Boulton AJM, Vinik AI, Arezzo JC et al. Diabetic neuropathies. Diabetes Care. 2005;28:956–62.

Butalia S, Palda VA, Sargeant RJ et al. Does this patient with diabetes have osteomyelitis of the lower extremity? JAMA. 2008;299:806–13.

England JD, Gronseth GS, Franklin G et al. Distal symmetric polyneuropathy: a definition for clinical research. Neurology. 2005;64:199–207.

Holman RR, Paul SK, Bethel A et al. 10-year follow up of intensive glucose control in type 2 diabetes. N Engl J Med. 2008;359:1577–89.

Kapoor A, Page S, LaValley M et al. Magnetic resonance imaging for diagnosing foot osteomyelitis. Arch Intern Med. 2007;167:125–32.

Mohamed Q, Gillies MC, Wong TY. Management of diabetic retinopathy: a systematic review. JAMA. 2007;298:902–16.

Nathan DM, Buse JB, Davidson, MB et al. Medical management of hyperglycemia in type 2 diabetes: a consensus algorithm for the initiation and adjustment of therapy. Diabetes Care. 2008;31:1–11.

Perkins BA, Olaleye D, Zinman B, Bril V. Simple screening tests for peripheral neuropathy in the diabetes clinic. Diabetes Care. 2001;24:250–56.

Saudek CD, Derr RL, Kalyani RR. Assessing glycemia in diabetes using self-monitoring blood glucose and hemoglobin A1c. JAMA. 2006;295:1688–97.

The Action to Control Cardiovascular Risk in Diabetes Study Group. Effects of intensive glucose lowering in type 2 DM. N Engl J Med. 2008;358:2545–59.

The ADVANCE Collaborative Group. Intensive blood glucose control and vascular outcomes in patients with type 2 diabetes. N Engl J Med. 2008;358:2560–72.

The Diabetes Control and Complications Trial Research Group. The effect of intensive treatment of diabetes on the development and progression of long-term complication in insulin-dependent diabetes mellitus. N Engl J Med. 1993;329:977–86.

UK Prospective Diabetes Study (UKPDS) Group. Intensive blood-glucose control with sulphonylureas or insulin compared with conventional treatment and risk of complications in patients with type 2 diabetes. (UKPDS 34) UK Prospective Diabetes Study Group. Lancet. 1998;352:837–53.

# I have a patient with acute diarrhea. How do I determine the cause?

## CHIEF COMPLAINT

**PATIENT** ▽1

Mr. C is a 35-year-old man who comes to your outpatient office complaining of 1 day of diarrhea.

☑ **What is the differential diagnosis of diarrhea? How would you frame the differential?**

## CONSTRUCTING A DIFFERENTIAL DIAGNOSIS

Although the presence of diarrhea is actually defined by stool weight, it is more useful to define acute diarrhea clinically. Diarrhea can be thought of as bowel movements of a looser consistency than usual that occur more than 3 times a day. Acute diarrhea develops over a period of 1–2 days and lasts for less than 4 weeks. (This chapter will not address chronic or intermittent diarrhea.) The differential diagnosis below uses the pivotal point of presenting symptoms to organize diagnoses into three categories: noninfectious, gastroenteritis, and infectious colitis. This structure is easy to remember, focuses history taking, allows prognosticating, and is also a good framework on which to consider therapy See Fig. 12–1.

Noninfectious diarrhea is recognized by the lack of constitutional symptoms. Infectious diarrhea that presents with large volume (often watery) stool, constitutional symptoms, nausea and vomiting, and often abdominal cramps can be categorized as gastroenteritis. Infectious colitis presents with fever, tenesmus, and dysentery (stools with blood and mucus). Many organisms can cause both gastroenteritis and inflammatory diarrhea.

A. Noninfectious diarrhea
   1. Medications and other ingestible substances (some with osmotic effect)
      a. Sorbitol (gum, mints, pill fillers)
      b. Mannitol
      c. Fructose (fruits, soft drinks)
      d. Fiber (bran, fruits, vegetables)
      e. Lactulose
   2. Magnesium-containing medications
      a. Nutritional supplements
      b. Antacids
      c. Laxatives
   3. Malabsorption
      a. Lactose intolerance
      b. Pancreatitis

   4. Medications causing diarrhea through nonosmotic means
      a. Metformin
      b. Antibiotics
      c. Colchicine
      d. Digoxin
      e. Selective serotonin reuptake inhibitor antidepressants
B. Infectious diarrhea: gastroenteritis
   1. Viral (most common)
      a. Caliciviruses (Norovirus, formally Norwalk virus)
      b. Rotovirus
   2. Bacterial (commonly food-borne)
      a. *Vibrio cholera*
      b. *Escherichia coli*
      c. *Shigella* species
      d. *Salmonella* species
      e. *Campylobacter* species
      f. *Yersinia enterocolitica*
   3. Toxin-mediated
      a. *Staphylococcus aureus*
      b. *Clostridium perfringens*
      c. *Bacillus cereus*
      d. *E coli*
C. Infectious diarrhea: inflammatory colitis
   1. Bacterial
      a. *Shigella* species
      b. *E coli*
      c. *Campylobacter* species
      d. *Salmonella* species
      e. *Y enterocolitica*
   2. Antibiotic-associated
      a. *Clostridium difficile*
      b. *Klebsiella oxytoca*
      c. Non-*C difficile*–related

▽1

The first symptom the patient noted was a poor appetite while eating breakfast. He was unable to finish his usual cup of coffee and a bowl of cereal. During his 20-minute drive to work he developed nausea and
(Continued)

diaphoresis. Upon arriving at work he developed low-grade fever, abdominal cramping, and vomiting. Over the next 12 hours, diarrhea developed. He describes the stool being watery and brown without any blood.

 At this point, what is the leading hypothesis, what are the active alternatives, and is there a must not miss diagnosis? Given this differential diagnosis, what tests should be ordered?

## PRIORITIZING THE DIFFERENTIAL DIAGNOSIS

Mr. C seeks medical attention within about 24 hours of the onset of diarrhea. The pivotal points in his history are acute onset of symptoms over about 60 minutes, early predominance of nausea, and watery brown stool. This presentation certainly speaks for an infectious cause. The low-grade fever and absence of dysentery make it likely that the diagnosis is in the category of gastroenteritis. Table 12–1 lists the differential diagnosis.

Mr. C is otherwise in good health. He reports no recent illnesses or antibiotic exposures. There have been no recent changes in his diet, and he has eaten only food prepared at home for the last week. He lives with his wife and reports no known sick contacts. He works as a bus driver.

**Table 12–1.** Diagnostic hypotheses for Mr. C.

| Diagnostic Hypotheses | Clinical Clues | Important Tests |
|---|---|---|
| **Leading Hypothesis** | | |
| Norovirus virus | Hyperacute onset Vomiting usually present | Resolution in 24–48 hours |
| **Active Alternative** | | |
| Toxin-mediated gastroenteritis, such as *Staphylococcus aureus* | Common food poisoning Onset 1–8 hours after exposure Vomiting is predominant | Rapid resolution, within 12 hours |
| Bacterial gastroenteritis, such as *Salmonella* infection | Usually food-borne Fairly specific clinical syndromes High fevers possible | Stool cultures can be diagnostic |
| **Other Alternative** | | |
| Rotavirus | Contact with children Vomiting common and constitutional signs present | Resolution in 24–72 hours |

He has not traveled from New York City, where he lives and works.

The physical exam is notable for temperature, 38.2°C; BP is 110/80 mm Hg and pulse is 100 bpm while lying down; BP is 90/72 mm Hg and pulse is 126 bpm while standing; RR, 12 breaths per minute. Sclera and conjunctiva are normal. The abdomen is soft and diffusely tender with hyperactive bowel sounds. The rectal exam shows brown, heme-negative stool.

 Is the clinical information sufficient to make a diagnosis? If not, what other information do you need?

## Leading Hypothesis: Norovirus

### Textbook Presentation

Acute vomiting is usually the presenting symptom. Mild diarrhea begins after the vomiting. Mild abdominal cramping is common. Low-grade fever and dehydration are usually present. All symptoms resolve completely by 3 days.

### Disease Highlights

A. Caliciviruses, of which Norovirus and closely related viruses such as Sapovirus are the most common, account for about 80% of adult nonbacterial gastroenteritis.

B. Most commonly occurs in winter.

C. Transmission may be person-to-person or may be food-borne. Norovirus is the most common cause of food-borne infection.

D. High attack rate (up to 50% of exposed individuals)

E. Incubation period is 1–2 days.

### Evidence-Based Diagnosis

A. There are no diagnostic tests available for routine clinical use.

B. Diagnosis is made by clinical presentation.

### Treatment

A. Supportive care

1. Most patients with acute diarrhea require only supportive care. Supportive care is meant to provide rehydration and symptom relief.

2. Rehydration

   a. Oral rehydration is the most important means of rehydration.

   b. For patients with mild diarrhea and little volume depletion, any oral fluids (such as the commonly prescribed Gatorade, pedialyte, chicken soup) are appropriate rehydration.

   c. For patients with more significant volume depletion, oral rehydration solutions should contain NaCl, KCl, $HCO_3$ or citrate, and glucose. The World Health Organization oral rehydration solution has the following composition:

      (1) Sodium: 75 mmol/L

      (2) Chloride: 65 mmol/L

**(3)** Glucose: 75 mmol/L

**(4)** Potassium: 20 mmol/L

**(5)** Citrate: 10 mmol/L

  **d.** If this solution is not available, patients can be instructed to mix the following in 1 L of water

    **(1)** One-half teaspoon of salt

    **(2)** One-quarter teaspoon of baking soda

    **(3)** 8 teaspoons of sugar

  **e.** IV fluids (lactated Ringer solution or normal saline) are reasonable until the patient can take fluid orally.

**3.** Antidiarrheals (such as loperamide) are safe and effective for patients without dysentery. Using antidiarrheals in a patient with dysentery is not safe because they can:

  **a.** Cause prolonged fever

  **b.** Cause toxic megacolon and perforation

  **c.** Possibly increase the risk of hemolytic uremic syndrome (HUS) in patients with *Shiga* toxin–producing *E coli* (STEC).

Antidiarrheals are very effective for control of symptoms. They should never be used for patients with dysentery or signs of invasive infection (tenesmus, blood or mucus in stool, high fever, and severe abdominal pain).

**4.** Antiemetics

**5.** Diet

  **a.** BRAT diet (banana, rice, applesauce, toast) is often recommended.

  **b.** Avoid dairy products (see below).

**B.** Antimicrobial therapy

**1.** Treatment other than supportive care is not necessary for Norovirus-like illnesses.

**2.** Empiric antimicrobial therapy is recommended for diarrheal infections only in limited circumstances. These circumstances never occur in patients with noninfectious diarrhea and almost never in patients with gastroenteritis. Specific circumstances are discussed throughout the chapter; general circumstances include the following:

  **a.** Severe disease (profuse diarrhea with hypovolemia)

  **b.** High fever

  **c.** Severe abdominal pain

  **d.** Dysentery

  **e.** High band count

Empiric antimicrobial therapy for diarrhea is reasonable for patients with severe symptoms.

## MAKING A DIAGNOSIS

At the time of the patient's visit he was feeling better than he had previously. He still noted an "upset stomach"

and was having soft watery diarrhea every 2–3 hours. He had not had any vomiting in about 6 hours and was therefore able to keep down fluids.

Have you crossed a diagnostic threshold for the leading hypothesis, Norovirus? Have you ruled out the active alternatives? Do other tests need to be done to exclude the alternative diagnoses?

Unlike most clinical situations an exact diagnosis in a patient with diarrhea often need not be made. The clinical syndrome in Mr. C is consistent with viral gastroenteritis. By recognizing this syndrome, you are able to reassure him that he should be better in the next 24–48 hours. Even if a diagnostic test for Norovirus were available for routine use in clinical practice, the usefulness would be low because treatment is only supportive.

Most evaluations for diarrhea are negative. Most studies report positive cultures in at most 5% of patients. Ova and parasite tests are even less likely to be positive.

In most patients with an acute diarrheal illness, diagnostic testing is not helpful to the patient but may be important from a public health standpoint.

## Alternative Diagnosis: Toxin-Mediated Gastroenteritis

### Textbook Presentation

The presentation of this syndrome, most commonly caused by *Staphylococcus aureus* or *C perfringens*, is usually acute, with vomiting and crampy abdominal pain. Vomiting is the predominant symptom with diarrhea being mild and watery and fever being low grade. Because of the very short lag between ingestion and illness (2–8 hours), the culpable meal is usually the last one eaten. Recovery is very rapid (12–48 hours).

### Disease Highlights

**A.** Toxin-mediated gastroenteritis caused by *S aureus*, *C perfringens*, or *B cereus* is essentially always food-borne. These organisms are not the most common causes of food-borne infection, in fact, they may account for only 1% of food-borne infections.

**B.** Viral causes probably account for about 60% of all food-borne infections. *Salmonella*, *Campylobacter*, *Shigella*, and *Cryptosporidium* are the most common bacterial and parasitic causes of food-borne infections according to the most recent data from the Centers for Disease Control and Prevention (CDC) (Table 12–2).

**C.** *S aureus*, *C perfringens*, and *B cereus* can often be recognized through the clinical and exposure history.

  **1.** This recognition can enable the physician to provide prognosis, avoid unnecessary testing, and prevent further infection from a common source.

  **2.** Table 12–3 describes the clinical syndromes of these infections.

**Table 12–2.** Bacterial causes of food-borne illness.

| Organism | Approximate % Total Food-Borne Infections, 2006 | % Infections with a Given Organism That Are Food-Borne |
|---|---|---|
| Salmonella | 38 | 95 |
| Campylobacter | 33 | 80 |
| Shigella | 16 | 20 |
| Cryptosporidium | 5 | 10 |
| STEC | 5 | 85 |
| Yersinia | 1 | 90 |
| Vibrio | 1 | 65 |
| Listeria | 1 | 99 |

STEC, Shigella toxin–producing *Escherichia coli*.

 Illnesses presenting with the acute onset of vomiting and constitutional symptoms, often with abdominal cramping, are usually caused by viruses or bacteria that elaborate toxins.

### Evidence-Based Diagnosis

A. There are no diagnostic tests available for routine clinical use.

B. Diagnosis is by clinical presentation, and these infections should be considered in any patient with acute gastrointestinal symptoms and recent, suspect food intake.

### Treatment

Treatment is supportive care and outlined above.

## Alternative Diagnosis: Gastroenteritis caused by *Salmonella* Species

### Textbook Presentation

The onset of disease is usually subacute with nausea, fever, and diarrhea. Fever and nausea often resolve over 1–2 days while diarrhea persists for 5–7 days. Patients usually have watery diarrhea with 6–8 bowel movements each day. Dysentery is possible. Bacteria commonly remain in the stool for 4–5 weeks. Salmonella gastroenteritis may cause higher fevers than viral or preformed toxin disease.

### Disease Highlights

A. *Salmonella* species cause 3 major types of disease.

   1. Diarrheal illnesses

      a. Gastroenteritis

      b. Dysentery (discussed later in the chapter)

   2. Bacteremia with the potential for focal infectious complication.

      a. Usually a secondary complication of gastroenteritis

      b. Bacteremia develops in ~5% of patients, and focal infections develop in a small percentage of these patients.

   3. Typhoid fever

      a. A systemic illness characterized by fever and abdominal pain caused by *Salmonella typhi*

      b. Typhoid fever is distinct from gastroenteritis, which is caused by non-typhi *Salmonella* species.

      c. Although not generally considered a diarrheal illness, some patients may have diarrhea as a predominant symptom.

      d. Although typhoid fever is a major problem worldwide, it is seen predominantly in the United States in unvaccinated travelers.

      e. Should be considered in the differential diagnosis of a traveler with a febrile illness.

B. Gastroenteritis is the most common *Salmonella*-related disease in the United States. The incidence of *Salmonella* diarrhea in 2006 was 14.8 cases/100,000 persons.

C. *Salmonella* is transmitted by:

   1. Food

      a. Eggs and poultry are most common sources.

      b. There are reports of infection from almost any type of food.

   2. Fecal-oral contact with infected patients

      a. Person-to-person transmission is less common than infection from contaminated food.

      b. Patients shed bacteria for weeks after infection.

   3. Animals also carry salmonella (reptiles most classically).

**Table 12–3.** Clinical syndromes of toxin-mediated gastroenteritis.

| Organism | Pathogenesis | Incubation | Source | Clinical Syndrome |
|---|---|---|---|---|
| Staphylococcus aureus | Preformed toxin | 1–6 hours | Protein rich food | Acute onset Vomiting predominant Resolves within 2 hours |
| Clostridium perfringens | Elaborated toxin | 8–16 hours | Meats | Diarrhea with abdominal cramping Lasts 1–2 days |
| Bacillus cereus | Preformed toxin | 1–6 hours | Grains | Very similar to S aureus |

### Evidence-Based Diagnosis

**A.** The gold standard for diagnosis of salmonella gastroenteritis remains stool culture results. There are tests with greater sensitivity, but none are used in routine clinical practice.

**B.** The details of the decision-making regarding use of stool cultures are covered in case 2.

### Treatment

**A.** Prevention: Because salmonella is heat sensitive, cooking food well and good hand washing practices prevent most infections.

**B.** Treatment

    **1.** Most salmonella infections require no treatment.

    **2.** The patients who should receive therapy beyond supportive care are those who have

        **a.** Severe disease (dehydration, dysentery, high fever)

        **b.** Immunocompromised status, probably including the very elderly

        **c.** Elevated risk of focal infection

            **(1)** Bacteremia

            **(2)** Prosthetic joints or hardware

            **(3)** Sickle cell anemia

        **d.** Typhoid fever

    **3.** Although most patients shed bacteria for weeks after infection, antibiotics should not be used in attempts to prevent transmission. Antibiotics do not shorten the duration of carriage and may prolong it.

## CASE RESOLUTION

Mr. C was sent home with directions for oral rehydration. He reported sleeping for most of the afternoon and was well enough to return to work the next day. By the following day (day 4 of the presentation), the patient was completely better. He reported that none of his close contacts became ill.

The patient's symptoms lasted 48–72 hours. He required no specific therapy. There were no suspicious food exposures and nobody else became ill. The case is consistent with a viral gastroenteritis such as Norovirus. The lack of a suspicious diet history makes a toxin-induced food-borne illness less likely.

## FOLLOW-UP OF MR. C

Two weeks later Mr. C comes to see you again. He attributes his recovery to antibiotics that he took on the day he saw you. (The antibiotics were left over from a prescription he had not completed for a dental infection). About 5 days after his recovery, he began to feel poorly again. For the last 10 days he has had diarrhea, abdominal bloating, and belching. He denies fever, chills, nausea, vomiting, or tenesmus. There has been no blood in his stool.

At this point, what is the leading hypothesis, what are the active alternatives, and is there a must not miss diagnosis? Given this differential diagnosis, what tests should be ordered?

## PRIORITIZING THE DIFFERENTIAL DIAGNOSIS

There are three pivotal points in this presentation:

**1.** The patient has recently experienced what was almost certainly an infectious GI illness.

**2.** The patient has recently taken antibiotics.

**3.** The patient's symptoms have been present for 10 days.

Ten days is prolonged when considering acute infectious diarrhea so other diagnoses should be considered. These include a noninfectious cause, a recurrent gastroenteritis, or an antibiotic-associated diarrhea. The recent gastroenteritis should raise the possibility of lactose intolerance. Lactose intolerance is common after gastroenteritis due to injury to the small bowel mucosa. Another possibility would be recurrent infectious gastroenteritis, which can occur since many of the bacteria that cause diarrhea can persist in the stool after clinical symptoms have resolved. This prolonged bacterial shedding also accounts for spread of the illness. This is especially common with *Salmonella* and *Campylobacter.* Antibiotic-associated diarrhea is a common entity, complicating between 2% and 25% of courses of antibiotics. The level of risk varies with the specific antibiotic. The prolonged nature of the illness should prompt consideration of the less typical pathogens, such as parasites; could our initial diagnosis have been incorrect? Table 12–4 lists the differential diagnosis.

The patient describes 3–4 soft bowel movements a day. He also notes a fair amount of abdominal discomfort. There is no real pain, but there is bloating and belching. He says he goes to the bathroom 3 or 4 additional times each day just to pass gas.

The patient took 3 doses of amoxicillin on the day he first came to see you. He ran out after these 3 doses. He has not traveled since his infection and does not note any unusual exposures. He reports that his diet has been a little more simple than usual with a lot of cereal, rice, potatoes, and milk to "soothe his stomach."

Is the clinical information sufficient to make a diagnosis? If not, what other information do you need?

## Leading Hypothesis: Lactose Intolerance

### Textbook Presentation

Lactose intolerance most commonly presents as chronic symptoms in a person of susceptible ethnic background. The symptoms

***Table 12–4.*** Diagnostic hypotheses for Mr. C's repeat visit.

| Diagnostic Hypotheses | Clinical Clues | Important Tests |
|---|---|---|
| **Leading Hypothesis** | | |
| Lactose intolerance | Ethnic predisposition Recent illness Relation to diet | Resolution with dietary changes |
| **Active Alternative** | | |
| Antibiotic-associated diarrhea | Only caused by *Clostridium difficile* about 15–20% of time | Usually resolves with discontinuation of antibiotic Specific tests for *C difficile* toxin |
| Recurrent infection | Similar symptoms as initial illness Most common with bacterial pathogen | Stool cultures |
| **Other Alternative** | | |
| Parasitic infection | Exposure history common (often with travel) Consider especially in immunosuppressed patients | Stool ova and parasites may be diagnostic |

may be subacute or acute in the setting of infection or dietary changes. The predominant symptom may be belching, bloating, flatulence, diarrhea, or abdominal pain. A suspicious dietary history should be present.

### Disease Highlights

**A.** Lactose intolerance is very common.

**B.** Predictable by ethnic background, worsens with age

**C.** Episodes of small bowel infection can cause transient lactose intolerance in anyone but are more apt to cause symptoms in people with low levels of lactase activity at baseline.

**D.** Ethnic groups and native populations most likely to have low levels of lactase activity come from the following regions:

   **1.** Middle East and Mediterranean

   **2.** East Asia

   **3.** Africa

   **4.** Native American

**E.** Milk, ice cream, and yogurt have the highest levels of lactose.

**F.** Foods with high lactose and low fat (skim milk) tend to cause the most symptoms as these foods deliver lactose to the small intestine the fastest.

### Evidence-Based Diagnosis

**A.** The diagnosis of lactose intolerance is generally a clinical one based on a suspicious history in a patient with a susceptible background whose symptoms resolve on a lactose-free diet.

**B.** More definitive tests, the lactose tolerance test or lactose breath hydrogen test, can be performed in patients in whom the diagnosis is likely but not clear historically.

**C.** Because of the high prevalence of mild lactose intolerance and the frequent exacerbation following gastroenteritis, patients with acute gastroenteritis should be advised to avoid dairy products for 2 weeks after recovery.

### Treatment

**A.** In general, lactose intolerance is treated by decreasing lactose intake.

**B.** Because people have variable levels of lactase activity, levels of tolerance differ from person to person.

**C.** Enzyme supplements, available over the counter, are often helpful.

**D.** In acquired illness (eg, post gastroenteritis), lactase levels will eventually recover when the intestinal brush border regenerates.

**E.** It is usually reasonable to suggest waiting 2 weeks before reintroducing lactose-containing products.

## MAKING A DIAGNOSIS

On exam he appears well. Vital signs are all normal. His abdominal exam reveals hyperactive bowel sounds with minimal distention. It is soft and nontender. Rectal exam reveals soft, brown, heme-negative stool.

**Have you crossed a diagnostic threshold for the leading hypothesis, lactose intolerance? Have you ruled out the active alternatives? Do other tests need to be done to exclude the alternative diagnoses?**

The patient does not appear to have an infectious cause of his diarrhea—at least not a bacterial or viral cause. This fact makes recurrence of his previous infection very unlikely. Antibiotic-associated diarrhea or diarrhea caused by a parasitic infection are still possible.

## Alternative Diagnosis: Antibiotic-Associated Diarrhea

### Textbook Presentation

Patients with antibiotic-associated diarrhea usually have symptoms of gastroenteritis or dysentery during antibiotic therapy. Upper abdominal symptoms of nausea and vomiting are rare.

### Disease Highlights

**A.** There are really 2 distinct types of antibiotic-associated diarrhea: diarrhea related to an enteric pathogen (primarily *C difficile*) and diarrhea related to other effects of antibiotics.

**B.** The antibiotics most commonly responsible for both types of diarrhea are:

   **1.** Clindamycin

   **2.** Cephalosporins

   **3.** Ampicillin, amoxicillin, and amoxicillin-clavulanate

C. *C difficile*

1. Accounts for 10–20% of antibiotic-associated diarrhea

2. *C difficile* causes diarrhea via toxin-mediated effects on the large bowel. This can present as severe diarrhea, often with symptoms of colonic inflammation and a high WBC count.

3. Risk factors for *C difficile* include advanced age, hospitalization, and exposure to antibiotics.

4. *C difficile* has been reported up to 6 months after a course of antibiotics.

5. There are recent reports of a greater incidence of community-acquired *C difficile* and *C difficile* related to the use of proton pump inhibitors.

6. Recent reports also speak to the increasing severity of *C difficile* related to change in the genetics dictating toxin production.

D. *K oxytoca*

1. Newly recognized cytotoxin-producing bacteria capable of causing antibiotic-associated hemorrhagic colitis.

2. Much less common than *C difficile*.

E. Patients with antibiotic-associated diarrhea not related to *C difficile* usually have mild disease that occurs either during or immediately after a course of antibiotics. Possible causes of this type of diarrhea are numerous:

1. Change in intestinal flora

2. Nonantimicrobial effect of antibiotics such as the promotility effects of erythromycin

3. Enteric infections other than *C difficile*

### Evidence-Based Diagnosis

A. Certain features make the diagnosis of antibiotic-associated diarrhea not associated with *C difficile* likely.

1. History of previous antibiotic-associated diarrhea not associated with *C difficile*.

2. Mild to moderate symptoms

3. Negative work up for *C difficile*.

B. *C difficile* colitis

1. Diagnosed by identification of either the toxin in the stool or by demonstration of the classic pseudomembranous colitis on sigmoidoscopy or colonoscopy.

2. Culture, although highly sensitive and specific, is used less because there are nontoxin-producing strains of *C difficile* that are not clinically important.

3. The test characteristics of the toxin assay are listed below. Because of the lower sensitivity, 3 samples are recommended.

   a. Sensitivity, 70–95%; specificity, 95–99%

   b. LR+, 14–95; LR−, 0.05–0.32

C. If a clinical syndrome consistent with *C difficile* colitis persists despite negative toxin assay, sigmoidoscopic exam of the colon is recommended. If symptoms do not resolve and evaluation for *C difficile* is negative, stool cultures to rule out another antibiotic-associated enteric infection are reasonable.

### Treatment

A. Antibiotic-associated diarrhea not related to *C difficile* infection usually resolves with discontinuation of antibiotics. Other useful treatments include:

1. Probiotic agents such as yogurt

2. Antidiarrheals

B. The treatment of *C difficile* is as follows:

1. First-line treatment is oral metronidazole; second-line treatment is oral vancomycin.

2. Avoid antidiarrheals

3. Relapse complicates 20–25% of cases of treated *C difficile*.

## Alternative Diagnosis: *Giardia lamblia*

### Textbook Presentation

Giardiasis can present as either acute or chronic diarrhea. It usually occurs in patients with exposure to infected water supplies, although person-to-person transmission can occur. Symptoms usually include diarrhea, nausea, abdominal cramps, bloating, flatulence, and foul-smelling stools.

### Disease Highlights

A. *Giardia* is the most common cause of parasitic diarrhea in the United States.

B. Most infections in the United States result from ingestion of contaminated water (from streams and lakes).

C. Cases most commonly occur in children age 1–9 or adults age 30–39.

D. Incidence peaks annually during the summer and early fall when people most commonly participate in water sports and camping.

E. Although usually sporadic, there are occasional outbreaks related to contamination of bodies of water used for recreation and drinking supplies.

F. Common symptoms

1. Diarrhea occurs in 96% of cases.

2. Weight loss is present in 62% of cases.

3. Abdominal cramps occur in 61% of cases.

4. Greasy stools are present in 57% of cases.

5. Belching, flatulence, and foul-smelling stools are commonly reported.

G. Fever is uncommon.

H. Chronic infection occurs in about 10% of untreated patients.

I. If evaluation for *Giardia* is negative and there is no response to empiric therapy, other organisms should also be considered.

1. This is especially true in patients who are immunocompromised.

2. Other organisms commonly seen are:

   a. *Cryptosporidium*

   b. *Cyclospora cayetanensis*

   c. *Isospora belli*

### Evidence-Based Diagnosis

A. *G lamblia*

1. Sensitivity of stool ova and parasites for *Giardia* is 50–70% for 1 stool sample.

2. Sensitivity is over 90% for 3 samples.

3. Antigen assays sensitive to over 90%.

B. Other organisms
   1. *Cryptosporidium* can be identified on stool antigen assay.
   2. *C cayetanensis* and *I belli* can be identified on acid-fast stain.

### Treatment

A. The treatment of choice for *G lamblia* infection is oral metronidazole.
B. Empiric therapy is often recommended.

## CASE RESOLUTION

▽1

A lactose-free diet was recommended for the patient. Three stool samples were tested for *C difficile* toxin; results were negative. The suspicion for a recurrent bacterial infection or a parasitic infection was very low.

The patient began a lactose-free diet and was better within 3 days. After 2 weeks, he slowly reintroduced his usual diet without symptoms.

## CHIEF COMPLAINT

PATIENT ▽2

Ms. V is a 45-year-old woman who comes to see you in the office; she complains of 4 days of diarrhea. She reports feeling tired and weak. She is moving her bowels about 6–8 times a day. She says that she has significant abdominal pain. She came in today because she has begun to pass bloody stools.

On physical exam, her vital signs are temperature, 38.3°C; BP, 130/84 mm Hg; pulse, 90 bpm; RR, 12 breaths per minute. She is orthostatic.

Her abdomen has hyperactive bowel sounds. It is diffusely tender, without peritoneal signs. Her stool is a mixture of soft brown stool and blood.

At this point, what is the leading hypothesis, what are the active alternatives, and is there a must not miss diagnosis? Given this differential diagnosis, what tests should be ordered?

## PRIORITIZING THE DIFFERENTIAL DIAGNOSIS

The pivotal points in this case are the presence of bloody stools, abdominal pain, and fever. This symptom complex makes diarrhea caused by a bacterial infection likely. The organisms that commonly cause bloody diarrhea are *Shigella* species, *Campylobacter* species, and *E coli*. *Salmonella* species, *Y enterocolitica,* and *C difficile* also may cause bloody diarrhea. Noninfectious causes, such as ischemia or ulcerative colitis, should also be considered.

It is impossible to clinically differentiate between the bacterial diarrheas. That said, it is important to know organisms' recognizable symptom complexes because these can give clues to the causative organism. Because treatment decisions are often made before the specific organism is identified by culture, these clues can help guide appropriate therapy. Table 12–5 lists the differential diagnosis.

▽2

The patient's first symptoms, 4 days ago, were fever and lethargy. She felt terrible for the entire day and thought she was getting the flu. The following day, she began to have diarrhea and diffuse abdominal pain. Two days later, the day she comes to your office, she began to have blood in her stool.

She reports that her husband is also sick with similar symptoms. His diarrhea developed the day before hers did but he has not noticed blood in his stool. He refused to come in because he figured it was "just a virus."

**Table 12–5.** Diagnostic hypotheses for Ms. V.

| Diagnostic Hypotheses | Clinical Clues | Important Tests |
|---|---|---|
| **Leading Hypothesis** | | |
| Bacterial diarrhea caused by *Campylobacter* infection | Constitutional prodrome Diarrhea with significant abdominal pain Occasional dysentery | Stool culture |
| **Active Alternative** | | |
| Bacterial diarrhea, caused by infection with *Shigella* species | Varies by species but classically colonic predominant symptoms—dysentery | Stool culture High bandemia common |
| **Active Alternatives—Must Not Miss** | | |
| Bacterial diarrhea, caused by infection with *Shiga* toxin–producing *Escherichia coli* 0157 | Diarrhea, usually bloody Fever uncommon Right-sided abdominal pain | Stool culture for organism must be specifically requested Toxin can be identified |
| **Other Alternative** | | |
| Ulcerative colitis | Usually subacute to chronic | Endoscopic diagnosis |

Is the clinical information sufficient to make a diagnosis? If not, what other information do you need?

## Leading Hypothesis: *Campylobacter* Infection

### Textbook Presentation

Presenting symptoms of *Campylobacter* infection are usually diarrhea and abdominal pain. The diarrhea is often profuse and watery and the pain can be severe, often mimicking appendicitis or other abdominal disease that may require surgery. The fever usually resolves over the first 2 days of the illness, while the diarrhea and abdominal pain may last 4–6 days.

### Disease Highlights

A. *Campylobacter* species are among the most commonly isolated pathogens in patients with diarrhea and are a common cause of bloody stool.

B. The incidence of *Campylobacter* diarrhea in 2006 was 12.7 cases/100,000 persons.

C. In 1 recent study of patients arriving at emergency departments with bloody diarrhea, the breakdown of diagnoses were:

1. *Shigella* in 15.3% of patients

2. *Campylobacter* in 6.2% of patients

3. *Salmonella* in 5.2% of patients

4. *Shiga* toxin–producing *E coli* in 2.6% of patients

5. Other cause in 1.6% of patients

D. Common aspects of the presentation are

1. Constitutional symptoms before GI disease

2. Bloody diarrhea beginning after 2–3 days of watery diarrhea

E. There can be rare late complications.

1. Reactive arthritis

2. Guillain-Barré

F. Bacteria commonly remain in the stool for 4–5 weeks and reinfection might occur.

### Evidence-Based Diagnosis

A. Although stool cultures are most likely to be negative (even in patients with bloody diarrhea), they can be useful in some circumstances.

1. *Campylobacter* and *Shigella* infections clearly benefit from treatment.

2. Inappropriate treatment of salmonella (treating mild or moderate non-typhi infection) is not helpful and may lead to prolonged carriage.

3. Culture results can be very useful from a public health standpoint.

B. Stool cultures are really the only way to distinguish organisms.

1. A representative study that looked at the clinical characteristics of patients with diagnostic stool cultures showed the overlap of the clinical syndromes.

2. Table 12–6 lists the percentage of patients with various characteristics by organism.

C. The decision making regarding whether to send stool cultures mirrors that for treatment discussed above. In order to increase the yield of the cultures (both in terms of positive results and clinical usefulness), consider the following questions:

1. Is there a clinical suspicion for a specific disease that requires treatment?

   a. Severely ill patient (fever, dysentery, abdominal pain); about 30% of patients with dysentery have positive cultures (compared with 1–6% of all patients).

   b. Suspicious exposure (travel, high-risk sexual behavior, antibiotics)

**Table 12–6.** Percentages of patients with various clinical characteristic by organism.

| Characteristic | Organism | | | |
| --- | --- | --- | --- | --- |
| | *Shigella* | *Campylobacter* | *Salmonella* | *E coli* |
| Bloody diarrhea | 54.3% | 37.0% | 33.8% | 91.3% |
| Abdominal pain | 77.9% | 79.5% | 69.7% | 90.5% |
| Abdominal tenderness | 33.5% | 45.4% | 28.8% | 72.0% |
| Subjective fever | 78.6% | 58.7% | 72.0% | 35.0% |
| Objective fever | 69.4% | 50.9% | 69.4% | 41.4% |
| Visible blood in stool sample | 14.7% | 7.8% | 4.8% | 63.0% |
| Occult blood | 59.1% | 52.0% | 43.4% | 82.8% |
| Fecal leukocytes | 37.8% | 42.9% | 29.4% | 70.5% |
| Leukocytes > 10,000/mcL | 58.0% | 42.0% | 45.3% | 70.9% |

Modified from Slutsker L et al. *Escherichia coli* O157:H7 diarrhea in the United States: clinical and epidemiologic features. Ann Intern Med. 1997;126:505–513.

**(1)** Traveler's diarrhea (usually *E coli*) can usually be treated empirically.

**(2)** Other infections associated with travel (*Entamoeba histolytica, G lamblia*) benefit from treatment.

**2.** Does the patient have an underlying disease that makes treatment more necessary?

**a.** Immunosuppression

**b.** Inflammatory bowel disease

**3.** Are there public health reasons that a diagnosis needs to be made?

**a.** Possible outbreak of food-borne illness

**b.** Patient might potentially spread disease (healthcare worker, daycare worker, food handler).

**D.** Is there a reason not to culture?

**1.** Stool cultures and ova and parasite exams of hospitalized patients are particularly unrevealing.

**2.** Consider limiting in-hospital cultures to the following circumstances:

**a.** Onset of diarrhea within 3 days of admission

**b.** Onset > 3 days but

**(1)** Patient is older than 65 years and has comorbidities.

**(2)** Patient has HIV infection.

**(3)** Neutropenia is present.

**(4)** Extraintestinal manifestations are present.

**(5)** There is an outbreak of diarrhea in the hospital.

 Patients with more severe clinical presentations, including high fever, abdominal pain, and dysentery, should always have stool cultures taken.

**E.** Diagnostic tests other than stool cultures are useful in certain situations.

**1.** *C difficile* toxin for patients exposed to antibiotics or proton pump inhibitors

**2.** Shiga toxin to identify *E coli* 0157 in all patients with bloody diarrhea

**3.** Fecal leukocytes may be helpful in deciding which patients are more likely to have positive stool cultures.

**a.** Sensitivity, 73%; specificity, 84%

**b.** LR+, 4.56; LR–, 0.32

**4.** WBC

**a.** WBC is neither sensitive nor specific for the presence of invasive bacterial infections.

**b.** A marked left shift, at least if the band count is > neutrophil count, suggests bacterial etiology in general and *Shigella* in particular.

## Treatment

**A.** Severe diarrhea with bloody stool is often (and appropriately) treated empirically while cultures are pending.

**B.** Empiric therapy is generally with a quinolone.

**C.** Some very important caveats should be kept in mind when empirically treating suspected bacterial diarrhea or dysentery.

**1.** Antibiotics shorten the course of diarrhea caused by *Shigella* and *Campylobacter*.

**2.** There is quinolone resistance in some strains of *Campylobacter*, so empiric therapy should be broadened to include a macrolide if the suspicion for *Campylobacter* is high or if the patient is very ill.

**3.** Antibiotics should be withheld if the patient is at high risk for STEC (see below).

**4.** Antibiotics are only beneficial for salmonella infections in the case of typhoid or severe disease.

## MAKING A DIAGNOSIS

The patient is given IV fluids in the office. After receiving acetaminophen and 2 L of fluid she is feeling somewhat better. Stool cultures are sent. A CBC and Chem-7 are normal.

Have you crossed a diagnostic threshold for the leading hypothesis, *Campylobacter* infection? Have you ruled out the active alternatives? Do other tests need to be done to exclude the alternative diagnoses?

## Alternative Diagnosis: *Shigella* Infection

### Textbook Presentation

*Shigella* infection often begins with fever and constitutional symptoms. Diarrhea is initially watery and may become bloody. The diarrhea can be very frequent. Tenesmus is often prominent.

### Disease Highlights

**A.** Although there is a spectrum of disease (some *Shigella* species can cause milder disease), a patient who is systemically ill with classic dysentery (frequent bloody stools with tenesmus) is most likely to have *Shigella* infection.

**B.** Incidence in 2006 was 6.1 cases/100,000 people.

**C.** Table 12–6 lists some of the common symptoms in patients with *Shigella*.

**D.** *Shigella* is a highly infectious organism with as few as 10 organisms causing disease.

### Evidence-Based Diagnosis

**A.** Because of the highly invasive nature of *Shigella,* some of the tests that reveal colonic inflammation are more useful in detecting *Shigella* than other organisms.

**1.** Sensitivity of band count > 1% = 85%.

**2.** Sensitivity of fecal leukocytes is at least 70%.

**B.** Stool culture is gold standard.

### Treatment

**A.** *Shigella* dysentery clearly benefits from treatment.

**B.** The drug of choice is oral ciprofloxacin.

# Alternative Diagnosis: Shiga Toxin–Producing *E coli* (0157:H7) Infection

## Textbook Presentation

The presentation of *E coli* depends on the type. STEC usually presents with diarrhea and abdominal pain. The pain is often worse in the right lower quadrant. Bloody diarrhea is very common, while nausea, vomiting, and fever are not.

## Disease Highlights

A. The secreted *Shiga* toxin is primarily responsible for disease.

B. Symptoms include bloody diarrhea (seen in most infected patients), severe abdominal pain, and absence of fever.

C. Incidence in 2006 was 1.3 cases/100,000 people.

D. STEC is associated with HUS.

   1. HUS is the simultaneous presence of a microangiopathic hemolytic anemia, thrombocytopenia, and acute renal failure.

   2. HUS occurs mainly in children and effects 5–10% of children infected with STEC.

   3. About 5% of cases HUS/thrombotic thrombocytopenic purpura (TTP) in adults are related to STEC.

E. Other than STEC, there are 4 types of *E coli* that cause diarrheal illness in adults. Information about the *E coli* diseases other than STEC is listed in Table 12–7.

## Evidence-Based Diagnosis

A. Table 12–6 lists some common symptoms in patients with diarrhea secondary to STEC.

B. Patients infected with STEC are significantly more likely than patients infected with other pathogens to

   1. Report bloody diarrhea

   2. Provide visibly bloody specimens

   3. Not report fever

**Table 12–7.** Diarrhea-producing *E coli* other than Shiga toxin– producing *E coli*.

| Type | Common Abbreviation | Characteristics |
|------|---------------------|-----------------|
| Enterotoxigenic *Escherichia coli* | ETEC | Symptoms caused by toxin Watery diarrhea Common cause of traveler's diarrhea |
| Enteropathogenic E coli | EPEC | Common cause of diarrhea in adults and children |
| Enteroinvasive E coli | EIEC | Causes bloody diarrhea with tenesmus similar to *Shigella* |
| Enteroaggregative E coli | EAEC | Cause of traveler's diarrhea of secondary importance |

   4. Have abdominal tenderness

   5. Have a WBC > 10,000/mcL

C. If an organism is isolated from a patient with bloody diarrhea, it is most likely to be *Shigella* or *Campylobacter*. On the other hand, a patient infected with enterohemorrhagic *E coli* (EHEC) is more likely to have bloody diarrhea than a patient with *Shigella* or *Campylobacter* infection.

D. Positive culture and detected *Shiga* toxin are considered diagnostic.

E. Culture for STEC often must be specifically requested.

## Treatment

A. Treatment of STEC is controversial.

B. Studies have reported no effect, an increase in risk of HUS, and beneficial effects with antibiotics.

C. Antibiotics are generally thought to not be indicated in the treatment of STEC.

# CASE RESOLUTION

2

The patient was treated with supportive therapy. Antidiarrheals were withheld because of her bloody diarrhea. Ciprofloxacin was prescribed empirically. Her stool was sent for culture.
   Her stool cultures were negative, and her symptoms resolved within 3 days.

The resolution of this case is not surprising. The decision to treat the patient was based on 2 things: she appeared quite ill and the presentation was thought to be consistent with *Campylobacter* infection. Even though stool cultures have the highest yield in patients with bloody stool, about 67% of the cultures will still be negative. Also not surprising is her rapid improvement since this is generally the course of infectious diarrhea.

# REVIEW OF OTHER IMPORTANT DISEASES

## Travelers' Diarrhea

### Textbook Presentation

Patients with traveler's diarrhea usually become ill in the first 5 days of their trips from a temperate climate to a tropical one. They usually have mild symptoms of a gastroenteritis-like illness. Patients are often better by the time they return home.

### Disease Highlights

A. Up to 10 million cases yearly

B. The highest risk destinations for traveler's diarrhea are in Asia, Africa, and South and Central America.

C. Disease usually occurs in the first 5 days (with a peak onset at 4 days) and resolves in 1–5 days.

D. Symptoms are usually mild to moderate diarrhea but more severe symptoms can occur.

E. Although the predominant cause of traveler's diarrhea is enterotoxigenic *E coli* (ETEC), any bacteria, virus, or parasite can be causative. Enteroaggregative *E coli* (EAEC) seems to be another important cause.

**F.** It is important to consider infections particularly common in certain locations.

**1.** St. Petersburg: *G lamblia*

**2.** Wilderness streams in Western US: *G lamblia*

**3.** Nepal: *Cyclospora, G lamblia*

**4.** India: *E histolytica*

**G.** Because these infections usually occur far from the patient's physician, the doctor's role is usually advisory.

**1.** Prevention

  **a.** Ensure clean water

    **(1)** Boiled, filtered, or chemically purified local water.

    **(2)** Carbonated beverages and bottled water

  **b.** Bismuth before meals

    **(1)** Decreases risk of diarrhea

    **(2)** Need to balance against the risk of included salicylates

  **c.** Prophylactic antibiotics are not recommended unless traveler is at special risk.

  **d.** Gastric acidity is natural prevention; temporarily discontinue proton pump inhibitors or $H_2$-blockers, if safe.

  **e.** CDC website has very useful information for patients.

**2.** Advise patients of common mistakes.

  **a.** Ice and mixed drinks are often made with contaminated water.

  **b.** Ensure bottled water is sealed and not just bottled tap water.

  **c.** As the renowned parasitologist Dr. B. H. Kean once said, "The only way to clean lettuce is with a blowtorch."

  **d.** Any food heated for a prolonged time is potentially dangerous.

  **e.** Fruit is only safe if the traveler peels it.

  **f.** A recent study reported that among table top sauces collected from restaurants in Guadalajara and tested for diarrheogenic *E coli*, 4 of 43 contained ETEC and 14 of 32 contained EAEC.

## Treatment

**A.** Supportive care

**B.** Avoid antidiarrheals if dysentery is present.

**C.** Antibiotics are warranted.

  **1.** Ciprofloxacin, azithromycin, and rifamaxin are the preferred agents.

  **2.** Decrease symptoms (from 3 days to 1 day)

  **3.** Consider causes of traveler's diarrhea other than ETEC (such as giardiasis, amebiasis), which require different therapies.

## REFERENCES

Adachi JA, Mathewson JJ, Jiang ZD, Ericsson CD, DuPont HL. Enteric pathogens in Mexican sauces of popular restaurants in Guadalajara, Mexico, and Houston, Texas. Ann Intern Med. 2002;136(12):884–7.

Bartlett JG. Clinical practice. Antibiotic-associated diarrhea. N Engl J Med. 2002;346(5):334–9.

Brodsky RE, Spencer HC Jr, Schultz MG. Giardiasis in American travelers to the Soviet Union. J Infect Dis. 1974;130(3):319–23.

Guerrant RL, Van Gilder T, Steiner TS et al. Practice guidelines for the management of infectious diarrhea. Clin Infect Dis. 2001;32(3):331–51.

Hogenauer C, Langner C, Beubler E et al. *Klebsiella oxytoca* as a causative organism of antibiotic-associated hemorrhagic colitis. N Engl J Med. 2006;355(23):2418–26.

Mead PS, Slutsker L, Dietz V et al. Food-related illness and death in the United States. Emerg Infect Dis. 1999;5(5):607–25.

Musher DM, Musher BL. Contagious acute gastrointestinal infections. N Engl J Med. 2004;351(23):2417–27.

Preliminary FoodNet data on the incidence of infection with pathogens transmitted commonly through food-10 states, 2006. MMWR Morb Mortal Wkly Rep. 2007;56(14):336–9.

Slutsker L, Ries AA, Greene KD, Wells JG, Hutwagner L, Griffin PM. *Escherichia coli* O157:H7 diarrhea in the United States: clinical and epidemiologic features. Ann Intern Med. 1997;126(7):505–13.

Steffen R, Collard F, Tornieporth N et al. Epidemiology, etiology, and impact of traveler's diarrhea in Jamaica. JAMA. 1999;281(9):811–7.

Talan D, Moran GJ, Newdow M et al. Etiology of bloody diarrhea among patients presenting to United States emergency departments: prevalence of *Escherichia coli* O157:H7 and other enteropathogens. Clin Infect Dis. 2001;32(4):573–80.

Thielman NM, Guerrant RL. Clinical practice. Acute infectious diarrhea. N Engl J Med. 2004;350(1):38–47.

Yoder JS, Beach MJ. Giardiasis surveillance--United States, 2003-2005. MMWR Surveill Summ. 2007;56(7):11–8.

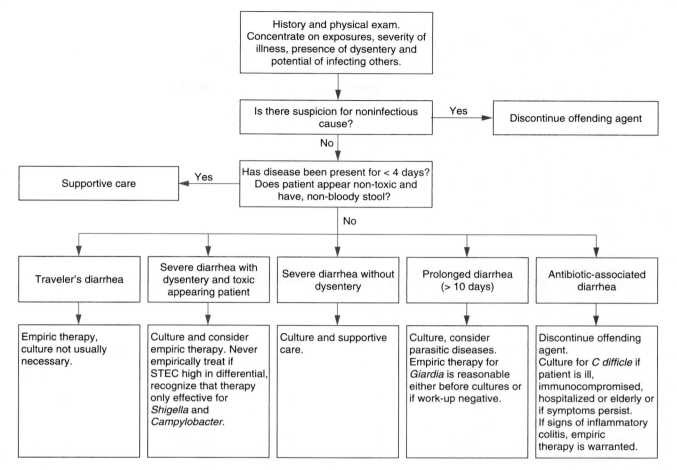

STEC, *Shiga* toxin–producing *Escherichia coli.*

***Figure 12–1.*** Diagnostic approach: diarrhea.

# 13

# I have a patient with dizziness.
# How do I determine the cause?

## CHIEF COMPLAINT

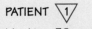

**PATIENT** ▽ 1

Mr. J is a 32-year-old man who comes to your office complaining of dizziness.

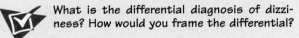

**What is the differential diagnosis of dizziness? How would you frame the differential?**

## CONSTRUCTING A DIFFERENTIAL DIAGNOSIS

The framework for dizziness recognizes that most patients who complain of dizziness are actually complaining of 1 of 4 distinct sensations (Figure 13–1):

1. Vertigo
2. Near syncope
3. Dysequilibrium
4. Nonspecific dizziness

The first pivotal step in evaluating the dizzy patient is to clarify the patient's symptom, since each of the above sensations has its own distinct differential diagnosis and evaluation. Therefore, the first and most important question is "What does it feel like when you are dizzy?" At this point, patients must be given enough time, *without interruptions or suggestions,* to describe their dizziness as clearly as possible. Commonly used descriptions, their precipitants, and differential diagnosis are listed in Table 13–1. The patient's description of the symptom and precipitant helps select the proper sensation, which is crucial to the remainder of the evaluation. The duration of the dizziness is also diagnostically useful.

## Differential Diagnosis of Dizziness

A. Vertigo is the most common cause of dizziness. Vertigo may arise from diseases of the inner ear (peripheral) or diseases of the brainstem (central). About 90% of patients with vertigo have a peripheral etiology.
  1. Peripheral
    a. Benign paroxysmal positional vertigo (BPPV)
    b. Labyrinthitis or vestibular neuritis
    c. Meniere disease
    d. Uncommon etiologies: head trauma, herpes zoster

2. Central
  a. Cerebrovascular disease
    (1) Vertebrobasilar insufficiency
    (2) Cerebellar or brainstem stroke
    (3) Cerebellar hemorrhage
    (4) Vertebral artery dissection
  b. Cerebellar degeneration
  c. Migraine
  d. Multiple sclerosis (MS)
  e. Alcohol intoxication
  f. Phenytoin toxicity
  g. Tumors of the brainstem or cerebellum
B. Near syncope is a common cause of severe dizziness, particularly in the elderly. (See Chapter 26, Syncope.)
C. Dysequilibrium. Etiologies include
  1. Multiple sensory deficits
  2. Parkinson disease
  3. Normal-pressure hydrocephalus
  4. Cerebellar disease (degeneration, tumor, infarction)
  5. Peripheral neuropathy (ie, diabetes)
  6. Dorsal column lesions
    a. $B_{12}$ deficiency
    b. Syphilis
    c. Compressive lesions
  7. Drugs (alcohol, benzodiazepines, anticonvulsants, aminoglycosides, antihypertensives, muscle relaxants, cisplatin)
D. Nonspecific dizziness. Etiologies include
  1. Psychological
    a. Major depression
    b. Anxiety, panic disorder
    c. Somatization disorder
  2. Recently corrected vision (new glasses, cataract removal)
  3. Medication side effect

▽ 1

Mr. J reports that when he is dizzy, it feels as though the room is spinning. His first episode occurred 3 days ago when he rolled over in bed. The spinning sensation was very intense, causing nausea and vomiting. It lasted less than 1 minute.

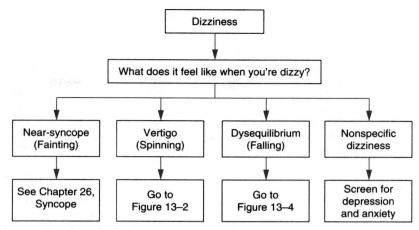

**Figure 13–1.** Diagnostic approach: dizziness.

 At this point, what is the leading hypothesis, what are the active alternatives, and is there a must not miss diagnosis? Given this differential diagnosis, what tests should be ordered?

## PRIORITIZING THE DIFFERENTIAL DIAGNOSIS

Clearly, Mr. J is describing vertigo, the most common complaint in patients with dizziness. Patients with vertigo complain that either they or their surroundings are spinning. Vertigo develops secondary to disorders in either the peripheral nervous system or

**Table 13–1.** Classification and characteristics of dizziness.

| | Vertigo | Near Syncope | Dysequilibrium | Nonspecific Dizziness |
|---|---|---|---|---|
| Chief complaint | Spinning or "merry-go-round" | Nearly fainting | Falling Loss of balance | Floating Vague |
| Typical precipitants | Turning over in bed Looking up to shelf | Standing | Walking | Stress |
| Important historical features | Attack duration *CNS signs or symptoms* (eg, dysarthria, ataxia, diplopia, headache, neck pain) Peripheral symptoms (eg, hearing loss, tinnitus) | CAD HF History of syncope Palpitations Medications Melena or rectal bleeding | Diabetes Neuropathy Visual problems Imbalance Medications | Multiple somatic complaints Feeling down or hopeless Anhedonia |
| Key physical exam findings | Cranial nerve exam Gait Finger-to-nose exam Dix-Hallpike maneuver | Orthostatic blood pressure and pulse Cardiac exam | Gait Sensation Position sense Cranial nerve exam Finger-to-nose exam | |
| Differential diagnosis | **Peripheral:** BPPV, Vestibular neuritis, Meniere disease **Central:** CVA, MS, cerebellar hemorrhage, migraine, brainstem tumors | Dehydration Hemorrhage Orthostatic hypotension Vasovagal Arrhythmias Hypoglycemia Aortic stenosis PE | Multiple sensory deficits Parkinson disease Cerebellar degeneration or stroke $B_{12}$ deficiency Tabes dorsalis Myelopathy | Depression Generalized anxiety disorder Panic attacks Somatization disorder |

BPPV, benign paroxysmal positional vertigo; CAD, coronary artery disease; CVA, cerebrovascular accident; HF, heart failure; MS, multiple sclerosis; PE, pulmonary embolism.

the CNS. Peripheral vertigo usually stems from disease in the semicircular canals and is far more common than central vertigo. Central vertigo occurs in patients with disorders involving the brainstem. While less common, central vertigo is serious and may be caused by stroke, hemorrhage, tumors, and MS. Therefore, the first **pivotal step** in the evaluation of a patient with vertigo is to distinguish peripheral from central vertigo. Features that suggest central vertigo include *CNS signs or symptoms, headache, significant imbalance,* and *cerebrovascular risk factors* (Figure 13–2). Central vertigo is suggested by abnormalities in the neurologic exam (particularly ataxia or cranial nerve abnormalities) and nystagmus that is vertical, downbeating or upbeating, persistent (> 1 minute), or fails to stop with repetition. Table 13–2 summarizes the differences between peripheral and central vertigo.

On further questioning, Mr. J reports that he had a similar episode 5 years ago. Other than nausea, he has no other symptoms. Specifically, he has not noticed any diplopia (double vision), imbalance, dysarthria (slurred

speech), ataxia, incoordination, or headaches. He has no risk factors for cerebrovascular disease (diabetes mellitus, hypertension, coronary artery disease, peripheral vascular disease). He has no prior history of neurologic complaints (eg, unilateral vision loss of optic neuritis or motor weakness). On physical exam, he appears anxious. His vital signs are BP, 110/70 mm Hg; RR, 16 breaths per minute; pulse, 84 bpm; temperature, 37.0°C. HEENT exam reveals extraocular muscles intact with 15 beats of horizontal nystagmus on left lateral gaze. This stops after repeating the maneuver several times. Optic disks are sharp and visual fields are intact to confrontation. Cardiac, pulmonary, and abdominal exams are normal. On neurologic exam, cranial nerves are intact (except for nystagmus). Hearing is grossly normal. Gait and finger-to-nose testing are normal.

**Is the clinical information sufficient to make a diagnosis? If not, what other information do you need?**

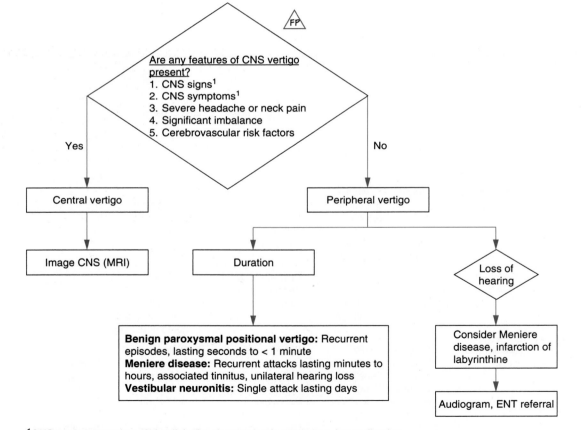

¹**CNS symptoms:** dysarthria, diplopia, abnormal gait, weakness, incoordination
**CNS signs:** cranial nerve abnormalities, ataxia, positive Romberg, abnormal nystagmus (eg, nystagmus seen on both leftward and rightward gaze does not fatigue with repetition of maneuver, lasts > 1 minutes, is not suppressed by visual fixation or is purely vertical or is downbeating)

*Figure 13–2.* Diagnostic approach: vertigo.

***Table 13–2.*** Features distinguishing central from peripheral vertigo.

| Finding | Peripheral Vertigo | Central Vertigo |
|---|---|---|
| CNS symptoms and signs (eg, dysarthria, diplopia [double vision], ataxia, cranial nerve palsies) | Rare | Common |
| Imbalance | Mild to moderate[1] | Severe |
| Nystagmus characteristics | Inhibited by fixation<br>Unidirectional<br>Horizontal with torsional component<br>Lasts < 1 minute<br>Fatigues with repetition | Not inhibited by fixation<br>May change direction<br>May be purely vertical, downbeating or torsional<br>Lasts > 1 minute<br>Does not fatigue |
| Duration of single episode | Depends on etiology | Depends on etiology |
| Risk factors for vascular disease | May be present or absent | Commonly present |
| Nausea and vomiting | Severe | Variable, may be minimal |
| Severity of vertigo | Severe | Less severe to none |
| Hearing loss | May be present in otosclerosis, Meniere disease | Uncommon. May occur in labyrinth infarctions |

[1]Patients with peripheral lesions can usually walk, whereas those with central lesions may have great difficulty.

Fortunately, Mr. J does not have any CNS symptoms or neurologic signs to suggest central vertigo. You strongly suspect peripheral vertigo. The leading hypothesis is BPPV. Vestibular neuritis and Meniere disease are active alternatives (Table 13–3).

***Table 13–3.*** Diagnostic hypotheses for Mr. J.

| Diagnostic Hypotheses | Clinical Clues | Important Tests |
|---|---|---|
| **Leading Hypothesis** | | |
| Benign paroxysmal positional vertigo | Vertigo lasts seconds, precipitated by rolling over in bed or looking up to shelf<br>Peripheral type nystagmus | Thorough neurologic history and physical exam (to exclude CNS lesions) |
| **Active Alternatives—Most Common** | | |
| Vestibular neuritis | Vertigo lasts for days<br>Peripheral type nystagmus | Thorough neurologic history and physical exam (to exclude CNS lesions) |
| Meniere disease | Vertigo lasts for minutes to hours<br>Tinnitus, intermittent hearing loss<br>Peripheral type nystagmus | Thorough neurologic history and physical exam<br>Audiogram |

## Leading Hypothesis: Benign Paroxysmal Positional Vertigo (BPPV)

### Textbook Presentation

BPPV typically presents with abrupt onset of severe dizziness. Patients often describe it as feeling like the room is spinning. They often note that the symptoms began when they rolled over in bed, looked up (to get something out of a closet), or bent down to tie their shoe. Each episode is *brief* (lasting 10-20 seconds) rather than *persistent* (as in vestibular neuritis). However, since the episodes occur in clusters, patients often complain of vertigo that occurs for days or weeks. A careful history can help make this distinction. Symptoms may recur years later.

 Determining the duration of a single episode of vertigo is critical to establish the correct diagnosis.

### Disease Highlights

A. Most common cause of vertigo

B. Vertigo precipitated by positional changes

C. Vertigo is brief, usually lasting < 15 seconds but may last as long as 90 seconds.

D. Patients typically have clusters of attacks over several weeks to 1 month and then remission. Recurrent clusters occur in about half of patients.

E. Secondary to free-floating canalith usually within posterior semicircular canal. The precipitant is usually unknown, although BPPV may follow labyrinthitis or head trauma.

### Evidence-Based Diagnosis

**A.** Patients with all 4 of the following criteria usually have BPPV (88% sensitive, 92% specific; LR+ 11, LR− 0.13):

    **1.** Recurrent vertigo

    **2.** Duration of attack < 1 minute

    **3.** Symptoms invariably provoked by changing head position

        **a.** Lying down or turning over in bed *or*

        **b.** 2 of the following: Reclining the head, rising from supine, or bending forward

    **4.** Not attributable to another disorder

**B.** One study reported the following symptoms in patients with BPPV:

    **1.** All patients with BPPV complained that the vertigo was provoked by turning over in bed.

    **2.** 50% of patients complained of imbalance but falling was rare (only 1/61) and should raise the concern for another disorder.

**C.** Positional nystagmus has a mixed rotary and horizontal component and can be precipitated by the Dix-Hallpike maneuver (Figure 13–3).

    **1.** Nystagmus usually begins after a few seconds, is brief (< 30 seconds), and fatigues with repetition of maneuver.

    **2.** Sensitivity, 42-78%; specificity 94%

    **3.** Nystagmus that begins immediately, lasts longer than 1 minute or fails to fatigue suggests a central (brainstem) disorder.

**D.** CNS imaging should be performed in patients with findings that suggest central disease and in patients with *atypical* findings for BPPV.

### Treatment

**A.** Most patients recover regardless of therapy; however, spontaneous resolution can take weeks to months.

**B.** The Epley maneuver is a complex rotational maneuver that repositions the canalith and is 85–95% effective at stopping vertigo.

**C.** Vestibular suppressants (meclizine and benzodiazepines) may delay CNS adaptation and should be used only when necessary for patients with frequent intolerable spells.

**D.** Surgical options are available for patients with refractory symptoms but are rarely necessary.

## MAKING A DIAGNOSIS

>
>
> Mr. J's history is characteristic of BPPV. At this point, the Dix-Hallpike maneuver should be performed to evaluate positional nystagmus.
>
> Mr. J reports intense vertigo with the maneuver. Horizontal nystagmus with a rotary component is noted, which lasts for 20 seconds. After repeating the maneuver, the nystagmus disappears.

---

> Have you crossed a diagnostic threshold for the leading hypothesis, BPPV? Have you ruled out the active alternatives? Do other tests need to be done to exclude the alternative diagnoses?

The clinical history, exam, and lack of risk factors for CNS disease all point to peripheral rather than central vertigo. The brief episodes strongly suggest BPPV. Other peripheral causes of vertigo should be considered.

## Alternative Diagnoses: Acute Vestibular Neuritis

### Textbook Presentation

Acute vestibular neuritis typically presents abruptly with severe *constant* vertigo and nausea made worse by head turning that lasts for days. Subsequently, patients may complain of *intermittent* vertigo that occurs for weeks to months and is precipitated by head movement.

### Disease Highlights

**A.** Acute vestibular neuritis may follow viral infection involving the vestibular nerve and the labyrinth.

**B.** Patients often have spontaneous vestibular nystagmus that is unilateral, horizontal, or horizontal and torsional and suppressed by visual fixation.

**C.** Nausea and vomiting are common.

**D.** Gait instability may be present, but patients maintain the ability to ambulate.

**E.** Severe vertigo typically lasts 2-3 days and may last up to 1 week.

**F.** Hearing may be impaired.

**G.** Ramsay Hunt syndrome is a variant of vestibular neuritis.

    **1.** Varicella zoster reactivation involving cranial nerves VII and VIII produces vestibular neuritis *with* hearing loss and facial weakness.

    **2.** Vesicles are seen in the external auditory canal.

### Evidence-Based Diagnosis

**A.** Diagnosis is usually made clinically.

**B.** Cerebellar infarction may present like vestibular neuritis and needs to be carefully considered (see below).

**C.** Perform MRI or magnetic resonance angiography (MRA) to evaluate patients with persistent vertigo for cerebellar infarction if any of the following features are present:

    **1.** Headache

    **2.** Weakness

    **3.** Dysmetria

    **4.** Inability to ambulate

    **5.** Cranial nerve findings

    **6.** Skew deviation[1]

    **7.** Nystagmus which is not suppressed by visual fixation

    **8.** Risk factors for vascular disease

    **9.** Persistence of severe vertigo beyond a few days

---

[1]In skew deviation, the eyes move in different directions with upward gaze; this suggests a central lesion.

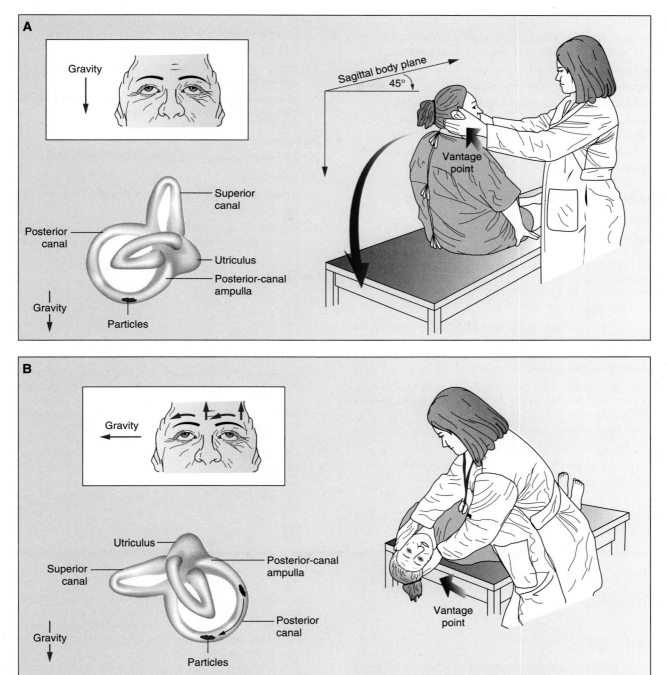

***Figure 13–3.*** The Dix-Hallpike test of a patient with benign paroxysmal positional vertigo affecting the right ear. **A:** The examiner stands at the patient's right side and rotates the patient's head 45 degrees to the right to align the right posterior semicircular canal with the sagittal plane of the body. **B:** The examiner moves the patient, whose eyes are open, from the seated to the supine right-ear-down position and then extends the patient's neck slightly so that the chin is pointed slightly upward. The latency, duration, and direction of nystagmus, if present, and the latency and duration of vertigo, if present, should be noted. The red arrows in the inset depict the direction of nystagmus in patients with typical benign paroxysmal positional vertigo. The presumed location in the labyrinth of the free-floating debris thought to cause the disorder is also shown. (Reproduced, with permission, from Furman JM, Cass SP. Benign paroxysmal positional vertigo. N Engl J Med. 1999;341(21):1590–6.)

## Treatment

A. Meclizine (antihistamine), dimenhydrinate, and scopolamine (anticholinergic) are drugs of choice in most patients.

B. Promethazine (especially for severe nausea, vomiting)

C. Benzodiazepines have also been used.

D. Medications are sedating. Driving should be avoided.

E. Corticosteroids have been demonstrated to improve vestibular recovery, although the impact on symptoms is unclear.

F. Vestibular rehabilitation using exercises that stimulate the labyrinth can promote CNS adaptation.

## Alternative Diagnosis: Meniere Disease

### Textbook Presentation

Patients complain of intermittent spells of vertigo. They may note associated ear fullness, unilateral hearing loss, and tinnitus. Spells typically last for minutes to hours (rarely longer than 4-5 hours) and occasionally up to a day.

### Disease Highlights

Secondary to excess fluid in the endolymphatic spaces of the inner ear.

### Evidence-Based Diagnosis

A. Diagnostic criteria of the American Academy of Otolaryngology and Head and Neck Surgery requires the following for a definite diagnosis:

1. Two spontaneous episodes of vertigo lasting > 20 minutes

2. Confirmed sensorineural hearing loss

3. Tinnitus or perception of aural fullness, or both

B. Audiometry should be performed.

1. Early Meniere disease is characterized by low frequency sensorineural hearing loss.

2. Hearing can be normal between attacks.

C. Test should be done to rule out syphilis (fluorescent treponemal antibody absorption [FTA-Ab]).

D. Some authors recommend an MRI to rule out CNS lesions (tumors, Arnold-Chiari malformations, MS).

## Treatment

A. Specialty consultation is advised.

B. Low salt diet

C. Anecdotal evidence suggests restriction of caffeine and tobacco.

D. Diuretics reduce vertigo.

E. Surgical therapies are available for patients with refractory incapacitating symptoms.

## CASE RESOLUTION

1

Mr. J's history, physical exam, and response to Dix-Hallpike maneuver are entirely consistent with peripheral vertigo. There are no alarm features to suggest central vertigo. The duration of each vertiginous episode suggests BPPV rather than vestibular neuritis or Meniere disease. There is no tinnitus or hearing loss to suggest Meniere disease. Further testing is not indicated.

An Epley maneuver is performed resulting in resolution of Mr. J's symptoms. One month later he returns and is feeling well.

## CHIEF COMPLAINT

PATIENT 2

Mr. D. is a 29-year-old white man who complains of dizziness. Detailed questioning reveals that he has had a constant spinning sensation for the last several weeks. He has no history of similar episodes or hearing loss. Although head movement exacerbates the symptom, it is persistent even when he is still. He has not experienced diplopia, dysarthria, arm or leg weakness, or visual loss. He has no history of hypertension, diabetes, or cocaine use. He has a prior history of migraines for several years. Vertigo has never preceded or accompanied the headache. On physical exam his vital signs are BP, 126/82 mm Hg; pulse, 74 bpm; RR, 16 breaths per minute; temperature, 37.0°C. HEENT exam reveals horizontal nystagmus on leftward and rightward gaze that lasts 1-2 minutes. The nystagmus does not fatigue with repetition of the maneuver. Pupils are equal, round, react to light and accommodation. Cardiac, pulmonary, and abdominal exams are normal. Neurologic exam reveals normal gait, motor strength, sensation, negative Romberg, and intact cranial nerves with the exception of the nystagmus noted above.

**At this point, what is the leading hypothesis, what are the active alternatives, and is there a must not miss diagnosis? Given this differential diagnosis, what tests should be ordered?**

## PRIORITIZING THE DIFFERENTIAL DIAGNOSIS

Again, the first task in evaluating the dizzy patient is to properly identify whether the patient has vertigo, near syncope, dysequilibrium, or nonspecific dizziness. Mr. D is clearly suffering from vertigo. Our next step is to determine whether the disease process is central or peripheral. Mr. D's persistent vertigo, lasting weeks, argues strongly for a central cause. BPPV and Meniere disease are not associated with vertigo of such long duration. Vestibular neuritis can last for days and occasionally weeks. However, Mr. D's prolonged nystagmus, which does not fatigue and is bidirectional, is a pivotal finding and strongly suggests a central process. Central processes that may cause vertigo include migraine, cerebrovascular disease, vertebrobasilar insufficiency, vertebral artery dissection, cerebellar hemorrhage, MS, and CNS tumors. The patient's age and absence of hypertension or diabetes makes cerebrovascular disease, vertebrobasilar insufficiency, or CNS tumor unlikely. The prior history of headaches and the patient's young age make migraine the leading hypothesis. Table 13–4 summarizes the differential diagnosis.

 Is the clinical information sufficient to make a diagnosis? If not, what other information do you need?

## Leading Hypothesis: Migraine & Vertigo

### Textbook Presentation

Classically, migraine sufferers complain of intermittent attacks of severe unilateral throbbing headache associated with photophobia, phonophobia, nausea and vomiting (see Chapter 18, Headache). Headaches may be preceded by a visual aura (scotoma or scintillating lights). Occasionally, an associated symptom is vertigo. This discussion will be limited to migraine and vertigo.

### Disease Highlights

A. Suggested criteria for definite migrainous vertigo include:
1. Recurrent episodic vertigo
2. Current or prior history of migraine
3. One of the following symptoms during at least 2 vertiginous attacks:
   a. Migrainous headache
   b. Photophobia
   c. Phonophobia
   d. Visual or other auras
4. Other causes ruled out by appropriate diagnostic studies

B. Vertigo may last several hours or days and may be spontaneous or positional.

C. Brainstem signs are rare.

### Evidence-Based Diagnosis

A. In patients with vertigo due to migraine, vertigo may precede, be concurrent with, or temporally unrelated to headache.

B. Vertigo was regularly associated with headache in 45% of patients and occurred with *and* without headache in 48% of patients. In 6% of patients, vertigo and migraine did not occur together.

C. In patients with a history of migraine and vertigo but without a clear temporal association of the two, other diagnoses should still be explored. Findings that suggest migraine as a *possible* etiology include
1. Typical migraine precipitants cause vertigo
2. Migraine medications alleviate vertigo

### Treatment
See Chapter 18, Headache.

## MAKING A DIAGNOSIS

 Have you crossed a diagnostic threshold for the leading hypothesis, migraine? Have you ruled out the active alternatives? Do other tests need to be done to exclude the alternative diagnoses?

Although Mr. D's history suggests a *migraine* disorder, there is no temporal association of Mr. D's vertigo and migraine. Furthermore, the continuous vertigo lasting for weeks is atypical for migraine, and the abnormal neurologic exam (nonfatiguing, bidirectional nystagmus) raises the possibility of a serious CNS disorder such as a cerebellar hemorrhage, vertebral artery dissection, or MS.

## Alternative Diagnosis: Cerebellar Hemorrhage

### Textbook Presentation

The textbook presentation of cerebellar hemorrhage is the abrupt onset of headache associated with vomiting, ataxia, and vertigo. The hemorrhage may occur with exertion or at rest. Patients may have incoordination and ataxia. Brainstem compression may produce weakness, cranial nerve abnormalities, coma, and death. Patients with cerebellar infarctions have similar symptoms.

### Disease Highlights

A. Cerebellar hemorrhage accounts for 5-16% cases of intracerebral hemorrhages.

B. Etiologies are heterogeneous:
1. Most common: Hypertensive hemorrhage, subarachnoid hemorrhage, amyloid angiopathy, and arteriovenous malformations
2. Less common: Blood dyscrasias, hemorrhagic infarction, septic emboli, anticoagulant and thrombolytic therapy, neoplasms, herpes simplex virus encephalitis, cocaine and amphetamine use

C. Demographics
1. Mean age is 61–73 years
2. Frequency of intracranial hemorrhage: Asians > Blacks > Hispanics > Whites
3. 36% of patients have diabetes mellitus
4. 32-73% of patients have hypertension
5. 14% of patients have coagulation disorders
6. 16% of patients have liver disease

D. Presentation
1. Headache is the initial symptom in 80% of patients.

 Cerebellar hemorrhage must be considered in patients who complain of acute headache and vertigo.

2. 60% of patients are comatose at presentation.
3. Rapid progression within minutes to hours is common.

    **a.** 38% of patients demonstrate an increase in the hematoma on repeat CT scan 3 hours after the initial scan.

    **b.** Hematoma expansion is associated with a 5× increase in poor outcomes and death.

  **4.** Neck stiffness, facial weakness, and gaze palsy may be seen.

**E.** Complications

  **1.** Hydrocephalus (48%)

  **2.** Chronic disability

  **3.** Herniation and death (42%)

  **4.** Other: Pneumonia, myocardial infarction, ventricular arrhythmias

**F.** Poor prognostic factors include

  **1.** Marked hydrocephalus

  **2.** Deteriorating consciousness

  **3.** Stupor and coma (100% mortality without surgery)

  **4.** Fever (correlates with ventricular extension of bleeding)

### Evidence-Based Diagnosis

**A.** Brainstem findings are common (100% in 1 small study).

**B.** Laboratory evaluation should include CBC, platelet count, INR, partial thromboplastin time, basic metabolic panel, ECG, chest radiograph, glucose and toxicology screen in young and middle-aged patients.

**C.** Cross sectional imaging is critical.

  **1.** Noncontrast CT and MRI/MRA scans are the tests of choice.

  **2.** MRI with MRA can demonstrate saccular aneurysms and arteriovenous malformations but is not always readily available or feasible in sick, unstable patients who need intensive monitoring.

    **a.** Consider aneurysms and arteriovenous malformations in patients with cerebellar hemorrhage who are younger than age 60, do not have a convincing history of hypertension, or have a history of cocaine use.

    **b.** Abnormal results on MRA can be evaluated with cerebral angiography.

  **3.** Prompt imaging is vital.

### Treatment

**A.** Cerebellar hemorrhages can compress vital brainstem structures and surgical evacuation can be lifesaving, particularly in large hemorrhages (> 3 cm) or those with brainstem compression or hydrocephalus.

  **1.** Surgical evacuation of these hematomas is recommended.

  **2.** Emergent neurosurgical consultation is advised.

**B.** ICU monitoring is critical.

**C.** Anticoagulation should be reversed, if present.

**D.** Guidelines of potential therapies to treat intracerebral hemorrhage, the associated hypertension, and increased intracranial pressure were published in 2007.

> **2**
> Neither Mr. D's age nor absence of headache suggest cerebellar hemorrhage. You wonder about vertebral artery dissection.

## Alternative Diagnosis: Vertebral Artery Dissection (VAD)

### Textbook Presentation

Unlike patients with atherosclerotic disease, patients with VAD are usually younger (mean age 48) and complain of severe neck pain, occipital headache, and evolving neurologic symptoms due to progressive involvement of the brainstem. Numbness, hemiparesis, quadriparesis, coma, a locked-in syndrome, or death can result from this uncommon but devastating illness.

### Disease Highlights

**A.** The vertebral artery passes through the transverse process of C1-C6. As C1 rotates on C2, the vertebral artery can be stretched and can be injured initiating dissection and subsequent thrombosis or aneurysm formation (which may be complicated by subarachnoid hemorrhage). Thrombosis is more common and may extend to involve the basilar artery compromising the entire brainstem.

**B.** Pain (from the dissection) is a common feature.

**C.** Risk factors *differ* from patients with typical ischemic stroke. VAD may occur spontaneously or following trauma, catheterization, sporting activity, or chiropractic cervical manipulation. When secondary to chiropractic manipulation, symptoms develop within 1 hour of procedure in 85% of patients.

### Evidence-Based Diagnosis

**A.** Warning symptoms are present in 54% of cases; the most common are occipital headache and neck pain. These symptoms are usually sudden, severe, and persistent until other neurologic signs develop. Headache preceded other neurologic signs and symptoms by 1-14 days.

**B.** Signs and symptoms

  **1.** Pain (neck, head, or both) occurs in 85% of cases.

  **2.** Other common symptoms include vertigo (57%), nausea and vomiting (53%), unilateral facial numbness (46%), unsteadiness (42%), cerebellar findings (35%), diplopia (23%), limb weakness (11%).

  **3.** Isolated vertigo and headache are present in 12% of cases.

**C.** VAD can be visualized with MRA, CTA and conventional angiography.

  **1.** MRA and CTA are highly accurate.

  **2.** Ultrasound with color Doppler is less sensitive for VAD (66%).

**D.** Neuroimaging: Infarction is seen in 65% of scans.

### Treatment

**A.** For patients with VAD and thrombosis, anticoagulation is the currently recommended therapy. It has been associated with lower mortality than placebo in uncontrolled trials. For patients with aneurysm formation, endovascular repair and surgery have been used.

**B.** In various series, 20-50% of patients had no or minor residual defect, 10-56% had major sequelae, and 10-24% died.

 In patients who complain of vertigo *and headache*, diagnostic possibilities include migraine, subarachnoid hemorrhage, cerebellar hemorrhage, and vertebral artery dissection.

2

Mr. D reiterates that he has no history of headache or neck pain. Furthermore, he has no history of trauma or chiropractic manipulation of the neck. His only headaches have been those typical of his prior migraines (and do not suggest intracranial hemorrhage). These headaches have not been associated with vertigo.

Mr. D's nystagmus still suggests central vertigo. After reviewing his differential diagnosis (Table 13–4) and realizing that migraine, cerebellar hemorrhage, and VAD are unlikely, you wonder if Mr. D may have MS. Although less common in men than women, no other diagnosis is suggested by the clinical features and exam. You order an MRI.

**Have you ruled out the alternative diagnosis of MS?**

## Alternative Diagnosis: MS

### Textbook Presentation

MS typically affects young women of Northern European dissent who experience *intermittent* neurologic symptoms due to disease

**Table 13–4.** Diagnostic hypotheses for Mr. D.

| Diagnostic Hypotheses | Clinical Clues | Important Tests |
|---|---|---|
| **Leading Hypothesis** | | |
| Migraine | History of recurring throbbing headaches with or without aura Temporal association of headache and vertigo | Thorough neurologic history and physical exam (to exclude CNS lesions) MRI |
| **Active Alternatives—Most Common** | | |
| Cerebellar hemorrhage | *Risks:* Hypertension, cocaine use, warfarin therapy *Other symptoms:* Severe headache at onset, vomiting, ataxia | Head CT scan or MRI/MRA (see below) |
| Vertebral artery dissection | *Risks:* Trauma or spinal manipulation *Other symptoms:* Severe headache or neck pain at onset, progressive neurologic deficit with cranial neuropathies, ataxia, weakness | MRA or angiogram |
| **Active Alternatives—Must Not Miss** | | |
| Multiple sclerosis | CNS lesions developing at different times and places: prior episodes of visual loss (optic neuritis), weakness, diplopia | Brain MRI Oligoclonal bands in cerebrospinal fluid |

that develops at *different* times and at *different* locations in the CNS. The most common presenting form of MS is relapsing-remitting MS, characterized by attacks followed by remission with remyelination. In the majority of patients (58%), this form of the disease transforms into secondary progressive MS.

### Disease Highlights

A. Etiology: MS develops secondary to an inflammatory autoimmune disease with multifocal CNS demyelination. Axonal injury also occurs.

B. Women are affected 2–3 times more than men.

C. Patients are usually between 18 and 45-years-old at onset.

D. Symptoms worsen in warm environments (ie, in the shower and during exercise).

E. Several studies suggest that late infection with Epstein-Barr virus (ie, in adolescence) may predispose patients to MS.

F. Although MS evolves with time into a multifocal disease, 85% of patients present with one of several clinically isolated syndromes (CIS). Conversely, 30% of patients with isolated syndrome progress to MS. Common initial syndromes include:

1. Partial spinal cord syndromes

   a. Band like sensation

   b. Varying degrees of pain, light touch, and proprioceptive loss

   c. Bilateral sensory loss from a certain level downwards

   d. Weakness associated with spasticity, hyperreflexia, and clonus

   e. Electrical sensation from spine into the limbs that occurs with neck flexion (Lhermitte sign)

2. Optic neuritis

   a. Presenting complaint in 15–20% of patients in whom MS is subsequently diagnosed

   b. Patients complain of monocular visual loss, monocular visual field loss (scotoma), and difficulty discerning color that evolves over hours to days.

   c. Pain with extraocular movement is common (92%).

   d. Afferent pupillary defect (Marcus Gunn pupil) is almost always seen.

   e. Fundoscopic exam is normal in two-thirds of patients. Swelling of the optic nerve may be seen but hemorrhages are rare.

   f. With long-term follow-up, MS develops in up to 15–75% of patients with optic neuritis (50–80% if the MRI scan is abnormal vs 6–22% if the MRI scan lacks disseminated features of MS).

3. Intranuclear ophthalmoplegia (INO)

   a. The medial longitudinal fasciculus pathway in the brainstem coordinates conjugate eye movement.

   b. An INO develops when a lesion interrupts the medial longitudinal fasciculus pathway.

   c. On lateral gaze, adduction is impaired and nystagmus develops in the abducting eye.

   d. Convergence is maintained, distinguishing an INO from a third nerve palsy.

   e. INO is seen in 33–50% of patients with MS.

   f. INO is not specific for MS; it may develop secondary to vascular disease.

G. Vertigo is the presenting symptom in 5% of patients with MS and is reported in 30-50% of patients with MS; it is commonly associated with other cranial nerve dysfunction.

H. Other common symptoms include a variety of sensory symptoms, urinary incontinence, heat sensitivity, fatigue, depression, and cognitive dysfunction.

I. Prognosis at 10 years
   1. 50% of patients require a cane
   2. 15% of patients are wheelchair-dependent

### Evidence-Based Diagnosis

A. Diagnosis is primarily clinical, resting on the demonstration of ≥ 2 attacks separated in space and time. In patients with CIS, several tests results increase the likelihood that the patient will progress to MS. These include multiple white matter lesions on MRI or cerebrospinal fluid analysis that demonstrates oligoclonal bands. The exact sensitivity and specificity varies dependent on whether the patient has a CIS or multiple symptoms, the duration of follow-up and the criteria of a positive result. The Poser and McDonald criteria incorporate clinical data with results from MRI, cerebrospinal fluid analysis, and evoked responses.

B. Brain MRI test of choice
   1. Demonstrates periventricular white matter lesions (lesions may also be seen in other white matter locations).
   2. Sensitivity ≈81–90%, specificity 71–96%.
   3. Gadolinium enhancement suggests active plaques.
   4. Ischemia, systemic lupus erythematosus, Behçet syndrome, syphilis, HIV, sarcoidosis, and other vasculitides may look similar to MS on MRI.

C. Spinal MRI has similar sensitivity (75-83%) to brain MRI but is more specific (97%) than brain MRI.

D. Evoked potentials
   1. Visual evoked potentials are 65–85% sensitive but not specific for MS.
   2. Somatosensory evoked potentials
      a. 69–77% sensitive
      b. Abnormal in 50% of patients with MS without sensory signs or symptoms

E. Cerebrospinal fluid can be useful in patients in whom the diagnosis is uncertain
   1. Cell counts are usually normal.
   2. Immunoglobulin (oligoclonal bands) may be elevated.
      a. Elevated in 60–70% of patients with CIS and 85–95% of patients with MS; 92% specific
      b. LR+, 11.3; LR− 0.11
      c. 25% of patients with oligoclonal bands and 1 event progressed to MS, compared with 9% without bands (at 3 years)

F. Differential diagnosis includes other inflammatory CNS diseases ie, acute disseminated encephalomyelitis, transverse myelitis, CNS vasculitis, systemic lupus erythematosus, syphilis, HIV, human T lymphotrophic virus type I, neurosarcoidosis, cerebrovascular disease, antiphospholipid syndromes, Lyme disease, and migraine.

G. Clues to alternative etiology include
   1. Single CNS lesion
   2. Unusual age of presentation
   3. Spinal lesion in absence of intracranial disease

### Treatment

A. Corticosteroids are recommended for acute attacks with distressing symptoms or disability and have been demonstrated to be superior to placebo in hastening relapse recovery. For optic neuritis, IV methylprednisolone is preferred to oral therapy.

B. Disease modifying agents can slow the rate of progression and relapse in relapse-remitting MS and CIS suggestive of MS.
   1. First-line agents include interferons and glatiramer.
      a. Side effects of interferons include flu-like symptoms, increase in liver function tests (LFTs), and the development of neutralizing antibodies.
      b. LFT abnormalities are common, but serious hepatotoxicity is rare.
   2. Mitoxantrone is also used.

C. Anti-integrin antibodies (natalizumab) may also be useful in the therapy of MS but can be complicated by progressive multifocal leukoencephalopathy.

D. Neuropathic pain can be treated with gabapentin, carbamazepine, and valproic acid.

E. Bone mineral density should be monitored in patients with diminished activity and in those requiring corticosteroids.

F. Specialty consultation is advised.

## CASE RESOLUTION

▽2

Mr. D's MRI reveals multiple periventricular and brainstem white matter lesions strongly suggestive of MS. A lumbar puncture is performed and positive for oligoclonal bands. Although the patient has suffered from only 1 clinical event, you are reasonably confident that he has MS. Mr. D refuses initial therapy. He returns 6 months later with monocular visual loss and eye pain. A diagnosis of optic neuritis is made. This confirms the diagnosis of MS. Mr. D agrees to see a neurologist who initiates interferon therapy. One year later, he is doing well, without any new or persistent symptoms.

# CHIEF COMPLAINT

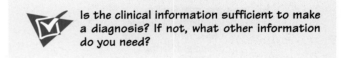

PATIENT 3

Mrs. P is an 85-year-old woman with diabetes who complains of dizziness. She reports that she has noticed dizziness for several years but that her symptoms seem to be progressing.

When asked to describe her symptoms in more detail, she reports that she feels (and worries) that she might fall. She reports no rotational or spinning sensation. She also reports no history of near or actual fainting.

At this point, what is the leading hypothesis, what are the active alternatives, and is there a must not miss diagnosis? Given this differential diagnosis, what tests should be ordered?

## PRIORITIZING THE DIFFERENTIAL DIAGNOSIS

Mrs. P is complaining of dysequilibrium. Dysequilibrium can arise from abnormalities of the brain, cerebellum, spinal cord, or peripheral nerves. Possible causes include Parkinson disease, normal-pressure hydrocephalus, cerebellar degeneration (ie, from alcohol), cerebellar stroke, vertebrobasilar insufficiency, $B_{12}$ deficiency, tabes dorsalis, and multiple sensory deficits. Finally, a multitude of drugs can cause dysequilibrium including benzodiazepines, tricyclic antidepressants, alcohol, and aminoglycosides. The neurologic exam is pivotal in such patients. The cranial nerve exam, gait, and sensory exams may provide critical clues to the diagnosis. Gait disturbances may suggest Parkinson disease (shuffling gait) or cerebellar disease (wide-based gait). Stocking glove sensory deficits are typical of diabetic neuropathy, whereas loss of proprioception suggests posterior column disease (ie, $B_{12}$ deficiency, tabes dorsalis, and some compressive spinal lesions) (A diagnostic approach is illustrated in Figure 13–4).

3

Mrs. P reports that her symptoms occur almost exclusively when she gets up from her bed during the night to go to the bathroom. She has stumbled twice but has never fallen. She reports a long history of cataracts (but has declined surgery). In addition, she has experienced tingling and numbness in her hands and feet for several years. She reports a history of hypertension but no known stroke. She fervently denies any history of sexually transmitted disease and was monogamous with her husband. She drinks alcohol rarely. Her medications include hydrochlorothiazide, metformin, triazolam (for sleep), and aspirin. On physical exam, her BP while sitting is 142/70 mm Hg and pulse is 76 bpm; while standing, her BP is 125/55 mm Hg and pulse is 82 bpm. She has bilaterally dense cataracts. Neurologic exam reveals decreased sensation to the monofilament in a stocking glove distribution. She has no resting or intention tremor. Her face is quite expressive. Gait is hesitant but not wide based. She is unsteady during Romberg testing. Finger-to-nose testing is normal. Cranial nerves are intact.

The **pivotal** features of Mrs. P's history and physical are her stocking glove neuropathy, diabetes mellitus, cataracts, and nocturnal pattern of symptoms (when the room is dark). In combination, these features suggest multiple sensory deficits, which should be the leading diagnosis. Active alternatives include medications, in particular the triazolam. The history of diabetes mellitus and hypertension increase the possibility of cerebellar stroke, and vertebrobasilar insufficiency (VBI) although her neurologic exam does not suggest this or Parkinson disease. Since treatment is available for $B_{12}$ deficiency and tabes dorsalis, they are "must not miss" possibilities. The differential diagnosis is summarized in Table 13–5.

Is the clinical information sufficient to make a diagnosis? If not, what other information do you need?

## Leading Hypothesis: Multiple Sensory Deficits

### Textbook Presentation

The typical patient is an elderly diabetic who complains of symptoms when arising from their bed during the night. Patients may fall or simply feel as though they are going to fall. Multiple sensory

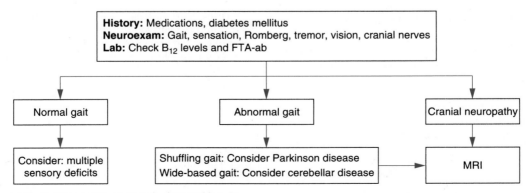

**Figure 13–4.** Diagnostic approach: dysequilibrium.

***Table 13–5.*** Diagnostic hypotheses for Mrs. P.

| Diagnostic Hypotheses | Clinical Clues | Important Tests |
|---|---|---|
| **Leading Hypothesis** | | |
| Multiple sensory deficits | Symptoms occur in dark environment Visual impairment (cataracts) Peripheral neuropathy Diabetes Orthopedic disorder | Careful neurologic exam |
| **Active Alternatives—Most Common** | | |
| Medications | Benzodiazepines Tricyclic antidepressants Aminoglycosides | Discontinue medication |
| Cerebellar stroke | *Risks:* Hypertension, diabetes mellitus, peripheral vascular disease, coronary artery disease, tobacco use, older age, atrial fibrillation, valvular heart disease *CNS signs:* Ataxia, dysmetria | MRI/MRA Transcranial Doppler angiogram |
| Vertebrobasilar insufficiency | *Risks:* Hypertension, diabetes mellitus, peripheral vascular disease, coronary artery disease, tobacco use, older age, atrial fibrillation, valvular heart disease *CNS signs or symptoms:* diplopia, dysarthria, weakness, ataxia | MRI/MRA CTA Transcranial Doppler angiogram |
| **Active Alternatives—Must Not Miss** | | |
| B$_{12}$ deficiency | Megaloblastic anemia Pancytopenia Vibratory and positional sensory deficits | See Chapter 6, Anemia Vitamin B$_{12}$ level MMA level |
| Tabes dorsalis | Vibratory and position sensory deficits History of primary syphilis (painless single ulcerated papule) secondary syphilis (rash involving palms and soles) | FTA antibody |

MMA = methylmalonic acid

losses and physical deconditioning create imbalance and an unsteady gait. Orthostatic hypotension (aggravated by many medications) and benzodiazepines for sleep may contribute to the symptoms.

### Disease Highlights

A. Multiple systems are involved.

B. Typically, at least 2 or more of the following are present:

1. Visual loss (secondary to myopia, presbyopia, cataracts, macular degeneration)

2. Proprioceptive loss (neuropathy from diabetes, myelopathy from cervical spondylosis)

3. Chronic bilateral vestibular damage (from ototoxic drugs)

4. Orthopedic disorder impairing ambulation

### Evidence-Based Diagnosis

A. Ataxia is uncommon (0/14 in one series).

B. Patients with significant ataxia or cerebellar findings should undergo MRI to exclude alternative diagnoses.

### Treatment

A multifaceted approach is often necessary; elements include:

A. Visual correction

B. Night lighting

C. Instructing patients to sit at the edge of the bed prior to standing

D. Modifying medications to minimize orthostatic hypotension (ie, α-blockers, diuretics)

E. When possible, eliminate benzodiazepines, neuroleptics, and any unnecessary medications.

F. Home visits can identify fall risks (electric and telephone cords, loose rugs, etc).

G. Lower limb strength training and balance training have been demonstrated to reduce falls.

H. Bisphosphonates reduce the risk of fractures in patients with osteoporosis.

## MAKING A DIAGNOSIS

Obtaining CNS imaging is often a matter of judgment in patients with dysequilibrium. Definite indications for MRI include cerebellar signs on physical exam (ataxia), cranial neuropathies, or history of cerebrovascular accident. Possible indications for CNS imaging include multiple risk factors for cerebrovascular disease. Given the Mrs. P's age, you remain concerned about cerebrovascular disease, in particular cerebellar stroke and vertebrobasilar insufficiency.

## Alternative Diagnosis: Cerebrovascular Disease

### Textbook Presentation

Cerebrovascular disease encompasses a multitude of diseases in which disordered blood supply results in CNS dysfunction. The neurologic symptoms may be transient (typically <1 h) if blood supply is reestablished quickly (transient ischemic attack [TIA]) or permanent if blood flow is not reestablished within this period (stroke). Patients with symptoms lasting > 1 hour but < 24 hours often have subclinical infarction. The location of ischemia within the brain and the mechanism of the event determine the type of symptoms, their rapidity of onset, and severity.

### Disease Highlights

A. Thrombosis

1. Large intracranial or extracranial vessels (ie, middle cerebral artery, carotid artery, vertebral artery)

a. Risk factors include older age, hypertension, tobacco use, and diabetes.

b. Occasionally, secondary to hypercoagulable states, heparin-induced thrombocytopenia, vasculitis (ie, Takayasu arteritis, giant cell arteritis), or sickle cell anemia

2. Small penetrating vessels: Small arteries that penetrate at right angles may be obstructed, resulting in small cavitary infarcts (lacunar infarcts—see below); usually involve basal ganglia, internal capsule, thalamus and pons.

3. May progress in stuttering manner

4. Unusual in patients younger than age 40

5. Headache *unusual* at onset of symptoms (< 20%)

B. Embolization

1. Sources include left atrium (particularly in patients with atrial fibrillation), left ventricle (myocardial infarction, heart failure), heart valves, aortic arch, and carotid or vertebral arteries.

2. Symptoms are maximal at onset and may involve multiple vascular territories.

C. Hemorrhage (≈20%)

1. Intraparenchymal

a. Usually secondary to hypertension

b. Other causes include trauma, amyloid angiopathy, bleeding diathesis (warfarin), vascular malformations or cocaine or methamphetamine use. (Cocaine may be associated with spasm and thrombosis or intracranial hemorrhage.)

c. Neurologic symptoms and headache progress over minutes to hours.

d. Headache is present at the onset of symptoms in 50–60% of cases.

e. Focal deficits common

2. Subarachnoid: (See Chapter 18, Headache)

D. Dissection of the carotid or vertebral arteries can cause ischemia due to thrombosis, embolization, or hemorrhage.

E. *Hypotension* may result in symmetric damage to watershed areas including occipital cortex (resulting in blindness), motor strips (resulting in shoulder and hip weakness).

## Evidence-Based Diagnosis

A. Initial evaluation should include serum glucose, CBC, prothrombin time, partial thromboplastin time, basic metabolic panel, an ECG (to look for atrial fibrillation or myocardial infarction), and neuroimaging.

B. Neuroimaging: MRI is far superior to CT scan for the diagnosis of ischemic stroke and almost identical for the diagnosis of hemorrhagic stroke (Table 13–6). The remainder of the

discussion will focus on the subset of cerebrovascular disorders (ie, VBI [thrombosis of the large basilar or vertebral arteries] and cerebellar infarction) that frequently involve the brainstem and cerebellum and may result in vertigo or imbalance.

## 1. Vertebrobasilar Insufficiency (VBI)

### Textbook Presentation

The classic presentation of VBI is an elderly patient with diabetes, hypertension, or both who complains of intermittent spells of vertigo associated with other neurologic symptoms, such as diplopia, dysphagia, dysarthria, weakness, or ataxia.

### Disease Highlights

A. Risk factors include diabetes, hypertension, increased age, coronary artery disease, peripheral vascular disease, tobacco use, and male sex.

B. Thrombosis and embolism (cardiac or artery to artery) are the most common causes.

C. Dizziness in patients with VBI may be described as tilting rather than spinning.

D. Symptoms usually last for minutes with VBI (but may persist in patients with stroke or cerebellar hemorrhage).

E. Basilar artery infarctions may result in cranial neuropathies, hemiparesis, and coma.

### Evidence-Based Diagnosis

A. 50% of patients have a normal neurologic exam between the episodes.

B. In most patients with VBI and vertigo, other CNS symptoms or signs (diplopia, ataxia, dysarthria, Horner syndrome, weakness, or crossed face and body numbness) are also present. However, in 7.5–20% of patients with VBI, isolated intermittent vertigo presents as the sole manifestation of basilar ischemia, which can be a harbinger of frank brainstem infarction.

 Basilar ischemia should be considered in patients with vertigo that is not clearly positional and who have significant cerebrovascular disease risk factors (ie, diabetes).

C. Most common symptom is visual dysfunction (eg, diplopia, visual field defects, hallucinations, and blindness).

D. Transcranial Doppler, MRA, CT angiography (CTA), and angiography have been used.

***Table 13–6.*** Sensitivity for diagnosis of acute stroke.

| | All Strokes | Ischemic Strokes | Hemorrhagic Strokes | Ischemic Strokes < 3 h |
|---|---|---|---|---|
| CT (noncontrast) | 26% | 16% | 93% | 12% |
| MRI | 83% | 83% | 85% | 73% |

1. MRI with MRA is procedure of choice.
   a. Noninvasive
   b. 95-97% sensitive and 99% specific for posterior circulation disorders
2. CTA can be used in patients with contraindications to MRI/MRA (ie, pacemakers).
3. Transcranial Doppler may be useful but is operator dependent.
4. Angiography is invasive, but it is the gold standard.
5. Echocardiography is used in patients with suspected embolic disease, particularly those without evidence of basilar or vertebral artery disease on neuroimaging and in those with infarcts in multiple vascular territories.

## Treatment

A. The treatment of patients with acute posterior circulation strokes is complex. If patients can be evaluated (including neuroimaging to exclude hemorrhage) and treated *within 3 hours of symptom onset*, options include intravenous tissue plasminogen activator (t-PA) and intra-arterial thrombolytic agents. *Guidelines for the use of rt-PA in stroke patients have been published and must be followed carefully to avoid intracranial hemorrhage.*

B. For secondary prevention, aspirin, clopidogrel, aspirin plus dipyridamole, and warfarin have been used.
   1. Warfarin is preferred for patients with stroke and atrial fibrillation.
   2. Some clinicians use warfarin for significant vertebral or basilar artery stenosis.
   3. Ticlopidine is a second-line drug due to the risk of hematologic toxicity.
   4. Angioplasty, stenting, and surgical reconstruction have been used in patients with vertebral artery and basilar artery stenosis who remain symptomatic despite medical therapy.
   5. Statin therapy is also recommended for patients with cerebrovascular atherosclerotic disease and low-density lipoprotein cholesterol levels > 70 mg/dL.

C. Modify risk factors

## 2. Lacunar Infarction of the Pons or Cerebellum

### Textbook Presentation

Typically, the presenting symptoms are rapid onset of hemiparesis, sensory symptoms, or ataxia.

### Disease Highlights

A. Small, deep, non-cortical white matter infarcts secondary to obstruction of the small penetrating arteries

B. Typically involves basal ganglia, internal capsule, thalamus, and pons

C. Cortical signs (aphasia, agnosia, apraxia and hemianopsia) are absent.

D. Symptoms depend on stroke location (Table 13–7).

E. Common causes of lacunar infarcts
   1. Hyalinosis of the small penetrating artery with subsequent thrombosis is the most common cause. The hyalinosis is a long-term complication of hypertension.
   2. The small penetrating arteries may also be obstructed by thrombosis or embolization arising from the parent artery (middle cerebral artery or basilar artery), which feeds the small penetrating artery. The recurrence rate in patients with parent arterial lesions is much higher than in patients without such lesions (16% vs 1%) and similar to patients with large artery infarcts (17%).
   3. Cardioembolism

F. Hypertension, diabetes, and smoking are risk factors.

G. Incidence in the black population is approximately twice that in the white population.

H. Vertigo in brainstem and cerebellar lacunar infarctions
   1. 48% of such infarctions were attributed to hypertension, 40% cardioembolic
   2. Concomitant cranial nerve findings and pronounced ataxia are common. However, 10% of cerebellar infarctions present without other cranial nerve findings and present similar to patients with vestibular neuritis with isolated, spontaneous, prolonged vertigo; nystagmus; and imbalance. Findings that suggest cerebellar infarction include significant imbalance or skew deviation:
      a. However, 29% of patients with cerebellar infarctions have imbalance mild enough that they maintain the ability to independently ambulate.
      b. Skew deviation suggests cerebellar infarction but is only 39% sensitive (100% specific); LR+ ∞, LR– 0.6
      c. The presence of any of the following features in a patient with persistent vertigo suggests that a patient may have cerebellar infarction and warrants an MRI/MRA:
         (1) Headache
         (2) Weakness

**Table 13–7.** Lacunar strokes: Location and associated symptoms.

| Name | Location | Typical Symptoms |
|------|----------|------------------|
| Pure motor stroke | Internal capsule, pons | Unilateral weakness, involves face, arm and leg without cortical findings |
| Pure sensory stroke | Thalamus | Unilateral sensory loss without cortical findings |
| Ataxia-hemiparesis | Pons | Ipsilateral weakness and limb ataxia, nystagmus and dysarthria may be seen |
| Dysarthria and clumsy hand syndrome | Pons or internal capsule | Facial weakness, dysarthria and slight hand weakness |

**(3)** Dysmetria

**(4)** Inability to ambulate

**(5)** Cranial nerve findings

**(6)** Skew deviation

**(7)** Nystagmus that is not suppressed by visual fixation

**(8)** Risk factors for vascular disease

## Evidence-Based Diagnosis

**A.** The sensitivity of the CT scan is low, at most 30-44%

**B.** MRI scan is 86% sensitive.

**C.** MRA is unable to visualize small vessel occlusion but can be useful to exclude occlusion of large feeding vessel and may be particularly useful in patients without typical risk factors for lacunar infarction.

**D.** Other tests may be useful

    **1.** Echocardiogram (to look for embolic etiology)

    **2.** Erythrocyte sedimentation rate (elevated in certain vasculitides).

## Treatment

**A.** Antihypertensive therapy reduces stroke 35-40%.

**B.** Recombinant tissue-type plasminogen activator (rt-PA) improves outcomes in *carefully selected* stroke patients *only if given within 3 hours of symptom onset. Guidelines for the use of rt-PA have been published and must be followed carefully to avoid intracranial hemorrhage.*

**C.** Secondary prevention with aspirin or other antiplatelet medication is recommended.

**D.** Risk factor management (control of diabetes mellitus, hypertension, dyslipidemia and smoking cessation)

The patient's symptoms of imbalance, occurring in the dark, and absence of vertigo or other neurologic symptoms is more consistent with multiple sensory deficits than with either VBI or cerebellar stroke. Nonetheless, given her age, an MRI is reasonable and reveals mild atrophy, appropriate to age without discrete evidence of prior infarction. Vitamin B$_{12}$ levels are normal and FTA-antibody testing for syphilis is negative.

## CASE RESOLUTION

Mrs. P's normal MRI effectively rules out cerebellar stroke as a cause of her dysequilibrium. She has no findings that suggest Parkinson disease (shuffling gait; resting, pill rolling tremor; bradykinesia; or masked facies) and her normal B$_{12}$ level and FTA-antibody exclude the diagnoses of B$_{12}$ deficiency and tabes dorsalis, respectively. You conclude that the dysequilibrium is caused by multiple sensory deficits.

---

Mrs. P's hydrochlorothiazide is reduced by half. In addition, the triazolam is discontinued, and she reluctantly agrees to cataract surgery. A home visit reveals multiple risk factors for falls (including loose rugs), which are removed. Nightlights are installed. One year later Mrs. P reports that she remains unsteady on standing but has not fallen or sustained a hip fracture.

## REVIEW OF OTHER IMPORTANT DISEASES

### Nonspecific Dizziness

#### Textbook Presentation

Patients with a variety of psychiatric disorders including panic disorder, generalized anxiety disorder, depression, and somatization disorder may complain of ill-defined dizziness. The dizziness is often of long duration (years) and poorly defined. Patients may complain of fogginess, feeling woozy, mental fuzziness, loss of energy, or a wobbly or a floating sensation. Patients may complain of other associated symptoms particularly if they have panic attacks including chest pain, shortness of breath, perioral paresthesias, tingling in the hands and feet, and lightheadedness.

#### Disease Highlights

**A.** 20-38% of patients attending a specialty dizzy clinic demonstrated panic disorder.

**B.** Psychiatric symptoms may develop without any identifiable organic cause or develop after episodes of true vertigo or syncope.

**C.** Symptoms are, in part, secondary to hyperventilation, which leads to hypocapnia resulting in decreased cerebral blood flow.

**D.** Patients may complain of lightheadedness or near syncope.

**E.** Depression is reviewed in Chapter 27, Involuntary Weight Loss

**F.** Milder variants of somatization disorder are more common than the full-blown entity. Such variants may be precipitated by stress or minor physiologic disturbances. Paradoxically, such patients are often disturbed by negative test results rather than reassured.

#### Evidence-Based Diagnosis

**A.** *Continuous sensation of vertigo > 1-2 weeks* without daily variation is likely psychogenic. This is to be distinguished from intermittent vertigo, recurring for weeks, precipitated by motion.

**B.** One study reported 62% of patients with hyperventilation had other significant psychiatric disorders.

**C.** Symptom reproduction by induced hyperventilation is nonspecific.

**D.** Care must be taken before ascribing dizziness to a psychiatric etiology.

    **1.** Multiple studies have demonstrated a high prevalence of anxiety (22-67%) among patients with well-defined *organic* etiologies of their dizziness.

    **2.** Anxiety scores were as high in patients with acute labyrinthine failure and vestibular dysfunction as among patients with no vestibular diagnosis.

    **3.** This suggests that dizziness from an organic etiology leads to significant psychiatric distress in many patients and that the psychiatric symptoms may be sequelae of the dizziness rather than the cause of the dizziness.

4. A fear response, symptom focus or abnormal mood that progresses to panic disorders, somatization disorders, or major depression may develop.

E. In some patients, an initial episode of vertigo or near syncope precipitates intense fear, which magnifies normal physiologic sensations. The history should review the first episode whenever possible.

F. Certain physical findings suggest a psychogenic disturbance.

1. Moment-to-moment fluctuations in impairment

2. Excessive slowness or hesitation

3. Exaggerated sway on Romberg, improved by distraction

4. Sudden buckling of knee, typically without falling

5. A cautious "walking on ice" pattern

## Treatment

A. Appropriate evaluation considers organic etiologies and evaluates appropriate possibilities.

B. Discuss patient's concerns and fears about the diagnosis.

C. Educate patient not to overly restrict physical activities since this impairs CNS compensation and may worsen the physical symptoms.

D. For patients with hyperventilation, breathing in and out of paper bag, increases inspired $PaCO_2$, and thereby arterial $PaCO_2$. This increases cerebral blood flow and improves symptoms.

E. Selective serotonin reuptake inhibitors (SSRIs) and benzodiazepines are used in patients with panic attacks and anxiety disorders. SSRIs are preferred due to potential problems with benzodiazepines (eg, dependence, tolerance, exacerbation of symptoms on discontinuation, sedation, interference with cognition in the elderly, and exacerbation of depression).

F. Cognitive and behavioral therapy have also been effective.

## REFERENCES

Balcer LJ. Clinical practice. Optic neuritis. N Engl J Med. 2006;354(12):1273–80.

Broderick J, Connolly S, Feldmann E et al. Guidelines for the management of spontaneous intracerebral hemorrhage in adults: 2007 update: a guideline from the American Heart Association/American Stroke Association Stroke Council, High Blood Pressure Research Council, and the Quality of Care and Outcomes in Research Interdisciplinary Working Group. Stroke. 2007;38(6):2001–23.

Chalela JA, Kidwell CS, Nentwich LM et al. Magnetic resonance imaging and computed tomography in emergency assessment of patients with suspected acute stroke: a prospective comparison. Lancet. 2007;369(9558):293–8.

Cnyrim CD, Newman-Toker D, Karch C, Brandt T, Strupp M. Bedside differentiation of vestibular neuritis from central "vestibular pseudoneuritis." J Neurol Neurosurg Psychiatry. 2008;79(4):458–60.

Furman JM, Cass SP. Benign paroxysmal positional vertigo. N Engl J Med. 1999;341(21):1590–6.

Gomez CR, Cruz-Flores S, Malkoff MD, Sauer CM, Burch CM. Isolated vertigo as a manifestation of vertebrobasilar ischemia. Neurology. 1996;47(1):94–7.

Lee H, Sohn SI, Cho YW et al. Cerebellar infarction presenting isolated vertigo: frequency and vascular topographical patterns. Neurology. 2006;67(7): 1178–83.

Neuhauser H, Leopold M, von Brevern M, Arnold G, Lempert T. The interrelations of migraine, vertigo, and migrainous vertigo. Neurology. 2001;56(4):436–41.

Rajajee V, Kidwell C, Starkman S et al. Diagnosis of lacunar infarcts within 6 hours of onset by clinical and CT criteria versus MRI. J Neuroimaging. 2008;18(1): 66–72.

Thacker EL, Mirzaei F, Ascherio A. Infectious mononucleosis and risk for multiple sclerosis: a meta-analysis. Ann Neurol. 2006;59(3):499–503.

van der Worp HB, van Gijn J. Clinical practice. Acute ischemic stroke. New England Journal of Medicine 2007;357(6):572–9.

# I have a patient with dyspnea.
# How do I determine the cause?

## CHIEF COMPLAINT

PATIENT ▽1

Mr. C is a 64-year-old man who comes to see you complaining of shortness of breath.

What is the differential diagnosis of dyspnea? How would you frame the differential?

## CONSTRUCTING A DIFFERENTIAL DIAGNOSIS

Heart disease, lung disease, and anemia are the most common causes of dyspnea. The simplest approach to the differential diagnosis is to consider the *anatomical* components of each of these systems. This in turn allows us to deduce a fairly comprehensive differential diagnosis of dyspnea. (Occasionally, neuromuscular disease and anxiety also cause dyspnea.)

## Differential Diagnosis of Dyspnea

A. Heart
 1. Endocardium: Valvular heart disease (ie, aortic stenosis [AS], aortic regurgitation [AR], mitral regurgitation [MR], and mitral stenosis)
 2. Conduction system
    a. Bradycardia (sick sinus syndrome, atrioventricular block)
    b. Tachycardia
       (1) Atrial fibrillation and other supraventricular tachycardias (SVTs)
       (2) Ventricular tachycardia
 3. Myocardium: Heart failure (HF)
    a. Systolic failure (coronary artery disease [CAD], hypertension, alcohol abuse)
    b. Diastolic failure (hypertension, AS, hypertrophic cardiomyopathy)
 4. Coronary arteries (ischemia)
 5. Pericardium (tamponade, constrictive pericarditis)
B. Lung
 1. Alveoli
    a. Pulmonary edema (HF or acute respiratory distress syndrome)
    b. Pneumonia

 2. Airways
    a. Suprathoracic airways (ie, laryngeal edema)
    b. Intrathoracic airways
       (1) Asthma
       (2) Chronic obstructive pulmonary disease (COPD) (see Chapter 28, Wheezing and Stridor)
 3. Blood vessels
    a. Pulmonary emboli
    b. Primary pulmonary hypertension
 4. Pleural
    a. Pneumothorax
    b. Pleural effusions
       (1) Transudative
          (a) HF
          (b) Cirrhosis
          (c) Nephrotic syndrome
          (d) Pulmonary embolism (PE)
       (2) Exudative
          (a) Tuberculosis
          (b) Cancer
          (c) Parapneumonic effusions
          (d) Connective tissue diseases
          (e) PE
 5. Interstitium
    a. Edema
    b. Inflammatory
       (1) Organic exposures (eg, hay, cotton, grain)
       (2) Mineral exposures (eg, asbestos, silicon, coal)
       (3) Idiopathic diseases (eg, sarcoidosis, scleroderma, systemic lupus erythematosus, Wegener granulomatosis)
    c. Infectious
C. Anemia

Despite this long list, certain symptoms, signs, and historical features can give pivotal clues to the diagnosis. Features that suggest HF include a history of myocardial infarction, CAD risk factors, long-standing hypertension, or alcohol abuse. Further, an $S_3$ gallop or jugular venous distention (JVD) are fingerprints for HF. Pulmonary embolism can be obvious or subtle and should be considered in patients taking exogenous estrogen and those with a history of cancer, recent immobilization, surgery, or leg swelling. A significant smoking history (≥ 20 pack years) raises the possibility of COPD. Wheezing—defined as a high-pitched sound on *exhalation*—suggests COPD or asthma, whereas stridor—defined as a high-pitched sound on *inspiration*—suggests upper airway obstruction. Menorrhagia or melena suggests anemia for which pale conjunctiva is virtually diagnostic. Fever and cough raise the possibility of pneumonia.

Certain tests are key in the evaluation of the patients with dyspnea. A chest radiograph, ECG and Hct are mandatory in the initial evaluation. In addition, echocardiography can reveal unsuspected HF or valvular heart disease. Pulmonary function tests can help determine whether the patient has obstructive, restrictive, or vascular lung disease (Table 14–1). Obstructive lung disease is characterized by decreased flows (forced expiratory volume in 1 second ($FEV_1$) and the fraction of expired air in the first second ($FEV_1/FVC$ or [$FEV_1\%$]), restriction by decrease volumes (total lung capacity [TLC]) and pulmonary vascular disease by decreased diffusing capacity of lung for carbon monoxide (DLCO). Figure 14–1 summarizes the approach to the patient with dyspnea.

Over the last 2 years, Mr. C has noticed worsening dyspnea on exertion. He complains of shortness of breath with minimal exertion. He is unable to walk around his

**Table 14–1.** Pulmonary function tests abnormalities in lung disease.

| Mechanism | Key PFT Abnormality | Other PFT Findings |
|---|---|---|
| Obstruction (all types) | ↓ Flows<br>↓ $FEV_1/FVC$ | TLC N/↑<br>RV ↑ |
| COPD (chronic bronchitis) | As above | |
| COPD (emphysema) | As above | DLCO ↓ |
| Asthma | Above and Bronchodilator produce an increase of ≥ 12% ↑ Methacholine produces a decrease of ≥ 20% ↓ | |
| Restriction (all types) | Volumes ↓, TLC ↓ | |
| Interstitium (eg, pulmonary fibrosis) | As above | RV ↓<br>DLCO ↓<br>$FEV_1\%$ N/↑ |
| Chest wall (eg, pleural effusion, obesity) | As above | DLCO WNL<br>RV N<br>$FEV_1\%$ N |
| Neuromuscular (eg, myasthenia) | As above | RV ↑, MVV ↓,<br>NIF ↓, PIF ↓ |
| Vascular (ie, pulmonary embolism) | DLCO ↓ | Other PFTs often nl |

DLCO, diffusing capacity of carbon monoxide; $FEV_1$, forced expiratory volume in 1 second; FVC, forced vital capacity; MVV, maximal minute ventilation; NIF, negative inspiratory force; PIF, positive inspiratory force; RV, residual volume; TLC, total lung capacity.

house without resting. Several years ago, Mr. C could walk several blocks without any difficulty. He notes that he is unable to sleep lying flat due to shortness of breath (orthopnea), and he sleeps on a recliner for the last 6 months. Occasionally, he awakes from sleep acutely short of breath (paroxysmal nocturnal dyspnea). He complains that his feet are swollen.

Always quantify the increase in dyspnea *from baseline*. Significant changes suggest serious disease and warrant thorough evaluations.

Past medical history is notable for a myocardial infarction 2 years ago. Vital signs are temperature, 37.0°C; RR, 24 breaths per minute; pulse, 110 bpm; BP, 120/78 mm Hg. His pulse is regular with an occasional irregularity. Cardiac exam reveals JVD to the angle of the jaw in the upright position, a grade II/VI systolic murmur at the apex, and a positive $S_3$ gallop. Lung exam reveals crackles half of the way up from the bases bilaterally. He has 2+ pretibial edema to the knees.

At this point, what is the leading hypothesis, what are the active alternatives, and is there a must not miss diagnosis? Given this differential diagnosis, what tests should be ordered?

## PRIORITIZING THE DIFFERENTIAL DIAGNOSIS

Although the differential diagnosis of dyspnea is broad, the patient has numerous signs and symptoms that point to a cardiac etiology. The JVD, $S_3$ gallop, and peripheral edema are all consistent with cardiac disease. The leading hypothesis with these signs and symptoms is HF secondary to his previous myocardial infarction. Alternative diagnoses include valvular heart disease (ie, MR, AS, or AR). This particular murmur is most consistent with MR. Mr. C's irregular pulse also raises the possibility of atrial fibrillation (AF). Finally, cardiac ischemia presenting as dyspnea rather than pain is a must not miss possibility. Table 14–2 lists the differential diagnosis.

Pursue highly specific positive physical findings (in this case the $S_3$ gallop and JVD); they should help drive the diagnostic search.

A chest radiograph, Hct, and ECG are performed.

Is the clinical information sufficient to make a diagnosis of HF? If not, what other information do you need?

**History and physical exam:** Quantify magnitude of change, time course, associated symptoms. Search for clues!

| | Diagnostic Hypothesis | Clinical Clues | | Tests |
|---|---|---|---|---|
| | | History | Physical | |
| **Cardiac Etiologies** | Valvular heart disease | Rheumatic heart disease | Significant murmur | Echocardiography |
| | Arrhythmia | Palpitations | Irregular pulse | ECG, holter, event monitor |
| | Heart failure | CAD or risk factors, hypertension, alcohol abuse, PND | S₃, JVD, crackles on exam | Chest radiography, BNP, echocardiography |
| | Acute coronary syndrome | Chest pain, CAD risk factors | S₃, JVD, crackles on lung exam | ECG, troponin, stress test, angiography |
| **Pulmonary Etiologies** | COPD | > 20 pack years tobacco | ↓ breath sounds, wheezing | Chest radiography, PFTs |
| | Asthma | Cold ± exercise → symptoms; +FH | Wheezing | PFTs, bronchodilator response, methacholine induced |
| | Pulmonary embolism | Sudden onset of dyspnea, pleuritic chest pain, cancer, surgery immobilization, estrogen therapy | Unilateral leg swelling | D-dimer CTA V̇/Q̇ scan Leg duplex |
| | Pneumonia (CAP, TB, PCP) | Fever, productive cough, high-risk sexual exposures, injection drug use | Crackles, fever thrush, Kaposi sarcoma, skin pop marks | Chest radiography HIV, CD4 (when appropriate) |
| | ILD | Known connective tissue disease, Raynaud phenomenon, vocational, occupational exposure | Diffuse lung crackles | PFTs, High resolution chest CT |
| | Anemia | Menorrhagia, melena, rectal bleeding | Pale conjunctiva | Hct |

**Baseline evaluation:** Chest radiograph, ECG, and Hct

**Supplemental evaluation:** Consider echocardiogram, PFTs, CTA

BNP, brain natriuretic peptide; CAD, coronary artery disease; CAP, community-acquired pneumonia; CTA, CT angiography; FH, family history; ILD, interstitial lung disease; JVD, jugular venous distention; PCP, *Pneumocystis jiroveci* pneumonia; PFTs, pulmonary function tests; PND, paroxysmal nocturnal dyspnea; TB, tuberculosis; V̇/Q̇, ventilation/perfusion.

*Figure 14–1.* Diagnostic approach: dyspnea.

## Leading Hypothesis: HF

### Textbook Presentation

Patients typically have fatigue, dyspnea on exertion, orthopnea, paroxysmal nocturnal dyspnea, and edema. Often, there is an antecedent history of either myocardial infarction or poorly controlled hypertension.

### Disease Highlights

A. Strictly speaking, HF refers to any cardiac pathology that impairs left ventricular filling or ejection, which may arise from disease of the pericardium, myocardium, or valves. The remainder of this discussion will focus on myocardial causes of HF. Valvular heart disease is discussed separately.

***Table 14–2.*** Diagnostic hypotheses for Mr. C.

| Diagnostic Hypothesis | Clinical Clues | Important Tests |
|---|---|---|
| **Leading Hypothesis** | | |
| Heart failure | History of myocardial infarction, poorly controlled hypertension S₃ gallop, JVD Crackles on lung exam Peripheral edema | Echocardiogram ECG BNP |
| **Active Alternatives-Most Common** | | |
| **Valvular disease** Mitral regurgitation | Blowing systolic murmur at apex radiating to axilla | Echocardiogram |
| Aortic stenosis | Systolic murmur at right upper sternal border radiating to neck Loss of A2 | Echocardiogram |
| Aortic regurgitation | Early diastolic murmur left sternal border | Echocardiogram |
| Atrial fibrillation | Irregularly irregular pulse | ECG Echocardiogram |
| **Active Alternatives-Must Not Miss** | | |
| Angina | Exertional symptoms History of CAD or risk factors (diabetes mellitus, male sex, tobacco use, hypertension, hypercholesterolemia) | ECG Stress test Coronary angiogram |

**B.** Pathophysiologic classification: HF may be secondary to systolic dysfunction, diastolic dysfunction, or both. HF may also be classified based on whether the primary process affects the left ventricle (LV) or the right ventricle (RV).

   **1.** Systolic heart failure

   **a.** Most common pathophysiology underlying HF.

   **b.** CAD accounts for 66% of all cases of HF.

   **c.** Other common causes include long-standing hypertension and alcohol abuse.

   **d.** Less common causes include viral cardiomyopathy, postpartum cardiomyopathy, drug toxicity (ie, adriamycin), and idiopathic cardiomyopathy.

   **2.** Diastolic heart failure

   **a.** Diastolic heart failure accounts for 20–60% of all HF cases.

   **b.** Diastolic *dysfunction* occurs when LV wall thickness increases and LV compliance decreases.

   **c.** Decreased LV compliance impairs LV filling and lowers cardiac output.

   **d.** Decreased LV compliance also results in increased LV pressure, which is transmitted to the pulmonary capillaries.

   **e.** The increasing pulmonary capillary pressures and decreased cardiac output cause dyspnea and fatigue.

   **f.** The mortality in patients with diastolic dysfunction and systolic dysfunction are similar.

   **g.** The most common cause of diastolic dysfunction is hypertension. Less common causes include AS and infiltrative cardiomyopathies (eg, hemochromatosis, amyloidosis).

   **3.** Right- versus left-sided HF

   **a.** HF may involve the LV, the RV, or both.

   **b.** Common causes of LV failure include CAD, hypertension, and alcoholic cardiomyopathy.

   **c.** Common causes of RV failure include severe pulmonary disease (especially COPD) and advanced LV failure.

   **d.** Peripheral edema, JVD, and fatigue may be seen in LV or RV failure, but pulmonary edema is seen only in LV failure.

   **4.** Progression

   **a.** Heart failure often triggers maladaptive neurohormonal changes including increased activation of the sympathetic nervous system and the angiotensin system.

   **b.** These neurohormonal responses promote sodium retention, increase afterload, and contribute to progressive HF.

   **c.** Therapies that interrupt these responses reduce mortality (see below).

**C.** Functional classification

   **1.** New York Heart Association: Descriptively useful. May be limited prognostically by the ability of patients to move from 1 class to another with therapy.

   **a.** Class I: Asymptomatic

   **b.** Class II: Symptoms on ordinary exertion (ie, climbing stairs)

   **c.** Class III: Symptoms with less than ordinary exertion (ie, walking on flat surface)

   **d.** Class IV: Symptoms at rest

   **2.** A more recent classification by the American College of Cardiology (ACC)/American Heart Association (AHA) recognizes 4 stages (A-D).

   **a.** Stage A: Patients are at risk for HF.

   **b.** Stage B: Patients have structural changes (ie, LV hypertrophy or decreased ejection fraction [EF]) but no symptoms.

   **c.** Stage C: Patients have structural changes and symptoms.

   **d.** Stage D: Patients have structural changes and refractory symptoms despite therapy.

**D.** Complications

   **1.** Electrical: Heart block, ventricular tachycardia, AF, sudden death

   **2.** Pulmonary edema

   **3.** Stroke and thromboembolism

   **a.** 2–4% annual incidence

   **b.** Risk increases if AF coexists

   **4.** MR (LV dilatation may lead to sufficient dilatation of the mitral annulus that it causes secondary MR [see below])

   **5.** Death

   **a.** Symptomatic mild to moderate HF: 20–30%/y

**b.** Symptomatic severe HF: up to 50%/y

**c.** Mechanism of death

**(1)** Sudden in 50% (secondary to ventricular tachycardia or asystole)

**(2)** Progressive HF in 50%

### Evidence-Based Diagnosis

**A.** The history should assess risk factors for HF, including hypertension, CAD, alcohol abuse, illicit drug use, and adriamycin as well as symptoms of HF.

**B.** Physical exam

**1.** Clinical signs and symptoms are affected by

**a.** Patient's *current* volume status

**b.** Chronicity. In *chronic* HF, signs and symptoms are frequently absent despite marked impairment of LV function *and* marked volume overload.

**2.** $S_3$ gallop

**a.** An $S_3$ gallop occurs when a large volume of blood rushes from the left atrium (LA) into the LV at the start of diastole (just after $S_2$).

/FP\ **b.** Virtually pathognomonic of volume overload and occurs most commonly in patients with decompensated HF.

**3.** $S_4$ gallop

**a.** Occurs when the LA contracts and sends blood into the LV (just before $S_1$).

**b.** An $S_4$ gallop may be heard in some normal patients and in many patients with hypertension and LV hypertrophy.

**c.** $S_4$ is *not* specific for HF.

**4.** JVD

**a.** Defined as > 3 cm of elevation above the sternal angle (Figure 14–2).

/FP\ **b.** Highly specific for HF (> 95%); may occur in RV or LV failure.

**5.** Table 14–3 summarizes the sensitivities, specificities, and LRs of clinical findings for HF in patients with dyspnea.

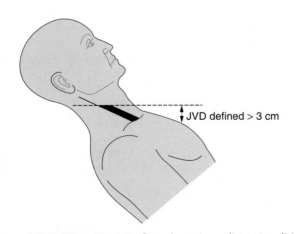

**Figure 14–2.** Measurement of jugular venous distention. (Modified from McGee S. Evidence Based Physician's Diagnosis, p. 402. Copyright © 2001. With permission from Elsevier.)

**Table 14–3.** Accuracy of clinical findings in heart failure.

| Finding | Sensitivity (%) | Specificity (%) | LR+ | LR− |
|---|---|---|---|---|
| Paroxysmal nocturnal dyspnea | 41 | 84 | 2.6 | 0.7 |
| Orthopnea | 50 | 77 | 2.2 | 0.65 |
| Dyspnea on exertion | 84 | 34 | 1.3 | 0.48 |
| $S_3$ | 13 | 99 | **11** | 0.88 |
| $S_4$ | 5 | 97 | 1.6 | 0.98 |
| Jugular venous distention | 39 | 92 | **5.1** | 0.66 |
| Crackles | 60 | 78 | 2.8 | 0.51 |
| Edema | 50 | 78 | 2.3 | 0.64 |

**a.** Classic signs and symptoms (orthopnea, paroxysmal nocturnal dyspnea, crackles, gallops and edema) are not sensitive for HF and their absence does not rule out HF. Indeed, even in severe chronic HF (mean EF 18%, pulmonary capillary wedge pressure (PCWP) > 22 mm Hg), 42% of patients did not have crackles, increased JVP, or edema.

**b.** However, certain findings are highly specific and significantly increase the likelihood of HF when present. An $S_3$ (but not an $S_4$) and JVD strongly suggest HF.

**c.** Other classic symptoms, like orthopnea, PND, and crackles, are not specific for HF.

**C.** Chest radiography

**1.** Cardiomegaly is the most sensitive finding (74%), and its absence modestly decreases the likelihood of HF (LR− 0.33).

**2.** Pulmonary venous congestion and interstitial edema are highly specific (96–97%) and when present strongly suggest HF (LR+ 12).

**3.** Pleural effusions are seen in 26% of patients with HF.

**a.** The effusions are usually small to moderate in size and unilateral or bilateral.

**b.** These effusions are transudative.

**c.** When due to HF, pleural effusions are usually accompanied by cardiomegaly, pulmonary vascular redistribution, or edema.

**d.** The absence of these findings or the presence of massive pleural effusions suggest some other etiology and warrants further evaluation.

**4.** Table 14–4 summarizes the accuracy of the chest radiograph in the diagnosis of HF.

**D.** ECG can provide evidence of prior myocardial infarction or LV hypertrophy. It can neither rule in nor rule out HF.

**E.** Brain natriuretic peptide (BNP)

**1.** Secreted by LV or RV in response to increased volume or pressure or both

***Table 14–4.*** Accuracy of chest radiography in heart failure.

| Finding | Sensitivity (%) | Specificity (%) | LR+ | LR– |
|---|---|---|---|---|
| Pulmonary venous congestion | 54 | 96 | 12.0 | 0.48 |
| Interstitial edema | 34 | 97 | 12.0 | 0.68 |
| Alveolar edema | 6 | 99 | 6 | 0.95 |
| Pleural effusions | 26 | 92 | 3.2 | 0.81 |
| Cardiomegaly | 74 | 78 | 3.3 | 0.33 |

**2.** May be elevated in systolic or diastolic HF

**3.** Levels increase proportionately to the degree of HF

**4.** Low BNP levels decrease the likelihood of HF in patients with dyspnea.

   **a.** BNP < 100 pg/mL

   **(1)** Sensitivity, 87–93%; specificity, 66–72%

   **(2)** LR–, 0.11–0.12; LR+, 2.7–3.1

   **b.** BNP < 50 pg/mL

   **(1)** Sensitivity, 97%; specificity, 62%

   **(2)** LR–, 0.05; LR+, 2.6

   **c.** May not rule out HF in patients with coexistent COPD

   **(1)** Sensitivity, 35%; specificity, 90%

   **(2)** LR–, 0.72; LR+, 3.5

**5.** High levels of BNP increase the likelihood of HF but are still not entirely specific.

   **a.** BNP ≥ 250 pg/mL

   **(1)** Sensitivity, 89%; specificity, 81%

   **(2)** LR+, 4.6; LR–, 0.14

   **b.** BNP is elevated in patients with right-sided HF (ie, due to cor pulmonale) and in many patients with PE.

   **(1)** A significant fraction of patients with PE are clinically stable but found to have RV dilatation on echocardiography as well as elevated BNP levels.

   **(2)** The BNP level in patients with stable PE was 88–487 pg/mL in 34% and 527–1300 pg/mL in 33%.

**6.** Some authorities use the following criteria to interpret BNP levels:

   **a.** < 100 pg/mL: HF unlikely

   **b.** 100–500 pg/mL: Indeterminate

   **c.** > 500 pg/mL: (LR+ 6) HF most likely diagnosis

**F.** Two-dimensional echocardiogram is the test of choice to diagnose HF.

   **1.** Systolic and diastolic function can be evaluated.

   **2.** Regional systolic dysfunction suggests an ischemic etiology.

   **3.** Valve function can be assessed.

**G.** Radionuclide tests can quantify EF but cannot access LV wall thickness or valvular abnormalities.

**H.** HF is frequently present but unsuspected in patients in whom COPD is diagnosed.

   **1.** Studies report unsuspected HF in ≈25% of patients with COPD. These patients had fewer pack years of tobacco use than patients without HF (9.6 vs 22.7).

   **2.** Pleural fluid, pulmonary revascularization, and edema were uncommon even in the subgroup with HF (9.1%) but when present strongly suggested HF (LR+ 9.1).

 Clinicians should have a low threshold for checking an echocardiogram in patients with COPD and dyspnea.

**Treatment**

**A.** Prevention: Hypertension therapy decreases the incidence of HF by 30–50%.

**B.** Initial laboratory tests: BUN, creatinine, electrolytes, CBC, TSH, fasting blood glucose or glycohemoglobin, lipid panel, and liver function tests

**C.** Routine chest radiograph, ECG and echocardiogram are recommended.

**D.** Coronary angiography or noninvasive imaging (ie, nuclear stress test) is recommended in patients with chest pain that may be cardiac, suspected CAD, or CAD risk factors.

**E.** Multiple therapies have been demonstrated to reduce morbidity and mortality in patients with *systolic* dysfunction and HF.

   **1.** ACE inhibitors

   **a.** Indicated in symptomatic and asymptomatic patients with reduced EF

   **b.** Angiotensin receptor blockers (ARBs) may be used in place of ACE inhibitors when a troublesome cough develops in patients taking ACE inhibitors.

   **c.** ARBs may cause angioedema in patients who had angioedema while taking ACE inhibitors.

   **2.** β-Blockers

   **a.** β-Blockers reduce morbidity and mortality in all stages of HF, including severe HF (EF < 25%).

   **b.** Indicated in symptomatic and asymptomatic patients with reduced EF

   **c.** Initiate therapy when patients are euvolemic.

   **d.** β-Blockers can precipitate fatal asthma even in patients with mild reactive airway disease. Some authorities advise against their use in any patient with asthma.

   **3.** Spironolactone

   **a.** Reduces mortality in patients with class IV HF and reduced EF.

   **b.** Contraindications include creatinine > 2.5 mg/dL in men and > 2.0 mg/dL in women, serum potassium level > 5.0 mEq/L, or cases in which patients cannot have their serum potassium adequately monitored.

   **4.** Hydralazine and nitrates, in addition to ACE inhibitors and β-blockers, have been demonstrated to reduce mortality in black patients with class III or IV HF. They may also be useful in patients who are unable to tolerate ACE inhibitors/ARBs.

F. Digoxin
   1. Reduces hospitalizations but not mortality.
   2. Low serum concentrations (0.5–0.8 mg/dL) are as effective as higher concentrations.
   3. ACC/AHA guidelines recommend digoxin only in *symptomatic* patients with reduced EF.
   4. Digoxin may *increase* mortality in women and is not advised for women by some authorities.

G. Diuretics (loop or thiazides)
   1. Mainstay of therapy to treat edema and pulmonary congestion (should be used in combination with salt restriction).
   2. The clinical assessment of volume status is critical. Increasing weight, edema, JVD, pulmonary edema, or an $S_3$ gallop suggests patients are volume overloaded.
   3. However, multiple studies demonstrate that patients with severe chronic HF and marked volume overload (by PCWP) may have no signs of HF.
   4. Therefore, patients with dyspnea should undergo aggressive diuresis while monitoring renal function.

H. Control of hypertension

I. Influenza and pneumococcal vaccination

J. Nonsteroidal antiinflammatory drugs and thiazolidinediones increase fluid retention and have been associated with worsening HF and precipitating HF and should be avoided. Thiazolidinediones are contraindicated in patients with class III or IV HF.

K. Cardiac resynchronization therapy (CRT): Some patients with HF have prolonged QRS intervals, which reflects prolonged and dyssynchronous depolarization. This nonuniform depolarization results in poorly organized contraction and contributes to LV dysfunction. In addition, it contributes to MR and LV remodeling.
   1. In cardiac resynchronization, wires are implanted in the atria and both ventricles to allow precise and coordinated depolarization of the atria and left and right ventricles.
   2. CRT improves EF, quality of life, and functional status, and it reduces hospitalizations and mortality in select patients.
   3. Indications include patients with class III or IV HF symptoms despite optimal medical therapy, an EF < 35%, and a QRS ≥ 0.12.

L. Implantable cardiac defibrillator (ICD)
   1. A substantial proportion of deaths in patients with HF are sudden (30% in dilated cardiomyopathy), presumably secondary to ventricular tachycardia and ventricular fibrillation.
   2. ICDs are indicated in select patients with HF, especially in patients who have survived cardiac arrest and in patients with unexplained syncope. ICDs are also recommended in patients without prior syncope or sudden cardiac death with NYHA class II or III HF and an EF < 35% as well as in patients with NYHA class I HF if it is ≥ 40 days after a myocardial infarction with an EF < 30%.

M. Heart transplantation is an option for a few patients with severe HF refractory to intensive medical therapy.

N. Therapy in patients with diastolic HF and normal EF
   1. Systolic and diastolic hypertension should be controlled.
   2. Diuretics can be used to treat pulmonary congestion or edema.

   3. Digoxin has no proven benefit.
   4. Control ventricular rate for patients with AF
   5. Coronary revascularization for patients with reversible ischemia
   6. The effectiveness of ACE inhibitors, β-blockers, or ARBs is less well established. Recent studies suggest ARBs decrease hospitalizations in patients with diastolic HF.

## MAKING A DIAGNOSIS

Mr. C has several features that are highly specific for HF. His history of prior myocardial infarction, orthopnea, and most importantly the clinical findings of JVD and an $S_3$ gallop are highly specific for HF.

**Have you crossed a diagnostic threshold for the leading hypothesis, HF? Have you ruled out the active alternatives? Do other tests need to be done to exclude the alternative diagnoses?**

## Alternative Diagnosis: Mitral regurgitation (MR)

### Textbook Presentation

Patients with MR may be identified due to an asymptomatic holosystolic murmur at the apex or during an evaluation of shortness of breath, dyspnea on exertion, orthopnea, and fatigue. Alternatively, it may be discovered during the evaluation of patients with AF.

### Disease Highlights

A. Trivial symptomatic MR is commonly discovered on echocardiogram. The remainder of the discussion will focus on patients with more significant regurgitation.

B. Etiologies: MR develops secondary to damaged mitral leaflets (primary) or a dilated mitral annulus (secondary).
   1. Primary MR
      a. Causes include mitral valve prolapse, rheumatic heart disease, and endocarditis.
      b. Although most patients with mitral valve prolapse never require valve replacement, it is the most common cause of MR and the need for valve replacement.
   2. Secondary MR
      a. HF: LV dilatation leads to mitral annular dilatation and MR.
      b. Ischemic MR: Leaflet tethering shortens the mitral apparatus, resulting in MR.

C. Pathophysiology
   1. Compensated MR: MR leads to LA dilatation, and compensatory LV dilatation. If systolic function is maintained, EF remains normal to high and LV end-systolic volume remains low because MR acts to reduce LV afterload.
   2. Decompensated MR: Systolic function may fail leading to increased LV end systolic volume, decreased stroke volume, and decreased EF. This may be irreversible.
   3. LA dilatation may lead to AF.

D. Disease progression is slow. Average delay from diagnosis to symptoms is 16 years. However, in patients with severe MR, the annual mortality is 5%.

E. Complications include dyspnea, pulmonary edema, AF, and sudden death.

## Evidence-Based Diagnosis

A. Physical exam: The typical murmur is a blowing, holosystolic murmur heard at the apex that radiates to the axilla. $S_2$ may be inaudible.

1. Grade 3 or louder systolic murmur

   a. 85% sensitive, 81% specific for moderate to severe MR

   b. LR+, 4.5; LR−, 0.19

2. $S_3$ gallop may be heard due to increased flow across the mitral valve.

B. ECG and chest radiograph may demonstrate LA enlargement or LV enlargement. Neither is sensitive or specific for the diagnosis.

C. Echocardiography is the test of choice to diagnose and quantify MR. Transesophageal echocardiography provides more precise details on valve anatomy and may help determine whether valve repair (versus replacement) is an option.

## Treatment

A. Serial echocardiography

1. Serial echocardiography is important to detect signs of *LV dysfunction, which may occur despite the absence of symptoms.*

2. Echocardiography is recommended annually or semiannually in patients with moderate to severe MR and after a change in signs or symptoms.

3. Serial echocardiography is not recommended for asymptomatic patients with mild MR with normal LV size and function.

B. Valve repair versus replacement

1. Valve repair is superior to valve replacement (when technically feasible).

2. Valve repair is associated with substantially decreased operative mortality (2% vs 6%), does not require subsequent anticoagulation, and is associated with a significantly better EF.

C. ACC/AHA guidelines for medical therapy and valve replacement are summarized in Table 14–5.

D. Treat underlying ischemia.

E. Anticoagulation

1. Patients are at increased risk for thromboembolism following mitral valve replacement or aortic valve replacement (AVR).

2. The risk varies depending on the location of the valve (mitral or aortic), type of valve (mechanical or bioprosthetic), and presence or absence of additional risk factors.

3. ACC/AHA guidelines are summarized in Table 14–6.

## Alternative Diagnosis: Chronic Aortic Regurgitation (AR)

### Textbook Presentation

Patients with chronic AR typically complain of progressive dyspnea on exertion or the sensation of a pounding heart. Alternatively, the

**Table 14–5.** ACC/AHA guidelines for medical therapy and valve replacement in patients with mitral regurgitation.

| MR Severity | Modifier | Treatment Recommendation |
|---|---|---|
| Severe | Symptoms | MV repair |
| Severe | Mild–moderate LV dysfunction (EF: 30–60%, LVESD > 40 mm) | MV repair |
| Severe | Associated with atrial fibrillation or pulmonary hypertension | MV repair |
| Severe | Likelihood of success > 90% | MV repair |
| Severe | Severe LV dysfunction (EF < 30%, LVESD > 55 mm) | ± MV repair[1] Optimize HF therapy |
| Any degree | No symptoms or LV dysfunction medical therapy | Observe No role for |
| | Secondary MR (due to HF) Diuretics β-Blockers CRT | ACE inhibitors |
| | Associated with hypertension Diuretics β-Blockers | ACE inhibitors |

ACC/AHA, American College of Cardiology/American Heart Association; CRT, cardiac resynchronization therapy; EF, ejection fraction; HF, heart failure; LV, left ventricular; LVESD, left ventricular end systolic diameter; MV, mitral valve.

patient may be asymptomatic, and the diagnosis may be suspected when an early diastolic murmur is detected by a careful examiner.

### Disease Highlights

A. Secondary to damaged aortic leaflets or dilated aortic root

B. Etiologies

1. Valvular abnormalities: Rheumatic carditis, bacterial endocarditis, congenital bicuspid valves, collagen vascular disease, fenfluramine and phentermine

2. Aortic root dilatation: Hypertension, ascending aortic aneurysm, Marfan syndrome, aortic dissection, syphilitic aortitis

C. Pathophysiology

1. Regurgitation results in LV remodeling and LV hypertrophy to maintain wall stress. LV end-diastolic volume increases to maintain effective stroke volume.

2. The increasing preload and afterload may eventually result in LV systolic dysfunction, and the LV end-systolic volume increases and EF decreases. LV end-diastolic pressure increases and pulmonary congestion and dyspnea result.

---

[1]The optimal approach to patients with MR & severe LV dysfunction is unclear. Surgery is beneficial in some and detrimental in others

***Table 14–6.*** ACC/AHA recommendations for anticoagulation following valve replacement.

| Valve Position | Valve Type | Risk factors[1] | Recommendation |
|---|---|---|---|
| Mitral | Bioprosthetic | Absent | Aspirin 75–100 mg |
| | | Present | Aspirin 75–100 mg and warfarin INR 2.5–3.5 |
| | Mechanical | Absent | Aspirin 75–100 mg and warfarin INR 2.5–3.5 |
| | | Present | Aspirin 75–100 mg and warfarin INR 2.5–3.5 |
| Aortic | Bioprosthetic | Absent | Aspirin 75–100 mg |
| | | Present | Aspirin 75–100 mg and warfarin INR 2–3 |
| | Mechanical | Absent | Aspirin 75 – 100 mg and warfarin INR 2.0–3.0[2] |
| | | Present | Aspirin 75–100 mg and warfarin INR 2.5–3.5 |

[1]Include atrial fibrillation, prior transient ischemic attack/cerebrovascular accident, heart failure, or hypercoagulable state.
[2]For Star Edwards valves or disk valves, an INR of 2.5–3.5 is recommended.
ACC/AHA, American College of Cardiology/American Heart Association.

**3.** Significant LV dysfunction can be irreversible. Valve replacement should be performed before irreversible LV dysfunction and HF develop (see below).

**4.** Progression to symptoms or LV dysfunction in patients with normal LV function develops in 4% of patients per year.

### Evidence-Based Diagnosis

**A.** The pulse pressure (the difference between the systolic and diastolic BP) is often wide in AR due to 2 processes. First, the large stroke volume increases the systolic BP and second, the regurgitation of blood back into the LV rapidly lowers the diastolic BP.

**1.** The wide pulse pressure causes many of the classic physical findings, such as bounding pulses and head bobbing.

**2.** Wide pulse pressures are not specific for AR. Other causes include anemia, fever, pregnancy, large arteriovenous fistula, cirrhosis, thyrotoxicosis, and patent ductus arteriosa.

**B.** Auscultation

**1.** May demonstrate an early decrescendo *diastolic* murmur following $S_2$. Best heard at the left sternal border.

**a.** Auscultation is more sensitive for moderate to severe AR.

**b.** Sensitivity is 0–64% among students and residents.

**c.** Sensitivity is 80–95% among experienced cardiologists.

**d.** Another study reported that the diastolic murmur of mild to moderate AR was rarely detected by attending non-cardiologists (sensitivity 4% mild AR, 14% moderate AR).

 **e.** However, the finding of a diastolic murmur is highly specific (98%).

**2.** A systolic murmur suggesting AS may be heard.

**a.** Regurgitation results in increasing end diastolic volumes.

**b.** Stroke volumes increase to maintain forward flow.

**c.** The increased cardiac output may exceed the capacity of even a normal aortic valve to accommodate flow, resulting in a high flow systolic murmur across the aortic valve. One study reported that 51% of patients with mild to moderate AR had a *systolic* murmur (86% in moderate AR and 50% in mild AR).

Although a diastolic murmur strongly suggests AR, *systolic* murmurs are often the *only* murmur heard in patients with AR.

**3.** Austin Flint murmur

**a.** Aortic regurgitant streams may impact the mitral valve leaflets during diastole resulting in functional mitral stenosis and a late diastolic murmur over the apex.

**b.** Sensitivity varies from 0% to 100%.

**C.** Doppler echocardiography is the test of choice.

**D.** Exercise testing can help access LV function during stress.

### Treatment

**A.** The key consideration in patients with AR is the appropriate timing of valve replacement (Table 14-7).

**1.** AV replacement (AVR) should be performed prior to the onset of *irreversible* LV dysfunction.

**2.** Serial echocardiography is important to detect signs of *LV dysfunction, which may occur in patients without symptoms.*

**B.** AVR is indicated in patients with severe AR associated with symptoms or LV dysfunction.

**C.** Replacement valves may be either mechanical or bioprosthetic (eg, porcine valves).

**1.** Mechanical valves are more durable and are often chosen for young patients to minimize the need for subsequent AVR. However, patients with mechanical valves require lifelong anticoagulation.

**2.** Bioprosthetic valves are used more often in older patients (> 70 years) with shorter life expectancies and patients with higher bleeding risks while receiving anticoagulation therapy.

**D.** Afterload reduction (with nifedipine or an ACE inhibitor) can reduce regurgitation, the rate of progression of cardiac enlargement, and the need for valve replacement. It should not be substituted for AVR in patients with an indication for valve replacement (Table 14–7).

**E.** β-Blockers are relatively contraindicated. Prolonged diastole increases regurgitation and accelerates progression.

**Table 14–7.** Treatment recommendations for patients with AR.

| Severity | Modifier | Treatment Recommendations |
|---|---|---|
| Severe | Symptomatic | AVR In patients who are not candidates for AVR, ACE inhibitors or nifedipine can be used to reduce progression |
| | LV dysfunction: EF ≤ 50% | AVR |
| | LV dilatation (without symptoms or dysfunction) | Afterload reduction or AVR if severe dilatation |
| Mild to moderate | Asymptomatic, normal EF, no hypertension | No therapy |
| Any degree | Hypertension Aortic root dilatation > 4.5–5 cm | Afterload reduction AVR |

AR, aortic regurgitation; AVR, aortic valve replacement; EF, ejection fraction; LV, left ventricular.

F. Patients are at increased risk for thromboembolic events following AVR and should receive prophylaxis. (see Table 14–6).

**Alternative Diagnosis: Aortic stenosis (AS)**

See Chapter 26, Syncope.

## Alternative Diagnosis: Atrial fibrillation (AF)

### Textbook Presentation

Classically, patients with AF seek medical care for palpitations. The abrupt onset often prompts patients to be seen emergently. Patients may also complain of shortness of breath and dyspnea on exertion. Occasionally, AF is detected during a routine office visit when an irregularly irregular pulse is noted and evaluated.

### Disease Highlights

A. AF is the most common clinical arrhythmia; its incidence increases with age (3.8% of patients ≥ 60 years old to 9% in those ≥ 80 years old).

B. May be episodic or persistent

C. Secondary to multiple wavelets of excitation that meander around the atria

D. Etiologies

1. Most common etiologies are hypertension, CAD, and HF.

2. Acute coronary syndrome: In 2–5% of patients presenting to the emergency department with new onset AF, it is secondary to an acute myocardial infarction.

3. Other etiologies include alcoholic heart disease, valvular heart disease, cor pulmonale, thyrotoxicosis, and PE.

E. Complications

1. Stroke: Stasis promotes thrombus formation within the atria. Subsequent embolization results in stroke and other systemic emboli.

   a. The annual stroke rate in AF patients not receiving anticoagulation is 4.1% per year. For the subgroup with a prior transient ischemic attack or stroke, the annual stroke rate increases to 13% per year.

   b. AF accounts for 1/6 of all strokes at an annual cost of $6.6 billion.

   c. Stroke is more common in patients with AF who have other clinical risk factors:

      (1) Valvular heart disease

      (2) Prior transient ischemic attack or stroke

      (3) Increasing age

      (4) Hypertension

      (5) Diabetes

      (6) HF

      (7) Gender (women affected 1.5–3.0 times more than men)

2. Worsening HF due to loss of atrial kick; especially important in patients with stiff LV (ie, diastolic dysfunction)

### Evidence-Based Diagnosis

A. Easily recognized on ECG (Figure 14–3)

B. Episodic AF can be detected with Holter monitoring or event recorders.

### Treatment

A. Evaluation

1. ECG can document AF, ischemia, bundle-branch block, a delta wave or short PR suggesting Wolff-Parkinson-White syndrome, or signs of right heart strain suggesting PE.

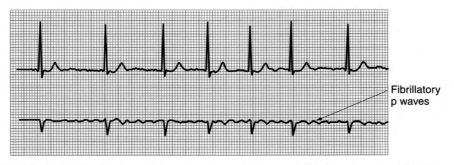

Fibrillatory p waves

**Figure 14–3.** ECG of atrial fibrillation demonstrating irregularly spaced QRS complexes and fibrillatory p waves.

**2.** Baseline echocardiogram to assess LV function and stroke risk

**3.** Obtain baseline thyroid function tests to rule out hyperthyroidism.

**4.** Electrolyte, BUN, and creatinine testing is recommended.

**5.** Consider evaluation for other etiologies (eg, PE).

**B.** Rhythm control versus rate control

  **1.** Cardioversion should be performed immediately in unstable patients.

  **2.** In stable patients, 2 options exist: rhythm control or rate control.

    **a.** Rhythm control attempts to restore normal sinus rhythm using cardioversion and antiarrhythmic agents.

    **b.** Rate control allows persistent AF. The *ventricular* response is controlled with atrioventricular nodal blocking agents (eg, β-blockers, diltiazem, verapamil, or digoxin). Anticoagulation is used to prevent stroke.

    **c.** Studies show that rhythm control and rate control results in similar mortality and stroke rates, even in patients with underlying HF.

    **d.** Rate control is the recommended strategy in most patients. (Patients with their first episode of AF or with symptoms or exercise intolerance may choose rhythm control.)

      **(1)** Uses β-blockers, diltiazem, verapamil, or digoxin

      **(2)** Verapamil and β-blockers should not be used concurrently in the same patient due to a high frequency of complications (bradycardia or HF).

      **(3)** β-Blockers, diltiazem, and verapamil should be avoided in patients with decompensated HF.

      **(4)** Digoxin

        **(a)** Less effective at controlling ventricular response during activity and in paroxysmal AF

        **(b)** Useful in patients with decreased LV function

        **(c)** Second-line drug

    **e.** Rhythm control therapy

      **(1)** Anticoagulation therapy is recommended for 3 weeks prior to cardioversion and 4 weeks after in certain patients who are at high risk for existing atrial thrombi and embolism including patients with AF for longer than 48 hours or of unknown duration as well as patients with mitral valve disease, heart failure, or prior embolism.

      **(2)** Low-risk patients (without the aforementioned risk factors) and AF of recent onset (< 48 hours) can be cardioverted without delay.

        **(a)** Heparin should be administered at presentation.

        **(b)** Alternatively, a transesophageal echocardiography can be performed in these patients, and cardioversion may be done if no thrombus is seen.

        **(c)** In either case, these patients should receive anticoagulation therapy for 4 weeks after cardioversion.

      **(3)** The probability of conversion to normal sinus rhythm decreases the longer the AF lasts.

      **(4)** Multiple antiarrhythmic drugs have been used to convert patients to normal sinus rhythm. Flecainide should be avoided in patients with a history of CAD or LV dysfunction. Cardiac consultation is advised.

**C.** The ACC/AHA have published guidelines for stroke prevention in persistent or paroxysmal AF.

  **1.** Warfarin and aspirin have been used to prevent strokes in patients with AF.

  **2.** Multiple studies suggest that warfarin is superior to aspirin at preventing stroke with an RR reduction of 64% versus 19% for aspirin. In the absence of contraindications, the benefit of warfarin usually outweighs the risk.

  **3.** The absolute benefit of warfarin increases as the risk of stroke increases.

    **a.** Warfarin reduces the absolute rate of stroke on average by 2.7% per year, but in patients with prior transient ischemic attack/cerebrovascular accident, the absolute risk reduction is 8.4% per year.

    **b.** AHA/ACC guidelines are summarized in Table 14–8.

  **4.** Two special groups are worth mentioning.

    **a.** Although physicians worry about bleeding complications in the elderly, studies show that the elderly patients with AF are at high risk for stroke and benefit from anticoagulation if they are carefully selected.

    **b.** Patients with lone AF (age < 60, no heart disease, hypertension or risk factors) are at the lowest risk for stroke (< 1% per year when treated with aspirin) and the absolute risk reduction from warfarin is very small and similar in magnitude to the risk of hemorrhage from warfarin.

      **(1)** The AHA/ACC does not recommend warfarin for these patients. However, physicians should still discuss the benefits and risks of warfarin therapy with these patients to decide between aspirin and warfarin therapy.

      **(2)** It is important to explain that although the risk of stroke (without warfarin) is low, the long-term

**Table 14–8.** Recommendations to prevent stroke in patients with persistent or paroxysmal atrial fibrillation.

| Risk Category | Definition | Therapeutic Recommendations |
|---|---|---|
| High risk | Prior TIA/CVA Valvular heart disease | Warfarin |
| Moderate risk | ≥ 2 risk factors[1] | Warfarin |
| Low risk | 1 risk factor | Warfarin or aspirin |
| Low risk | 2 of 3 less-validated risk factors: age 65–74, women, CAD | Warfarin or aspirin |
| Lone atrial fibrillation | Age ≤ 60, no heart disease, no hypertension or risk factors | Aspirin |

[1]Risk factors include history of hypertension, heart failure, age ≥ 75 years, diabetes mellitus.
CAD, coronary artery disease; TIA/CVA, transient ischemic attack/cerebrovascular accident.

consequences of stroke can be grave and are usually more permanent than those of hemorrhage.

5. Contraindications to warfarin therapy include recent GI or CNS hemorrhage, recent trauma or surgery, uncontrolled hypertension, noncompliance, syncope, or alcoholism.

## Alternative Diagnosis: CAD

See Chapter 8, Chest Pain.

## CASE RESOLUTION

Mr. C undergoes a transthoracic echocardiogram, which reveals marked systolic dysfunction and an EF of 18%. There are regional wall motion abnormalities. The anterior wall is very hypokinetic. There is no significant AS or AR. MR is mild.

Mr. C's echocardiogram confirms HF. The regional wall motion abnormalities suggest an ischemic etiology, likely secondary to his prior infarction. A stress test to rule out reversible ischemia would be appropriate. The echocardiogram rules out significant valvular heart disease as the primary etiology of his dyspnea.

A stress thallium study is performed. This reveals a large prior myocardial infarction but no reversible ischemia. The EF is 20%.

The stress test confirms prior myocardial infarction as the cause of Mr. C's HF without evidence of active ischemia.

Mr. C is admitted for treatment of his HF. He starts a salt-restricted diet and is given diuretics, ACE inhibitors, and β-blockers (when his HF is controlled). The diuresis results in a 20-pound weight loss, and his dyspnea on exertion improves markedly. His orthopnea resolves. He remains stable at follow-up 5 years later.

## CHIEF COMPLAINT

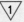

### PATIENT 2

Mrs. L is a 58-year-old woman who arrives at the emergency department with a chief complaint of shortness of breath. She reports that this has developed gradually over the last 3–6 months. Six months ago, she was able to walk as far as she wanted without any shortness of breath. Now she is experiencing dyspnea even walking around her house. She denies any episodes of acute shortness of breath, chest pain, or hemoptysis. She denies wheezing. She has no history of myocardial infarction, hypertension, or known heart disease. She smoked 1 pack of cigarettes per day for 10 years and quit when she was 28 years old. She drinks 1 glass of wine per week. She works as an accountant and spends her free time with her grandchildren. She has no unusual hobbies.

At this point, what is the leading hypothesis, what are the active alternatives, and is there a must not miss diagnosis? Given this differential diagnosis, what tests should be ordered?

## PRIORITIZING THE DIFFERENTIAL DIAGNOSIS

Mrs. L's shortness of breath is not only severe but markedly worse than baseline. Both of these features should prompt a thorough investigation. Unfortunately, the clinical information does not suggest a specific diagnosis. There is no history of CAD, hypertension, or alcohol abuse to suggest HF nor is there a significant tobacco history to suggest COPD. A careful exam is vital to look for helpful clues.

On physical exam, the patient appears comfortable at rest, but becomes markedly dyspneic with ambulation. Vital signs are BP, 140/70 mm Hg; pulse, 72 bpm; temperature, 37.1°C; RR, 20 breaths per minute. Conjunctiva are pink. Lung exam is clear to percussion and auscultation. There are no crackles or wheezes. Cardiac exam reveals a regular rate and rhythm. $S_1$ and $S_2$ are normal. There is no JVD, $S_3$, $S_4$, or murmur. There is only trace peripheral edema. Abdominal exam is normal. A chest radiograph, ECG, and CBC are normal.

Despite a thorough exam, the leading diagnosis is unclear. In such cases, it is particularly important to systematically review the differential diagnosis in order to arrive at the correct diagnosis. Each item on the list should be reviewed in light of the history and physical to determine whether it remains in the differential and should be explored further, or whether the existing information makes it highly unlikely.

Refer to the differential diagnosis listed at the beginning of the chapter. The absence of a murmur makes MR and AS unlikely, since the clinical exam is 85–90% sensitive for these conditions. The clinical exam is less sensitive for AR (see above). Therefore, AR remains on the differential diagnosis. An arrhythmia is essentially ruled out by the patient's normal heart rate during symptoms. HF is not particularly suggested by the history and physical exam, but it cannot be excluded given the low sensitivity of the $S_3$ gallop and JVD. The patient denies any history of chest pain, but dyspnea is occasionally an anginal equivalent, thus CAD remains a possibility. Alveolar diseases are unlikely given the normal chest radiograph. Pneumonia seems highly unlikely given the absence of cough, fever, or infiltrate on chest film. Asthma remains a possibility although this is not particularly suggested by the history or physical. COPD is effectively ruled out by the trivial smoking history. PE cannot be excluded by the current information and remains on the list, although the presentation is not particularly classic for PE. Since PE is associated with a high mortality, it should be considered a must not miss possibility. A significant pleural effusion or pneumothorax are ruled out by the normal chest radiograph, which also makes interstitial disease unlikely (although not impossible). Anemia is ruled out by the normal CBC. We can now focus on the clinical clues and diagnostic tests for these remaining possible diagnoses (AR, HF, CAD, asthma, and PE). Table 14–9 lists the differential diagnosis.

 A methodical approach to the differential diagnosis is vital whenever the leading diagnosis is unclear or when the leading hypothesis cannot be confirmed.

In terms of CAD, she denies any history of exertional chest pain or pressure and has minimal coronary risk factors. (Her last cholesterol level was normal [180 mg/dL] with an HDL of 70 mg/dL. She has no history of diabetes mellitus, no family history of CAD, and no recent

**Table 14–9.** Diagnostic hypotheses for Mrs. L.

| Diagnostic Hypothesis | Clinical Clues | Important Tests |
|---|---|---|
| **Active Alternatives—Most Common** | | |
| Heart failure | Poorly controlled hypertension or history of myocardial infarction S₃ gallop, JVD Crackles on lung exam Peripheral edema | Echocardiogram BNP |
| Coronary artery disease | History of symptoms with exertion (eg, chest pain, pressure) Risk factors for coronary artery disease | ECG Exercise stress tests |
| Aortic regurgitation | Early diastolic murmur left sternal border | Echocardiogram |
| Asthma | History of wheezing Chest tightness Worsening cough with cold, exercise, pets, mold | Peak flow Pulmonary function tests Methacholine challenge Response to treatment |
| **Active Alternatives—Must Not Miss** | | |
| Pulmonary embolism | Pleuritic chest pain Risk factors (immobilization, postoperative or postpartum states, estrogen therapy, cancer, thrombophilia) | CTA D-dimer Duplex leg exam Ventilation perfusion (V/Q) scan Pulmonary angiography |

CTA = CT angiography.

tobacco use.) With respect to asthma, she denies any history of wheezing or worsening cough associated with cold, exercise, pets, or dust. With respect to PE, she denies sudden onset of chest pain, chest pain with inspiration, hemoptysis, immobilization, cancer, surgery, family history of venous thromboembolism or leg swelling. She does take hormone replacement therapy (HRT).

An echocardiogram reveals normal LV function and a normal aortic valve. Pulmonary function tests reveal normal total lung capacity, FEV₁, and DLCO. A methacholine challenge test is also normal.

Considering each diagnosis in turn, the patient's physical exam and echocardiogram exclude HF and AR. The patient's pretest probability of CAD is quite low given her age, sex, and risk factors (3.2%; see Chapter 8, Chest Pain). In addition, the Framingham data suggest the likelihood of a coronary event in a female patient with these CAD risk factors to be < 1% over the ensuing 8 years. The history as well as the normal pulmonary function tests with methacholine challenge make asthma very unlikely. Although her history sounds atypical for PE, she is taking HRT, a known risk factor for venous thromboembolism. Given the exclusion of the other diagnoses, PE becomes more probable. You revise your differential diagnosis and make PE both your leading and must not miss diagnosis.

 **Is the clinical information sufficient to make a diagnosis of PE? If not, what other information do you need?**

## Leading Hypothesis: PE

### Textbook Presentation

Classically, patients with PE experience the sudden onset of shortness of breath and severe chest pain that increases with inspiration. Patients may complain of hemoptysis and associated leg swelling.

### Disease Highlights

A. Pathophysiology: Most commonly occurs when a lower extremity venous thrombosis embolizes to the lung. Upper extremity thrombi may also cause PE.

   **1.** 80% of patients with PE have deep venous thrombosis (DVT)

   **2.** 48% of patients with DVT have PE (often asymptomatic)

B. Symptoms vary markedly. Massive obstruction may result in RV failure and death, whereas lesser obstruction may be asymptomatic.

C. 3-month mortality is 17.5%

D. Risk factors for venous thromboembolism

   **1.** Age (2 × increased risk per decade)

   **2.** Estrogenic factors

     **a.** Obesity

     **b.** Oral birth control pill

     **c.** HRT

   **3.** Immobilization (including prolonged ground or air travel)

4. Postoperative or postpartum states (hip fracture surgery, and total hip or knee replacement create particularly high risk)

5. Cancer

6. History of venous thromboembolism

7. Thrombophilia

    **a.** Antiphospholipid antibodies: Present in 2–8.5% of patients with venous thromboembolism

    **b.** Factor V Leiden

        **(1)** Most common thrombophilia

        **(2)** Mutation in factor V causes resistance to cleavage by activated protein C

        **(3)** 11% of patients with DVT

        **(4)** Confers a 2.7 × increased risk of venous thromboembolism

        **(5)** Combined with oral birth control pill, mutation increases risk 35 times

    **c.** Prothrombin gene mutation

    **d.** Protein C or S deficiency (rare)

        **(1)** Protein C and S are naturally occurring anticoagulants

        **(2)** Deficiency is associated with hypercoagulability.

        **(3)** Synthesis of protein C and S requires vitamin K.

        **(4)** Warfarin decreases synthesis of both factors

        **(5)** Assays for protein C and S must be performed while patients are not taking warfarin.

    **e.** Antithrombin III deficiency (also rare): Assay must be done while patient is not taking heparin.

    **f.** Hyperhomocysteinemia: 3 × increased risk of venous thromboembolism

    **g.** Increased factor VIII: 6 × increased risk

## Evidence-Based Diagnosis

**A.** Symptoms

    **1.** A myriad of symptoms and signs may be seen in patients with PE.

    **2.** The prevalence of these findings is probably overestimated in the literature because much of these data came from older trials, which used angiography and included a large percentage (57%) of patients with massive PE.

**B.** Classic presentations

    **1.** Chest pain with dyspnea or chest pain, dyspnea, and hemoptysis are uncommon and may be seen in as few as 20–33% of patients.

    **2.** Between 12% and 25% of patients have isolated dyspnea, and about 80% of patients with PE have risk factors.

**C.** Studies have reported a range of prevalence of various symptoms in PE, in part dependent on the population (Table 14–10).

    **1.** The modest LRs (comparing patients in whom PE was considered and ruled in or ruled out respectively) suggest that signs and symptoms can neither rule in nor rule out the disease.

    **2.** Sudden onset of dyspnea and leg swelling favor PE whereas fever, cough, crackles, and wheezes do not.

**D.** Tachypnea has been reported in 54–85% of patients and an accentuated P2 in 15–57%.

***Table 14–10.*** Accuracy of symptoms and signs in PE.

| Symptoms and Signs | Sensitivity(%) | Specificity(%) | LR+ | LR– |
|---|---|---|---|---|
| Dyspnea | 59–84 | 51 | 1.7 | 0.3 |
| Dyspnea, sudden onset | 73–78 | 71 | 2.7 | 0.3 |
| Pleuritic chest pain | 32–74 | 70 | 1.5 | 0.8 |
| Cough | 11–51 | 85 | 0.7 | 1.0 |
| Hemoptysis | 9–30 | 95 | 1.8 | 1.0 |
| Syncope | 5–26 | 87 | 2.0 | 0.9 |
| Tachycardia | 24–70 | 77 | 1.0 | 1.0 |
| Crackles | 18–58 | 74 | 0.7 | 1.1 |
| Wheezes | 4–21 | 87 | 0.3 | 1.1 |
| Fever (>38°C) | 7 | 79 | 0.3 | 1.2 |
| Pleural rub | 3–18 | 96 | 1 | 1 |
| Leg swelling | 17–41 | 91 | 1.9 | 0.9 |

**E.** One study reported that 25% of patients with an unexplained exacerbation of COPD actually had a PE. Unexplained exacerbation was defined as the absence of signs of lower respiratory infection (increased sputum, purulence, fever, cold or sore throat) or patients who had parenchymal consolidation on chest radiograph without fever or chills.

The classic presentation of PE is actually the exception. Patients may have very few symptoms. A high index of suspicion must be maintained for the diagnosis of PE.

**F.** Chest film

    **1.** Normal in 50% of patients with PE

    **2.** May reveal focal oligemia (45%), wedge-shaped infiltrate (15%), or pleural effusions (45%)

**G.** ABG may demonstrate hypoxemia and hypocarbia, but findings are neither sensitive nor specific for PE.

    **1.** $PaO_2$ < 80 mm Hg: Sensitivity 58–74%; LR+ 1.2, LR– 0.8

    **2.** $PaCO_2$ < 36 mm Hg: Sensitivity 44%; LR+ 1.1, LR– 0.9

    **3.** $PaO_2$ and $PaCO_2$ do not differ between patients in whom PE is considered and ruled in or ruled out.

Patients with PE may *not* be hypoxic. Therefore, normal arterial oxygen does not rule out PE. (On the other hand, unexplained hypoxia, particularly in the company of a normal chest radiograph, should raise the suspicion of PE.)

**H.** ECG

    **1.** Useful to diagnose other conditions (ie, myocardial infarction)

2. Certain findings suggest PE but are unusual
   a. S1Q3T3 (19–50%)
   b. T wave inversions in V1–V4 are seen in 23–68% of patients with PE. This ECG pattern also suggests an acute coronary syndrome, but the additional presence of T wave inversions in both leads III and V1 strongly suggests PE (88% sensitive, 99% specific; LR+ 88, LR– 0.12).
   c. Transient right bundle-branch block (6–67%)

I. Troponin
   1. A marker of myocardial damage
   2. Elevated in up to 57% of patients with documented PE

J. D-dimers
   1. Fibrin breakdown products
   2. Elevated in many conditions: surgery, trauma, cancer, end-stage renal disease, and venous thromboembolism
   3. Nonspecific. Elevated levels do not diagnose venous thromboembolism
   4. Sensitivity to rule out venous thromboembolism depends on assay used.
      a. Enzyme-linked immunosorbent assay (ELISA) and quantitative rapid ELISA are more sensitive than other assays (95–98%; LR– 0.05–0.11).
      b. Other D-dimer assays are not sensitive enough to rule out venous thromboembolism.
      c. A negative quantitative rapid ELISA markedly decreases the likelihood of PE and effectively rules out PE in patients with a low to moderate pretest probability of PE.

K. CT angiography (CTA)
   1. Test of choice in moderate- to high-risk patients
   2. Noninvasive
   3. May demonstrate filling defects in proximal pulmonary arteries
   4. Positive findings highly specific for PE
   5. Makes alternative diagnosis in 25% of patients (lymphadenopathy, tumor, aortic dissection)
   6. A negative study effectively rules out PE in low- to moderate-risk patients

L. Ventilation-perfusion ($\dot{V}/\dot{Q}$) scan
   1. Radionuclear study used less frequently since advent of CTA
   2. Radio-isotope infused and inhaled
   3. ($\dot{V}/\dot{Q}$) images are compared. A variety of results may be seen.
   4. *High probability scan*
      a. Multiple areas of absent perfusion with normal ventilation
      b. Effectively rules in PE
         (1) 60% sensitive, 96% specific
         (2) LR+ 15, LR – 0.4
   5. *Normal or near normal perfusion scan* effectively rules out PE. (Normal scans are seen in 0–2% of patients with PE.)
   6. *Nondiagnostic scan (low or intermediate)*
      a. Matched areas of $\dot{V}/\dot{Q}$ abnormality
      b. 67% of patients who undergo $\dot{V}/\dot{Q}$ testing have this pattern
      c. Neither rules in or out PE

M. Angiography
   1. Gold standard
   2. Invasive and rarely used; serious complications occur in 0–3% of patients

N. Diagnostic Approach
   1. In order to select the best strategy, it is critical to assess the patient's pretest probability of PE first.
      a. The Wells score is a validated tool (Table 14–11). As the pretest probability of PE increases, more sensitive strategies must be used to effectively rule out PE.
      b. Figure 14–4 shows one algorithm.
   2. Low-pretest probability of PE
      a. Several studies have documented an excellent negative predictive value (NPV) (99–100%) in patients with a Wells score of ≤ 4 and a negative high-sensitivity D-dimer, effectively ruling out PE.
      b. A separate meta-analysis suggested this strategy for patients with a Wells score of < 2, but recommended a CTA in patients with a higher score.
      c. A negative CTA in low- to moderate-risk patients also effectively rules out PE.
   3. Moderate-high probability of PE (Wells score > 4).
      a. A negative D-dimer is no longer adequate to rule out PE.
      b. CTA
         (1) CTA alone has an excellent PPV (92–96%).
         (2) However, in high-risk patients (Wells score > 6), the negative PPV of CTA alone has varied from 60%, 75%, 89%, to 98%.
            (a) Additional testing is appropriate in high-risk patients with a negative CTA; options include duplex leg ultrasonography, indirect CT of the leg veins (CTV), V/Q scanning, and pulmonary angiography.

**Table 14–11.** Wells score in the diagnosis of PE.

| Criteria | Points |
|---|---|
| Clinical signs and symptoms of DVT (minimum of leg swelling and pain with palpation of the deep veins) | 3 |
| An alternative diagnosis is less likely than PE | 3 |
| Heart rate > 100 bpm | 1.5 |
| Immobilization or surgery in the previous 4 weeks | 1.5 |
| Previous DVT/PE | 1.5 |
| Hemoptysis | 1 |
| Malignancy (on treatment, treated in last 6 months or palliative) | 1 |

DVT/PE, deep venous thrombosis/pulmonary embolism.
Modified, with permission, from Wells PS et al. Derivation of a simple clinical model to categorize patients probability of pulmonary embolism: increasing the models utility with the SimpliRED D-dimer. Thromb Haemost. 2000;83:416–20.

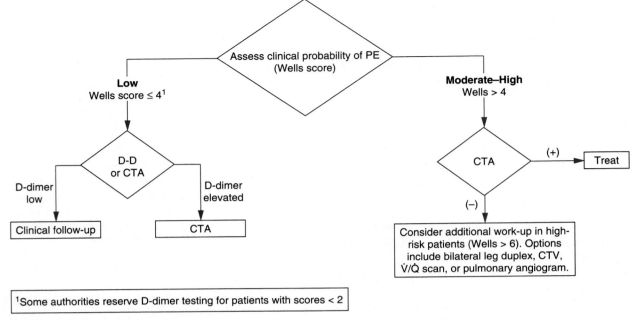

$^{1}$Some authorities reserve D-dimer testing for patients with scores < 2

CTA, CT angiography.

***Figure 14–4.*** Diagnostic algorithm for suspected pulmonary emboli.

**(b)** Since a diagnosis of DVT is taken as a surrogate marker for the diagnosis of PE, duplex leg ultrasonography is the most commonly used test in this situation.

**(c)** Another alternative to rule out DVT is CTV, which can be performed at the same time as CTA. However, some studies suggest that it is less sensitive than leg ultrasound (sensitivity 60–100%, specificity 93–100%).

**(d)** A combined strategy of CTA and duplex leg ultrasonography has an excellent NPV (≈100%) and is advisable for patients with a high likelihood of PE.

**c.** In patients with renal insufficiency and contrast allergy, V̇/Q̇ scanning can be considered in place of CTA.

**d.** Pulmonary angiography is rarely used.

## Diagnosis of DVT

**A.** Given the overlap of PE and DVT (and the same therapy), the diagnosis of DVT is often taken as evidence of concomitant PE.

**B.** Several clinical features modestly increase the likelihood of DVT including malignancy (LR+ 2.7), prior DVT (LR+ 2.3), immobilization (LR+ 2.0), and recent surgery (LR+ 1.8).

**C.** Signs and symptoms are not very helpful at ruling DVT in or out. Leg swelling is only 32% sensitive, LR+ 1.45, LR– 0.67; leg pain LR+ 1.08, LR– 0.9; Homan sign LR+ 1.4, LR– 0.87.

 The clinical exam is insensitive for the diagnosis of DVT. Clinicians must have a low threshold for ordering D-dimer or duplex studies.

**D.** Clinical prediction rule can help predict risk of DVT (Table 14–12).

**E.** D-dimer
   **1.** 88–92% sensitive, 45–72% specific
   **2.** In patients with a low clinical risk, the NPV of a negative D-dimer is 99%.

**F.** Duplex ultrasonography
   **1.** 89–96% sensitive for symptomatic proximal DVT, 94–99% specific; LR+, 24, LR–, 0.05
   **2.** Incidence of symptomatic DVT < 1% in patients with initial negative color duplex exam.
   **3.** Less sensitive for distal (below the knee) DVT 73–93%
   **4.** Patients with increasing symptoms should be reevaluated.

**G.** Other options include venography (invasive) and magnetic resonance direct thrombus imaging (accurate but costly).

**H.** Diagnostic strategy
   **1.** A recent meta-analysis suggested that patients with a low pretest probability of DVT could be evaluated with a high sensitivity D-dimer. A negative result effectively rules out DVT.
   **2.** For patients at moderate- to high-risk for DVT, those with a history of prior VTE, or those with comorbidities, an ultrasound is recommended (Figure 14–5).
   **3.** For patients with suspected calf DVT, a repeat study 1 week later can be useful to rule out proximal extension.

## Treatment of PE and DVT

**A.** Options include low-molecular-weight heparin (LMWH), unfractionated heparin, and fondaparinux.

**Table 14–12.** Clinical model for predicting the pretest probability of deep venous thrombosis.[1]

| Clinical Characteristic | Score |
|---|---|
| Active cancer (patient receiving treatment for cancer within the previous 6 mo or currently receiving palliative treatment) | 1 |
| Paralysis, paresis, or recent plaster immobilization of the lower extremities | 1 |
| Recently bedridden for 3 days or more, or major surgery within the previous 12 wk requiring general or regional anesthesia | 1 |
| Localized tenderness along the distribution of the deep venous system | 1 |
| Entire leg swollen | 1 |
| Calf swelling at least 3 cm larger than that of the asymptomatic side (measured 10 cm below tibial tuberosity) | 1 |
| Pitting edema confined to the symptomatic leg | 1 |
| Collateral superficial veins (nonvaricose) | 1 |
| Previously documented deep venous thrombosis | 1 |
| Alternative diagnosis at least as likely as deep venous thrombosis | −2 |

[1]A score of two or higher indicates that the probability of deep venous thrombosis is likely; a score of less than two indicates that the probability of deep venous thrombosis is unlikely. In patients with symptoms in both legs, the more symptomatic leg is used.
Modified, with permission, from Wells PS et al. Evaluation of D-dimer in the diagnosis of suspected deep-vein thrombosis. N Engl J Med. 2003;349:1227–35.

B. LMWH

1. Superior to unfractionated heparin at reducing mortality and bleeding in the treatment of DVT and at least equivalent in patients with hemodynamically stable PE

2. Easier to dose and more consistently therapeutic than unfractionated IV heparin.

3. Associated with a lower risk of heparin-induced thrombocytopenia than unfractionated heparin.

4. In obese patients and patients with renal insufficiency, the bioavailability of LMWH is difficult to predict. Consultation is recommended for such patients.

C. Oxygen should be administered to patients with hypoxemia.

D. Warfarin is started at the same time as heparin or LMWH.

1. The initial warfarin dose is 5–10 mg/day for the first 2 days and is adjusted based on the INR; 10 mg/day is superior to 5 mg/day in well-nourished outpatients not taking antibiotics.

2. The target INR is 2.0–3.0.

3. Heparin is coadministered for ≥ 5 days and discontinued when the INR has been therapeutic for 2 consecutive days.

4. Patients with venous thromboembolism secondary to the antiphospholipid syndrome may require more intensive anticoagulation. The optimal target INR is uncertain.

5. Patients with venous thromboembolism secondary to active cancer have a high rate of recurrence during warfarin therapy. Long-term LMWH is superior.

6. Long-term anticoagulation: Duration of therapy

a. Warfarin is effective *during* therapy. For many patients, the risk of recurrence increases when warfarin is discontinued.

b. The risk of recurrence varies depending on the precipitating risk factor for the initial venous thromboembolism. From lowest to highest risk:

(1) Postoperative or postpartum patients

(2) Other short-term risk factors (immobilization)

(3) Idiopathic venous thromboembolism (no clinical risk factors or thrombophilia)

(4) Thrombophilic states

(5) Antiphospholipid syndrome

(6) Active cancer

c. Persistent clot seen on duplex exam at the *completion* of anticoagulation therapy increases the risk of subsequent VTE (Table 14–10).

d. D-dimer elevation at the *completion* of therapy also increases the risk of recurrent VTE in patients with a single idiopathic VTE. Furthermore, restarting anticoagulation in these patients reduced the annual risk to 1.3% (Table 14–13).

e. Patients with venous thromboembolism secondary to postoperative or postpartum states should be treated for 3–6 months.

f. A meta-analysis concluded that therapy should be prolonged (> 12 months and perhaps indefinitely) in patients with venous thromboembolism that was not secondary to a short-term identified risk factor (ie, surgery, postpartum state). Extended duration and potentially indefinite anticoagulation should be considered in patients with venous thromboembolism and any of the following:

(1) Recurrent venous thromboembolism

(2) Cancer

(3) Thrombophilia

(4) Idiopathic venous thromboembolism

g. A meta-analysis suggested the RR of recurrence after discontinuation of warfarin was higher in men than women (RR 1.56).

h. Patients with symptomatic isolated calf vein thrombosis should be treated with anticoagulation for at least 6–12 weeks. If for any reason anticoagulation is not administered, serial noninvasive studies of the lower extremity should be performed over the next 10–14 days to assess for proximal extension of thrombus.

E. Inferior vena caval procedures

1. Inferior vena cava filters protect patients from PE but are associated with an increased risk of subsequent DVT.

2. Indications for placement

a. Contraindication or complications of anticoagulant therapy

b. Recurrent venous thromboembolism that occurs despite adequate anticoagulation

c. Chronic recurrent embolism or massive PE with pulmonary hypertension

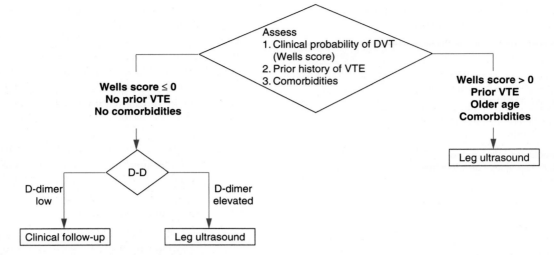

***Figure 14–5.*** Diagnostic algorithm for DVT.

**F.** For massive PE associated with hypotension, thrombolysis and catheter and surgical embolectomy have been used.

**G.** Compression stockings are recommended for patients older than 40 years with proximal DVT; patients should start wearing the stockings within 1 month of diagnosis and continue wearing them for ≥ 1 year to decrease the likelihood of post-thrombotic syndrome (NNT 4).

***Table 14–13.*** Annual recurrence rates of venous thromboembolism after completing warfarin therapy.

| Risk Category | Annual recurrence rate (%) | |
|---|---|---|
| Postpartum or postoperative state | 0 | |
| | Duplex[1] (−) | Duplex (+) |
| Short-term risk factor | 0 | 7.1 |
| Idiopathic VTE | 4.4 | 7.5 |
| Thrombophilic state | 10 | 23 |
| Cancer (on active therapy) | 18–34[2] | |
| D-dimer at completion of warfarin | | |
| Normal (no anticoagulation) | 4.4% | |
| Elevated (no anticoagulation) | 10.9% | |
| Elevated (anticoagulation restarted) | 1.3% | |

[1]Duplex result at the completion of 3 months of anticoagulation therapy.
[2]Recurrence rates were despite ongoing active therapy (18% for patients on LWMH and 34% for patients continuing on warfarin.)

**H.** *Primary* prevention of venous thromboembolism

   **1.** 25% of venous thromboembolic events are associated with hospitalization. At particularly high risk are patients undergoing hip fracture surgery, hip or knee replacement, and those with spinal cord injury.

   **2.** Hospitalized medical patients account for 50–75% of hospital-associated venous thromboembolism.

   **a.** Anticoagulation prophylaxis has been demonstrated to reduce fatal and nonfatal venous thromboembolism.

   **b.** At particularly high risk include patients who are older than 40 years, who are hospitalized for ≥ 3 days with limited mobility, and who have ≥ 1 of the following:

   **(1)** Acute infections disease

   **(2)** Class III or IV HF

   **(3)** Acute myocardial infarction

   **(4)** Cerebrovascular accident

   **(5)** Cancer

   **(6)** Acute respiratory disease

   **(7)** Rheumatic disease

   **(8)** Body mass index > 30

   **(9)** Recent surgery or trauma

   **(10)** Thrombophilia or prior venous thromboembolism.

   **3.** The intensity of the prophylaxis depends on the specific clinical situation. Options include compression stockings, pneumatic compression devices (particularly useful in patients who have active bleeding or are at high risk), and a variety of heparinoids. Guidelines are updated frequently by the American College of Chest Physicians.

**I.** Work-up for thrombophilia: Duration of therapy may be affected by presence of underlying thrombophilia. Clear guidelines for routine testing have not been determined. Consider tests for thrombophilic states in patients without clear precipitant of venous thromboembolism.

## MAKING A DIAGNOSIS

You review the patient's Wells score and assign her 3 points since PE is the most likely diagnosis. She also takes HRT, which is a risk factor for PE. Although there is some debate about the use of D-dimer to rule out PE in a patient with a score of 3, you elect to perform a CTA rather than a D-dimer because PE is the most likely diagnosis.

The CTA reveals multiple small pulmonary emboli.

 **Have you crossed a diagnostic threshold for the leading hypothesis, PE? Have you ruled out the active alternatives? Do other tests need to be done to exclude the alternative diagnoses?**

The CTA is highly specific for PE. At this point, PE is ruled in and further confirmation is unnecessary. There is no need for further testing to exclude alternative diagnoses.

## Alternative Diagnosis: Asthma

See Chapter 28, Wheezing and Stridor.

## Alternative Diagnosis: CAD

See Chapter 8, Chest Pain.

## CASE RESOLUTION

A hypercoagulable work-up is sent to assess future risk of recurrence (prior to heparin and warfarin therapy). Her HRT is stopped. Mrs. L is started on LMWH and warfarin. At follow-up 6 months later, she reports feeling better. Her anticoagulation therapy has been uncomplicated.

## REFERENCES

American College of Cardiology; American Heart Association Task Force on Practice Guidelines (Writing Committee to revise the 1998 guidelines for the management of patients with valvular heart disease); Society of Cardiovascular Anesthesiologists, Bonow RO, Carabello BA, Chatterjee K et al. ACC/AHA 2006 guidelines for the management of patients with valvular heart disease: a report of the American College of Cardiology/American Heart Association Task Force on Practice Guidelines (writing committee to Revise the 1998 guidelines for the management of patients with valvular heart disease) developed in collaboration with the Society of Cardiovascular Anesthesiologists endorsed by the Society for Cardiovascular Angiography and Interventions and the Society of Thoracic Surgeons. J Am Coll Cardiol. 2006;48(3):e1–148.

Battaglia M, Pewsner D, Juni P, Egger M, Bucher HC, Bachmann LM. Accuracy of B-type natriuretic peptide tests to exclude congestive heart failure: systematic review of test accuracy studies. Arch Intern Med. 2006;166(10):1073–80.

Bell WR, Simon TL, DeMets DL. The clinical features of submassive and massive pulmonary emboli. Am J Med. 1977;62(3):355–60.

European Heart Rhythm Association; Heart Rhythm Society, Fuster V, Rydén LE, Cannom DS et al; American College of Cardiology; American Heart Association Task Force on Practice Guidelines; European Society of Cardiology Committee for Practice Guidelines; Writing Committee to Revise the 2001 Guidelines for the Management of Patients With Atrial Fibrillation. ACC/AHA/ESC 2006 guidelines for the management of patients with atrial fibrillation--executive summary: a report of the American College of Cardiology/American Heart Association Task Force on Practice Guidelines and the European Society of Cardiology Committee for Practice Guidelines (Writing Committee to Revise the 2001 Guidelines for the Management of Patients With Atrial Fibrillation). J Am Coll Cardiol. 2006;48(4):854–906.

Goodacre S, Sutton AJ, Sampson FC. Meta-analysis: The value of clinical assessment in the diagnosis of deep venous thrombosis. Ann Intern Med. 2005;143(2):129–39.

Hart RG, Pearce LA, Aguilar MI. Meta-analysis: antithrombotic therapy to prevent stroke in patients who have nonvalvular atrial fibrillation. Ann Intern Med. 2007;146(12):857–67.

Heidenreich PA, Schnittger I, Hancock SL, Atwood JE. A systolic murmur is a common presentation of aortic regurgitation detected by echocardiography. Clin Cardiol. 2004;27(9):502–6.

Hunt SA, Abraham WT, Chin MH et al. ACC/AHA 2005 Guideline Update for the Diagnosis and Management of Chronic Heart Failure in the Adult: a report of the American College of Cardiology/American Heart Association Task Force on Practice Guidelines (Writing Committee to Update the 2001 Guidelines for the Evaluation and Management of Heart Failure): developed in collaboration with the American College of Chest Physicians and the International Society for Heart and Lung Transplantation: endorsed by the Heart Rhythm Society. Circulation. 2005;112(12):e154–235.

Marcus GM, Gerber IL, McKeown BH et al. Association between phonocardiographic third and fourth heart sounds and objective measures of left ventricular function. JAMA. 2005;293(18):2238–44.

Miniati M, Prediletto R, Formichi B et al. Accuracy of clinical assessment in the diagnosis of pulmonary embolism. Am J Respir Crit Care Med. 1999;159(3):864–71.

Oudega R, Moons KG, Hoes AW. Limited value of patient history and physical examination in diagnosing deep vein thrombosis in primary care. Fam Pract. 2005;22(1):86–91.

Page RL. Clinical practice. Newly diagnosed atrial fibrillation. N Engl J Med. 2004;351(23):2408–16.

Qaseem A, Snow V, Barry P et al. Current diagnosis of venous thromboembolism in primary care: a clinical practice guideline from the American Academy of Family Physicians and the American College of Physicians. Ann Fam Med. 2007;5:(1):57–62.

Segal JB, Streiff MB, Hofmann LV, Thornton K, Bass EB. Management of venous thromboembolism: a systematic review for a practice guideline. Ann Intern Med. 2007;146(3):211–22.

Snow V, Qaseem A, Barry P et al. Management of venous thromboembolism: a clinical practice guideline from the American College of Physicians and the American Academy of Family Physicians. Ann Intern Med. 2007;146(3):204–10.

Tillie-Leblond I, Marquette CH, Perez T et al. Pulmonary embolism in patients with unexplained exacerbation of chronic obstructive pulmonary disease: prevalence and risk factors. Ann Intern Med. 2006;144(6):390–6.

Stein PD, Willis PW 3rd, DeMets DL. History and physical examination in acute pulmonary embolism in patients without preexisting cardiac or pulmonary disease. Am J Cardiol. 1981;47(2):218–23.

Tapson VF. Acute pulmonary embolism. N Engl J Med. 2008;358(10):1037–52.

Wang CS, FitzGerald JM, Schulzer M, Mak E, Ayas NT. Does this dyspneic patient in the emergency department have congestive heart failure? JAMA. 2005;294(15):1944–56.

Wells PS, Owen C, Doucette S, Fergusson D, Tran H. Does this patient have deep vein thrombosis? JAMA. 2006;295(2):199–207.

# I have a patient with edema. How do I determine the cause?

## CHIEF COMPLAINT

PATIENT 1

Mrs. V is 62-year-old woman with leg edema for the past 2 weeks.

What is the differential diagnosis of edema? How would you frame the differential?

## CONSTRUCTING A DIFFERENTIAL DIAGNOSIS

Edema is defined as an increase in the interstitial fluid volume and is generally not clinically apparent until the interstitial volume has increased by at least 2.5–3 L. It is useful to review some background pathophysiology before discussing the differential diagnosis:

A. Distribution of total body water

　1. 67% intracellular; 33% extracellular

　2. Extracellular water: 25% intravascular; 75% interstitial

B. Regulation of fluid distribution between the intravascular and interstitial spaces

　1. There is constant exchange of water and solutes at the arteriolar end of the capillaries

　2. Fluid is returned from the interstitial space to the intravascular space at the venous end of the capillaries and via the lymphatics.

　3. Movement of fluid from the intravascular space to the interstitium occurs through several mechanisms

　　a. Capillary hydrostatic (hydraulic) pressure pushes fluid out of the vessels

　　b. Interstitial oncotic pressure pulls fluid into the interstitium

　　c. Capillary permeability allows fluid to escape into the interstitium

　4. Movement of fluid from the interstitium to the intravascular space occurs when opposite pressures predominate

　　a. Intravascular (plasma) oncotic pressure from plasma proteins pulls fluid into the vascular space

　　b. Interstitial hydrostatic pressure pushes fluid out of the interstitium

　5. In skeletal muscle, the capillary hydrostatic pressure and the intravascular oncotic pressure are the most important.

　6. There is normally a small gradient favoring filtration out of the vascular space into the interstitium; the excess fluid is removed via the lymphatic system.

C. Edema formation occurs when there is

　1. An increase in capillary hydrostatic pressure (for example, increased plasma volume due to renal sodium retention)

　2. An increase in capillary permeability (for example, burns, angioedema)

　3. An increase in interstitial oncotic pressure (for example, myxedema)

　4. A decrease in plasma oncotic pressure (for example, hypoalbuminemia)

　5. Lymphatic obstruction

Although it is possible to construct a pathophysiologic framework (Figure 15–1) for the differential diagnosis of edema, it is more useful clinically to combine anatomic, pathophysiologic, and organ/system frameworks:

A. Generalized edema due to a systemic cause and manifested by bilateral leg edema, with or without presacral edema, ascites, pleural effusion, pulmonary edema, periorbital edema

　1. Cardiovascular

　　a. Systolic or diastolic dysfunction, or both

　　b. Constrictive pericarditis

　　c. Pulmonary hypertension

　2. Hepatic (cirrhosis)

　3. Renal

　　a. Advanced renal failure of any cause

　　b. Nephrotic syndrome

　4. Anemia

The most common systemic causes of edema are cardiac, renal, and hepatic diseases as well as anemia.

　5. Nutritional deficiency

　6. Medications

　　a. Antidepressants: Monoamine oxidase inhibitors

　　b. Antihypertensives

　　　(1) Calcium channel blockers, especially dihydropyridines

　　　(2) Direct vasodilators (hydralazine, minoxidil)

　　　(3) β-Blockers

　　c. Hormones

　　　(1) Estrogens/progesterones

　　　(2) Testosterone

　　　(3) Corticosteroids

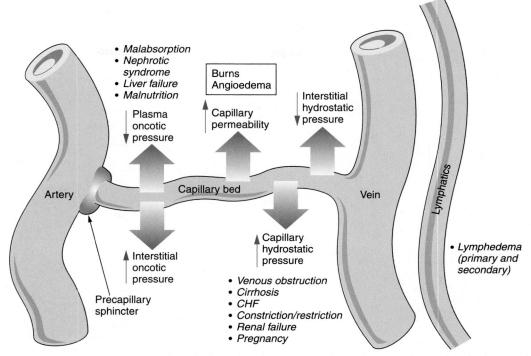

***Figure 15–1.*** Pathophysiology of edema. (Adapted with permission from Cho S et al. Peripheral edema. Am J Med. 2002;V113:581. Copyright © 2002 *Excerpta Medica,* Inc.)

**d.** Nonselective nonsteroidal antiinflammatory drugs (NSAIDs) and cyclooxygenase-2 inhibitors

**e.** Rosiglitazone, pioglitazone

**8.** Refeeding edema

**9.** Myxedema

**B.** Limb edema due to a venous or lymphatic cause, manifested by unilateral or bilateral edema

**1.** Venous disease

**a.** Obstruction

**(1)** Deep venous thrombosis (DVT) (see Chapter 14, Dyspnea for a full discussion of lower extremity DVT)

**(2)** Lymphadenopathy

**(3)** Pelvic mass

**b.** Insufficiency

**2.** Lymphatic obstruction (lymphedema)

**a.** Primary (idiopathic, often bilateral)

**(1)** Congenital

**(2)** Lymphedema praecox (onset in puberty) or tarda (onset after age 20)

**b.** Secondary (more common, generally unilateral)

**(1)** Neoplasm

**(2)** Surgery (especially, following mastectomy)

**(3)** Radiation therapy

**(4)** Miscellaneous (tuberculosis, recurrent lymphangitis, filariasis)

**C.** Localized edema

**1.** Burns

**2.** Angioedema, hives

**3.** Trauma

**4.** Cellulitis, erysipelas

Figure 15–2 outlines the diagnostic approach to edema.

Mrs. V was well until a couple of months ago when she began feeling a bit more tired than usual, despite continuing to sleep well. She has had no shortness of breath or chest pain. She has noted intermittent vague abdominal pain, not related to eating, position, or bowel movements. She has been a bit constipated and feels bloated. Over the last 2 weeks, she has noted swelling in her feet and lower legs and has not been able to wear her regular shoes. As she tells you this, you note that she is wearing house slippers, and that her socks have produced a significant indentation above her ankles.

Her past medical history is notable for hypertension and diabetes, both well controlled. She had a blood transfusion during a cholecystectomy 25 years ago. Her current medications include hydrochlorothiazide, lisinopril, rosiglitazone, simvastatin, and aspirin. She has no history of heart or kidney disease, or tobacco or alcohol use.

 **At this point, what is the leading hypothesis, and what are the active alternatives? What other tests should be ordered?**

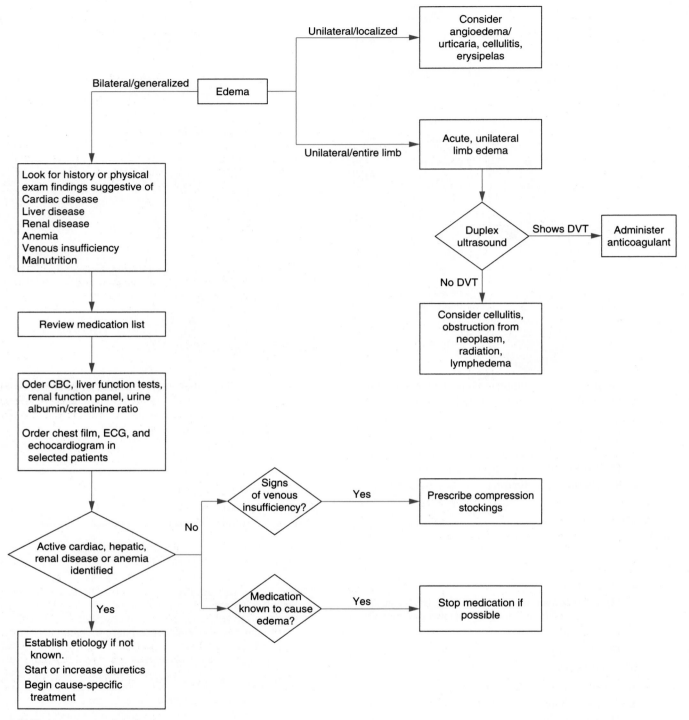

DVT, deep venous thrombosis.

***Figure 15–2.*** Diagnostic approach: edema.

## PRIORITIZING THE DIFFERENTIAL DIAGNOSIS

Even before examining Mrs. V, you can see that she has significant bilateral leg edema, a pivotal point in her presentation. Although there are some local diseases that can present with bilateral leg edema, the first step in such patients is always to look for systemic causes. While the history and physical are often not sensitive or specific enough to make a diagnosis, they are a good starting point for organizing the differential. So the first question to ask is, "Does Mrs. V have any signs or symptoms pointing to a cardiac, hepatic, or renal cause of her edema?" The answers to this question would be additional pivotal points. Mrs. V's history of a blood transfusion puts her at risk for chronic hepatitis and cirrhosis, and her vague abdominal complaints raise the possibility of ascites, more commonly seen with cirrhosis than heart failure (HF) or renal failure. She is certainly at risk for both cardiac and renal disease because of her history of hypertension and diabetes. While most patients with heart failure complain of shortness of breath, some describe only fatigue. Medication should be considered as a cause, since rosiglitazone frequently causes edema; hypothyroidism does not cause pitting edema, and so is not likely. Finally, although it is uncommon for obstruction to cause bilateral edema, you should think about ovarian cancer causing malignant ascites and venous obstruction, either via extrinsic compression or due to associated DVT formation. Table 15–1 lists the differential diagnosis.

**Table 15–1.** Diagnostic hypotheses for Mrs. V

| Diagnostic Hypotheses | Clinical Clues | Important Tests |
|---|---|---|
| **Leading Hypothesis** | | |
| Cirrhosis | Hepatitis risk factors<br>Ascites<br>Spider angiomata<br>Gynecomastia<br>Normal or low JVP<br>Splenomegaly | Ultrasound<br>Bilirubin<br>Liver enzymes<br>Prothrombin time<br>Albumin<br>Liver biopsy |
| **Active Alternatives—Must Not Miss** | | |
| Heart failure | Cardiovascular risk factors<br>Dyspnea<br>Elevated JVP<br>Crackles<br>$S_3$ | ECG<br>Chest radiograph<br>Echocardiogram |
| Renal disease (insufficiency or nephrotic syndrome) | Malaise<br>Nausea<br>Dyspnea<br>Edema | BUN/creatinine<br>Urinalysis<br>Albumin/creatinine ratio |
| **Active Alternatives—Most Common** | | |
| Medication | History | History |
| **Other Hypotheses** | | |
| Ovarian cancer | Abdominal pain or bloating<br>Increased abdominal girth<br>Family history | Transvaginal ultrasound<br>CA-125 |

JVP, jugular venous pressure.

 Always look for systemic causes of edema in patients with bilateral leg edema.

In general, Mrs. V appears fatigued. Her BP is 100/60 mm Hg, pulse is 92 bpm, and RR is 16 breaths per minute. Sclera are anicteric, jugular venous pressure is normal, and lungs are clear. On cardiac exam, she has a normal $S_1$ and $S_2$, a soft $S_4$, and no $S_3$ or murmurs. Her abdomen is slightly distended, but soft and nontender; there is a fluid wave. Her liver is not enlarged, but the spleen is palpable. Rectal exam shows hemorrhoids and guaiac-negative stool. She has 2+ edema bilaterally.

**Is the clinical information sufficient to make a diagnosis? If not, what other information do you need?**

## Leading Hypothesis: Cirrhosis

### Textbook Presentation

Patients with cirrhosis can be asymptomatic or have mild symptoms, such as fatigue. Some patients have the classic manifestations of portal hypertension: ascites, edema, variceal bleeding, encephalopathy, or hypersplenism.

### Disease Highlights

A. Etiology

  1. Most common causes

    a. Alcohol

    b. Chronic hepatitis B or C

    c. Nonalcoholic fatty liver disease (NAFLD)

    d. Hemochromatosis

    e. Primary or secondary biliary cirrhosis

  2. Less common causes

    a. Drugs and toxins (isoniazid, methotrexate, amiodarone)

    b. Autoimmune hepatitis

    c. Genetic metabolic diseases (Wilson, $\alpha_1$-antitrypsin deficiency, glycogen storage diseases, porphyria)

    d. Infections (schistosomiasis, echinococcosis, brucellosis)

    e. Cardiac

The 2 most common causes of cirrhosis in the United States are alcoholic liver disease and chronic hepatitis C.

B. Pathophysiology

  1. Advanced fibrosis, or cirrhosis, causes architectural distortion of the hepatic vasculature, leading to shunting of the blood coming into the liver via the portal vein directly to the hepatic vein outflow system, which causes

    a. Impaired hepatocyte function due to loss of normal sinusoids

b. Increased intrahepatic resistance, or portal hypertension

c. Increased risk of hepatocellular carcinoma due to increased regenerative activity

2. Consequences of cirrhosis and portal hypertension include

a. Formation of portosystemic collaterals (ie, varices)

b. Splanchnic vasodilation

c. Renal vasoconstriction and hypoperfusion of the kidneys, causing salt and water retention

d. Increased cardiac output

e. Decreased production of albumin and clotting factors

f. Increased capillary hydrostatic pressure resulting in ascites; hypoalbuminemia and salt and water retention also contribute to ascites formation

C. Prognosis

1. Risk factors for developing cirrhosis in patients with hepatitis C include age over 50, regular alcohol consumption, and male sex; for those with NAFLD, risk factors include older age, obesity, insulin resistance, hypertension, and hyperlipidemia.

2. Decompensation rates are 4%/year for hepatitis C cirrhosis and 10%/year for hepatitis B; patients with alcoholic cirrhosis who continue to drink decompensate rapidly.

3. 5-year mortality approaches 85% after decompensation if transplantation is not performed.

4. The Childs-Pugh-Turcotte classification of cirrhosis severity predicts prognosis (see Chapter 17, GI Bleeding).

## Evidence-Based Diagnosis

A. Cirrhosis is a pathologic diagnosis definitively made only by examining the entire liver at autopsy or after liver transplantation.

B. The traditional gold standard is percutaneous liver biopsy, although due to sampling error, the sensitivity has been reported to be as low as 70–80%.

C. The clinical presentation is variable, making clinical diagnosis difficult.

1. Patients may have physical findings suggestive of chronic liver disease (see below), constitutional symptoms, asymptomatic liver enzyme or radiologic abnormalities, manifestations of portal hypertension (see below), or no symptoms at all. Cirrhosis is sometimes diagnosed at autopsy in patients in whom the disease never manifested.

2. Physical findings associated with chronic liver disease include

a. Spider angiomata

b. Palmar erythema

c. Dupuytren contracture (alcoholic cirrhosis only)

d. Gynecomastia

e. Testicular atrophy

f. Jaundice

g. Ascites

h. Peripheral edema

i. Hepatomegaly

j. Splenomegaly

k. Caput medusae

l. None of these are sensitive or specific enough to diagnose cirrhosis, although multiple findings in combination do increase the pretest probability of cirrhosis.

3. Patients who show manifestations of portal hypertension (see below) are assumed to have cirrhosis.

D. Several noninvasive models and techniques have been developed to predict cirrhosis *in patients with chronic hepatitis C,* although they are not currently used in place of biopsy.

1. Ultrasound-based elastography, which measures mean hepatic stiffness (sensitivity 87%, specificity 91% for cirrhosis; sensitivity 70% and specificity 84% for advanced fibrosis)

2. AST (SGOT) to platelet ratio index (APRI)

a. $$\frac{(\text{AST level/Upper limit of normal AST}) \times 100}{\text{platelet count}}$$

b. For APRI > 0.5, the sensitivity is 81% and specificity 50% for significant fibrosis

c. For APRI > 1, the sensitivity is 76% and specificity 71% for cirrhosis

3. Fibrotest is a commercial product that combines the results of several assays into a predictive score.

a. It has a sensitivity of 75% and specificity of 85% for significant fibrosis.

b. It is 95% accurate in identifying patients with minimal or no fibrosis.

E. Test characteristics of ultrasound to diagnose cirrhosis are variable (LR+, 2.5–11.6; LR−, 0.13–0.73).

F. MRI has sensitivity and specificity as high as 93% and 82%, respectively.

## Treatment

The treatment of cirrhosis depends on the underlying cause. Treatments for selected causes of cirrhosis are discussed in Chapter 22, Jaundice and Abnormal Liver Enzymes.

# Manifestations of Portal Hypertension

Once it has been determined that the patient probably or definitively has cirrhosis, it is important to determine the specific cause of the cirrhosis (see Chapter 22, Jaundice and Abnormal Liver Enzymes) and to determine whether the patient has manifestations of portal hypertension: variceal bleeding, ascites and its complications, hepatic encephalopathy, and hypersplenism.

## 1. Variceal Bleeding

See Chapter 17, GI Bleeding.

## 2. Ascites

### Textbook Presentation

The patient complains of an inability to fasten her pants due to increasing abdominal girth, sometimes accompanied by dyspnea and edema.

### Disease Highlights

A. Epidemiology

1. Ascites develops over 5 years in 30% of patients with compensated cirrhosis, defined as the absence of manifestations of portal hypertension.

**2.** 1-year survival rates drop significantly once ascites develops.

**B.** Complications of ascites

   **1.** Respiratory compromise due to compression of lung volumes

   **2.** Hepatorenal syndrome (HRS)

   **a.** Diagnostic criteria

   **(1)** Cirrhosis with ascites

   **(2)** Serum creatinine > 1.5 mg/dL

   **(3)** Serum creatinine stays above 1.5 mg/dL after at least 2 days of diuretic withdrawal and volume expansion with albumin

   **(4)** Absence of shock

   **(5)** No current or recent treatment with nephrotoxic drugs

   **(6)** Absence of parenchymal kidney disease (< 500 mg/day of proteinuria, < 50 RBC/hpf, abnormalities on renal ultrasound)

   **b.** Clinical syndromes

   **(1)** Acute renal failure (type 1 HRS): serum creatinine doubles or increases to > 2.5 mg/dL in less than 2 weeks

   **(2)** Refractory ascites (type 2 HRS): serum creatinine 1.25–2.5 mg/dL with a steady or slowly progressive course

   **c.** Incidence in patients with cirrhosis and ascites is 18% at 1 year and 39% at 5 years

   **d.** The prognosis is poor (Figure 15–3)

   **e.** Precipitants of type 1 HRS include bacterial infections (especially spontaneous bacterial peritonitis), GI bleeding, alcoholic hepatitis, overdiuresis, and large volume paracentesis.

**f.** HRS is due to peripheral vasodilation which causes decreased systemic vascular resistance, resulting in renal arteriolar vasoconstriction, decreased renal blood flow, and a reduced glomerular filtration rate (GFR).

**g.** Treatment of HRS

   **(1)** Liver transplantation is the definitive treatment for both types of HRS.

   **(2)** There are limited data regarding the use of transvenous intrahepatic portosystemic shunts (TIPS) and vasopressin derivatives to treat type 1 HRS.

   **(3)** The treatment of refractory ascites will be discussed below.

**3.** Spontaneous bacterial peritonitis (SBP)

   **a.** Prevalence of 10–30% in hospitalized cirrhotic patients, with 1-year recurrence rate of 70% and mortality rate of about 20%; 96% of patients with SBP have a Childs-Pugh-Turcotte grade of B or C

   **b.** Overgrowth of intestinal bacterial and increased intestinal permeability lead to movement of bacteria into mesenteric lymph nodes; the bacteria can then enter the systemic circulation and colonize the ascitic fluid.

   **c.** The 3 most common isolates are *Escherichia coli, Klebsiella pneumoniae,* and pneumococci.

   **d.** Symptoms include fever (50–75% of patients), abdominal pain (27–72%), chills (16–29%), nausea/vomiting (8–21%), mental status changes (up to 50%), and decreased renal function (33%); about 13% of patients are asymptomatic.

   **e.** Risk factors for SBP include ascitic fluid total protein level ≤ 1 g/dL, upper GI bleeding, prior episode of SBP

   **f.** Diagnosis of SBP

   **(1)** Criteria for performing a diagnostic paracentesis in patients with cirrhosis and ascites:

   **(a)** Admission to the hospital

   **(b)** Change in clinical status (fever, abdominal pain, mental status changes, ileus, septic shock)

   **(c)** Development of leukocytosis, acidosis, or renal failure

   **(d)** Active GI bleeding

   **(2)** Always inoculate blood culture tubes at the bedside to maximize yield of ascitic fluid cultures.

   **(3)** Interpretation of ascitic fluid cell counts and cultures (Table 15–2)

 Consider secondary peritonitis if more than 1 organism is cultured from the ascitic fluid.

   **(4)** Other ascitic fluid findings that increase the likelihood of SBP included WBC count > 1000 cells/mcL (LR+ = 9.1), pH < 7.35 (LR+ = 9.0), and blood-ascitic fluid pH gradient ≥ 0.1 (LR+ = 11)

   **g.** Treatment of SBP

   **(1)** Empiric treatment should be started prior to return of culture results

   **(2)** IV cefotaxime is the best-studied antibiotic for SBP; amoxicillin-clavulanic acid has also been studied.

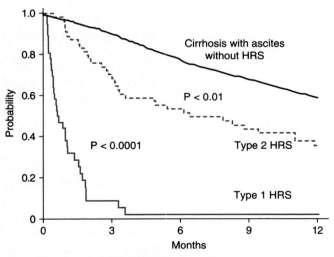

Salerno: Gut, Volume 56(9). September 2007.1310–1318

***Figure 15–3.*** Survival in hepatorenal syndrome. (Reproduced, with permission, from Salerno F et al. Diagnosis, prevention and treatment of hepatorenal syndrome in cirrhosis. Gut. 2007 Sep; 56(9):1310–18.)

**Table 15–2.** Interpretation of ascitic fluid results.

| Condition | Polymorphonuclear Count (cells/mcL) | Culture Results |
|---|---|---|
| Spontaneous bacterial peritonitis | ≥ 250 | Single organism |
| Culture-negative neutrophilic ascites | ≥ 250 | Negative |
| Monomicrobial nonneutrocytic bacterascites | < 250 | Single organism |
| Secondary bacterial peritonitis | ≥ 250 | Polymicrobial |
| Polymicrobial bacterascites | < 250 | Polymicrobial |

(3) Intravenous albumin has been shown to reduce mortality and development of renal impairment.

(4) All patients who recover from SBP should receive secondary prophylaxis with oral norfloxacin.

(5) Since 2-year survival after SBP is only about 30%, liver transplantation should be considered in patients who recover from SBP.

## Evidence-Based Diagnosis

A. Physical exam: See Chapter 22, Jaundice and Abnormal Liver Enzymes

B. Peritoneal fluid analysis

1. Serum-ascites albumin gradient

   a. In portal hypertension, ascites occurs due to transudation, without changes in permeability that would allow albumin to leak into the ascitic fluid.

   b. Therefore, the albumin content of ascitic fluid is low relative to serum.

   c. This is in contrast to exudative types of ascites, such as ascites from infection or malignancy, in which albumin can leak into the ascitic fluid.

   d. A serum-ascites albumin gradient (serum albumin-ascitic fluid albumin) of ≥ 1.1 mg/dL has a LR+ of 4.6 for the diagnosis of ascites due to portal hypertension; a serum ascites-albumin gradient of < 1.1 mg/dL has a LR– of 0.06 for the diagnosis of portal hypertension.

2. Ascitic fluid total protein

   a. Also based on the principle that ascites due to cirrhosis is transudative and should have a low protein content relative to serum

   b. Using a cut point of 2.5 mg/dL of ascitic fluid total protein to distinguish an exudate from a transudate had an accuracy of only 56%.

 Serum-ascites albumin gradient is the best test for distinguishing between ascites due to portal hypertension and ascites due to other causes.

## Treatment

A. Sodium restriction (sodium intake < 2 g/d) is commonly recommended, but there are no clinical trials showing that it leads to improved outcomes; fluid restriction of 1000–1500 mL/day is recommended if the serum sodium is < 130 mEq/L.

B. Spironolactone is the diuretic of choice to treat the aldosterone driven salt and water retention seen in cirrhosis.

1. 75% of patients respond

2. Furosemide or other loop diuretics can be added in patients who do not respond to spironolactone alone; 90% of patients respond to sodium restricted diets, spironolactone, and loop diuretics.

3. In order to avoid hypovolemia and renal impairment, the rate of weight loss should not exceed 0.5 kg/d in the absence of peripheral edema or 1 kg/d in the presences of edema.

 Aspirin and NSAIDs blunt the natriuretic effect of diuretics and should be avoided in patients with ascites.

C. Large volume paracentesis with volume expansion (dextran or albumin) for patients unresponsive to diuretics

D. TIPS

1. Creates a shunt between the high-pressure portal vein and the low-pressure hepatic vein, leading to improved hemodynamics and a decrease in ascites

2. Complications include bleeding, shunt stenosis or thrombosis, right-sided heart failure, and encephalopathy in 30% of patients.

E. Liver transplantation

F. When should ascites be treated with measures beyond sodium restriction?

1. Not in grade 1 ascites (detectable only by ultrasound)

2. Grade 2 (moderate) and grade 3 (severe) ascites are generally treated due to patient discomfort and respiratory compromise.

   a. Grade 2 should be treated with diuretics.

   b. Grade 3 should be treated with paracentesis, followed by diuretics.

3. Refractory ascites (ascites not responsive to maximal tolerated medical therapy) should be treated with repeated paracentesis or TIPS, or both.

## 3. Encephalopathy

### Textbook Presentation

The classic presentation of hepatic encephalopathy is a patient with known cirrhosis who has mental status changes or is in a coma.

### Disease Highlights

A. Present in 50–70% of patients with chronic liver disease

B. The clinical manifestations range from subtle abnormalities detectable only on neuropsychological testing to coma (Table 15–3).

C. Can be precipitated by a wide variety of insults including

1. Increased ammonia production due to

   a. Excess dietary protein

**Table 15–3.** Grading system for hepatic encephalopathy.

| Grade | Level of Consciousness | Clinical Symptoms | Neurologic Signs | EEG Abnormalities |
|---|---|---|---|---|
| 0 | Normal | None | None | None |
| Subclinical | Normal | Normal | Abnormal neuropsychological testing | None |
| 1 | Sleep-wake reversal, restlessness | Forgetfulness, agitation, irritability, mild confusion | Tremor, apraxia, incoordination | Present |
| 2 | Lethargy, slow responses | Disorientation, amnesia, inappropriate behavior | Asterixis, dysarthria, ataxia, hypoactive reflexes | Present |
| 3 | Somnolence, confusion | Disorientation, aggressive behavior | Asterixis, hyperactive reflexes, positive Babinski sign, muscle rigidity | Present |
| 4 | Coma | Unresponsive | Decerebration | Present |

b. Constipation

c. GI bleeding

d. Infection

e. Azotemia

f. Hypokalemia

g. Systemic alkalosis

2. Reduced metabolism of toxins because of hepatic hypoxia due to

a. Dehydration

b. Arterial hypotension

c. Anemia

3. Increased central nervous depressant effect with use of benzodiazepines or other psychoactive drugs

4. Reduced metabolism of toxins because diversion of portal blood, due to surgical or intrahepatic shunts

 Always look for the underlying cause of worsening hepatic encephalopathy.

## Evidence-Based Diagnosis

A. There is some correlation between the degree of elevation of ammonia (either arterial or venous) and the severity of the encephalopathy, but the ammonia level cannot be used to determine the presence or absence of hepatic encephalopathy.

B. Diagnosis is based on history and exclusion of other causes of encephalopathy in a patient with significant liver dysfunction.

## Treatment

A. Treatment focuses on reduction of intestinal production of ammonia.

B. Lactulose removes both dietary and endogenous sources of ammonia through its cathartic action; it also lowers pH, which reduces the population of urease-producing bacteria, and traps ammonia as ammonium ions in the gut lumen.

1. Frequently used in clinical practice, although most studies showing an improvement in encephalopathy are of poor quality

2. Daily dose should be titrated to result in 2–4 soft stools/day.

3. Complications include hypovolemia and hypernatremia.

C. Antibiotics reduce the population of urease-producing bacteria.

1. Rifaximin may be superior to lactulose.

2. Neomycin is equivalent to lactulose but has the potential to cause ototoxicity and nephrotoxicity with long-term use.

D. Consideration of liver transplantation is indicated in patients with hepatic encephalopathy.

## 4. Hypersplenism

### Textbook Presentation

Cytopenias are found on routine blood testing in a patient with cirrhosis.

### Disease Highlights

A. Splenomegaly is found in 36–92% of patients with cirrhosis; 11–55% have the clinical syndrome of hypersplenism, defined as the presence of leukopenia or thrombocytopenia (or both) with splenomegaly.

B. There is a rough correlation between spleen size and degree of decrease in blood cells.

C. Blood cell abnormalities in liver disease

1. Thrombocytopenia is due to platelet sequestration in the spleen, impaired bone marrow production, and decreased platelet survival.

2. Leukopenia is due to sequestration in the spleen and is rare compared with thrombocytopenia (1 series found 64% of cirrhotic patients had thrombocytopenia, but only 5% had leukopenia).

3. Although not part of the syndrome of hypersplenism, anemia often occurs in patients with cirrhosis and is due to increased destruction in the spleen as well as iron or folate deficiency; there is also reduced erythropoietin production.

### Evidence-Based Diagnosis

A. Hypersplenism is a clinical syndrome without a specific set of diagnostic criteria.

B. Hypersplenism is manifested by splenomegaly and a significant reduction in 1 or more cellular elements of the blood, in the presence of normal or hypercellular bone marrow.

## Treatment

**A.** Treatment is usually not necessary.

**B.** Splenectomy or partial splenic embolization is sometimes done for severe thrombocytopenia with bleeding complications.

**C.** Granulocyte-macrophage colony-stimulating factor (GM-CSF) and erythropoietin are rarely used.

**D.** TIPS does not correct thrombocytopenia.

## MAKING A DIAGNOSIS

Initial laboratory test results follow: WBC, 9700/mcL; Hgb, 10.5 g/dL; Hct, 31%; MCV, 86 mcm³; platelet, 123,000 mcL; electrolytes normal; BUN, 8 mg/dL; creatinine, 0.4 mg/dL; glucose, 97 mg/dL; albumin, 2.1 g/dL; alkaline phosphatase, 95 units/L; total bilirubin, 1.2 mg/dL; ALT, 102 units/L; AST, 66 units/L; PT/PTT normal; urinalysis, 2+ protein with no cells or casts.

Have you crossed a diagnostic threshold for the leading hypothesis, cirrhosis and portal hypertension? Have you ruled out the active alternatives? Do other tests need to be done to exclude the alternative diagnoses?

Mrs. V's physical exam suggests that she has splenomegaly, ascites, and edema, without pulmonary findings or an elevated jugular venous pressure, making HF unlikely. Her laboratory results are notable for elevation of transaminases and hypoalbuminemia—all consistent with chronic liver disease. However, the findings of proteinuria and hypoalbuminemia are also consistent with nephrotic syndrome.

## Alternative Diagnosis: Nephrotic Syndrome

### Textbook Presentation

Patients with nephrotic syndrome classically have edema (often periorbital), hypertension, hypoalbuminemia, hyperlipidemia, and at least 3.5 g/24 hour of proteinuria.

### Disease Highlights

**A.** Etiology

  **1.** Primary glomerular diseases

    **a.** Etiology uncertain but probably immune mediated

    **b.** Most common pathologies found in adults are membranous and focal glomerulosclerosis (33% each)

    **c.** Less common pathologies found in adults are minimal change disease (15%), IgA nephropathy (10%), and membranoproliferative glomerulonephritis (2–5%)

  **2.** There are many systemic diseases associated with nephrotic syndrome

    **a.** Diabetes is the most common cause in the United States.

    **b.** Systemic lupus erythematosus (SLE) generally causes an inflammatory nephritis, but sometimes a noninflammatory, membranous pathology.

    **c.** Amyloidosis and multiple myeloma should be considered in patients over 40.

    **d.** Infections commonly associated with nephrotic syndrome include HIV, hepatitis B, hepatitis C, syphilis, and malaria.

    **e.** Malignancies, especially lung, breast, and colon cancer, and Hodgkin lymphoma are associated with nephrotic syndrome; occasionally nephrotic syndrome is the presentation of the malignancy

    **f.** Many drugs, including NSAIDs, captopril, and heroin, can cause nephrotic syndrome.

**B.** Clinical consequences

  **1.** Primary sodium retention by the kidney causes edema and hypertension.

  **2.** Albumin excretion leads to hypoalbuminemia, which also contributes to edema formation.

  **3.** Alterations in lipoprotein production and catabolism lead to elevations of low-density lipoprotein and sometimes triglycerides.

  **4.** Immunoglobulin excretion causes increased susceptibility to infection.

  **5.** Thromboembolic complications

    **a.** Due to increased procoagulatory factors and fibrinogen, altered fibrinolytic system, urinary loss of antithrombin III, and increased platelet activity

    **b.** The annual incidence of venous thromboses (eg, renal vein thrombosis, pulmonary embolism, DVT) is 1.02%, with an annual incidence of 1.48% for arterial thromboembolism (ATE); in the first 6 months after diagnosis, the incidence for venous thromboembolism (VTE) is 9.85% and for ATE 5.52%.

      **(1)** Risk factors for VTE include serum albumin < 2.0–2.5 mg/dL, protein excretion > 8 g/24 h; GFR and traditional risk factors predict ATE

      **(2)** The role of prophylactic anticoagulation is unclear, but it should be considered in high-risk patients.

### Evidence-Based Diagnosis

**A.** Nephrotic syndrome is defined by the presence of urinary protein excretion of at least 3.5 g/24 hours, measured with either a 24-hour specimen or a spot albumin/creatinine ratio > 3000–3500 mcg/mg.

**B.** Laboratory evaluation should include

  **1.** CBC

  **2.** Comprehensive metabolic panel (renal and liver function, including serum albumin)

  **3.** Fasting glucose and $HbA_{1c}$

  **4.** Antinuclear antibody (ANA)

  **5.** HIV

  **6.** Hepatitis B serology (surface antigen, core antibody)

  **7.** Hepatitis C antibody

  **8.** Serum and urine protein electrophoresis

**C.** Renal biopsy is often necessary.

### Treatment

**A.** Loop diuretics are used to treat the edema; high doses are often needed due to the primary sodium retention by the kidney.

B. ACE inhibitors reduce proteinuria in both hypertensive and normotensive patients.

   1. The antiproteinuric effect becomes maximal in 28 days.

   2. The effect can be increased by a low-salt diet, diuretic treatment, or both.

   3. Proteinuria is further reduced when an angiotensin receptor blocker is added to the ACE inhibitor.

C. Corticosteroids and other immunosuppressives are used in selected patients.

## CASE RESOLUTION

Mrs. V's hepatitis C antibody is positive, with negative hepatitis B serologies. Her total cholesterol is 145 mg/dL, and her 24-hour urinary protein excretion is 1.4 g. An abdominal CT scan demonstrates a small, nodular liver; splenomegaly; and ascites. You schedule an esophagogastroduodenoscopy to screen for varices, start spironolactone because of the discomfort she is having from the edema, and refer her to a hepatologist.

## CHIEF COMPLAINT

PATIENT

Mrs. E is a 62-year-old woman with a long history of hypertension that is well controlled with hydrochlorothiazide, atenolol, and amlodipine. She comes in today with a new complaint of swelling in her legs and feet for several weeks. It is generally most noticeable late in the day and is often absent when she first gets up in the morning. She has no history of liver or kidney disease or alcohol use. She has no chest pain and no shortness of breath, although notes she finds it tiring to climb stairs or walk more than a few blocks. She smoked a few cigarettes a day for 20 years, but quit 20 years ago.

Her physical exam is notable for a BMI of 38, clear lungs, an $S_4$ with no $S_3$ or murmurs, and a normal abdomen. Her legs show 1+ edema to the knees bilaterally. She has a long-standing goiter that is unchanged from previous exams. It is difficult to identify her jugular venous pressure due to the shape of her neck.

At this point, what is the leading hypothesis, what are the active alternatives, and is there a must not miss diagnosis? Given this differential diagnosis, what tests should be ordered?

## PRIORITIZING THE DIFFERENTIAL

Once again, given the pivotal finding of bilateral edema, the first step is to look for systemic causes, focusing first on cardiac, hepatic, and renal causes. Mrs. E's long-standing history of hypertension raises the possibility of diastolic dysfunction, and the lack of physical exam findings does not rule this out. There are no clinical clues to suggest liver or kidney disease, but these are easy to test for and should always be ruled out. Amlodipine commonly causes edema, but she has taken it for years without symptoms. "Dependent edema," edema that is worsened by standing and improves or resolves with leg elevation, is consistent with, but not specific for, venous insufficiency. A final consideration would be pulmonary hypertension. Patients with pulmonary hypertension

commonly complain of dyspnea in addition to edema, and the tired feeling she experiences with exertion could represent dyspnea. Additionally, she is overweight, putting her at risk for obstructive sleep apnea and consequent pulmonary hypertension. Table 15–4 lists the differential diagnosis.

Initial laboratory test results include BUN, 15 mg/dL; creatinine, 0.9 mg/dL; albumin/creatinine, ratio 5 mcg/mg; normal liver enzymes, albumin, and prothrombin time.

The ECG and chest radiograph are normal. An echocardiogram shows normal left ventricle size and function, elevated pulmonary pressures consistent with moderate pulmonary hypertension (estimated mean PAP 40 mm Hg), mild tricuspid regurgitation, and normal right ventricular size and function.

Is the clinical information sufficient to make a diagnosis? If not, what other information do you need?

There is no evidence of renal disease, liver disease, or diastolic dysfunction. However, the echocardiogram shows the somewhat unexpected finding of pulmonary hypertension. This necessitates revising the original set of diagnostic hypotheses: the leading hypothesis is now pulmonary hypertension, and venous insufficiency is the remaining active alternative.

## Leading Hypothesis: Pulmonary Hypertension

### Textbook Presentation

Patients commonly complain of long-standing dyspnea that progresses over months or years. Syncope, exertional chest pain, and edema occur with more severe pulmonary hypertension and impaired right heart function.

### Disease Highlights

A. Definition

   1. The normal mean pulmonary artery pressure (PAP) is 12 mm Hg.

***Table 15–4.*** Diagnostic hypotheses for Mrs. E.

| Diagnostic Hypotheses | Clinical Clues | Important Tests |
|---|---|---|
| **Leading Hypothesis** | | |
| Diastolic dysfunction | History of hypertension Dyspnea Edema Elevated JVP S₃ | Echocardiogram |
| **Active Alternatives—Most Common** | | |
| Venous insufficiency | Dependent edema Varicose veins Typical skin changes (see description below) | Physical exam Duplex ultrasound |
| **Active Alternatives—Must Not Miss** | | |
| Renal and liver disease | See Table 15–1 | See Table 15–1 |
| **Other Hypotheses** | | |
| Pulmonary hypertension | Dyspnea, often long-standing Edema Syncope | Echocardiogram Right heart catheterization |

JVP, jugular venous pressure.

2. Pulmonary hypertension is defined as a mean PAP > 25 mm Hg, with a mean pulmonary arterial occlusion pressure < 15 mm Hg; severe pulmonary hypertension is defined as a mean PAP of at least 50 mm Hg.

B. Pathophysiology: the increased pulmonary vascular resistance is due to 3 factors:

1. Vascular remodeling with vascular inflammation and endothelial cell proliferation

2. Platelet dysfunction and thrombosis

3. Vasoconstriction due to 2 factors

    a. Endothelial dysfunction resulting in overproduction of vasoconstrictors such endothelin-1 and underproduction of vasodilators such as nitric oxide, prostacyclin, and vasoactive intestinal peptide

    b. Abnormal voltage-gated potassium channels

C. The clinical classification was revised in 2003 and is organized using a pathophysiologic framework

1. Pulmonary arterial hypertension (PAH)

    a. Idiopathic PAH

    b. Familial PAH

    c. PAH associated with

        (1) Collagen vascular disease (especially scleroderma, SLE, and mixed connective tissue disease)

        (2) Congenital systemic-pulmonary shunts

        (3) Portal hypertension (1–6% of patients)

        (4) HIV infection (0.5% of patients)

        (5) Drugs or toxins (dexfenfluramine or fenfluramine containing appetite suppressants, amphetamine, methamphetamine, cocaine)

    d. PAH associated with significant venous or capillary involvement (pulmonary veno-occlusive disease or capillary hemangiomatosis)

2. Pulmonary hypertension with left heart disease (ventricular, atrial, valvular)

3. Pulmonary hypertension associated with lung disease or hypoxemia

    a. Chronic obstructive pulmonary disease

    b. Interstitial lung disease

    c. Sleep disordered breathing

    d. Alveolar hypoventilation

    e. Chronic exposure to high altitude

4. Pulmonary hypertension due to chronic thromboembolic disease (proximal or distal pulmonary arteries)

5. Miscellaneous (sarcoidosis; compression of pulmonary vessels due to adenopathy, tumor, fibrosing mediastinitis)

**Evidence-Based Diagnosis**

A. History

1. In 1 series of patients with PAH, initial symptoms included dyspnea (60%), fatigue (19%), chest pain (7%), syncope (8%), edema (3%).

2. At the time these patients were given the diagnosis of PAH and were enrolled in the study, 98% had dyspnea, 73% fatigue, 47% chest pain, 36% syncope, 37% edema, and 33% palpitations.

B. Physical exam

1. Characteristic findings include

    a. An accentuated pulmonary component of $S_2$

    b. Sustained left lower parasternal movement

    c. An early systolic click

    d. Increased jugular a and v waves

    e. Tricuspid regurgitation murmur

    f. Hepatojugular reflux

    g. Pulsatile liver

    h. Elevated jugular venous pressure

    i. Edema

2. Sustained left lower parasternal movement for detecting a mean PAP > 50 mm Hg: sensitivity, 71%; specificity, 80%; LR+, 3.6; LR–, 0.4

3. A palpable $P_2$ for detecting a mean PAP > 50 mm Hg (studied in patients with mitral stenosis): sensitivity, 96%; specificity, 73%; LR+, 3.6; LR–, 0.05

C. ECG

1. Expected findings include right axis deviation, right ventricular hypertrophy, and P-pulmonale pattern (right atrial enlargement).

2. Not sensitive or specific enough to diagnosis pulmonary hypertension (sensitivity, 51%; specificity, 86%; LR+, 3.6; LR–, 0.56)

D. Chest film

1. Expected findings include enlargement of pulmonary arteries and right ventricular enlargement.

**2.** Not sensitive or specific enough to diagnose pulmonary hypertension (sensitivity, 46%; specificity, 63%)

**E.** Transthoracic echocardiogram

    **1.** Most common noninvasive way to estimate pulmonary pressure

    **2.** Echocardiogram estimates often correlate fairly well with invasively determined PAPs, but differences as large as 38 mm Hg have been reported in individual patients.

    **3.** Sensitivity ranges from 79% to 100%.

    **4.** Specificity ranges from 60% to 98%.

**F.** Right heart catheterization is the gold standard for diagnosing pulmonary hypertension, and all patients with suspected pulmonary hypertension need a right heart catheterization to confirm the finding.

### Treatment

**A.** Depends on underlying etiology

**B.** Correct underlying cause when possible

    **1.** For obstructive sleep apnea, administer continuous positive airway pressure.

    **2.** For chronic thromboembolism, begin anticoagulation and consider thromboendarterectomy.

    **3.** For valvular disease, replace the valve.

    **4.** For congenital heart disease, repair surgically.

    **5.** For left ventricular dysfunction, optimize medical regimen.

**C.** Oxygen therapy for patients with hypoxemia ($PO_2$ < 55 mm Hg at rest, oxygen saturation < 85% with exercise)

**D.** Most patients require loop diuretics.

**E.** Most medication trials showing improvement in hemodynamics and/or exercise capacity have included patients with idiopathic, fenfluramine-associated, and connective tissue disease–associated pulmonary hypertension

    **1.** Currently available drugs include oral endothelin antagonists such as bosentan, oral phosphodiesterase-5 inhibitors such as sildenafil, and prostacyclins such as epoprostenol (parenteral) or iloprost (inhaled).

    **2.** Calcium blockers are effective in a few patients.

## MAKING A DIAGNOSIS

Mrs. E has a normal physical exam, ECG, and chest radiograph, normal right ventricular function on echocardiogram, and the isolated finding of moderately elevated PAP seen on an echocardiogram. The echocardiogram estimate of PAP alone is not specific enough to make the diagnosis of pulmonary hypertension, and Mrs. E has no other findings supporting the diagnosis of pulmonary hypertension. Furthermore, Mrs. E's dyspnea is minimal, suggesting that she has neither significant pulmonary hypertension nor pulmonary disease.

You explain the puzzling finding to Mrs. E. She does not want to undergo a right heart catheterization to verify the PAP. She reports that she is able to walk a mile every morning without shortness of breath, and that her edema is most noticeable when she has been on her feet for a long time.

Have you crossed a diagnostic threshold for the leading hypothesis, pulmonary hypertension? Have you ruled out the active alternatives? Do other tests need to be done to exclude the alternative diagnoses?

## Alternative Diagnosis: Venous Insufficiency

### Textbook Presentation

Venous insufficiency can be asymptomatic or manifested just by small visible, but nonpalpable veins. In more severe cases, the patient has large varicose veins and skin changes ranging from edema to fibrosing panniculitis to ulceration. Symptoms include leg fullness or heaviness, aching leg pain, and nocturnal leg cramps.

### Disease Highlights

**A.** Anatomy (Figure 15-4)

    **1.** The superficial saphenous veins join the deep system at the knee (popliteal vein) and the groin (femoral vein).

    **2.** Perforating veins directly connect the saphenous veins and the deep veins at various points along their parallel courses.

    **3.** Valves within the veins prevent reflux back toward the feet.

**B.** Pathophysiology and epidemiology

    **1.** Chronic venous disease is due to venous hypertension caused by reflux through incompetent valves, venous outflow obstruction, or lack of calf muscle pumping due to obesity or immobility.

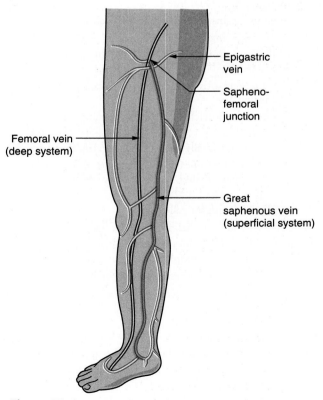

***Figure 15–4.*** Anatomy of the superficial venous system.

**a.** Reflux occurs in the superficial system in about 45% of patients, both the superficial and deep systems in about 40%, and in the deep system only in the remainder of patients

**b.** Prolonged standing leads to marked increases in venous pressure in all people; while those with competent valves quickly lower the venous pressure with walking, individuals with incompetent valves have only slight decreases in pressure with walking.

**2.** Varicose veins are found in 25–33% of women and 10–20% of men.

**3.** Prevalence of skin changes is 3–11%; prevalence of skin ulcers is 0.3–1%.

**4.** Risk factors for venous insufficiency include advancing age, obesity, a history of phlebitis or venous thrombosis, serious leg trauma, pregnancy, prolonged standing, and greater height.

**5.** Postthrombotic syndrome (venous insufficiency after a DVT) occurs in 35–69% of patients at 3 years and in 49–100% of patients at 5–10 years; incidence is reduced to 8% if patients are treated with adequate anticoagulation, early mobilization, and long-term use of compression stockings.

**C.** Classification

**1.** Class 1: telangiectasias or reticular veins (nonpalpable subdermal veins up to 4 mm in diameter)

**2.** Class 2: varicose veins (palpable, subcutaneous veins > 4 mm in diameter)

**3.** Class 3: edema without skin changes

**a.** Initially present just at the end of day but can become persistent and massive

**b.** Can be unilateral initially

**c.** Often begins around medial malleolus

**4.** Class 4: skin changes

**a.** Pigmentation due to breakdown of extravasated RBCs

**b.** Stasis dermatitis: itching, weeping, scaling, erosions, and crusting

**c.** Lipodermatosclerosis or fibrosing panniculitis

**(1)** Induration initially at medial ankle, spreading circumferentially round the entire leg, up to mid calf

**(2)** The skin is heavily pigmented and fixed to subcutaneous tissues, with brawny edema above the fibrosis and in the foot below

**(3)** High risk for cellulitis

**5.** Classes 5 and 6: healed or nonhealed ulcers

**a.** Usually low on the medial ankle or along the path of the long or short saphenous vein

**b.** Never above the knee or on the forefoot

**c.** Chronic and recurrent, often lasting for months or even years

**Evidence-Based Diagnosis**

**A.** Diagnosis is often made based on the appearance of the leg.

**B.** Venography is the gold standard.

**C.** Duplex ultrasonography is the best noninvasive test.

**1.** Should be done if the diagnosis is in doubt (especially to rule out DVT), in patients with atypical symptoms or presentations, or if surgery is being considered

**2.** For diagnosing valvular incompetence, the sensitivity is 84%, specificity is 88%, LR+ = 7, and LR− = 0.18.

**3.** For diagnosing severe venous insufficiency, the sensitivity is 77%, specificity is 85%, LR+ = 5.1, and LR− = 0.26.

**D.** Because many patients have both arterial and venous insufficiency, concurrent arterial disease must be ruled out with the ankle brachial index (ABI).

**Treatment**

**A.** Compression stockings are the most important treatment modality.

**1.** Have been shown to reduce risk of postthrombotic syndrome, to accelerate ulcer healing, and to prevent recurrent ulceration

**2.** Classified into several grades, based on degree of compression at the ankle

**a.** 20–30 mm Hg: for patients with varicose veins, edema, leg fatigue (Classes 2 and 3)

**b.** 30–40 mm Hg: for patients with severe varicosities or moderate disease (Classes 4–6)

**c.** 40–50 mm Hg: for patients with recurrent ulceration

**3.** Knee high stockings are better tolerated than thigh high stockings.

**4.** Compliance often poor due to skin irritation, discomfort, and difficulty putting on the stockings.

 Compression stockings should not be used in patients with peripheral arterial disease or with invasive infection at an ulcer site.

**5.** Alternative ways to provide compression include elastic wraps and intermittent pneumatic compression pumps.

**6.** Ulcers should be covered with a dressing before putting on the compression device.

**B.** Diuretics are ineffective for the edema unless given with compression therapy.

**C.** Treatment of venous insufficiency ulcers

**1.** Occlusive dressing

**2.** Leg elevation and compression

**3.** Aspirin, 325 mg daily, might accelerate healing.

**4.** Pentoxifylline might accelerate healing.

**5.** Topical antibiotics have no role.

**6.** Systemic antibiotics indicated only if cellulitis or other invasive infection is present.

**D.** Interventional therapies

**1.** Sclerotherapy for spider veins, venous lakes, varicose veins 1–4 mm in diameter

**2.** Endovenous radiofrequency ablation and laser: alternative to vein stripping for great saphenous vein reflux

**3.** Iliac vein stenting for venous outflow abnormalities

**4.** Vein stripping and ligation

a. Usually involves removing the saphenous vein with high ligation of the saphenofemoral junction

b. Shown to result in significant improvement in symptoms in patients with Class 2–6 disease

c. Surgery plus compression is better than compression alone for preventing ulcer recurrence (12% combined therapy vs. 28% compression alone).

## CASE RESOLUTION

You decide that Mrs. E's symptoms are more consistent with venous insufficiency than with pulmonary hypertension. Duplex ultrasonographic scans confirm valvular incompetence, and you recommend that Mrs. E wear compression stockings. She returns in 3 months reporting that she has no edema when she wears the stockings, and that she continues to walk 1 mile daily without any dyspnea.

## CHIEF COMPLAINT

### PATIENT 3

Mrs. K is a 64-year-old woman who had a right mastectomy 2 years ago for breast cancer. She was treated with adjuvant radiation therapy and has been taking tamoxifen since completing the radiation. She has had no evidence of recurrent disease but has had some right arm swelling for at least 18 months. She comes to see you now because 2 days ago the swelling of her right arm worsened, with associated pain and redness. This morning her temperature was 37.9°C.

At this point, what is the leading hypothesis, what are the active alternatives, and is there a must not miss diagnosis? Given this differential diagnosis, what tests should be ordered?

## PRIORITIZING THE DIFFERENTIAL

Mrs. K has chronic lymphedema due to disruption of her lymphatic drainage by her previous surgery and radiation therapy. This is a pivotal point in her history since patients with lymphatic disruption and lymphedema are at high risk for skin and subcutaneous infections. Pathophysiologically, the edema found in cellulitis is due to a localized increase in capillary permeability due to inflammation; however, patients with underlying limb abnormalities will often present with more diffuse edema. The other primary consideration in *any* patient with unilateral limb swelling is DVT. Mrs. K has several risk factors for this, including history of cancer, possible venous scarring secondary to radiation, and use of tamoxifen (a drug associated with a relative risk for DVT of about 3). Table 15–5 lists the differential diagnosis.

Always think about DVT in a patient with unilateral limb swelling.

### 3

On physical exam, Mrs. K is clearly uncomfortable. Her temperature is 38.3°C, pulse 102 bpm, RR 16 breaths

per minute, and BP 125/80 mm Hg. Her right upper arm and chest are bright red, hot, and tender. The border of the erythema is sharply demarcated, and the area of erythema feels indurated. She has eczema of all of her fingers, with multiple areas of cracked skin.

 Is the clinical information sufficient to make a diagnosis? If not, what other information do you need?

## Leading Hypothesis: Cellulitis & Erysipelas

### Textbook Presentation

A painful, red, hot, and swollen limb develops acutely in a patient with underlying venous or lymphatic disease.

**Table 15–5.** Diagnostic hypotheses for Mrs. K.

| Diagnostic Hypotheses | Clinical Clues | Important Tests |
|---|---|---|
| **Leading Hypothesis** | | |
| Cellulitis or erysipelas | Edema<br>Erythema<br>Pain<br>Fever<br>Entry site for infection<br>Underlying venous insufficiency or lymphedema | Clinical exam |
| **Active Alternative—Must Not Miss** | | |
| Upper extremity DVT | Unilateral arm/neck swelling<br>Feeling of fullness or heaviness<br>DVT risk factors (especially indwelling intravenous catheter) | Duplex ultrasound<br>CT<br>MRA<br>Venography |

DVT, deep venous thrombosis.

## Disease Highlights

**A. Definitions**

  **1.** Cellulitis is an infection of the dermis and subcutaneous tissue.

  **2.** Erysipelas is a superficial cellulitis with prominent lymphatic involvement.

**B. Cellulitis highlights**

  **1.** Risk factors for the development of cellulitis

    **a.** Lymphedema

    **b.** Peripheral edema

    **c.** Venous insufficiency

    **d.** Obesity

    **e.** Diabetes

    **f.** History of cellulitis

    **g.** Breast cancer treatment

      **(1)** Cellulitis of the ipsilateral arm is seen in women in whom lymphedema of the arm develops after mastectomy.

      **(2)** Cellulitis of the ipsilateral breast is seen in women in whom localized lymphedema develops after lumpectomy, axillary node dissection, and radiation therapy.

  **2.** Often an entry site for infection can be identified (leg ulcer, trauma, tinea pedis, eczema, subcutaneous abscess)

  **3.** Clinical presentation

    **a.** Presence of systemic symptoms (eg, fever, chills, myalgias) is unusual and suggest concomitant bacteremia or a more serious infection such as necrotizing fasciitis.

    **b.** Physical findings

      **(1)** Nonpalpable, confluent erythema with indistinct margins

      **(2)** Generalized swelling

      **(3)** Warmth and tenderness of involved skin

      **(4)** Tender regional adenopathy sometimes found

      **(5)** Lymphangitis and abscess formation sometimes seen

      **(6)** In women who have been treated for breast cancer and have arm lymphedema, the humeral area of the ipsilateral extremity is most often involved, with extension to the shoulder and forearm.

      **(7)** In breast cellulitis, the infection starts at the lumpectomy site and can extend to the remainder of the breast, the anterior shoulder, back, and ipsilateral upper extremity.

  **4.** Microbiology

    **a.** β-Hemolytic streptococci and *Staphylococcus aureus* are the most common organisms.

      **(1)** Community-acquired methicillin-resistant *S aureus* (MRSA), usually the USA300 genotype, is increasingly common; it is now the most common pathogen cultured from skin and soft tissue infections in urban emergency departments

      **(2)** The following groups are at risk for having community-acquired MRSA:

        **(a)** Household contacts

        **(b)** Soldiers

        **(c)** Children

        **(d)** Men who have sex with men

        **(e)** Incarcerated persons

        **(f)** Athletes

        **(g)** Native Americans, Pacific Islanders

        **(h)** Injection drug users

        **(i)** Patients with a previous community-acquired MRSA infection

      **(3)** Many patients with community-acquired MRSA have none of these risk factors

      **(4)** Skin abscesses, often with central necrosis, are a very common manifestation of community-acquired MRSA; patients often think they have been bitten by a spider or other insect.

      **(5)** Other manifestations include cellulitis, necrotizing pneumonia, pleural empyema, necrotizing fasciitis, septic thrombophlebitis, myositis, and severe sepsis

    **b.** A variety of other organisms may be seen with specific exposures or sites of infection (Table 15-6)

**C. Erysipelas highlights**

  **1.** Risk factors for development of erysipelas

**Table 15–6.** Microbiology of cellulitis.

| Cellulitis Syndrome | Location/ Key Point | Likely Organisms |
|---|---|---|
| Periorbital | Periorbital | *Staphylococcus aureus*, pneumococcus, group A streptococcus (GAS) |
| Orbital | Emergent because of potential to affect oculomotor function and visual acuity | Staphylococcus, streptococcus |
| Perianal | Evaluate for underlying abscess | GAS |
| Breast cancer treatment | See text | Non-group A hemolytic streptococcus |
| Saphenous vein harvest | Ipsilateral leg | GAS or non-group A streptococcus |
| Injection drug use | Extremities, neck | Staphylococcus, streptococcus (groups A, C, F, G), gram-negative organisms, anaerobes |
| Crepitant cellulitis | Trunk, extremities; consider necrotizing fasciitis | GAS, anaerobes, *Clostridia* |
| Salt water exposure | Exposed body part | *Vibrio vulnificus* |
| Fresh water exposure | Exposed body part | *Aeromonas hydrophilia* |
| Hot tub exposure | Bathing suit distribution | *Pseudomonas aeruginosa* |

**a.** Similar to those for cellulitis

**b.** Lymphedema and an identified portal of entry (primarily tinea pedis) are the 2 strongest risk factors in 1 study.

 Always treat tinea pedis in a patient with cellulitis, erysipelas, or risk factors for developing those infections.

**2.** Clinical presentation

    **a.** Sudden onset of fever (85% of patients), erythema, edema, and pain

    **b.** Physical findings

        **(1)** Palpable plaque of erythema that extends by 2–10 cm/day

        **(2)** **Sharply demarcated border**

        **(3)** Leg is the most common site (90%), then the arm (5%), and then the face (2.5%).

        **(4)** Regional adenopathy and lymphangitis sometimes seen

    **c.** Recurrence rate of 10% at 6 months and 30% at 3 years is usually due to untreated local factors.

    **d.** Patients should respond to antibiotic therapy in 24–72 hours.

**3.** Microbiology

    **a.** Streptococci are the causative organisms in 90% of cases (group A in about 58–67% of cases caused by streptococci, group B in 3–9%, and group C or G in 14–25%)

    **b.** *S aureus* is also found in 10% of cases, although it is unclear whether it is contributing to the infection or just colonizing.

## Evidence-Based Diagnosis

**A.** Both cellulitis and erysipelas are clinical diagnoses.

**B.** Blood cultures are positive in 2–5% of patients.

**C.** Skin biopsy cultures are positive in 5-40% of patients, but are rarely necessary.

**D.** Aspiration of the leading edge of erythema is sometimes done, but the yield is low.

**E.** Toe web cultures are sometimes helpful in patients with tinea pedis.

**F.** If there is a skin abscess associated with the cellulitis, it should be drained and the fluid cultured.

 Cultures are rarely helpful in cellulitis or erysipelas without an associated abscess.

## Treatment

**A.** Cellulitis

    **1.** Initial therapy is usually empiric.

    **2.** Must cover staphylococcus and streptococcus

    **3.** Purulent cellulitis is more likely to be caused by *S aureus;* nonpurulent cellulitis is often due to a combination of staphylococci and streptococci.

    **4.** Because of the emergence of community-acquired MRSA, antibiotics previously used for cellulitis (such as cephalexin or dicloxicillin) may not be effective.

        **a.** Local susceptibility patterns can guide choices.

        **b.** Oral drugs to which community-acquired MRSA is commonly sensitive include clindamycin, trimethoprim-sulfamethoxazole, and tetracyclines.

            **(1)** Streptococci are often resistant to trimethoprim-sulfamethoxazole and tetracyclines.

            **(2)** 10–20% of MRSA isolates that are sensitive to clindamycin, but resistant to erythromycin, develop inducible clindamycin resistance due to the presence of the *erm* gene.

            **(3)** Clindamycin sensitive/erythromycin resistant isolates should undergo the "D-Zone Test" to look for inducible resistance (Figure 15–5).

    **5.** A reasonable choice for cellulitis would be clindamycin or a β-lactam antibiotic (such as dicloxicillin or amoxicillin/clavulanate) plus trimethoprim-sulfamethoxazole.

    **6.** Should treat for 10–14 days

**B.** Erysipelas

    **1.** Penicillin G or amoxicillin is effective in > 80% of patients with erysipelas.

    **2.** Other drugs that have been studied include macrolides and fluoroquinolones

    **3.** Should treat for 10–20 days

**C.** Uncomplicated, slowly progressive infection in a well-appearing patient can be treated with oral antibiotics if

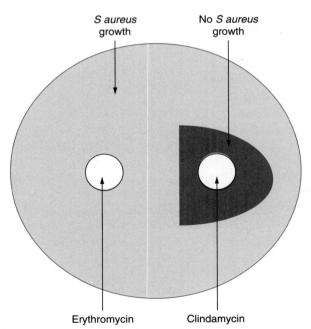

When there is inducible clindamycin resistance, the zone of clindamycin inhibition is blunted on the side next to the erythromycin disk, resulting in a "D" shaped area of no growth surrounding the clindamycin disk. If there is no inducible resistance, the no growth area around the clindamycin disk will be a more symmetric circle

***Figure 15–5.*** D-Zone test.

1. The patient has no GI upset
2. The limb can be elevated
3. Serial exams are feasible

D. Patients who appear ill, who have rapidly progressive infection, are immunocompromised, or who might not be able to follow treatment instructions should be admitted for IV antibiotics, generally including vancomycin.

E. Obtain infectious disease and surgical consultations for patients with rapidly progressive infections, especially if progression occurs while they are receiving appropriate antibiotics.

## MAKING A DIAGNOSIS

Initial laboratory tests include the following: WBC 11,700/mcL, 83% PMNs, 10% basophils, 7% lymphocytes; Hgb, 13.5 g/dL; glucose, 88 mg/dL; creatinine, 0.8 mg/dL.

 Have you crossed a diagnostic threshold for the leading hypothesis, cellulitis or erysipelas? Have you ruled out the active alternatives? Do other tests need to be done to exclude the alternative diagnoses?

## Alternative Diagnosis: Upper Extremity DVT (UEDVT)

### Textbook Presentation

Patients can be asymptomatic, but generally arm, shoulder, or neck discomfort or fullness as well as arm swelling are the presenting symptoms.

### Disease Highlights

A. Classification

1. Primary UEDVT (20% of cases)

   a. Idiopathic

   b. Effort thrombosis, also known as Paget-Schroetter syndrome

   (1) Occurs in young men after strenuous exercise, which causes microtrauma to the veins

   (2) May or may not find compression by hypertrophied muscles or a cervical rib

2. Secondary UEDVT (80% of cases) (Table 15–7)

   a. Indwelling central venous catheter–associated UEDVT (up to 70% of cases)

   (1) UEDVT occurs more often with large catheters than with smaller ones.

   (2) Risk increases with duration of catheter use, being negligible within 6 days and increasing significantly after 2 weeks.

   (3) Risk is higher with polyvinyl chloride-coated catheters than with silicone ones.

   b. Malignancy (> 40% of cases); patients with cancer and an indwelling catheter are at especially high risk.

**Table 15–7.** Risk factors for upper extremity deep venous thrombosis.

| Risk Factor | Adjust Odds Ratio (95% CI) |
|---|---|
| Indwelling central venous catheter (CVC) | 9.7 (7.8–12.2) |
| CVC plus inherited coagulation disorder | ~30 |
| Cancer | 18.1 (9.4–35.1) |
| Metastatic vs localized cancer | 11.5 (1.6–80.2) |
| Cancer plus CVC | 43.6 (25.5–74.6) |
| Oral contraceptives plus factor V Leiden or prothrombin G20210A mutation | 13.6 (2.7–67.3) |
| Upper extremity surgery | 13.1 (2.1–80.6) |
| Upper extremity plaster cast | 7.0 (1.7–29.5) |

   c. Hypercoagulable states

   d. Other miscellaneous causes (surgery, infection, immobility, concurrent lower extremity DVT)

B. Sites

1. Subclavian in 18–69% of cases

2. Axillary in 5–42% of cases

3. Internal jugular in 8–29% of cases

4. Brachial in 4–13% of cases

5. Multiple veins are often involved, but bilateral UEDVT is rare.

C. Clinical features

1. Pain is present in ~40% of patients.

2. Edema is present ~80% of patients in some series, but patients with catheter-related UEDVT often do not have edema.

3. Patients may note numbness, heaviness, paresthesias, pruritus, and coldness.

4. Dilated cutaneous veins sometimes visible.

D. Complications

1. Pulmonary embolism occurs in up to 36% of cases and is more often seen with secondary UEDVT, especially catheter-related.

 UEDVT can cause pulmonary embolism.

2. Recurrent thrombosis occurs in up to 10% of patients.

3. Postthrombotic syndrome is seen in up to 4–34% of patients in different series.

### Evidence-Based Diagnosis

A. Venography is the gold standard.

B. Duplex ultrasonography is the most commonly used noninvasive test.

1. Disadvantages include a blind spot caused by the clavicle and difficulties interpreting the study if there are collateral veins.

**2.** Sensitivity ranges from 56% to 100%, and specificity from 94% to 100%

**3.** Magnetic resonance angiography and CT are sometimes done; sensitivity and specificity are unknown.

## Treatment

**A.** Anticoagulation with heparin, followed by at least 3 months of warfarin; patients with cancer or chronic indwelling central venous catheters should receive anticoagulation therapy indefinitely.

**B.** Thrombolysis with or without stent placement is sometimes done, especially in patients who require permanent indwelling catheters.

## CASE RESOLUTION

▽3

Mrs. K's presentation of a sharply demarcated, erythematous plaque, fever, and leukocytosis is diagnostic of erysipelas. The portal of entry is the eczematous, cracked skin on her hands. Although she has some risk factors for UEDVT, it is not necessary to test for it at this point. Because of the extent of infection, Mrs. K is admitted to the hospital and treated with IV cefazolin. One of 2 blood cultures grows group A β-hemolytic streptococci. She improves rapidly and is switched to oral penicillin and is discharged.

## REFERENCES

Angeli P, Merkel C. Pathogenesis and management of hepatorenal syndrome in patients with cirrhosis. J Hepatol. 2008;28:S93–S103.

Baarslad HJ, van Beek EJR, Koopman MMW, Reekers JA. Prospective study of color duplex ultrasonography compared with contrast venography in patients suspected of having deep venous thrombosis of the upper extremities. Ann Intern Med. 2002;136:865–72.

Bergan JJ, Schmid-Schonbein GW, Smith PD, Nicolaides AN, Boisseau MR, Eklof B. Chronic venous disease. N Engl J Med. 2006;355:488–98.

Bernardi E, Pesavento R, Prandoni P. Upper extremity deep venous thrombosis. Semin Thromb Hemost. 2006;32:729–36.

Bonnetblanc JM, Bedane C. Erysipelas. Am J Clin Dermatol. 2003;4:157–63.

Chin KM, Rubin LJ. Pulmonary arterial hypertension. J Am Coll Cardiol. 2008;51:1527–38.

Daum RS. Skin and soft tissue infections caused by methicillin-resistant *Staphylococcus aureus*. N Engl J Med. 2007;357:380–90.

Eberhardt RT, Raffetto JD. Chronic venous insufficiency. Circulation. 2005;111:2398–2409.

Madaio MP, Harrington JT. The diagnosis of glomerular diseases. Arch Intern Med. 2001;161:25–34.

Mahmoodi BK, ten Kate MK, Waanders F et al. High absolute risks and predictors of venous and arterial thromboembolic events in patients with nephrotic syndrome: results from a large retrospective cohort study. Circulation. 2008;117:224–30.

McGee S. Evidence based physical diagnosis. W.B. Saunders; 2001:435, 457.

McGoon M, Gutterman D, Steen V et al. Screening, early detection, and diagnosis of pulmonary hypertension. Chest. 2004;126:14S–34S.

Mustafa BO, Rathbun SW, Whitsett TL, Raskob GE. Sensitivity and specificity of ultrasonography in the diagnosis of upper extremity deep vein thrombosis. Arch Intern Med. 2002;162:401–4.

Rich S, Dantzker Dr, Ayres SM et al. Primary pulmonary hypertension: a national prospective study. Ann Intern Med. 1987;107:216–23.

Rogers RL, Perkins J. Skin and soft tissue infections. Primary Care: Clinics in Office Practice. 2006;33:697–710.

Schuppan D, Afdhal NH. Liver cirrhosis. Lancet. 2008;371:838–51.

Sheer TA, Runyon BA. Spontaneous bacterial peritonitis. Dig Dis. 2005;23:39–46.

Swartz MN. Cellulitis. N Engl J Med. 2004;350:904–12.

Wong CL et al. Does this patient have bacterial peritonitis or portal hypertension? JAMA. 2008;299:1166–78.

# I have a patient with fatigue.
# How do I determine the cause?

## CHIEF COMPLAINT

**PATIENT** 1

Mrs. M is a 42-year-old woman who has had fatigue for the past 6 months.

 **What is the differential diagnosis of fatigue? How would you frame the differential?**

## CONSTRUCTING A DIFFERENTIAL DIAGNOSIS

Before considering the differential diagnosis, it is important to understand what the patient means by fatigue, which is conventionally defined as a sensation of exhaustion after usual activities, or a feeling of insufficient energy to begin usual activities. Most people consider the terms fatigue, tiredness, and lack of energy synonymous. However, patients sometimes use these terms when they are actually experiencing other symptoms, especially excessive sleepiness, weakness, or dyspnea on exertion.

 Always ask patients what they mean when they report fatigue. Always ask directly about weakness, excessive sleepiness, and dyspnea.

Acute fatigue is common in conjunction with a variety of acute illnesses, ranging from uncomplicated viral infections to exacerbations of heart failure (HF). Fatigue is also a prominent symptom in some chronic diseases, such as multiple sclerosis and cancer. This chapter will not discuss fatigue in such patients but will focus on evaluating the symptom of fatigue lasting weeks to months in patients without already diagnosed conditions known to cause fatigue.

The differential diagnosis of fatigue is extremely broad and best organized with an organ/system approach.

A. Psychiatric
   1. Depression
   2. Anxiety
   3. Somatization disorder
   4. Substance abuse
B. Sleep disorders
   1. Insomnia
   2. Obstructive sleep apnea
   3. Periodic leg movements
   4. Narcolepsy
C. Endocrine
   1. Thyroid disease
   2. Diabetes
   3. Hypoadrenalism
D. Medications (Table 16–1)
E. Hematologic or oncologic
   1. Anemia
   2. Cancer
F. Renal: renal failure
G. GI: liver disease
H. Cardiovascular: chronic heart disease
I. Pulmonary: chronic lung disease
J. Neuromuscular: myositis, multiple sclerosis
K. Infectious: chronic infections
L. Rheumatologic: autoimmune diseases
M. Fatigue of unknown etiology
   1. Chronic fatigue syndrome
   2. Idiopathic chronic fatigue: fatigue for which no medical, psychiatric, or sleep pattern explanation can be found.

Figure 16-1 outlines the evaluation of fatigue in an algorithm.

 The most common causes of fatigue are psychiatric disorders, sleep disorders, and medication side effects.

1

Mrs. M reports that she is tired all the time, beginning first thing in the morning and lasting all day. She also reports frontal headaches several mornings per week, intermittent lower abdominal pain relieved by bowel movements, and low back pain. She does not complain of any trouble sleeping.

Her past medical history is notable for menorrhagia and iron deficiency anemia when she was in her 20s and is otherwise unremarkable. Currently, her menses occur every 30 days, with bleeding for 3–4 days. Her family history is notable for thyroid disease in her mother and breast cancer in her paternal grandmother.

She takes no medications, does not smoke, and does not drink alcohol. She has never used illicit drugs. She works as a teacher, and her husband is a security guard. They have 2 children, ages 9 and 12.

***Table 16-1.*** Medications that affect sleep.

| Medications that cause insomnia | Antihypertensives: Clonidine, methyldopa, reserpine, propranolol, atenolol |
| --- | --- |
| | Anticholinergics: Ipratropium |
| | CNS stimulants: Methylphenidate |
| | Hormones: Oral contraceptives, thyroid hormone, corticosteroids, progesterone |
| | Sympathomimetic amines: Albuterol, theophylline, phenylpropanolamine, pseudoephedrine |
| | Antineoplastics: Leuprolide, goserelin, pentostatin, interferon alfa |
| | Miscellaneous: Phenytoin, nicotine, levodopa, quinidine, caffeine, alcohol |
| Medications that cause drowsiness | Tricyclic antidepressants: Amitriptyline, imipramine |
| | Opioids |
| | Benzodiazepines |
| | Nonsteroidal antiinflammatory drugs |
| | Anticonvulsants: Gabapentin |
| | Alcohol |

 At this point, what is the leading hypothesis, what are the active alternatives, and is there a must not miss diagnosis? Given this differential diagnosis, what tests should be ordered?

## PRIORITIZING THE DIFFERENTIAL DIAGNOSIS

A specific causative medical disease that explains fatigue is found in less than 10% of patients who seek medical attention from their primary care physician. Up to 75% of patients with fatigue have psychiatric symptoms. Sleep disorders are also common in patients with fatigue, and in one referral clinic, 80% of patients with fatigue had sleep disorders. Patients with several somatic complaints, such as Mrs. M, are particularly likely to have psychiatric causes for fatigue, as are patients who feel tired constantly. Because sleep disorders are so common, either in association with psychiatric disorders or alone, they are always an active alternative in patients with fatigue. Patients often do not spontaneously describe sleep disturbances and psychiatric symptoms, so it is important to ask about them directly.

 All patients with fatigue need a detailed psychosocial and sleep history.

Although most patients with fatigue do *not* have anemia, hypothyroidism, or diabetes, they are important and treatable, and so are generally considered "must not miss" diagnoses. Anemia and hypothyroidism are somewhat likely in Mrs. M because of her previous history of anemia and her family history of thyroid disease. Finally, on occasion, fatigue may be the presenting symptom in patients with surprisingly severe cardiac, pulmonary, renal, or liver disease. Table 16–2 lists the differential diagnosis.

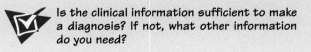 Despite the rarity of positive results, most patients with fatigue need basic laboratory testing consisting of a blood count, chemistry panel (including glucose, electrolytes, BUN, creatinine, and liver function tests), and TSH.

Mrs. M does not lack interest in her usual activities or feel depressed. She has not lost or gained weight. She worries about money and her family but has never had a panic attack and does not consider herself excessively nervous or anxious.

On physical exam, she appears healthy and her affect is normal. HEENT exam is normal. There is no thyromegaly or adenopathy. Lungs are clear. There are no breast masses. Cardiac and abdominal exams are normal, and there is no edema. Her CBC, glucose, electrolytes, BUN, creatinine, liver function tests, and TSH are all normal.

Is the clinical information sufficient to make a diagnosis? If not, what other information do you need?

## Leading Hypotheses: Depression & Anxiety

See Chapter 27, Involuntary Weight Loss.

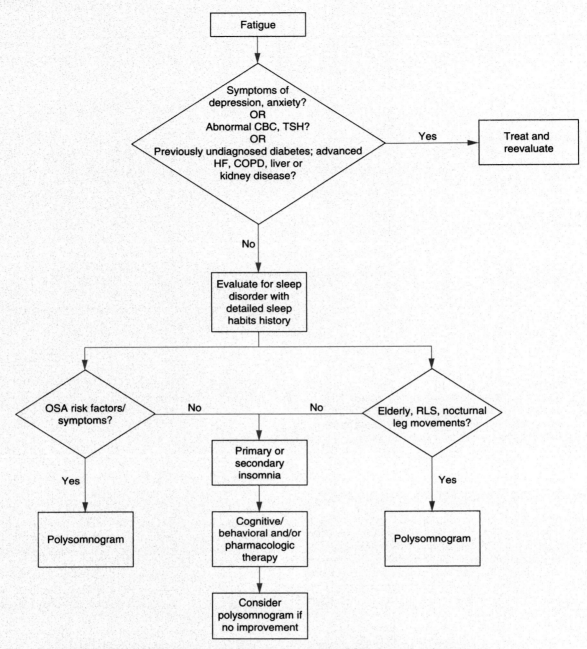

COPD, chronic obstructive pulmonary disease; HF, heart failure; OSA, obstructive sleep apnea; RLS, restless legs syndrome.

***Figure 16-1.*** Diagnostic approach: fatigue.

## MAKING A DIAGNOSIS

Mrs. M does not meet DSM criteria for anxiety or depression. It is therefore necessary to consider the alternative diagnoses.

Mrs. M works as a teacher, rising at 6 AM, leaving her house at 7 AM, and returning home about 5 PM. She then prepares dinner for her family, helps her 2 children with their homework, and grades papers until 9:30 PM. She watches a little television, and then goes to sleep about 10:00 PM. Her husband works from 3 PM to 11 PM, and she often wakes up when he gets home at midnight. He needs

***Table 16-2.*** Diagnostic hypotheses for Mrs. M.

| Diagnostic Hypotheses | Clinical Clues | Important Tests |
|---|---|---|
| **Leading Hypotheses** | | |
| Depression | History of loss<br>Prior depression<br>Postpartum state<br>Family history<br>> 6 somatic symptoms<br>Positive depression screen | History |
| Anxiety | Multiple somatic symptoms<br>Anxiety<br>Panic attacks | History |
| **Active Alternatives—Most Common** | | |
| Insomnia | Fatigue | History |
| Sleep apnea | Daytime sleepiness | Polysomnogram |
| Periodic limb movements | Daytime sleepiness<br>Restless leg syndrome | History<br>Polysomnogram |
| Narcolepsy | Sudden episodes of daytime sleep | Multiple sleep latency test |
| **Active Alternatives—Must Not Miss** | | |
| Anemia | Fatigue<br>Dyspnea<br>Symptoms of blood loss | CBC |
| Hypothyroidism | Fatigue<br>Constipation<br>Cold intolerance | TSH |
| Diabetes | Family history<br>Obesity<br>Hypertension<br>Ethnic group<br>Polyuria<br>Polydipsia | Fasting plasma glucose |
| **Other Hypotheses** | | |
| Advanced renal disease | Fatigue<br>Anorexia<br>Nausea<br>Edema | BUN<br>Creatinine |
| Advanced liver disease | Fatigue<br>Anorexia<br>Nausea<br>Edema | AST (SGOT)<br>ALT (SGPT)<br>Bilirubin |
| Advanced cardiac disease | Dyspnea<br>Orthopnea<br>PND<br>Edema | ECG<br>Echocardiography<br>Stress test |
| Advanced pulmonary disease | Dyspnea<br>Cachexia | Pulmonary exam<br>Pulmonary function tests<br>Chest radiograph |

some time to "wind down" before he goes to sleep, so they often talk and watch TV in bed for an hour or so. After her husband dozes off, she often cannot fall back asleep, and will sit in bed "surfing" the Internet on her laptop for an hour or two.

 **Is the clinical information sufficient to make a diagnosis? If not, what other information do you need?**

## Revised Leading Hypothesis: Insomnia

### Textbook Presentation

Patients with insomnia sometimes have trouble falling asleep, sometimes fall asleep easily but wake up during the night, or both.

### Disease Highlights

A. Primary insomnia

1. Pathogenesis unknown, but may be due to a state of hyper-arousal (demonstrated on positron emission tomography (PET) scans and by measurements of adrenal hormones)

2. Three types

   a. Idiopathic: arises in childhood; persistent

   b. Psychophysiologic

   (1) Due to a maladaptive response in which the patient associates the bed environment with arousal rather than sleep

   (2) Often begins due to a precipitant of acute insomnia, such as a death of a family member, but persists after the precipitant resolves

   c. Paradoxical: a mismatch between the patient's perception of the duration of sleep and objective findings on polysomnography

B. Secondary insomnia

1. Adjustment insomnia: associated with active psychosocial stressors

2. Inadequate sleep hygiene: associated with lifestyle habits than impair sleep

3. Due to an active psychiatric disorder, such as anxiety or depression

4. Due to a medical condition, such as chronic pain, dyspnea, cough, hot flashes

5. Due to a drug or substance, such as alcohol, caffeine, medication, or an illicit drug

C. Although not officially considered insomnias, other disorders such as shift-work sleep disorder (seen in patients whose work shift varies), and delayed sleep phase syndrome (a delay in sleep period of > 2 hours relative to conventional times) should also be considered in patients with insomnia.

### Evidence-Based Diagnosis

A. Obtaining a thorough history helps establish the diagnosis of insomnia. Initial screening questions include the following:

1. Difficulty initiating sleep, staying asleep, or both?

2. Early awakening?

3. Non-restorative sleep?

4. Daytime consequences? (Lack of daytime fatigue or sleepiness suggests the insomnia is not clinically significant.)

5. Frequency and duration?

B. Follow-up questions

1. Precipitating events, progression, ameliorating or exacerbating factors?

2. Sleep-wake schedule?

3. Cognitive attitude toward sleep?

   a. Negative expectations regarding the ability to sleep and distortions about the effects of insomnia lead to perpetuation of the insomnia.

   b. Attitudes toward previous treatments are also important.

4. Psychiatric disorder present?

5. Substance misuse or medication use?

6. Medical illness with nocturnal symptoms?

7. Symptoms of sleep apnea, restless legs? (See discussion below.)

### Treatment

A. Behavioral therapy

1. Stimulus control therapy

   a. Also known as sleep hygiene

   b. Based on premise that insomnia is a conditioned response to temporal and environmental cues

   c. Has been shown to be effective for sleep onset and maintenance

   d. Principles of sleep hygiene

   (1) Go to bed only when sleepy.

   (2) Use the bedroom only for sleep and sex, not reading, watching television, eating, or working.

   (3) If unable to sleep after 20 minutes in bed, get out of bed, go into another room, read or listen to quiet music, and then return to bed when sleepy.

   (4) Maintain a consistent sleep-wake schedule; go to bed and get up at the same time each day.

   (5) Avoid daytime napping; if napping is necessary, limit the nap to less than 30 minutes and take the nap no later than the early afternoon.

   (6) Avoid caffeine, alcohol, and other stimulants (such as decongestants).

   (7) Exercise regularly, but not in the late evening.

2. Relaxation therapy

   a. Methods include progressive muscle relaxation, biofeedback to reduce somatic arousal, imagery training, and meditation.

   b. Useful for both sleep onset and maintenance

   c. Often requires practice with a trained professional

3. Sleep restriction therapy

   a. Decreases the amount of time spent in bed in order to increase the percentage of time in bed spent sleeping

   b. Usually keep waking time constant and make bedtime later, with progressive moving up of bedtime as sleep improves

   c. Effective for sleep onset and maintenance

B. Cognitive therapy involves identifying dysfunctional beliefs about sleep and then substituting more functional attitudes that can reduce anxiety.

C. Combination therapy: combining cognitive and behavioral therapy has been shown to be superior to relaxation therapy alone.

D. Pharmacotherapy

1. Most studies of pharmacologic agents are short (12 days to 6 months), so data about long-term effects are lacking.

2. Basic principles for using pharmacotherapy to treat chronic insomnia

   a. Use agents with shorter half-lives to minimize daytime sedation.

**b.** Use the lowest effective dose.

**c.** Try to dose intermittently, such as 2–4 times per week, rather than daily.

**d.** Try to limit daily use to a maximum of 3–4 weeks.

**e.** Discontinue medication gradually.

**f.** Monitor for rebound insomnia when medications are stopped.

**4.** Categories of medications (Table 16–3)

    **a.** Benzodiazepines

      **(1)** Effective in initiating and maintaining sleep

      **(2)** Efficacy may decrease with duration of administration, although one 8-week study of temazepam did not demonstrate any tolerance.

      **(3)** Can develop marked rebound insomnia lasting 1–3 nights when triazolam is stopped; intermediate acting benzodiazepines cause only mild rebound insomnia, and rebound is rare with long duration benzodiazepines.

      **(4)** Side effects (daytime drowsiness, cognitive impairment, and potential for delirium) are all greater with longer-acting drugs and are more common in elderly patients.

    **b.** Benzodiazepine receptor agonists

      **(1)** Nonbenzodiazepine compounds that bind to only 1 type of benzodiazepine receptor

      **(2)** Zolpidem, zaleplon, and eszopiclone are effective in initiating sleep; zolpidem is possibly more effective than zaleplon in maintaining sleep.

      **(3)** Because of its extremely short half-life, zaleplon can be taken during the night.

      **(4)** No tolerance, dependence, or rebound insomnia has been reported.

      **(5)** Little or no daytime drowsiness

      **(6)** No evidence of cognitive impairment with zaleplon; zolpidem may cause mild impairment.

      **(7)** Zolpidem can be used intermittently (3–5 times/week) in patients with chronic insomnia.

    **c.** Antihistamines

      **(1)** Should not be used as sleeping aids due to minimal effectiveness and impairment of sleep quality.

      **(2)** Daytime drowsiness is common.

      **(3)** Commonly cause delirium in elderly patients

    **d.** Antidepressants

      **(1)** Trazodone is frequently used for sleep; limited data suggest that trazodone is better than placebo but inferior to zolpidem.

      **(2)** Low-dose tricyclic antidepressants, such as amitriptyline, are sometimes used; one 4-week study of doxepin showed beneficial effects on sleep latency and total sleep time.

        **(a)** Elimination half-lives are long, often leading to daytime sedation.

        **(b)** Potential for anticholinergic side effects, even at low doses

**E.** Pharmacologic therapy versus cognitive behavioral therapy

  **1.** Data comparing pharmacotherapy with behavioral and cognitive therapy are limited.

    **a.** Overall, treatment effects are similar.

    **b.** Perhaps more rapid improvement with pharmacotherapy

    **c.** Perhaps more sustained improvement with behavioral therapy

  **2.** Studies of combined cognitive behavioral and pharmacologic therapy versus cognitive behavioral therapy alone show that the cognitive behavioral therapy alone group maintained results at 10–24 months, but the combined group did not.

## CASE RESOLUTION

Mrs. M is reassured that her laboratory tests are normal. She realizes that she often gets 6 hours of sleep or less a night. After listening to you explain the principles of sleep hygiene, she decides to talk with her husband about ways they could spend time together without interrupting her sleep so often.

When she returns 6 months later, she reports that she is still tired because she values the time she spends with her husband at night. However, she now asks him to sleep in the guest room when she feels exceptionally fatigued, so she can have a few nights of uninterrupted sleep. She has also found that a 15-minute nap at lunchtime helps.

**Table 16-3.** Medications used to treat insomnia.

| Medication | Dose range (mg) | Half-life of drug and active metabolites (hrs) |
|---|---|---|
| **Benzodiazepines** | | |
| Triazolam[1] | 0.125–0.25 | 2–5 |
| Temazepam[1] | 7.5–30 | 8–15 |
| Estazolam[1] | 0.5–2 | 10–24 |
| Lorazepam | 0.5–4 | 8–24 |
| Clonazepam | 0.5–2 | 19–60 |
| **Benzodiazepine receptor agonists (BZRAs)** | | |
| Zaleplon[1] | 5–20 | 1 |
| Zolpidem[1] | 5–10 | 3 |
| Eszopiclone[1] | 1–3 | 5–7 |
| **Melatonin receptor agonist** | | |
| Ramelteon[1] | 8 | 2–5 |
| **Miscellaneous** | | |
| Diphenhydramine | 25–50 mg | 2.4–9.3 |
| Trazodone | 25–100 | 5–9 |

[1]Approved by the US Food and Drug Administration for treatment of insomnia.

# REVIEW OF OTHER IMPORTANT DISEASES

## Obstructive Sleep Apnea (OSA)

### Textbook Presentation

Patients with OSA often complain of daytime sleepiness or fatigue. Bed partners often note snoring or actual apneic episodes. Most patients are obese.

### Disease Highlights

A. Present in up to 24% of men and 9% of women

B. An obstructive apnea is at least 10 seconds of cessation of ventilation; a hypopnea is at least a 30% reduction in air flow for 10 seconds or longer with at least a 4% reduction in oxygen saturation.

C. The apnea-hypopnea index (AHI) is the total number of apneas plus hypopneas per hour.

  1. OSA is defined as an AHI ≥ 5 with daytime somnolence, or an AHI ≥ 15 regardless of symptoms.

  2. Mild OSA is an AHI of 5–14; moderate is an AHI of 15–30, and severe is an AHI > 30.

D. Pathophysiology

  1. There are normal decreases in tonic pharyngeal muscle tone and compensatory reflex dilators during sleep.

  2. Patients with OSA have smaller upper airways due to increased parapharyngeal fat, tongue prominence, elongated palate, or thickened lateral pharyngeal walls, and are unable to maintain airway stability.

  3. During inspiration, the negative upper airway pressures close these narrowed airways, resulting in apneas or hypopneas.

E. Risk factors

  1. Obesity

    a. A 1 SD increase in body mass index (BMI) is associated with 4.5-fold increased risk of OSA.

    b. Visceral and truncal fat, and neck circumference correlate more with OSA than BMI alone.

  2. Smoking (RR = 3).

  3. Nighttime nasal congestion is associated with OSA (RR = 1.8).

  4. Anesthesia, sedative/hypnotic medications, and sleep deprivation can promote apneic episodes.

F. Consequences of OSA

  1. Increased rate of motor vehicle accidents (RR = 2.5)

  2. Hypertension (RR = 2.89); some studies have shown a reduction in BP of 10 mm Hg when OSA is treated.

  3. HF (RR = 2.38); treatment of OSA in patients with HF improves left ventricular ejection fraction by 5–8%.

  4. Atrial fibrillation is twice as likely to recur after cardioversion in patients with untreated OSA.

  5. An association with impaired glucose tolerance has been observed.

  6. Long-standing, severe OSA can lead to cor pulmonale.

### Evidence-Based Diagnosis

A. History and physical exam

  1. The complaint of sleepiness has traditionally been thought to suggest the diagnosis of an intrinsic sleep disorder.

  2. One study of patients with OSA showed that patients more often reported fatigue, tiredness, or lack of energy than sleepiness.

    a. When patients were asked to choose 1 of these symptoms, they chose lack of energy most often.

    b. Severity of sleep apnea did not correlate with choice of symptom terminology.

  3. Since no 1 historical or physical exam finding can reliably predict OSA, several clinical decision rules have been developed, but none is widely used in clinical practice.

B. Polysomnography

  1. Records electroencephalogram, electromyelogram, ECG, heart rate, respiratory effort, airflow, and oxygen saturation during sleep

  2. Gold standard for diagnosis of OSA

  3. One study found a sensitivity of 66% for the first night study in patients who underwent 2 consecutive night studies; the sensitivity increased by 25% after the second night.

  4. The more severe the OSA, the less variability in the night-to-night polysomnogram results.

### Treatment

A. Risk factor modification

  1. Weight loss, smoking cessation, avoiding alcohol before bedtime

  2. A 10% weight loss leads to a 25% reduction in the AHI.

B. Nasal therapies (external dilator strips, internal nasal dilators, lubricants): limited data, generally not sufficient treatment

C. Continuous positive airway pressure (CPAP)

  1. Pneumatically splints the upper airway throughout the respiratory cycle

  2. The pressure must be determined during polysomnography (a "CPAP titration") and is set to eliminate, or at least reduce, apneas and hypopneas.

  3. Has been shown to reduce symptoms, and improve both hypertension and heart failure

D. Oral appliances

  1. Designed to advance the mandible, pulling the tongue forward and opening the pharyngeal airway

  2. Not consistently effective

E. Surgery

  1. Uvulopalatoplasty (UPPP)

    a. Excision of the uvula, part of the soft palate, and tonsils

    b. Significant postoperative pain and the potential for nasal reflux and voice changes

    c. < 50% of patients achieve an AHI < 10

    d. Sometimes combined with maxillomandibular advancement, which has been effective in 60% of the patients reported

  2. Laser and radiofrequency ablation of the oropharyngeal tissues not effective

  3. Tracheostomy, which is curative, is sometimes necessary for patients with severe OSA who cannot tolerate CPAP.

# Periodic Limb Movement Disorder (PLMD)

## Textbook Presentation

The patient complains of daytime sleepiness or fatigue, and the bed partner complains that the patient is very restless, even kicking the bed partner.

## Disease Highlights

A. Periodic episodes of repetitive and stereotyped limb movements occurring during non-REM sleep, generally consisting of big toe extension in combination with partial flexion of the ankle, knee, and hip.

B. The movements recur at regular intervals of 20–40 seconds and cause arousal, although the patient is usually unaware.

C. Rare in persons younger than 30 years; found in 5% of persons aged 30–50, and in 44% of persons older than 65 years.

D. Primary cause of insomnia in 17% of patients

E. Can be unmasked after successful treatment of OSA

F. Accompanied by restless leg syndrome (RLS) in 25% of patients

   1. Diagnostic criteria for RLS

      a. The urge to move the legs, accompanied by uncomfortable or unpleasant sensations, often described as "creeping" or "crawling"

      b. Worsening of symptoms when inactive

      c. Partial symptom relief with movement

      d. Presence of symptoms only in the evening or at night, or worsening of daytime symptoms in the evening

   2. Found in 2–15% of the general population, and 10–35% of patients over 65

   3. Accompanied by PLMD in 85% of cases

   4. Can be primary or secondary to iron deficiency anemia, renal failure, or peripheral neuropathy

## Evidence-Based Diagnosis

A. PLMD is diagnosed by polysomnography

B. RLS is a clinical diagnosis

## Treatment of PLMD

Effective medications include dopamine agonists (pramipexole or ropinirole) and clonazepam.

# Hypothyroidism

## Textbook Presentation

Patients with hypothyroidism commonly complain of fatigue, constipation, or cold intolerance.

## Disease Highlights

This discussion focuses on primary hypothyroidism in nonpregnant adults.

A. Epidemiology

   1. Prevalence of overt hypothyroidism is 0.1–2% (see below for a discussion of subclinical hypothyroidism)

   2. Prevalence increases with age

   3. 10 times more common in women than men

B. Etiology

   1. Primary hypothyroidism: failure of the thyroid gland to produce adequate thyroid hormone

      a. Most common cause in iodine sufficient areas is chronic autoimmune (Hashimoto) thyroiditis

         (1) Both cell-mediated and antibody-mediated destruction of the thyroid gland

         (2) Autoantibodies against thyroid peroxidase, thyroglobulin, and TSH receptor

         (3) Patients may or may not have a goiter on presentation

      b. Iodine deficiency is a common cause worldwide; patients have large goiters

      c. Thyroidectomy or radioactive iodine therapy both cause hypothyroidism

         (1) Patients with partial thyroidectomy may not need replacement but should be monitored annually

         (2) Postablative hypothyroidism develops several weeks after the radioactive iodine therapy

      d. Can develop years later in patients who have undergone external neck radiation

      e. Amiodarone and lithium commonly cause hypothyroidism

      f. Less common etiologies include infiltrative diseases, such as sarcoidosis, and thyroid agenesis

   2. Central hypothyroidism: reduction in TSH due to pituitary or hypothalamic disorder

      a. Pituitary adenoma is the most common cause

      b. Granulomatous diseases, especially sarcoidosis, can infiltrate the hypothalamus

C. Clinical manifestations

   1. Metabolic: Decreased metabolism that can lead to weight gain, cold intolerance, and increased total and LDL cholesterol (due to decreased clearance)

   2. Cardiac: Reduction in myocardial contractility and heart rate

   3. Skin: Nonpitting edema, due to accumulation of glycosaminoglycans; dry skin; coarse, fragile hair

   4. CNS: fatigue, delayed relaxation phase of the deep tendon reflexes

   5. Pulmonary: hypoventilation seen with severe hypothyroidism

   6. GI: reduced intestinal motility causes constipation

   7. Reproductive: menstrual abnormalities, reduced fertility, increased risk of miscarriage.

## Evidence-Based Diagnosis

A. The signs and symptoms of hypothyroidism all lack sensitivity and specificity.

B. The TSH is the best screening test for both primary hypothyroidism and hyperthyroidism; it is not necessary to measure thyroid hormone levels initially unless central hypothyroidism is suspected.

C. If the TSH is normal, no further testing is necessary.

D. If the TSH is elevated, the free $T_4$ or free thyroxine index (FTI) should be ordered next.

   1. Most of $T_4$ is bound to thyroxine-binding globulin and albumin.

2. The levels of these binding proteins are affected by a variety of medical conditions, thus altering the level of total $T_4$.

3. Free $T_4$ better reflects the patient's thyroid function than total $T_4$; free $T_4$ can be measured directly or can be calculated and is then called the FTI.

 To assess thyroid function, order a TSH followed by a measurement of free $T_4$; do not order a total $T_4$ ($TT_4$).

E. If the TSH is elevated, and the free $T_4$ is decreased, the patient has overt hypothyroidism and should be treated.

F. If the TSH is elevated and the free $T_4$ is normal, the patient may have subclinical hypothyroidism.

1. The TSH and free $T_4$ should be repeated to confirm the diagnosis.

2. The most common cause is chronic autoimmune (Hashimoto) thyroiditis.

3. The overall prevalence is 4–8% but is up to 20% in women over 60.

4. The progression rate to overt hypothyroidism is 2–5%/year; patients with higher levels of TSH and positive thyroid antibodies are more likely to progress.

5. It is not clear whether subclinical hypothyroidism leads to symptoms or cardiovascular consequences, and there is little or no evidence that treating subclinical hypothyroidism improves patient well being.

## Treatment

A. Overt hypothyroidism

1. All patients should be treated with levothyroxine ($T_4$).

2. The full replacement dose is 1.6 mcg/kg/day, but in older patients or those with underlying coronary disease, it is preferable to start with a lower of dose of 25–50 mcg/day.

3. Levothyroxine is best absorbed on an empty stomach, with a 40% reduction in absorption if taken with food; calcium, iron, antacids, proton pump inhibitors, and anticonvulsants also interfere with absorption.

4. The half-life of levothyroxine is 7 days, so steady state concentration is reached in about 6 weeks.

5. The TSH level should be checked 6 weeks after every dose adjustment, with the goal of increasing the dose until the TSH is within the normal range.

6. Once the dose is stable, it is sufficient to check the TSH annually.

B. Subclinical hypothyroidism

1. Experts agree that patients with a TSH > 10 mcU/mL should be treated; some experts would also treat patients with positive thyroid antibodies.

2. There is controversy regarding treating patients with mildly elevated TSH levels (< 10 mcU/mL); if the patient has symptoms consistent with hypothyroidism, it is reasonable to prescribe a several month trial of levothyroxine with monitoring of symptoms.

## REFERENCES

Devdhar M, Ousman YH, Burman KD. Hypothyroidism. Endocrinol Metab Clin North Am. 2007;36:595–615.

Neubauer DN. Insomnia. Prim Care. 2005;32:375–88.

Olson EJ, Park JG, Morgenthaler TI. Obstructive Sleep Apnea-Hypopnea Syndrome. Prim Care. 2005;32:329–59.

Pang KP, Terris DJ. Screening for obstructive sleep apnea: an evidence-based analysis. Am J Otolaryngol. 2006;27:112–18.

Sateia MJ, Nowell PD. Insomnia. Lancet. 2004;364:1959–73.

Silber MH. Chronic insomnia. N Engl J Med. 2005;353:803–10.

Surks MI, Ortiz E, Daniels DH, et al. Subclinical thyroid disease. JAMA. 2004;291:228–38.

White DP. Sleep apnea. Proc Am Thorac Soc. 2006;3:124–28.

Wolkove N, Elkholy O, Baltzan M, Palayew M. Sleep and aging: sleep disorders commonly found in older people. CMAJ. 2007;176:1299–1304.

# I have a patient with GI bleeding. How do I determine the cause?

## CHIEF COMPLAINT

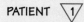

PATIENT 1

Mr. T is a 66-year-old man who arrives at the emergency department with bloody stools and dizziness. His symptoms started 2 hours ago.

 What is the differential diagnosis of GI bleeding. How would you frame the differential?

## CONSTRUCTING A DIFFERENTIAL DIAGNOSIS

The approach to GI bleeding is similar to the approach to other potentially life-threatening illnesses. Patient stabilization, specifically, hemodynamic stabilization is the first step in management. In a patient with GI bleeding, management precedes diagnosis, usually made by colonoscopy or esophagogastroduodenoscopy (EGD).

Initial management takes a very regimented course. The patient must be hemodynamically stabilized, preparation must be made in case of further bleeding, and initial diagnostic tests must be completed.

A. Hemodynamic stabilization
   1. Clinically assess volume status.
      a. Signs of shock may be seen with 30–40% volume depletion.
      b. Orthostasis can be seen with 20–25% volume depletion.
      c. Tachycardia may be present with 15% volume depletion.
   2. Calculate necessary replacement (weight in kg × 0.6 (lean body weight made up of water) × % volume depletion).
   3. Replace fluid losses initially with normal saline or Ringers solution.
   4. Administer typed (or O–) blood if there has been a large degree of blood loss.
B. Preparation for further bleeding
   1. All patients should have their blood typed and be cross-matched for at least 2 units.
   2. Patients may initially have normal Hcts that drop only with fluid replacement.

 It is common for a patient with a significant GI bleed to have a normal Hct at presentation.

3. Remember that the physical exam is insensitive for anemia (see Chapter 6, Anemia).
4. Two large bore IVs
   a. IVs should be 16 gauge or greater.
   b. Flow = $\Delta P\ (\pi r^4/8\mu)$ where $\Delta P$ is the pressure differential, r is the radius of the IV, $\mu$ is the viscosity of the fluid, and L is the length of the IV.
   c. Flow can therefore be maximized by
      (1) Increasing the pressure behind the fluid being infused (squeezing the bag).
      (2) Decreasing the length of the IV.
      (3) Increasing the gauge of the IV (the most effective as the flow goes up by the fourth power of any increase).
   d. Large gauge IVs (16 and larger) are much more effective than central lines for volume resuscitation.

 Always make sure your patient has 2 usable large bore IVs, so you do not have to worry about IV access should life-threatening bleeding develop.

   e. In large bleeds, a Foley catheter can help monitor fluid status.
C. Initial diagnostic tests
   1. CBC and platelet count
   2. Basic metabolic panel (chem-7)
   3. Liver function tests (LFTs) (Abnormal LFTs raise the risk of underlying severe liver disease and thus coagulopathy and varices.)
   4. Prothrombin time and partial thromboplastin time
   5. Upright chest radiograph
      a. Can diagnose perforated viscus
      b. May provide clues to other diagnoses
   6. Possibly nasogastric (NG) tube placement, which may help localize the source and acuity of blood loss

The differential diagnosis of GI bleeding is based on an anatomic framework. Upper GI bleeds originate proximal to the ligament of Treitz, while lower GI bleeds are distal and primarily colonic. The causes of upper and lower GI bleeding are arranged in the approximate order of frequency. Bleeding from a small bowel source is less common. The last category is anorectal bleeding. These are generally smaller bleeds with limited potential to cause hemodynamic instability.

A. Upper GI bleeds
   1. Common

    **a.** Peptic ulcer disease

    **b.** Varices

    **c.** Mallory-Weiss tear

  **2.** Less common

    **a.** Angiodysplasia

    **b.** Gastritis

    **c.** Malignancy

    **d.** Esophagitis

    **e.** Dieulafoy lesion

**B.** Lower GI bleeds

  **1.** Common

    **a.** Diverticulosis

    **b.** Malignancy or polyp

    **c.** Colitis

      **(1)** Inflammatory

      **(2)** Infectious

      **(3)** Ischemic

    **d.** Angiodysplasia

  **2.** Less common small bowel sources

    **a.** Angiodysplasia

    **b.** Ulcers

    **c.** Malignancy

    **d.** Crohn disease

    **e.** Meckel diverticulum

**C.** Anorectal bleeding

  **1.** Hemorrhoids

  **2.** Anal fissures

Mr. T was well until this morning. Abdominal cramping developed while he was eating breakfast. He did not have nausea. He went to the bathroom and passed a large bowel movement of stool mixed with blood. Afterward, he felt better and went to lie down. About 30 minutes later, he had the same sensation and this time passed what he described as "about a pint" of bright red blood. While getting up from the toilet, he became dizzy and had to sit on the bathroom floor for 15 minutes before he could crawl to the phone to dial 911.

**At this point, what is the leading hypothesis, what are the active alternatives, and is there a must not miss diagnosis? Given this differential diagnosis, what tests should be ordered?**

## PRIORITIZING THE DIFFERENTIAL DIAGNOSIS

The lack of nausea, vomiting, or abdominal pain, and the presence of bright red blood per rectum are pivotal points in this case and make a lower GI source most likely. Cramping is often seen with GI bleeds, caused by blood passing through the bowel. The volume of blood makes hemorrhoids or fissures unlikely, so bleeding from

**Table 17–1.** Diagnostic hypotheses for Mr. T.

| Diagnostic Hypotheses | Clinical Clues | Important Tests |
|---|---|---|
| **Leading Hypothesis** | | |
| Diverticular bleed | Brisk self-limited bleeds History of diverticuli | Colonoscopy |
| **Active Alternative** | | |
| Angiodysplasia | Brisk lower GI bleeds More common with end-stage renal disease | Colonoscopy or small bowel endoscopy |
| **Other Alternative** | | |
| Peptic ulcer disease | Often asymptomatic May present with epigastric pain or weight loss | Esophagogastro-duodenoscopy |
| **Active Alternative—Must Not Miss** | | |
| Colon cancer | History of anemia or changing bowel habits | Colonoscopy |

diverticuli, colitis, malignancy, or angiodysplasia have to be considered most likely. Whether he has had recent change in bowel habits, weight loss, or previous bloody stools is unknown; all these factors would heighten suspicion for colitis or malignancy. Upper sources of bleeding must also be considered. A brisk bleed from an upper source can present with bright red blood per rectum. Assuming there is no history of liver disease, peptic ulcer disease would be the most likely cause. Table 17–1 lists the differential diagnosis.

Blood is a cathartic. A brisk bleed from an upper source can present with bright red blood per rectum.

Mr. T reports no recent illness or change in bowel habits. He reports no family history of colon cancer, and he has never had a colonoscopy. He has a fifty-pack year smoking history and quit about 6 years ago. He reports drinking 2–4 beers each night.

On physical exam, Mr. T looks anxious but is otherwise well. While sitting, his BP is 120/92 mm Hg and his pulse is 100 bpm. While standing, his BP is 100/80 mm Hg and his pulse is 122 bpm. His temperature is 37.0°C and his RR is 16 breaths per minute. There is no conjunctival pallor. Lungs and heart exams are normal. There are hyperactive bowel sounds but the abdomen is soft, nontender, and with no organomegaly. Rectal exam reveals bright red blood.

**Is the clinical information sufficient to make a diagnosis? If not, what other information do you need?**

## Leading Hypothesis: Diverticular Bleed

### Textbook Presentation

The typical presentation is an episode of bright red blood per rectum in an older patient. There may be abdominal cramping but no real pain. A history of previously diagnosed diverticuli (on a screening colonoscopy, for instance) and possibly a previous, self-limited hemorrhage is often present.

### Disease Highlights

**A.** Most common cause of lower GI bleeding
  1. Prevalence of causes of GI bleeding varies from study to study.
  2. One large review gave the following data:
     **a.** Diverticulosis: 33%
     **b.** Colonic malignancy or polyp: 19%
     **c.** Inflammatory bowel disease (IBD) or ulcers: 18%
     **d.** Angiodysplasia: 8%
     **e.** Anorectal cause: 4%

**B.** The risk of diverticular hemorrhage in a patient with diverticuli is not known but is estimated to be 3–15%.

**C.** Although diverticuli are most commonly left sided, right-sided lesions seem to cause the heaviest bleeds.

**D.** Bleeding occurs as a vessel is stretched over the dome of a diverticulum. Luminal trauma likely leads to bleeding from the weakened vessel.

**E.** Spontaneous cessation and only moderate blood loss is the rule, but recurrence is common.
  1. ≈ 75% of patients experience spontaneous cessation of hemorrhage.
  2. Nearly all patients require less than 4 units of packed RBCs.
  3. ≈ 40% of patients will have recurrent bleeding.

**F.** Diverticular hemorrhage carries a poor short-term prognosis.
  1. In general, lower GI bleeding carries a better overall prognosis than upper GI bleeding with about half the mortality rate.
  2. Mortality rates for diverticular hemorrhage are higher (11% at 1 year and 20% at 4 years) although the cause of death is rarely related to the GI hemorrhage.

 Although diverticular hemorrhage seldom causes death, it is a marker for a relatively poor, short-term prognosis.

### Evidence-Based Diagnosis

The first step in making the diagnosis of any GI bleed is to determine whether the source of the bleeding is the upper or lower tract.

**A.** History
  1. Certain historical features may point to a specific diagnosis (Table 17–2).
     **a.** These features should be sought in every patient with GI bleeding.
     **b.** They are, however, only suggestive and by no means diagnostic.

**Table 17–2.** DHistorical features in the diagnosis of GI bleeding.

| Historical Feature | Suggested Diagnosis |
| --- | --- |
| NSAID use | Peptic ulcer disease |
| Severe vascular disease | Ischemic colitis |
| Pelvic radiation | Radiation colitis |
| Febrile illness | Infectious colitis |
| Aortic graft | Aortoenteric fistula (duodenal most common) |
| Liver disease or alcohol history | Esophageal varices |
| Retching preceding hematemesis | Mallory-Weiss tear |
| Recent colonic polypectomy | Post polypectomy bleeding |
| Severe constipation | Stercoral ulcer |

NSAID, nonsteroidal antiinflammatory drug.

  2. A physician's assessment of the appearance of stool is somewhat predictive of the site of bleeding (Table 17–3).
  3. Certain features suggest upper GI bleeds
     **a.** Nausea and vomiting
     **b.** Hematemesis or coffee-ground emesis
     **c.** Melena (80% sensitivity, 84% specificity; LR+ = 5.1, LR− = 0.23)
     **d.** BUN/creatinine ratio > 30 (39% sensitivity, 94% specificity; LR+ = 6.5, LR− = 0.64)
  4. Lower GI bleeds
     **a.** Hematochezia generally suggests a lower GI source of bleeding.
     **b.** 10–15% of patients with hematochezia have an upper GI source. These patients are more likely to be older and to have duodenal ulcers.
  5. Patients, as well as nurses and doctors, overestimate blood volume when seeing blood in a toilet.

**Table 17–3.** DTest characteristics of physician assessment of stool appearance.

| Physician descriptor and corresponding bleeding site | Sensitivity | Specificity | LR+ | LR− |
| --- | --- | --- | --- | --- |
| Bright red blood for lower GI bleeding | 46% | 90% | 4.6 | 0.6 |
| Black stool for upper GI bleeding | 71% | 88% | 5.92 | 0.33 |

Adapted from Zuckerman GR, Trellis DR, Sherman TM, Clouse RE. An objective measure of stool color for differentiating upper from lower gastrointestinal bleeding. *Dig Dis Sci.* 1995;40:1614–1621 with kind permission from Springer Science and Business Media.

B. Physical exam
   1. Aids in the localization of GI bleeding by identifying related diseases.
      a. Look for stigmata of chronic liver disease, cancer-related cachexia, or extraintestinal manifestations of IBD.
      b. Patients who are volume depleted, orthostatic, or hypotensive are about twice as likely to have an upper GI bleed than a lower GI bleed.
   2. An NG tube is a minimally invasive way to assess the acuity of bleeding and to help localize its source.
      a. An NG tube should usually be placed unless the patient is stable and an EGD will soon be performed or there is an obvious lower GI source.
      b. After placement, the contents of the stomach are withdrawn, and the tube is flushed until the return is clear.
      c. A bloody return, after a non-traumatic tube placement, is essentially diagnostic of an upper GI bleed (LR+ ≈ 11.0).
      d. A negative lavage does not exclude an upper GI source.
      e. The test characteristics for NG aspiration diagnosing an actively bleeding upper GI source are
         (1) Sensitivity, 79%; specificity, 55%
         (2) LR+, 1.76; LR−, 0.38

 A positive NG is diagnostic of upper GI bleeding, although not necessarily active bleeding.

C. Endoscopy
   1. In a patient with GI bleeding, EGD is usually recommended as the first procedure unless the suspicion for a lower GI bleed is very high (based on history and a negative NG tube aspirate). This recommendation is based partly on the higher potential for severe blood loss from upper GI bleeds.
   2. Colonoscopy
      a. The diagnosis of diverticular hemorrhage is usually made on colonoscopy.
      b. It is important to realize that this diagnosis is usually presumptive (87% of the time in some studies) based on seeing diverticuli and blood in that region of the colon.
      c. Less commonly, a definitive diagnosis is made when active bleeding or stigmata of recent bleeding in a diverticulum is seen.
D. Tagged RBC scan
   1. Usually uses Tc 99m-labeled RBCs.
   2. Can detect bleeds as slow as 0.1 mL/min.
   3. Most commonly used for detecting the source of bleeding in patients with persistent bleeding and normal endoscopy.
   4. Test characteristics are not very good.
      a. In a recent, representative study only 39% of patients had positive scans (sensitivity = 39%).
      b. In this study of patients who had further evaluation of their bleeding, 48% were found to have bleeding at the sight of the positive scan and 10% were found to have bleeding at a different site.

      c. Scans in patients who recently required transfusion are most likely to be positive. Those that turn positive quickly are best at localizing bleeding ≈ 95%).
E. Angiography
   1. Requires bleeding at a rate of about 0.5 mL/min to detect active bleeding.
   2. Sensitivity is about 50% but depends greatly on selection of patients.
   3. In diverticular bleeding, angiography is very useful at localizing the site of bleeding before surgery.

**Treatment**

A. Management of blood loss
   1. All GI bleeds call for similar treatment of a patient who has lost, or has the potential to lose, a significant amount of blood.
   2. Monitoring
      a. Clinically: Is there recurrent bleeding, increasing tachycardia, or orthostasis?
      b. Laboratory: Is the Hct falling?
         (1) Typically, patients have a CBC checked every 6 hours until stability has been achieved.
         (2) Intensity of monitoring varies with risk of rebleeding.
   3. Transfusion
      a. Transfusion is generally initiated when Hct < 20% or < 25% in patients with cardiopulmonary disease.
      b. In the setting of acute hemorrhage, transfusion needs to be used more liberally in order to address the expected falls in blood counts.
      c. Transfusion is recommended for blood loss of > 30% ≈ 1 L).
      d. Alternatively, it is recommended when the Hct is ≈ 24% in a patient who is actively bleeding or when Hct is ≈ 30% in a patient with cardiopulmonary disease who is actively bleeding.
      e. In general, there should be a very low threshold for giving a transfusion to a patient who is orthostatic and actively bleeding.
B. Management of diverticular hemorrhage
   1. Specific treatment is seldom necessary because most diverticular hemorrhages stop spontaneously.
   2. Endoscopic treatment, primarily clipping but also thermocoagulation or sclerotherapy, is occasionally used.
   3. Angiographic intervention, with vasoconstrictor agents or embolization, can also be used. Occasionally, local vasopressin infusion may be a temporizing measure.
C. Colectomy
   1. Curative therapy for diverticular bleeding is removal of the portion of the colon containing the diverticuli.
   2. Recommended for either persistent, large bleeds (over 4 units in 24 hours or 10 units during the course of a single bleed) or for frequent recurrences.

 The diagnosis of diverticular hemorrhage is often presumptive. Localization of the bleeding site before surgery must be as definitive as possible.

## MAKING A DIAGNOSIS

Mr. T was given 1 L of normal saline. While in the emergency department, he again passed a large amount of bright red blood.

Initial laboratory tests are normal. Important values are BUN, 12 mg/dL; creatinine, 1.1 mg/dL; Hgb, 13.9 g/dL; Hct, 39%. NG tube lavage did not reveal any blood, but there was no bilious return. The patient was admitted to the medical ICU.

Have you crossed a diagnostic threshold for the leading hypothesis, diverticular bleed? Have you ruled out the active alternatives? Do other tests need to be done to exclude the alternative diagnoses?

Mr. T weighs 75 kg. His orthostasis suggests 20% volume depletion. Given this weight, his fluid deficit is about 9 L (75 kg × 20% volume depletion × 60%). Assuming this deficit is all from the GI bleed, it is very likely that his Hct will fall once he is hydrated.

His history, normal BUN/creatinine ratio, and clear NG tube lavage are suggestive of a lower GI bleed. The patient was admitted to an ICU bed because, although he is relatively young and without comorbidities, he is orthostatic and has shown evidence of active bleeding. Following stabilization, initial endoscopy with either colonoscopy or EGD would be reasonable.

## Alternative Diagnosis: Angiodysplasia

### Textbook Presentation

Bleeding from angiodysplasia can look like any other cause of lower GI bleeding. It is seen almost exclusively in older adults and can present with anything from hematochezia to occult blood loss. In general, hemorrhage from angiodysplasia tends to be less brisk than that from diverticuli.

### Disease Highlights

A. Angiodysplasia, also called arteriovenous malformations, are dilated submucosal veins that are most commonly seen in the right colon of adults over age 60.

B. Present in < 5% of patients over age 60.

C. Most patients with angiodysplasias do not bleed.

D. Angiodysplasia has historically been associated with various other diseases (eg, aortic stenosis and cirrhosis).

1. These relationships have not been proved.

2. Angiodysplasia is a common cause of bleeding in patients with end-stage renal disease.

### Evidence-Based Diagnosis

A. Similar to the diagnosis of diverticular hemorrhage, colonoscopy, tagged RBC scan, and angiography are all used.

B. Colonoscopy is the most common tool. It allows good visualization of the cecum, which is the site of most angiodysplasias.

C. Angiography can provide evidence of a diagnosis even without active bleeding if suspicious vascular patterns are seen.

D. As in diverticular hemorrhage, the diagnosis is often presumptive, made on the basis of visualizing nonbleeding angiodysplasia in a patient with GI bleeding.

### Treatment

A. Both acute and chronic bleeding is generally treated endoscopically with thermal or laser ablation. This method can be repeated for recurrent bleeding.

B. Angiographic intervention, with vasoconstrictor agents or embolization, is rarely used.

C. Surgical management (right hemicolectomy) is sometimes required for frequent, recurrent bleeding.

D. Hormonal therapy with estrogen has been used to prevent recurrent bleeding in angiodysplasia, but a recent study suggests that this is not very effective.

E. Whenever possible, long-term antiplatelet therapy should be discontinued.

## Alternative Diagnosis: Colon Cancer

### Textbook Presentation

A typical presentation is iron deficiency anemia and constipation in a middle-aged patient. Physical exam may reveal anemia and fullness in the left lower quadrant.

### Disease Highlights

A. The most common presenting symptoms in patients with colon cancer are listed below. It should be noted that these data are from 1991. Colon cancer screening has become more widespread since this time, presumably reducing the proportion of cases that present with acute GI bleeding.

1. Acute GI bleeding: 34%

2. Abdominal pain: 22%

3. Screening: 12%

4. Anemia: 11%

5. Large bowel obstruction: 4%

B. Unlike colon cancer, colonic polyps are an unlikely cause of acute bleeding. Colonic polyps are most likely to bleed when they are removed. GI bleeding after polypectomy is not uncommon, occurring after about 1 in 200 procedures.

### Evidence-Based Diagnosis

A. Colon cancer and colonic polyps are diagnosed either by barium enema, colonoscopy, or CT colonography (virtual colonoscopy). All tests effectively detect large tumors but test characteristics vary for adenomas of around 1 cm.

1. Colonoscopy is generally considered the gold standard. Sensitivity is about 95% overall and is close to 100% for polyps > 1 cm but lower for cecal polyps.

2. Barium enema: sensitivity ≈ 50%

3. CT colonography

    a. In CT colonography, data from CT scans are used to generate displays of the interior of the colon.

    b. In a study using the most advanced techniques and experienced radiologists, CT colonography was equivalent to traditional colonoscopy in finding large polyps.

B. Definitive diagnosis is made by obtaining a biopsy specimen, usually endoscopically.

## Treatment

Surgical excision is the mainstay of treatment for colon cancer with chemotherapy indicated for those patients with more advanced disease.

## CASE RESOLUTION

Six hours and 3 L of normal saline after his initial Hct of 39%, a repeat Hct was 30%. He was given 2 units of packed RBCs. Given the clinical suspicion of a lower GI bleed, colonoscopy was done about 6 hours after admission. There were multiple left-sided diverticuli and a right-sided diverticulum with a nonbleeding visible vessel. A diagnosis of a diverticular hemorrhage was made.

Following the 2 units of packed RBCs and 3 L of normal saline, Mr. T was clinically euvolemic and his Hct stabilized at 31%. He remained in the hospital for about 48 hours during which there was no recurrent bleeding and his Hct remained stable.

## CHIEF COMPLAINT

PATIENT 2

Mr. M is a 39-year-old man who arrives at the emergency department after vomiting blood. He reports waking the morning of admission with an "upset stomach." He initially attributed this to a hangover. After about an hour he vomited "a gallon of blood" with no other stomach contents. Almost immediately afterward, he had a second episode of hematemesis and called 911.

At this point, what is the leading hypothesis, what are the active alternatives, and is there a must not miss diagnosis? Given this differential diagnosis, what tests should be ordered?

## PRIORITIZING THE DIFFERENTIAL DIAGNOSIS

Mr. M is having an upper GI bleed. The hematemesis is a pivotal point in this case and localizes the source of the bleeding to above the ligament of Treitz. Peptic ulcer disease and gastritis are the most common causes of upper GI bleeding. Although not always present, preceding symptoms of abdominal distress are common with peptic ulcer disease and gastritis. Esophageal varices should be considered in the differential diagnosis given the patient's history of alcohol use. The details of the patient's alcohol use are still unknown, so we cannot predict his risk for portal hypertension. A Mallory-Weiss tear is also possible, but the patient would report vomiting before the onset of bleeding. Table 17–4 lists the differential diagnosis.

2

On further history, the patient reports no previous episodes of GI bleeding. He reports occasional stomach upset, usually following drinking binges. He denies NSAID use. Mr. M says that he has been drinking heavily since his late teens. He drinks at least a fifth of hard liquor and a 6-pack of beer daily for the last 20 years. He reports that he has not seen a doctor since his pediatrician.

**Table 17–4.** Diagnostic hypotheses for Mr. M.

| Diagnostic Hypotheses | Clinical Clues | Important Tests |
|---|---|---|
| **Leading Hypothesis** | | |
| Peptic ulcer disease | Abdominal pain NSAID use Relationship to eating | Esophagogastroduodenoscopy (EGD) |
| **Active Alternative** | | |
| Gastritis | Often asymptomatic prior to hemorrhage | EGD |
| **Active Alternative—-Must Not Miss** | | |
| Esophageal varices | History of portal hypertension, usually due to cirrhosis Stigmata of chronic liver disease | EGD |
| **Other Alternative** | | |
| **Mallory-Weiss tear** | Hematemesis preceded by vomiting, especially with retching | EGD |

On physical exam, Mr. M is anxious and appears tired. He smells of alcohol. While sitting, his BP is 140/80 mm Hg and his pulse is 100 bpm. While standing, his BP is 100/80 mm Hg and his pulse is 130 bpm. His temperature is 37.0°C and RR is 16 breaths per minute. Sclera are slightly icteric. Lungs are clear and heart is tachycardic but regular. Abdomen is soft without hepatomegaly. There is no ascites but the spleen is palpable about 2 cm below the costal margin.

Given the alcohol history, scleral icterus, and splenomegaly, (all pivotal points) a hemorrhage from esophageal varices needs to move above peptic ulcer disease on the differential diagnosis.

Is the clinical information sufficient to make a diagnosis? If not, what other information do you need?

## Leading Hypothesis: Esophageal Variceal Hemorrhage

### Textbook Presentation

A patient with known cirrhosis presents with heavy upper GI bleeding (hematemesis or melena). There are stigmata of chronic liver disease and frequently a history of previous hemorrhages. Laboratory data demonstrate LFTs consistent with cirrhosis and thrombocytopenia.

### Disease Highlights

A. Esophageal varices are portosystemic collaterals that dilate when portal pressures exceed 12 mm Hg.

B. Although varices are the second most common cause of upper GI bleeding, they account for 80–90% of GI bleeds in patients with cirrhosis.

C. Gastroesophageal varices are present in about 50% of patients with cirrhosis.

   1. The prevalence of varices depends on the severity of the cirrhosis.

   2. The Child-Turcotte-Pugh system classifies patients based on the severity of their cirrhosis. The system takes into account the presence of encephalopathy, ascites, hyperbilirubinemia, hypoalbuminemia, and clotting deficiencies (Table 17–5).

   3. 40% of patients with Child-Turcotte-Pugh grade A disease have varices, while 85% of patients with Child-Turcotte-Pugh grade C disease have varices.

D. Approximately 33% of patients with varices will experience hemorrhage.

E. Varices may develop from cirrhosis of any cause.

F. Varices carry the worst prognosis of GI bleeds.

   1. Nearly 33% of patients die at the time of their first variceal hemorrhage.

   2. Up to 70% of survivors have recurrent bleeding in the first year.

   3. A variceal bleed carries a 32–80% 1-year mortality.

Esophageal varices are by far the most lethal type of GI bleeding.

### Evidence-Based Diagnosis

A. Of all causes of GI bleeding, varices are probably the easiest to predict. One study has the sensitivity and specificity of physicians predicting variceal hemorrhage at 82% and 96%, respectively, much better than for other diagnoses.

B. The gold standard for the diagnosis of varices is endoscopy.

### Treatment

A. Prophylactic treatment

   1. Because variceal bleeding carries such a high mortality, the goal is to predict bleeding and treat prophylactically.

   2. All patients with cirrhosis should undergo screening endoscopy every other year.

      a. Patients without splenomegaly or thrombocytopenia are at the lowest risk for having varices (≈ 4%). Endoscopy may be delayed in these patients.

      b. Patients who continue to drink, have poor liver function, and have various endoscopic markers have the highest chance of bleeding.

   3. Once diagnosed, β-blockers (usually propranolol or nadolol) and nitrates are prescribed to decrease portal pressures.

      a. Nitrates reduce portal pressure but are inferior to β-blockers in reducing rate of first bleed.

      b. Shunt procedures reduce bleeding rates at the cost of more frequent encephalopathy and higher mortality rates.

   4. Patients with the highest risk of bleeding or those who are intolerant of β-blockers should undergo band ligation of the varices.

   5. Liver transplantation is the definitive therapy.

B. Treatment of acute hemorrhage

   1. Even more than other GI bleeds, achievement of hemodynamic stability in variceal bleeds is of primary importance because the hemorrhage is potentially massive.

   2. Transfuse to a target Hct of 25–30%; overexpansion of blood volume increases portal pressure and the risk of rebleeding.

   3. IV octreotide should be given as soon as variceal hemorrhage is suspected. It achieves cessation of variceal bleeding in about 80% of patients.

   4. Endoscopic banding or sclerotherapy are done initially and if bleeding persists.

   5. Other therapies include balloon tamponade of varices and transvenous intrahepatic portosystemic shunting (TIPS).

   6. Surgical intervention is seldom called for as the mortality is extremely high.

   7. Cirrhotic patients with upper GI bleeding are at high risk for bacterial infections. Administration of norfloxacin for 7 days has been shown to decrease both the rate of bacterial infections and mortality.

***Table 17–5.*** Child-Turcotte-Pugh classification.

| Parameter | 1 point | 2 points | 3 points |
| --- | --- | --- | --- |
| Ascites | Absent | Slight | Moderate |
| Bilirubin mg/dL | ≤ 2 | 2–3 | > 3 |
| Albumin, g/dL | > 3.5 | 2.8–3.5 | < 2.8 |
| INR | < 1.7 | 1.8–2.3 | > 2.3 |
| Encephalopathy | None | Grade 1–2 | Grade 3–4 |

Grade A (well-compensated disease, 2-year survival 85%): 5–6 points
Grade B (significant functional compromise, 2-year survival 60%): 7–9 points
Grade C (decompensated disease, 2-year survival 35%): 10–15 points

## MAKING A DIAGNOSIS

NG tube lavage in the emergency department revealed bright red blood that did not clear with flushing. The patient was admitted to the ICU and received 1 L of normal saline and 2 units of O– packed RBCs. A Foley catheter was placed for close monitoring of volume status. After another large episode of hematemesis, Mr. M was intubated for airway protection. IV octreotide was begun, and the GI service was called to perform urgent endoscopy.

**Have you crossed a diagnostic threshold for the leading hypothesis, variceal hemorrhage? Have you ruled out the active alternatives? Do other tests need to be done to exclude the alternative diagnoses?**

The patient is having a large upper GI bleed and is clearly actively bleeding. Initial management is aimed at hemodynamic stabilization. The decision to place the patient in the ICU was based on his hemodynamic instability, active bleeding, and need for close monitoring. Given the alcohol history, the volume of the bleed, and the lack of previous abdominal symptoms, esophageal varices is highest on the differential diagnosis, and empiric therapy has begun with octreotide. Peptic ulcer disease is the most common cause of upper GI bleeding, and we do not yet know whether this patient has cirrhosis. Dieulafoy lesions can also cause large upper GI bleeds.

## Alternative Diagnosis: Peptic Ulcer Disease

The details of peptic ulcer disease are given in Chapter 27, Involuntary Weight Loss. This section will only deal with hemorrhage from peptic ulcers.

### Textbook Presentation

The classic presentation is a middle-aged person with chronic dyspepsia, long-term use of nonsteroidal antiinflammatory drugs (NSAIDs), or *Helicobacter pylori* infection who has an episode of hematemesis or melena, or both.

### Disease Highlights

A. Most common cause of GI bleeds.

    1. Upper GI bleeds are 4–8 times more common than lower GI bleeds.

    2. Peptic ulcer disease accounts for at least 50% of upper GI bleeds.

B. Bleeding occurs when an ulcer erodes into a vessel in the stomach or duodenal wall.

C. About 50% of patients with bleeding or perforation have had no previous symptoms.

D. Causative factors are long-term use of NSAIDs, *H pylori* infection, or stress from critical illness.

E. Similar to diverticuli, most cases are self-limited ($\approx$ 80%).

**Table 17–6.** Approximate rates for recurrent bleeding by endoscopic finding.

| Lesion | Rebleeding Rate |
|---|---|
| Actively oozing vessel | 55% |
| Nonbleeding visible vessel | 45% |
| Adherent clot | 15–35% |
| Clean based ulcer | 5% |

### Evidence-Based Diagnosis

A. Except in rare cases, all patients with GI bleeding in whom an ulcer is suspected undergo endoscopy. Endoscopy is useful from diagnostic, prognostic, and therapeutic standpoints.

B. Endoscopy has a 92% sensitivity for ulcers and allows for exclusion of malignancy as a cause of the ulcer.

C. Endoscopy is also useful because it gives information about a patient's risk of recurrent bleeding and thus enables discharge planning. Table 17–6 gives approximate rates for recurrent bleeding by endoscopic finding.

D. Other endoscopic findings associated with high-risk are ulcer size > 2 cm and arterial bleeding.

E. Clinical factors such as transfusion requirements, age, comorbid conditions, and hemodynamic stability must also be taken into account.

### Treatment

A. Hemodynamic stabilization

B. Endoscopy

    1. Early endoscopy achieves hemostasis in > 94% of patients and decreases length of hospital stay.

    2. There are many different modes of controlling bleeding endoscopically, including thermocoagulation, sclerotherapy, and argon plasma coagulation.

    3. Repeat endoscopy is effective in the 15–20% of patients who have a recurrence of bleeding.

C. Medication

    1. IV $H_2$-blockers are probably only minimally effective in treating gastric ulcers.

    2. Recent studies have demonstrated the effectiveness of IV proton pump inhibitors in treating patients with ulcers who are actively bleeding, reducing the risk of rebleeding and the need for surgery.

D. Although surgical therapy is less frequently necessary than it once was, it does still play a role for patients whose severe bleeding cannot be controlled endoscopically.

## Alternative Diagnosis: Mallory-Weiss Tear

### Textbook Presentation

Mallory-Weiss tear is typically seen in patients with vomiting of any cause in whom hematemesis develops acutely.

### Disease Highlights

A. Mallory-Weiss tears are mucosal tears at the gastroesophageal junction.

**B.** It is a common misconception that Mallory-Weiss tears always follow retching when in fact a history of retching preceding hematemesis is present in about 33% of cases.

### Evidence-Based Diagnosis

Diagnosis is routinely made on upper endoscopy.

### Treatment

Mallory-Weiss tears seldom require specific treatment. Rebleeding is quite rare.

## CASE RESOLUTION

Emergency endoscopy was performed in the ICU. Mr. M was found to have large esophageal and gastric varices. A clear bleeding source was found and treated with

banding. Although there was no clinically significant rebleeding, other complications developed. He remained intubated for 5 days for presumed aspiration pneumonia, and his recovery was delayed by alcohol withdrawal and mild encephalopathy.

During the hospitalization he was found to have Child-Turcotte-Pugh grade B cirrhosis. At the time of discharge, he was taking propranolol, isosorbide mononitrate, and lactulose. Follow-up in an outpatient alcohol program and the hepatology practice was scheduled. He did not come to any follow-up visits.

Mr. M's emergent endoscopy was indicated by the severity of the bleeding. His bleeding was controlled with a combination of medical and endoscopic management. The complicated hospital course is not surprising given the comorbid conditions frequently present in patients with varices. Mr. M had advanced cirrhosis and alcohol dependence.

## CHIEF COMPLAINT

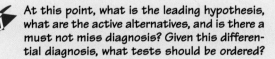

Ms. S is a 35-year-old woman who comes to the outpatient clinic for an initial visit. She is well and is without complaints. On review of systems, she notes that she occasionally passes bright red blood per rectum. This has happened about 4 times over the past 5 years. It is never associated with pain. She sometimes sees the blood on the toilet paper and sometimes in the bowl.

At this point, what is the leading hypothesis, what are the active alternatives, and is there a must not miss diagnosis? Given this differential diagnosis, what tests should be ordered?

## PRIORITIZING THE DIFFERENTIAL DIAGNOSIS

Ms. S has recurrent, lower GI bleeding that has occurred intermittently over a number of years without obvious negative health effects. This type of bleeding can be categorized as benign sounding anorectal bleeding. It is bleeding in a young patient without "red flags" for serious disease such as anemia, change in bowel habits, weight loss, or diarrhea. Between 10% and 20% of the population will have this type of bleeding. The goal is to diagnose these patients appropriately without missing occasional serious lesions and without subjecting excessive numbers of patients to unpleasant evaluation. The pivotal points in this case are the patient's young age, the small volume of blood loss, and the absence of "red flags."

The differential diagnosis includes hemorrhoidal bleeding and bleeding from anal fissures. Anal fissures are usually painful so

hemorrhoids are the more likely diagnosis in this case. IBD, especially ulcerative colitis, could cause similar symptoms, but the intermittent nature of symptoms makes IBD less likely. We need to know more about the patient's bowel habits. Diverticuli and colonic angiodysplasia could account for the patient's symptoms but would be very unusual in a patient this age. Colon or rectal cancer are also rare in this age group but should be considered. Table 17–7 lists the differential diagnosis.

**Table 17–7.** Diagnostic hypothesis for Ms. S.

| Diagnostic Hypotheses | Clinical Clues | Important Tests |
|---|---|---|
| **Leading Hypothesis** | | |
| Hemorrhoids | Painful or painless bright red blood per rectum | Anoscopy |
| **Active Alternative—Most Common** | | |
| Anal fissures | Bright red blood per rectum, often associated with severe pain | External inspection and anoscopy |
| **Active Alternative—Must Not Miss** | | |
| Ulcerative colitis | Usually associated with diarrhea | Colonoscopy |
| Colon cancer | History of anemia or changing bowel habits | Colonoscopy |

On further history Ms. S reports no recent change in bowel habits, no weight loss, and says she feels well. She does report that although the bleeding has never been associated with pain, it is sometimes associated with constipation. She has never used any treatment.

 **Is the clinical information sufficient to make a diagnosis? If not, what other information do you need?**

## Leading Hypothesis: Hemorrhoidal Bleeding

### Textbook Presentation

Hemorrhoidal bleeding typically presents with severe rectal pain and bleeding. The pain is worst with bowel movements, straining, or sitting. Occasionally, hemorrhoids can present with painless bleeding.

### Disease Highlights

A. Hemorrhoids are generally classified as internal or external.

  1. External hemorrhoids

     a. Occur below the dentate line.

     b. Present either as painless bleeding; engorged, painful, swollen perianal tissue; or with thrombosis. Thrombosed hemorrhoids are purple, extremely painful, and may bleed.

  2. Internal hemorrhoids

     a. Occur above the dentate line.

     b. Symptoms can be a feeling of internal fullness, painless bleeding, or prolapse. Prolapse is usually painful and sometimes associated with bleeding.

B. Both internal and external hemorrhoids will be most symptomatic with sitting, straining, and constipation.

 A physician should always verify a patient's self-diagnosis of hemorrhoids. Many patients refer to all perianal symptoms as hemorrhoids.

### Evidence-Based Diagnosis

A. Hemorrhoidal bleeding is diagnosed by direct observation.

  1. This may be accomplished visually in patients with external hemorrhoids.

  2. Patients with internal hemorrhoids require anoscopy to see hemorrhoids.

B. An important question is "When does benign sounding anorectal bleeding need a more extensive evaluation than an anal exam with or without anoscopy?"

  1. One study looked at 201 patients who had the complaint of rectal bleeding elicited on a review of symptoms.

     a. 24% of these patients were found to have serious disease. The diseases were polyps in 13%, colon cancer in 6.5%, and IBD in 4% of patients.

     b. Factors associated with risk of serious disease were age, short duration of bleeding, and blood mixed with stool.

     c. No cancers were found in patients younger than 50.

     d. 6 of the 37 patients who had a clear source of anorectal bleeding (fissures or hemorrhoids) also had polyps or cancer.

  2. Another study found only 10 polyps among 314 patients under 40 with rectal bleeding compared with 27 polyps and 1 case of cancer among 256 patients between the ages of 40 and 50.

C. In general, if a young patient with rectal bleeding does not have a clear anorectal source or if the bleeding continues despite treatment of the anorectal source, a more complete evaluation (with colonoscopy) should be done. Patients over 40 should always be evaluated.

 Although serious disease is rare among young people with rectal bleeding, it does occur.

### Treatment

A. Most hemorrhoids and anal fissures can be treated conservatively with general recommendations for perianal well being.

  1. Sitz baths to relax anal sphincter.

  2. Analgesia with acetaminophen, topical creams or short-term topical corticosteroids. A doughnut cushion is sometimes helpful for prolonged sitting.

  3. Soften stool with increased fluid intake, a high-fiber diet, and docusate sodium or mineral oil.

  4. Avoid anything that may lead to constipation.

  5. Avoid prolonged sitting, especially on the toilet.

B. Internal hemorrhoids that prolapse or continue to bleed usually require surgical removal.

C. Thrombosed, irreducible internal hemorrhoids and thrombosed external hemorrhoids require rapid surgical treatment.

## MAKING A DIAGNOSIS

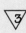

Ms. S has a normal general physical exam. External anal exam and digital rectal exam are normal. Anoscopy reveals 1 large, nonbleeding internal hemorrhoid. A CBC is normal.

 **Have you crossed a diagnostic threshold for the leading hypothesis, hemorrhoidal bleeding? Have you ruled out the active alternatives? Do other tests need to be done to exclude the alternative diagnoses?**

The patient has an internal hemorrhoid on exam. This is almost certainly, but not definitely, the cause of her bleeding. Because she is currently asymptomatic, it would be reasonable to postpone further work-up for now.

## Alternative Diagnosis: Anal Fissures

### Textbook Presentation

Patients typically have severe rectal pain with bowel movements and bright red blood on the toilet paper. On physical exam, a fissure can be found at the midline, posterior to the anal opening.

### Disease Highlights

**A.** Anal fissures occur secondary to trauma to the mucosa of the anal canal, most commonly by hard stool.

**B.** Fissures usually present as acute onset, painful defecation, usually with bleeding.

**C.** Fissures can become chronic.

   **1.** Pain causes anal sphincter spasm that, in turn, causes recurrent trauma.

   **2.** Chronic fissures can be associated with sentinel piles.

**D.** Fissures are present at the midline.

   **1.** Fissures are usually posterior in men and can be posterior or anterior in women.

   **2.** Other diagnoses, such as Crohn disease or sexually transmitted diseases, should be considered when fissures are lateral to the anal opening.

### Evidence-Based Diagnosis

**A.** Fissures are diagnosed by direct observation.

**B.** Physical exam is sometimes difficult since patients are often in pain.

### Treatment

**A.** In most cases, general supportive recommendations outlined above for the treatment of hemorrhoids will bring relief of symptoms in days to weeks.

**B.** More chronic fissures often need therapy to relax the anal sphincter.

   **1.** Topical nitrates and injected botulinum toxin are effective.

   **2.** Surgical sphincterotomy is almost always effective but carries a small risk of permanent fecal incontinence.

## CASE RESOLUTION

▽3

One year later Ms. S returns to the clinic with recurrent bleeding. Anoscopy revealed a bleeding internal hemorrhoid. Symptoms resolve with supportive care, but bleeding recurs 1 month later. Colonoscopy is performed and reveals only internal hemorrhoids. The patient declines definitive therapy and continues to experience rare episodes of hemorrhoidal bleeding.

The patient's history of recurrent bleeding is quite common. Many patients with hemorrhoids will have occasional flares. The decision to perform colonoscopy was a difficult one. Although her young age and presence of an abnormality on anoscopy makes serious disease unlikely, evaluation of any patient with recurrent rectal bleeding is appropriate.

## REVIEW OF OTHER IMPORTANT DISEASES

### Occult GI Bleeding

### Textbook Presentation

Occult GI bleeding presents in 1 of 2 ways: either in a patient with newly discovered iron deficiency anemia or in a patient with positive fecal occult blood tests.

### Disease Highlights

**A.** Generally a disease of older patients; average age in most studies is the early 60s.

**B.** Upper GI lesions cause occult GI bleeding slightly more commonly than lower GI lesions.

**C.** Common upper and lower GI tract diseases account for most causes of occult GI bleeding.

   **1.** Upper

      **a.** Esophagitis

      **b.** Peptic ulcer disease

      **c.** Gastritis or duodenitis

      **d.** Angiodysplasia

      **e.** Gastric cancer

   **2.** Lower

      **a.** Colonic adenomas

      **b.** Colonic carcinoma

      **c.** Colitis

      **d.** Angiodysplasia

**D.** Long-term aspirin, NSAID, or alcohol use is found in about 40% of patients with an upper GI tract lesion.

**E.** A small percentage of patients, $\approx$ 5%, have lesions of both the upper and lower GI tract.

### Evidence-Based Diagnosis

**A.** All patients with occult GI bleeding need evaluation of the GI tract.

**B.** All patients with iron deficiency anemia need to have cause of the iron deficiency identified.

   **1.** Iron deficiency is usually due to chronic blood loss. Rarely, it is due to poor iron intake or iron malabsorption.

   **2.** Menstrual and GI blood loss are the most common sources.

   **3.** All men, all women without menorrhagia, and all women over 50 (even those with menorrhagia) need to have an evaluation of the GI tract.

   **4.** Women under age 40 with menorrhagia do not necessarily need further GI evaluation, unless they have GI symptoms or a family history of early colon cancer.

   **5.** Women between 40 and 50 years of age with menorrhagia need to be managed carefully. They should be asked about minimal GI symptoms (celiac sprue causes iron deficiency through malabsorption and the symptoms can be easily attributed to irritable bowel syndrome). There should be a low threshold for recommending colonoscopy in this subset of patients.

**Always** determine the source of blood loss in occult GI bleeding and iron deficiency anemia.

C. Evaluation of the GI tract in patients with occult GI bleeding should be done as follows:

1. If the patient is older than 40 years or has a family history of colon cancer, evaluation should begin with colonoscopy.

2. If there are symptoms of upper GI disease, evaluation should begin with an EGD.

3. If neither of the above is true, evaluation should begin with colonoscopy.

4. If the first test is unrevealing, the other test should be done.

5. Evaluation should end after the first positive test.

6. If no diagnosis is made after both EGD and colonoscopy, most experts recommend small bowel imaging with either a radiographic small bowel follow through or video capsule endoscopy.

   a. Video capsule endoscopy appears to be more accurate than radiologic methods of imaging the small bowel.

   b. After being swallowed, the capsule transmits 2 images per second to a receiving device worn by the patient.

   c. Initial data suggest diagnostic yields of 40–80%.

## Obscure GI Bleeding

### Textbook Presentation

Obscure GI bleeding refers to GI bleeding with normal upper and lower endoscopy and small bowel evaluation by radiographic procedure or capsule endoscopy. Included in the diagnosis are patients with occult bleeding, as discussed above, who have had a normal evaluation but persistent bleeding and those patients with acute GI bleeding and an unrevealing initial evaluation.

### Disease Highlights

A. Obscure GI bleeding may be either overt or occult.

B. About 50% of the patients with obscure GI bleeding have an upper or colonic source. Peptic ulcer disease or ulcers within hiatal hernias are the most common diagnoses.

C. A small bowel source of bleeding is rare, accounting for < 5% of patients with GI bleeding.

D. In patients with a small bowel source, angiodysplasia is the most common diagnosis followed by ulcers, malignancy (accounting for about 10% of small bowel bleeding), Crohn disease, and Meckel diverticula, among others.

### Evidence-Based Diagnosis

A. A directed history may provide clues to the source of obscure GI bleeding. Ask about use of medications that can cause mucosal damage (eg, NSAIDs, bisphosphonates) as well as a history of diseases that predispose patients to GI bleeding (HIV, neurofibromatosis).

B. In patients who are actively bleeding, the first step in evaluation is usually repeat endoscopy, looking for lesions that were missed on the initial evaluation.

C. If repeated upper and lower endoscopy are negative, various means of endoscopically visualizing the small bowel may be used.

1. Enteroscopy is usually the next procedure recommended.

   a. In enteroscopy, a long endoscope (often a colonoscope) is passed orally.

   b. Visualization of 40–60 cm of jejunum is common.

   c. Diagnostic yields of 40–75% have been reported.

2. Double balloon enteroscopy, available at some centers, may improve yields by allowing visualization of the entire small bowel.

3. In rare cases, endoscopy of the small bowel can be done at the time of exploratory laparotomy. This yields diagnoses 70–90% of the time but the invasive nature limits its usefulness.

D. Meckel diverticulum scan uses a nuclear tracer that binds to parietal cells.

1. Sensitivity is between 75% and 100%.

2. Diagnosis only really considered when obscure bleeding occurs in a patient younger than 30.

### Treatment

The treatment of obscure bleeding varies by the cause of bleeding.

## REFERENCES

Cuellar RE, Gavaler JS, Alexander JA et al. Gastrointestinal tract hemorrhage. The value of a nasogastric aspirate. Arch Intern Med. 1990;150(7):1381–4.

Helfand M, Marton KI, Zimmer-Gembeck MJ, Sox HC Jr. History of visible rectal bleeding in a primary care population. Initial assessment and 10-year follow-up. JAMA. 1997;277(1):44–8.

Junquera F, Feu F, Papo M et al. A multicenter, randomized, clinical trial of hormonal therapy in the prevention of rebleeding from gastrointestinal angiodysplasia. Gastroenterology. 2001;121(5):1073–9.

Lewis JD, Shih CE, Blecker D. Endoscopy for hematochezia in patients under 50 years of age. Dig Dis Sci. 2001;46(12):2660–5.

Madhotra R, Mulcahy HE, Willner I, Reuben A. Prediction of esophageal varices in patients with cirrhosis. J Clin Gastroenterol. 2002;34(1):81–5.

McGuire HH Jr. Bleeding colonic diverticula. A reappraisal of natural history and management. Ann Surg. 1994;220(5):653–6.

Ohmann C, Thon K, Stoltzing H, Yang Q, Lorenz W. Upper gastrointestinal tract bleeding: assessing the diagnostic contributions of the history and clinical findings. Med Decis Making. 1986;6(4):208–15.

Olds GD, Cooper GS, Chak A, Sivak MV Jr, Chitale AA, Wong RC. The yield of bleeding scans in acute lower gastrointestinal hemorrhage. J Clin Gastroenterol. 2005;39(4):273–7.

Pickhardt PJ, Choi JR, Hwang I et al. Computed tomographic virtual colonoscopy to screen for colorectal neoplasia in asymptomatic adults. N Engl J Med. 2003;349(23):2191–200.

Sharara AI, Rockey DC. Gastroesophageal variceal hemorrhage. N Engl J Med. 2001;345(9):669–81.

Speights VO, Johnson MW, Stoltenberg PH, Rappaport ES, Helbert B, Riggs M. Colorectal cancer: current trends in initial clinical manifestations. South Med J. 1991;84(5):575–8.

Witting MD, Magder L, Heins AE, Mattu A, Granja CA, Baumgarten M. ED predictors of upper gastrointestinal tract bleeding in patients without hematemesis. Am J Emerg Med. 2006;24(3):280–5.

Zuckerman GR, Trellis DR, Sherman TM, Clouse RE. An objective measure of stool color for differentiating upper from lower gastrointestinal bleeding. Dig Dis Sci. 1995;40(8):1614–21.

# I have a patient with headache. How do I determine the cause?

## CHIEF COMPLAINT

## CONSTRUCTING A DIFFERENTIAL DIAGNOSIS

Headache is one of the most common physical complaints. Because less than 1% of all headaches are life-threatening, the challenge is to reassure and treat patients with benign headaches appropriately while finding the rare, life-threatening headache without excessive evaluation.

Headaches are classified as primary or secondary. Primary headaches are syndromes unto themselves rather than signs of other diseases. Although potentially disabling, they are reliably not life-threatening. Secondary headaches are symptoms of other illnesses. Unlike primary headaches, secondary headaches are potentially dangerous.

The distinction of primary and secondary headaches is useful diagnostically. Primary headaches are diagnosed clinically, sometimes using diagnostic criteria (the most commonly used are published by the International Headache Society, IHS). Traditional diagnostic studies cannot verify the diagnosis. Secondary headaches often can be definitively diagnosed by recognizing the underlying disease.

Clinically, primary and secondary headaches can be difficult to distinguish. The single most important question when developing a differential diagnosis for a headache is, "Is this headache new or old?" Chronic headaches tend to be primary, while new-onset headaches are usually secondary. This is the first and most important pivotal point in diagnosing headaches. This distinction is not perfect. There are some chronic headaches that are secondary headaches and even classic, primary headaches (such as migraines) can present as a new headache. The differentiation of old versus new also depends on how rapidly a patient brings his or her symptoms to medical attention. This being said, the following breakdown provides a clinically useful way of organizing headaches.

A. Old headaches
 1. Primary
  a. Tension headaches
  b. Migraine headaches
  c. Cluster headaches
 2. Secondary
  a. Cervical degenerative joint disease
  b. Temporomandibular joint syndrome
  c. Headaches associated with substances or their withdrawal
   (1) Caffeine
   (2) Nitrates
   (3) Analgesics (often presenting as chronic daily headaches)
   (4) Ergotamine
B. New headaches
 1. Primary
  a. Benign cough headache
  b. Benign exertional headache
  c. Headache associated with sexual activity
  d. Benign thunderclap headache
  e. Idiopathic intracranial hypertension (pseudotumor cerebri)
 2. Secondary
  a. Infectious
   (1) Upper respiratory tract infection
   (2) Sinusitis
   (3) Meningitis
  b. Vascular
   (1) Temporal arteritis
   (2) Subarachnoid hemorrhage (SAH)
   (3) Parenchymal hemorrhage
   (4) Malignant hypertension
   (5) Cavernous sinus thrombosis
  c. Space occupying lesions
   (1) Brain tumors
   (2) Subdural hematoma
  d. Medical morning headaches
   (1) Sleep disturbance
   (2) Night-time hypoglycemia

month. The headaches are so severe that he is unable to work while experiencing one. He describes them as a throbbing pain behind his right eye. (When describing the headache, he places the base of his hand over his eye with his fingers wrapping over his forehead.) The headaches are often associated with nausea and, in the last few months, he has occasionally vomited with them.

 At this point, what is the leading hypothesis, what are the active alternatives, and is there a must not miss diagnosis. Given this differential diagnosis, what tests should be ordered?

## PRIORITIZING THE DIFFERENTIAL DIAGNOSIS

The severity and chronicity of the headaches are pivotal points in this case. Although Mr. M's headaches are terribly severe, they have to be classified as old headaches since they have been occurring for years. This fact is reassuring, meaning that his headaches are most likely a primary headache. In a young healthy person with chronic headaches, migraines and tension headaches are most likely. Given the severity of the headaches, migraines are more likely than tension headaches. Given the severe, throbbing nature of the headaches, a vascular cause should at least be considered. An intracranial aneurysm could cause similar symptoms, but the chronicity makes this less likely. Table 18–1 lists the differential diagnosis.

 Severity is less important than quality in distinguishing a new headache from an old headache. A severe headache that is identical in quality to chronic headaches is less worrisome than a mild headache that is dissimilar to any previous headache.

**Table 18–1.** Diagnostic hypotheses for Mr. M.

| Diagnostic Hypotheses | Clinical Clues | Important Tests |
|---|---|---|
| **Leading Hypothesis** | | |
| Migraine headache | Moderate to severe, unilateral throbbing headache, sometimes associated with aura | Diagnostic criteria and exclusion of secondary headaches |
| **Active Alternative—Most Common** | | |
| Tension headache | Chronic, pressure-type headache of mild to moderate intensity | Diagnostic criteria and exclusion of secondary headaches |
| **Active Alternative—Must Not Miss** | | |
| Intracranial aneurysm | Acute or subacute headache Headache features are nonspecific | CT scan MR angiography or traditional angiography |

 Mr. M has used ibuprofen in the past with good response, but this is no longer working well. His past history is remarkable only for severe car-sickness as a child.

 Is the clinical information sufficient to make a diagnosis? If not what other information do you need?

## Leading Hypothesis: Migraine Headaches

### Textbook Presentation

Migraines most often first present in women in their teens or 20s. The headaches are unilateral and throbbing and are severe enough to make it impossible to do work during an attack. They are occasionally preceded by about 20 minutes of flickering lights in a visual field (aura). Patients usually find it necessary to lie in a dark, quiet room.

### Disease Highlights

A. The description of migraine headaches adopted by the IHS is, "Recurring headache disorder manifesting in attacks lasting 4–72 hours. Typical characteristics of headache are unilateral location, pulsating quality, moderate or severe intensity, aggravation by routine physical activity and association with nausea, and/or photophobia and phonophobia."

B. Migraine headaches are a chronic headache syndrome caused by a neurovascular disorder. Neural events lead to intracranial vasodilatation.

C. They may begin at any age but most commonly begin during adolescence.

D. They are 2–3 times more common in women than men.

E. Auras frequently accompany migraines.

   1. Somewhere between 33% and 75% of patients with migraines have auras. Of all people with migraine,

      a. 18% always have auras

      b. 13% sometimes have auras

      c. 8% have auras without headaches.

   2. Auras are usually visual, precede the headache, and last for about 20 minutes.

   3. Descriptions of auras

      a. Frequently, patients will initially describe a blind spot.

      b. Auras usually involve 1 portion of the visual field.

      c. Auras may vary. The frequency of some types of aura is given in Table 18–2.

      d. Scintillating scotoma often occur. These are often described as flashing lights, spots of light, zigzag lines, or squiggles.

### Evidence-Based Diagnosis

A. Migraine headaches are among the most severe of all the recurrent headache syndromes. (Cluster headaches are the other primary headache that causes severe pain.)

   1. They should be considered in any patient with headaches severe enough to be the chief complaint at a doctor visit.

**Table 18–2.** Qualities of migraine auras.

| Types of aura | Prevalence |
|---|---|
| Zigzags | 56% |
| Stars or flashes | 83% |
| Scotoma | 40% |
| Hemianopsia | 7% |
| Sensory aura | 20% |
| Aphasia | 11% |
| Motor aura | 4% |
| **Duration of aura** | **Prevalence** |
| < 30 minutes | 70% |
| 30-60 minutes | 18% |
| > 60 minutes | 7% |

2. Of initial visits for headaches in the primary care setting, 90% meet criteria for migraines.

The diagnosis of migraine headache should be seriously considered in any patient who has recurrent headaches that cause disability.

B. As with other primary headaches, diagnosis is guided by the IHS's diagnostic criteria rather than by diagnostic tests.

C. The criteria for migraines are divided into migraines with and without aura.

1. Migraine without aura

    a. A patient must have at least 5 attacks that last 4–72 hours

    b. The headache must have 2 of the following qualities:

        (1) Unilateral pain

        (2) Pulsating pain

        (3) Moderate to severe (must limit activity)

        (4) Aggravated by routine physical activity

    c. And have 1 of the following associated symptoms:

        (1) Nausea and/or vomiting

        (2) Photophobia or phonophobia

2. Migraine with aura

    a. Definition: "Recurring disorder manifesting in attacks of reversible focal neurological symptoms that usually develop gradually over 5–20 minutes and lasting less than 60 minutes." A migraine type headache usually follows the aura symptoms. Less commonly, auras can be followed by a headache that lacks migrainous features or auras can occur with no subsequent headache.

    b. A patient must have at least 2 attacks.

D. It is important to remember that diagnostic criteria, although helpful, need to be used carefully when applied to an individual patient. A patient who clearly has the disease in question may not perfectly fit the criteria. Consider these data about some of classic migraine symptoms:

1. 50% of patients with migraines have nonpulsatile headaches.

2. 40% have bilateral headaches.

Diagnostic criteria are more helpful for research than patient care. They should be used cautiously with individual patients.

E. Other less common types of migraine occur.

1. These include headaches with aura lasting longer than 60 minutes and migraine aura without a headache.

2. These syndromes are difficult to diagnose and require exclusion of other diseases (such as cerebrovascular accident, transient ischemic attack, or retinal detachment) that could cause similar symptoms.

F. Besides the diagnostic criteria, there are many other aspects of the history that are suggestive of migraine headaches.

1. A recent, systematic review suggested the mnemonic POUNDing as a diagnostic test for migraines.

    a. Is the headache **p**ulsatile?

    b. Does it last between 4 and 72 h**o**urs without medications?

    c. Is it **u**nilateral?

    d. Is there **n**ausea?

    e. Is it **d**isabling?

2. If 4 or 5 questions are answered with "Yes," the LR+ is 24, which rules in the diagnosis of migraine headache.

3. Another recent review provided test characteristics for various headache qualities in distinguishing migraines from tension headaches. Table 18–3 shows those characteristics that have at least a moderate effect on posttest probability.

**Table 18–3.** Characteristics for symptoms of migraine.

| Criteria | Sensitivity (%) | Specificity (%) | LR+ | LR– |
|---|---|---|---|---|
| Nausea | 82 | 96 | 23.2 | 0.19 |
| Photophobia | 79 | 87 | 6.0 | 0.24 |
| Phonophobia | 5.2 | 3.7 | 5.2 | 0.38 |
| Exacerbated by physical activity | 81 | 78 | 3.7 | 0.24 |
| Unilateral | 66 | 78 | 3.1 | 0.43 |
| Throbbing | 76 | 77 | 3.3 | 0.32 |
| Precipitated by chocolate | 22 | 95 | 4.6 | 0.82 |
| Precipitated by cheese | 38 | 92 | 4.9 | 0.68 |

4. When differentiating migraines from tension headaches, nausea is an important clue to migraines.

5. Interestingly, some commonly considered characteristics, such as headache duration and relationship of headache to stress, weather, menses, fatigue, and odors, were not helpful in differentiating migraines from tension headaches.

6. Presence of a family history was helpful in making the diagnosis with an LR+ of 5.0.

7. Patients with migraines are also more likely to have had vomiting attacks as children and to have suffered from motion sickness.

G. Given the severity of migraine, a common issue is when does a patient with a probable migraine need neuroimaging? The following are predictors of abnormal neuroimaging and are generally agreed upon indications for imaging in people with headaches.

    1. Abnormal neurologic exam or symptoms that are atypical for aura, especially dizziness, lack of coordination, numbness or tingling, or worsening of headache with the Valsalva maneuver

    2. Increasing frequency of headaches or a change in headache quality or pattern

    3. Headaches that awaken patients from sleep

    4. New headaches in patients over 50

    5. First headache, worst headache, or abrupt-onset headache

    6. New headache in patients with cancer, immunosuppression, or pregnancy

    7. Headache associated with loss of consciousness

    8. Headache triggered by exertion

    9. Special consideration should be given to a person who is receiving warfarin therapy.

## MAKING A DIAGNOSIS

> Mr. M's physical exam, including a detailed neurologic exam, is completely normal.

Mr. M's headaches fulfill the criteria for migraine headaches. They are pulsatile, unilateral, disabling, and associated with nausea, thus fulfilling 4 of the POUNDing criteria. The history of motion sickness provides another clue. The increasing frequency and severity of the headaches is somewhat worrisome, and neurologic imaging would be reasonable but not entirely necessary given the high positive likelihood of the POUNDing criteria.

### Treatment

A. Treatment of migraines is either abortive or prophylactic.

B. Abortive therapy

    1. Abortive therapy should be used at the very first sign of a migraine. Patients should be advised not to wait until they "are sure it is a migraine."

    2. Effective drugs are outlined in Table 18–4 with the individual considerations mainly from the consensus comments from the US Headache Consortium.

**Table 18–4.** Recommended treatments for migraine.

| Drug | Considerations |
|---|---|
| NSAIDs | First-line therapy; may be used with antiemetics |
| Acetaminophen plus aspirin plus caffeine | Another first-line therapy; may also be used with antiemetics |
| Triptans (SQ, PO, IN) | For moderate to severe migraines, combination with NSAIDS probably more effective that monotherapy |
| Dihydroergotamine (SQ, IV, IM, IN) | For moderate to severe migraines; maybe used with antiemetics |
| Antiemetics (prochlorperazine maleate or metoclopramide) | Used as adjuncts as above |
| Opioids | For moderate to severe migraine—rescue therapy. Limit use due to risk of rebound and medication overuse |
| Corticosteroids | Rescue therapy for intractable migraines |
| Butalbital plus aspirin plus caffeine | Occasional use for moderate and severe migraines |
| Acetaminophen, dichloralphenazone, and isometheptene | Occasional use for mild to moderate migraines |

IM, intramuscular; IN, intranasal; IV, intravenous; NSAIDs, nonsteroidal antiinflammatory drugs; PO, oral; SQ, subcutaneous.

C. Prophylactic therapy

    1. Prophylactic therapy is instituted when patient and doctor agree that the migraines are frequent enough, severe enough, or persistent enough to warrant regular medications.

    2. Prophylactic therapy does not need to be used every day. It can be used only around the times that migraines predictably occur (such as perimenstrually).

    3. The most effective medications are:

        a. β-Blockers

            (1) Propranolol

            (2) Timolol

        b. Divalproex

        c. Amitriptyline

 Have you crossed a diagnostic threshold for the leading hypothesis, migraine headaches? Have you ruled out the active alternatives? Do other tests need to be done to exclude the alternative diagnoses?

## Alternative Diagnosis: Tension Headaches

### Textbook Presentation

Tension headaches are the most common type of headache. They generally occur a few times each month and are described as bilateral and squeezing. They are usually relieved with over-the-counter analgesics and are seldom severe enough to cause real disability.

## Disease Highlights

A. The IHS definition of episodic tension type headache is, "Recurrent episodes of H/A lasting minutes to days. The pain is typically pressing/tightening in quality, of mild or moderate intensity, bilateral in location and does not worsen with routine physical activity. Nausea is absent, but photophobia or phonophobia may be present."

B. Most common type of headache, it is 1 of the only conditions discussed in this book that is more likely to be present than not, the 1-year prevalence of tension headaches is 63% in men and 86% in women.

C. The IHS criteria differentiate headaches as episodic or chronic and with or without associated tenderness of pericranial muscles.

D. The pathophysiology of tension headaches is still a topic of debate.

1. Episodic tension headaches are likely related to tenderness and spasm in the pericranial muscles while chronic tension headaches are related to changes in the CNS caused by the chronic pain of tension headaches.

2. There is evidence to suggest that people who suffer from more frequent tension headaches have higher levels of perceived stress and lower pain thresholds than those without headaches.

E. Tension headaches can be troublesome but are seldom disabling.

## Evidence-Based Diagnosis

A. Because tension headaches are the most common form of headaches, they are the default diagnosis in almost every patient with a mild to moderate headache syndrome.

B. A detailed history and physical exam is required to exclude other headache syndromes that require specific treatment.

C. Special attention should be given to excluding migraines.

D. The IHS diagnostic criteria for episodic tension headaches are:

1. At least 10 previous headaches

2. Duration of 30 minutes to 7 days

3. 2 of the following

   a. Pressing or tightening (nonpulsating) quality

   b. Mild to moderate in severity (inhibits but does not prevent activity)

   c. Bilateral

   d. Not aggravated by routine activity

4. No nausea or vomiting

5. Photophobia or phonophobia may be present, but not both

E. Chronic tension type headaches often develop from the more common episodic headaches. These are similar in quality but occur at least 15 days of the month.

## Treatment

A. Episodic tension headaches

1. Usually treated by patients without the input of a physician.

2. Simple analgesics (acetaminophen or nonsteroidal antiinflammatory drugs [NSAIDs]) are the basis of most treatment.

3. For more severe headaches, combinations that include caffeine or codeine can be used.

4. In patients with frequent, but still episodic tension headaches, efforts at stress reduction are helpful.

B. Chronic tension headaches

1. These are often quite difficult to treat especially if they have been caused by medication overuse.

2. Chronic tension headaches are one of the chronic daily headaches. This category includes a number of daily headache syndromes including medication overuse headaches.

3. One of the first interventions in treating chronic tension headaches should almost always be "detoxification" from the patient's regimen of pain medications.

   a. Long-term use of many headache medications has the potential to cause or exacerbate chronic tension headaches.

   b. The most common culprit medications are ergotamine, NSAIDs, caffeine, and opioids.

   c. Detoxification can be difficult and occasionally requires hospitalization.

4. While all previous medications are being withdrawn, the addition of tricyclic antidepressants (TCAs) and stress management, either alone or in combination, are effective.

   a. TCAs work faster than stress management.

   b. Even a combination of both TCAs and stress management only reduce headache frequency and severity by about 50%.

## Alternative Diagnosis: Headache due to Unruptured CNS Aneurysm

### Textbook Presentation

The classic presentation of a headache caused by a CNS aneurysm is a unilateral and throbbing headache that is new in a middle-aged patient.

### Disease Highlights

A. CNS aneurysm may present in 3 ways

1. Asymptomatic detection: This commonly occurs when a patient has a ruptured aneurysm and another, nonruptured aneurysm is found during the evaluation.

2. Acute rupture or acute expansion (discussed later in the chapter)

3. Chronic headache

B. The studies of the chronic headaches caused by unruptured aneurysms are, by their nature, somewhat flawed since they must be retrospective.

### Evidence-Based Diagnosis

A. The headaches of unruptured aneurysms are nonspecific.

1. One study looked retrospectively at the symptoms of 111 patients referred for therapy of unruptured aneurysms; 54 of the patients had symptoms referable to the aneurysm at the time of diagnosis.

2. Of the 54 patients with symptoms, 35 (65%) had chronic symptoms.

3. In 18 of these 35 patients, the chronic symptom was headache without other neurologic sign.

4. Patient's headaches were divided equally between unilateral and bilateral.

**B.** Neuroimaging

1. Contrast-enhanced CT and magnetic resonance angiography (MRA) are very sensitive means of detecting CNS aneurysms.

   **a.** Sensitivity for aneurysms > 1 cm in diameter is probably 100%.

   **b.** Sensitivity for all aneurysms is lower (62% for CT and 45% for MRI).

      **(1)** Aneurysms < 1 cm can, rarely, cause symptoms. These symptoms may include chronic headaches.

      **(2)** Repair of aneurysms < 1 cm in a patient who has not had a previous rupture is generally not recommended since the rupture rates are so low.

2. Traditional angiography

   **a.** Considered the gold standard for diagnosis

   **b.** Usually required prior to repair

   **c.** There are case reports of small aneurysms being missed on traditional angiography and being seen on CT and MRA.

**Treatment**

**A.** The treatment of CNS aneurysms can be accomplished with neurosurgical or endovascular procedures.

**B.** Management decisions are difficult in a patient with a small aneurysm and a suspicious headache because there is no definitive way to know whether the aneurysm is causing the headache prior to surgery.

## CASE RESOLUTION

Because the quality of Mr. M's headaches had not changed at all, the decision was made not to image his brain. He was given long-acting propranolol at 80 mg/d as a prophylactic medication and prescribed oral sumatriptan to be used as needed as abortive therapy. At a 1-month follow-up, the patient reported only a single mild headache for which he used ibuprofen.

The decision to forgo imaging was difficult. Although the likelihood of finding another cause of headaches was small, the patient's headaches had changed. His complete response to migraine prophylaxis is diagnostic.

## CHIEF COMPLAINT

PATIENT 2

Mrs. L is a 65-year-old woman who comes to an outpatient clinic complaining of headaches. She reports waking up almost every morning with a moderate to severe, bitemporal headache. She reports never having headaches of any consequence in the past but has been quite troubled for the last 2 months.

At this point, what is the leading hypothesis, what are the active alternatives, and is there a must not miss diagnosis? Given this differential diagnosis, what tests should be ordered?

## PRIORITIZING THE DIFFERENTIAL DIAGNOSIS

Mrs. L's headaches are of concern because she is older and the headaches are new. Her age and the acuity of the headaches are pivotal features. Both these features raise the likelihood that the headaches are secondary and, therefore, potentially dangerous. Morning headaches are classically associated with brain tumors. Edema forms around the CNS lesion while the patient is supine at night leading to headaches from increased intracranial pressure in the morning. Further history is needed, as brain tumors are most likely in patients with other types of cancer.

Morning headaches are also a fairly common symptom of many habits, diseases, and exposures. Headaches associated with substances or their withdrawals are a common cause of morning headaches. Alcohol, caffeine, and carbon monoxide are probably the most common. Other common causes of morning headaches can be grouped as "medical morning headaches." These are headaches caused by diseases that are active at night or that disturb sleep. Nighttime hypoglycemia and obstructive sleep apnea (OSA) are common causes of headaches in this category. Tension headaches should always be in the differential of headaches and may, on occasion, cause morning headaches.

The presence of a new, bitemporal headache in an older patient should raise the possibility of temporal arteritis. Although these headaches are not classically morning headaches, they should still be considered. Temporal arteritis will be discussed later in the chapter. Table 18–5 lists the differential diagnosis.

Even more than with most headaches, an extensive history is necessary in a patient with morning headaches.

Mrs. L reports otherwise feeling well. She says the headaches occur nearly every morning, irrespective of day of the week or whether she has slept at home or at her weekend house. She denies neurologic symptoms such as focal numbness, weakness, or visual disturbances. She denies snoring or excessive daytime somnolence. She read on an Internet site that new-onset, morning headaches are classic for brain tumors, and she is very nervous.

*Her medical history is notable only for noninsulin-dependent diabetes mellitus, which has always been under good control. She reports no recent change in her diet, weight, or medication. Medications are 325 mg/d of aspirin, 10 mg/d orally of atorvastatin, and 5 mg of oral glyburide taken twice daily.*

**Is the clinical information sufficient to make a diagnosis? If not, what other information do you need?**

Many patients seeking care for a headache believe they have a brain tumor. It is important to recognize this—a little definitive reassurance can go a long way.

## Leading Hypothesis: Intracranial Neoplasms

### Textbook Presentation

Brain tumors classically present with progressive morning headaches associated with focal neurologic deficits.

### Disease Highlights

A. Brain tumors are classified as metastatic, primary extra-axial, and primary intra-axial.

***Table 18–5.*** Diagnostic hypotheses for Mrs. L.

| Diagnostic Hypotheses | Clinical Clues | Important Tests |
|---|---|---|
| **Leading Hypothesis** | | |
| Brain tumor | History of malignancy Focal neurologic deficit | CNS imaging |
| **Active Alternative** | | |
| Substance exposure or withdrawal | *Caffeine:* Worst when sleeping late, often worst on vacations or weekends | Response to caffeine |
| | *Alcohol:* Occurs following intoxication | Relation only to alcohol use |
| | *Carbon monoxide poisoning:* Headache that occurs in an exposed cohort and resolves upon leaving site of exposure | Carboxyhemo-globin levels |
| **Medical morning headaches** | *Nighttime hypoglycemia:* Most common in diabetics with recent medication or diet changes. | 2 AM finger stick |
| | *Obstructive sleep apnea:* Obesity and daytime somnolence | Polysomnogram |
| Tension headaches | Chronic, pressure-type headache of mild to moderate intensity | Diagnostic criteria and exclusion of secondary headaches |

B. The relative frequency of types of tumors within each type are listed below:

1. Metastatic
   a. Lung, 37%
   b. Breast, 19%
   c. Melanoma, 16%

2. Primary extra-axial
   a. Meningioma, 80%
   b. Acoustic neuroma, 10%
   c. Pituitary adenoma, 7%

3. Primary intra-axial
   a. Glioblastoma, 47%
   b. Astrocytoma, 39%

C. Metastatic tumors are about 7 times more common than primary tumors. Thus, a patient with known malignancy and new headaches should undergo imaging.

D. Intracranial neoplasms generally present with focal signs, including seizure, or signs of increased intracranial pressure such as headache.

E. Although the presenting symptoms vary with type of tumor, the most common symptoms are:

1. Headache (about 50% of the time)
2. Seizure
3. Hemiparesis
4. Change in mental status

### Evidence-Based Diagnosis

A. History

1. The history of a patient's headache is not particularly helpful in making a diagnosis of intracranial neoplasms.

2. One very good report retrospectively studied 111 patients with brain tumors. The symptoms were nonspecific.

   a. Only 48% of patients had headaches.
   b. Only 17% had classic brain tumor headache (defined as severe, worse in the morning and associated with nausea and vomiting).
   c. 77% of patients met the criteria for tension headaches.
   d. 9% of patients had migraine-like headaches.
   e. The most common qualities were
      (1) Intermittent, 62%
      (2) Frontal, 68%
      (3) Bilateral, 72%

Brain tumor headaches are nonspecific. A patient with a new headache and a preexisting cancer that could potentially metastasize to the CNS should undergo imaging.

B. Neuroimaging

1. Contrast-enhanced CT
   a. A reasonable choice for screening patients in whom there is a low suspicion.
   b. The sensitivity of a contrast-enhanced CT for intracranial neoplasm is around 90%.

**2.** MRI with contrast is the procedure of choice for imaging brain tumors. The sensitivity of MRI is nearly 100%, and the detail provided often suggests a likely pathology.

## Treatment

**A.** The treatment of brain tumors depends on the pathology.

**B.** Importantly, patients with signs of increased intracranial pressure or seizure should be hospitalized immediately enabling both rapid diagnosis and treatment.

## MAKING A DIAGNOSIS

Mrs. L's physical exam, including a detailed neurologic exam, is normal. Laboratory tests done on the day of the visit revealed a normal CBC, normal chem-7, and a glycosylated Hgb of 5.9% (down from 7% 3 months earlier). A noncontrast head CT done on the day of the visit was normal. The patient was asked to set her alarm and check a finger-stick glucose at 2 AM. Her reading was 42 mg/dL.

Have you crossed a diagnostic threshold for the leading hypothesis, intracranial neoplasms? Have you ruled out the active alternatives? Do other tests need to be done to exclude the alternative diagnoses?

Given that intracranial neoplasms are relatively rare in patients without preexisting cancers and the presence of morning headaches is a nonspecific finding, it is unlikely that the patient has a brain tumor. The noncontrast head CT was probably a reasonable test to do. It essentially rules out a tumor and, given the patient's concern, it was an effective method of calming her.

After the negative CT and unrevealing laboratory test results, attention must be turned to possible exposures or the "medical morning headaches." The patient's marked drop in her glycosylated Hgb and early morning hypoglycemia are suggestive of a diagnosis.

## Alternative Diagnosis: Medical Morning Headaches

### Textbook Presentation

Various diseases can cause headaches that occur predominantly in the morning. The headaches are generally worst upon awakening and then improve as the day progresses. Classically, the more common symptoms of the underlying disease (daytime hypoglycemia with overly controlled diabetes mellitus or daytime somnolence with OSA) are present.

### Disease Highlights

**A.** The most rigorously defined morning headaches are those caused by disturbed sleep. The sleep disturbance can be of almost any etiology.

   **1.** Primary sleep disturbance

   **a.** OSA

   **b.** Periodic leg movement of sleep (PLMS)

   **2.** Abnormal sleep duration

   **a.** Excessive sleep

   **b.** Interrupted sleep

   **c.** Sleep deprivation

   **3.** Secondary to another disease

   **a.** Chronic pain

   **b.** Depression

**B.** Hypoglycemia that occurs while asleep or awake can cause headaches.

### Evidence-Based Diagnosis

**A.** The diagnosis of medical morning headaches depends on recognition of the underlying disease, its treatment, and the response of the presenting headache.

**B.** Recognition of the OSA and nighttime hypoglycemia can be difficult since clinical clues are nonspecific.

   **1.** Nighttime hypoglycemia should be considered in any patient treated for diabetes and morning headaches. Abnormal nocturnal glucose readings and resolution of headaches with achievement of euglycemia are diagnostic.

   **2.** Clinical predictors of OSA are poor (See Chapter 16, Fatigue). Polysomnography is diagnostic and will also provide information about PLMS and, sometimes, insomnia related to chronic pain.

A sleep study is a reasonable diagnostic test in a patient with morning headaches and no readily apparent cause.

### Treatment

The treatment of medical morning headaches depends on the cause.

**A.** Nighttime hypoglycemia: improved management of diabetes

**B.** OSA: Continuous positive airway pressure

**C.** PLMS: Carbidopa and levodopa

**D.** Pain syndromes: Improved pain control

## Alternative Diagnosis: Headaches Associated with Substances or Their Withdrawal

### Textbook Presentation

These are headaches that occur in close temporal relation to substance exposure or substance withdrawal. They resolve when culprit substance is no longer used.

### Disease Highlights

**A.** Many substances can cause headaches acutely, with long-term use, or after their withdrawal.

   **1.** Acute exposure

   **a.** Nitrites ("hot dog headache")

   **b.** MSG ("Chinese restaurant syndrome")

   **c.** Carbon monoxide

   **2.** Long-term exposure (analgesics)

   **3.** Withdrawal from acute exposure (alcohol)

**4.** Withdrawal from chronic exposure

    **a.** Caffeine

    **b.** Opioids

**B.** Of these headaches, caffeine withdrawal, hangovers, and carbon monoxide poisoning are probably the most common causes of morning headaches.

### Evidence-Based Diagnosis

**A.** Caffeine withdrawal headaches

  **1.** The IHS criteria require that:

    **a.** Patients have a headache that is bilateral or pulsating or both.

    **b.** Patients drink ≥ 200 mg of caffeine daily for > 2 weeks.

    **c.** The headaches occur within 24 hours of the last caffeine intake and are relieved within 1 hour by 100 mg of caffeine.

    **d.** That the headache resolves within 7 days of total caffeine withdrawal.

  **2.** An average cup of coffee contains about 100 mg of caffeine.

  **3.** Premium coffees may contain significantly more. A 12-oz coffee at Starbucks contains 375 mg of caffeine.

  **4.** The average adult American ingests approximately 280 mg of caffeine each day.

  **5.** Caffeine withdrawal should be suspected if headaches seem to occur when coffee intake changes, such as on weekends and during vacations.

 Caffeine withdrawal should be considered when headaches occur when patients sleep later than usual or occur mainly on weekends or vacations.

**B.** Carbon monoxide poisoning

  **1.** Presentation runs the spectrum from mild headache to headache with nausea, vomiting, and anxiety to coma and cardiovascular collapse.

  **2.** Various aspects of a patient's history increase suspicion of this diagnosis.

    **a.** A patient's headache only occurs in a single location and resolves when the patient is removed from this setting.

    **b.** Multiple family members or roommates have similar symptoms.

    **c.** Carbon monoxide poisoning is most common in the winter.

  **3.** An elevated carboxyhemoglobin level makes the diagnosis. ABG measurement and pulse oximetry do not detect carbon monoxide poisoning.

 Because carbon monoxide poisoning is potentially life-threatening, the diagnosis should be considered whenever a patient has a potentially consistent history.

### Treatment

**A.** Treatment of headaches associated with substances or their withdrawal depends on the substance.

**B.** Patients with headaches from carbon monoxide poisoning should be removed from their house while the source is repaired.

**C.** Patients with caffeine withdrawal headaches should either be weaned off caffeine or counseled on the need to continue regular use (an option generally preferred by medical students).

## CASE RESOLUTION

A tentative diagnosis of morning headaches due to nocturnal hypoglycemia was made. The patient was advised not to take the evening dose of glyburide; her headaches resolved the next day. At her next visit, the patient's medications were inspected. The label on the bottle was correct, but inspection of the pills revealed that 10-mg pills had been mistakenly dispensed, doubling her dose.

Adverse effects of medications are common. Although most commonly intrinsic to the medication, they can also be related to inappropriate prescribing or incorrect dispensing.

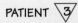

## CHIEF COMPLAINT

PATIENT

Mr. J is a 27-year-old man who arrives at his primary care physician's office complaining of a headache. He has a long history of mild tension-type headaches managed with acetaminophen. Three days ago, a severe headache suddenly developed while he was weight lifting. He describes this headache as the "worst headache of his life." The headache slowly resolved over about 2 hours. He is now feeling completely well. He has been afraid to exercise since this headache.

At this point, what is the leading hypothesis, what are the active alternatives, and is there a must not miss diagnosis? Given this differential diagnosis, what tests should be ordered?

## PRIORITIZING THE DIFFERENTIAL DIAGNOSIS

Both the acuity and severity of this headache are worrisome and pivotal. The onset during exercise is also concerning. This type of headache, one that begins at its peak intensity, is referred to as a thunderclap headache.

SAH is the leading hypothesis and must not miss diagnosis for this type of headache. His designation of the headache as the "worst headache of his life" is classic for SAH, although the resolution of the pain is not typical. Other headaches can present in similar fashion. Benign thunderclap headaches are clinically indistinguishable from SAH. Headaches due to cough, exertion, and sexual activity are primary headache syndromes that may mimic SAH. A parenchymal hemorrhage is possible but unlikely given the patient's age and absence of a history of hypertension.

There are some rare diseases that can occasionally present with a thunderclap headache; these include cerebral venous sinus thrombosis, pituitary apoplexy, carotid dissection, and spontaneous intracranial hypotension from cerebrospinal fluid (CSF) leaks. Table 18–6 lists the differential diagnosis.

Assume that a thunderclap headache is caused by a SAH until proven otherwise.

 A headache that starts abruptly and is reaches its maximal severity within seconds (a thunderclap headache) should be assumed to be caused by a subarachnoid hemorrhage until proven otherwise.

Mr. J's past medical history is notable only for mild asthma for which he uses albuterol as needed.

On physical exam, he appears well and not in any distress. His vital signs are temperature, 36.9°C; pulse, 82 bpm; BP, 112/82 mm Hg; RR, 14 breaths per minute. His neck is supple and detailed neurologic exam is also normal.

**Is the clinical information sufficient to make a diagnosis? If not, what other information do you need?**

**Table 18–6.** Diagnostic hypotheses for Mr. J.

| Diagnostic Hypotheses | Clinical Clues | Important Tests |
|---|---|---|
| **Leading Hypothesis** | | |
| Subarachnoid hemorrhage (SAH) | "Worst headache of life" Acute onset | Noncontrast head CT scan Lumbar puncture |
| **Active Alternative** | | |
| Cough, exertional, and sexual headaches | Acute headaches associated with cough, exertion, or sexual activity | History CNS imaging |
| Benign thunderclap headaches | Indistinguishable from SAH | Noncontrast head CT scan Lumbar puncture |
| Intracerebral hemorrhage | Headache with focal neurologic signs | Noncontrast head CT scan |

## Leading Hypothesis: SAH

### Textbook Presentation

A middle-aged patient experiences "the worst headache of his life." Soon after the headache begins, the patient experiences vomiting and then focal neurologic symptoms. Soon after presentation the patient loses consciousness. If the patient is alert at the time of medical assessment, focal neurologic signs and meningismus are present on the physical exam.

### Disease Highlights

A. SAH is primarily caused by rupture of a saccular aneurysm in or near the circle of Willis (≈ 85%).

B. Aneurysms are present in about 4% of the population.

C. Largest aneurysms (> 1 cm) rupture at a rate of about 0.5%/year.

D. The vast majority of ruptures occur in persons 40–65 years old.

E. SAH carries a mortality of about 50%.

F. It is generally accepted that anywhere from 10% to 50% of patients will have a warning or sentinel headache in the weeks preceding the SAH.

   1. Likely caused by expansion or a small leak from an aneurysm.

   2. This headache is usually the same sort of abrupt onset (thunderclap) headache as SAH but resolves within 24 hours.

   3. About 50% of patients with warning headaches actually seek medical care at the time of their headache.

### Evidence-Based Diagnosis

A. Pretest probability

   1. SAH accounts for 1–4% of headaches presenting to the emergency department.

   2. Among headaches presenting to the emergency department, SAH accounts for

      a. 12% of patients with the "worst headache of my life"

      b. 25% of patients with the "worst headache of my life" and neurologic findings

   3. The prevalence of the various possible symptoms of SAH vary from study to study. Some of the more common symptoms are listed below (with prevalence figures from 1 large review).

      a. Headache, 90%

      b. Stiff neck, 74%

      c. Change in mental status, 60%

      d. Stupor or coma, 27%

B. Diagnostic tests

   1. The initial diagnostic test is a noncontrast head CT. The sensitivity of this test varies with the time since the onset of symptoms.

      a. First 12 hours, 97%

      b. 12–24 hours, 93%

      c. Falls to as low as 80% after 2 weeks.

   2. Next to angiography, CSF exam for RBC and xanthochromia (the result of first oxyhemoglobin and later bilirubin) from deteriorating RBCs is the most accurate diagnostic method.

      a. RBCs are seen immediately in the CSF in 100% of patients. The specificity, however, can be limited by traumatic lumbar punctures.

   **b.** Sensitivity of RBCs begins to fall after about 24 hours.

   **c.** Spectrophotometric detection of xanthochromia is 100% specific for SAH.

   **d.** Most experts suggest delaying the lumbar puncture for 6–12 hours after the onset of a headache in a patient with a suspicious headache and negative CT scan as it takes 12–24 hours for the sensitivity to reach nearly 100%.

   **e.** The sensitivity of xanthochromia remains at 100% for over 1 week.

   **3.** In all patients with documented SAH, angiography is performed to assist in surgical planning. Angiography might also be done for patients in whom the diagnosis is unclear even after lumbar puncture.

**C.** Importance of correct diagnosis

   **1.** About 25% of patients with SAH are initially misdiagnosed.

   **2.** Patients with less severe clinical presentations are most commonly misdiagnosed.

   **3.** Patients who are initially misdiagnosed are only about half as likely to have a good or excellent outcome.

All patients in whom SAH is suspected should undergo a noncontrast head CT. Lumbar puncture should be done in a patient with a normal head CT and even only minimal suspicion of a SAH.

## Treatment

**A.** Prevention of rebleeding

   **1.** The primary treatment of a SAH is to occlude the culprit aneurysm to prevent rebleeding.

   **2.** This is usually accomplished by deploying platinum coils via arterial catheters within the aneurysm to cause occlusion.

   **3.** Neurosurgical clipping of aneurysms is now second-line therapy.

**B.** Prevention of cerebral vasospasm and resulting ischemia

   **1.** The cause of cerebral vasospasm is poorly understood but is predicted by the volume of blood lost in hemorrhage and loss of consciousness at the time of hemorrhage.

   **2.** Calcium antagonists, primarily nimodipine, decrease the risk of vasospasm.

**C.** Management of hydrocephalus

## MAKING A DIAGNOSIS

The patient had a thunderclap headache that he describes as the worst headache of his life, which mandates urgent evaluation.

Mr. J is referred from clinic for a noncontrast head CT. The results are normal.

Have you crossed a diagnostic threshold for the leading hypothesis, SAH? Have you ruled out the active alternatives? Do other tests need to be done to exclude the alternative diagnoses?

## Alternative Diagnoses: Primary Cough Headache, Primary Exertional Headache, and Headache Associated with Sexual Activity

### Textbook Presentation

These headaches are primary headaches precipitated by cough, exertion (usually involving the Valsalva maneuver), and sexual activity (peaking at orgasm). They may mimic SAH.

### Disease Highlights

**A.** Cough headaches

   **1.** Most common in men ($\approx$ 3:1)

   **2.** More common in older patients (mean age, 67)

   **3.** Last < 1 minute

**B.** Exertional headaches

   **1.** Most common in men ($\approx$ 90%)

   **2.** Occurs in young people (mean age, 24)

   **3.** Often bilateral and throbbing

   **4.** Sometimes related to migraines (some patients may induce migraines with physical activity)

   **5.** Lasts from 5 minutes to 24 hours

**C.** Sexual headaches

   **1.** Also most common in men ($\approx$ 85%)

   **2.** Mean age, 41

   **3.** Lasts < 3 hours

   **4.** Can occur as 3 types

      **a.** Dull type: dull headache worsening with sexual excitement

      **b.** Explosive type: SAH-like headache occurring at orgasm

      **c.** Postural type: postural headache developing after coitus

### Evidence-Based Diagnosis

**A.** Although these headaches may be indistinguishable from more concerning headaches, the clinical presentation can sometimes help identify the diagnosis.

**B.** They should be considered when the headache starts with cough, sexual activity, or exercise.

**C.** One review suggested other distinguishing features.

   **1.** Cough headaches

      **a.** Either represented the primary headache syndrome or symptoms of an Arnold-Chiari type I malformation in which the cerebellar tonsils protrude out of the base of the skull

      **b.** Those headaches lasting > 30 minutes were usually secondary to a Chiari type I malformation.

      **c.** Patients with Chiari type I malformations were younger than those with primary cough headaches (mean age, 39 vs 67)

   **2.** Sexual headaches

      **a.** Almost always (93%) benign

      **b.** The only sexual headache not part of the primary syndrome was a SAH.

      **c.** Patients with benign sexual headaches tended to have multiple episodes of the headache.

3. Exertional headaches

   **a.** Either represented the primary headache syndrome or secondary headache including SAH and brain tumor.

   **b.** The primary and secondary headaches were generally indistinguishable.

 Exertional headaches are clinically indistinguishable from SAH.

### Treatment

**A.** Cough headaches are effectively treated with cough suppression and NSAIDs.

**B.** Exertional headaches are treated by avoiding strenuous activity, especially in hot weather or at high altitudes or by using preexertion ergotamine, β-blockers, or NSAIDs.

**C.** Sexual headaches are effectively treated with prophylactic β-blockers.

## Alternative Diagnosis: Benign Thunderclap Headache

### Textbook Presentation

Benign thunderclap headaches present in a way indistinguishable from SAH. The diagnosis is made after normal results are obtained on CT scan and lumbar puncture. These headaches occasionally recur in an unpredictable way.

### Disease Highlights

**A.** Primary headache syndrome

**B.** Clinically indistinguishable from SAH but lacks any associated neurologic symptoms or signs.

**C.** Headaches frequently recur over 1–2 weeks and then intermittently over years.

**D.** In the best study of these headaches:

   **1.** SAH developed in none of the 71 patients studied.

   **2.** Headaches generally lasted from 8 to 72 hours.

   **3.** 51 (72%) of the patients had their headaches unrelated to cough, sexual activity, or exertion.

   **4.** 17% of the patients had recurrent, similar headaches.

### Evidence-Based Diagnosis

**A.** Benign thunderclap headaches are diagnosed when there is a suspicious clinical presentation and SAH is ruled out.

**B.** Given the poor prognosis of SAH, CT scan and lumbar puncture should be performed in all patients prior to the diagnosis.

 Because benign thunderclap headaches are clinically indistinguishable from SAH, they can only be diagnosed after SAH has been ruled out.

### Treatment

**A.** Treatment is challenging because these headaches are short-lived and very intermittent.

**B.** As-needed analgesics are probably the only reasonable therapy.

## Alternative Diagnosis: Intracerebral Hemorrhage

### Textbook Presentation

Intracerebral hemorrhage generally presents in older, hypertensive patients with acute-onset headache and focal neurologic symptoms and signs.

### Disease Highlights

**A.** Intracerebral hemorrhage accounts for about 10% of strokes, being less common than embolic and thrombotic strokes.

**B.** Hypertension is the most common cause, followed by amyloid angiopathy, saccular aneurysm rupture, and arteriovenous malformation rupture.

**C.** Among patients with hypertension, Asians and blacks have the highest risk of hemorrhagic cerebrovascular accidents.

**D.** The incidence of hypertension-related intracerebral hemorrhage has declined over the last 3 decades with better control of hypertension.

**E.** In young patients without hypertension, diseases such as arteriovenous malformation, aneurysm rupture, and drug use should be considered.

**F.** Arteriovenous malformations are present in 0.01% to 0.05% of the population and usually present in persons between the ages of 20 and 40 years.

   **1.** Presentation may be with hemorrhage, seizure, or headache.

   **2.** About 50% of patients with arteriovenous malformation will experience bleeding. Patients with hypertension or a previous hemorrhage have the highest rate of bleeding.

### Evidence-Based Diagnosis

**A.** Patients with intracerebral hemorrhage usually have headache and focal neurologic signs.

**B.** A thunderclap-type headache is the presenting sign in nearly 60% of patients.

**C.** Vomiting is present in about 50% of patients, and seizures are present in about 10%.

**D.** Noncontrast CT and MRI are equally accurate in making this diagnosis with sensitivities of nearly 100%. MRI may be better at detecting hemorrhagic transformation of ischemic strokes.

### Treatment

See the Treatment section under Cerebellar Hemorrhage in Chapter 13, Dizziness.

## CASE RESOLUTION

Given the acute-onset during exercise, the normal neurologic exam, and the lack of symptoms during the intervening 3 days, the patient was thought to have primary exertional headache. A sentinel headache, preceding an SAH, however, was thought a must not miss alternative. Given this, the patient underwent lumbar puncture that revealed no RBCs and no xanthochromia. He subsequently experienced a similar headache 2 weeks later with exercise. He was then treated with preexercise propranolol with good response.

The evaluation of this patient was reasonable. Although he was feeling well at the time of the visit, the test threshold for SAH needs to be very low given the severity of disease. SAH tends to be misdiagnosed in patients with the mildest symptoms. This is because the physician's suspicion is lowest in these patients and probably because the CT scan may be less sensitive in people with presumably small hemorrhages. Accurate diagnosis of these patients is highly desirable as they potentially have the best outcomes.

With a normal CT scan and a negative lumbar puncture, the diagnosis becomes either benign thunderclap headache or benign exertional headache. The difference is likely semantic, but the headache's onset and recurrence during exercise makes benign exertional headache the diagnosis. Intracerebral bleed from an arteriovenous malformation was a possibility but was ruled out with the normal CT scan.

## CHIEF COMPLAINT

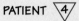

PATIENT

Mrs. T is an 80-year-old woman who comes to your office complaining of headaches for the past 3 months. She reports always having had mild headaches that never troubled her enough to see a doctor. This headache has been persistent, bilateral, band-like, and throbbing.

At her present visit, she reports no visual changes, no recent head trauma, and no neurologic deficits. She does report fatigue and says that she has lost about 15 lbs over the last month. She denies jaw symptoms.

Her past medical history is notable for hypertension for which she takes hydrochlorothiazide and a breast mass noted 2 years before. The mass was thought to be low suspicion for malignancy and the patient declined work-up.

 At this point, what is the leading hypothesis, what are the active alternatives, and is there a must not miss diagnosis? Given this differential diagnosis, what tests should be ordered?

## PRIORITIZING THE DIFFERENTIAL DIAGNOSIS

This presentation is of concern because the patient is elderly, she has a new headache, and she has experienced weight loss. The differential diagnosis must take into account these pivotal points of age, subacute onset, and constitutional symptoms. The persistence of the headache probably excludes diagnoses such as intracerebral hemorrhage or infections.

Temporal arteritis and malignancy are both possible given the patient's age and subacute presentation. The throbbing nature of the pain and weight loss could certainly be consistent with either of these types of headache. The history of a breast mass has to make metastatic disease a real consideration. Subdural hematoma is possible, but the lack of a history of head trauma makes this less likely. Although a diagnosis of tension headaches should be given with extreme caution in an elderly person with new headaches, the persistent band-like description raises this possibility. Table 18–7 lists the differential diagnosis.

4

Soon after the headache began (3 months prior to her current presentation), she went to an emergency department and cervical osteoarthritis was diagnosed. She was given ibuprofen, muscle relaxants, and a referral to a rheumatologist. She saw the rheumatologist about 2 weeks later. An ESR done at that visit was 56 mm/h.

Is the clinical information sufficient to make a diagnosis? If not, what other information do you need?

## Leading Hypothesis: Temporal Arteritis

### Textbook Presentation

Temporal arteritis classically presents in white women over age 50 as a bilateral, throbbing headache. Jaw pain and fatigue with chewing (jaw claudication) may be present. There may be a history of polymyalgia rheumatica or consistent symptoms (shoulder and hip girdle pain) and the physical exam can reveal beading and tenderness of the temporal arteries. The erythrocyte sedimentation rate (ESR) is usually elevated.

***Table 18–7.*** Diagnostic hypotheses for Mrs. T.

| Diagnostic Hypotheses | Clinical Clues | Important Tests |
|---|---|---|
| **Leading Hypothesis** | | |
| Temporal arteritis | Throbbing headache Symptoms of polymyalgia rheumatica Temporal artery abnormalities | Erythrocyte sedimentation rate (ESR) Temporal artery biopsy |
| **Active Alternative—Most Common** | | |
| Tension headache | Chronic, pressure-type headache of mild to moderate intensity | Diagnostic criteria and exclusion of secondary headaches |
| **Active Alternative** | | |
| Brain tumor | History of malignancy Focal neurologic deficit | CNS imaging |
| **Other Alternative** | | |
| Subdural hematoma | Elderly patients with a history of falls | Noncontrast head CT scan |

## Disease Highlights

**A.** Temporal (or giant cell) arteritis is a corticosteroid-responsive vasculitis of large arteries.

**B.** Primarily involves the vessels of the aortic arch, particularly the external carotid.

**C.** Affects persons over age 50, women more commonly than men.

**D.** Although the most common presentation is a new headache, temporal arteritis can present with nonspecific manifestations of a chronic inflammatory disorder.

   **1.** Fever

   **2.** Anemia

   **3.** Fatigue

   **4.** Weight loss

   **5.** Elevated ESR or C-reactive protein

**E.** It can also present with specific complications of the disease.

   **1.** Jaw claudication

   **2.** Blindness (secondary to ophthalmic artery vasculitis)

**F.** Related to polymyalgia rheumatica

   **1.** 15% of patients with polymyalgia rheumatica have temporal arteritis.

   **2.** As many as 40% of patients with temporal arteritis have polymyalgia rheumatica.

**F.** Rapid diagnosis and treatment are critical to prevent vasculitis-associated thrombosis in the effected vessels.

## Evidence-Based Diagnosis

**A.** Clinical findings

   **1.** The clinical signs and symptoms of temporal arteritis are not highly predictive.

   **2.** Two recent systematic reviews presented test characteristics for many of the commonly cited findings. These are outlined in Table 18–8.

   **3.** A few combinations of signs and symptoms have been found to have very high positive LRs.

     **a.** Headache and jaw claudication: LR+ 8.0

     **b.** Scalp tenderness and jaw claudication: LR+ 17.0

**Table 18–8.** Positive LRs for signs and symptoms of temporal arteritis.

| Symptom or Sign | LR+ |
|---|---|
| Jaw claudication | 4.2–6.7 |
| Diplopia | 3.4–3.5 |
| Beaded temporal artery | 4.6 |
| Enlarged temporal artery | 4.3 |
| Scalp tenderness | 3.0 |
| Temporal artery tenderness | 2.6 |
| Any temporal artery abnormality | 2.0 |

**4.** Reflecting the poor performance of these clinical predictors, only 30–40% of patients referred for temporal artery biopsy have the disease.

 Because the clinical signs and symptoms of temporal arteritis are not highly predictive, temporal artery biopsy should be used in any patient in whom the clinical suspicion is even moderate.

**B.** ESR has been used to "rule out" temporal arteritis.

   **1.** The sensitivity of an abnormal ESR is 96–99%.

   **2.** The test characteristics of the ESR at various cut points are shown below. (A normal ESR is usually considered to be < age/2 in men and (age + 10)/2 in women.)

     **a.** Abnormal: LR+, 1.1–1.2; LR–, 0.025-0.2

     **b.** ESR > 50 mm/h: LR+, 1.2; LR–, 0.35

     **c.** ESR > 100 mm/h: LR+, 1.9; LR–, 0.8

**C.** Temporal artery ultrasound

   **1.** Ultrasound has been used as a diagnostic tool

   **2.** Inflamed arteries have a hypoechoic halo around the lumen.

   **3.** Most studies have found this finding to be insensitive and not specific enough to avoid biopsy.

**D.** Temporal artery biopsy

   **1.** Considered the gold standard for diagnosing temporal arteritis.

   **2.** Given the difficulty of clinically diagnosing temporal arteritis and the common side effects of the treatment, temporal artery biopsy is always recommended to establish the diagnosis of temporal arteritis.

   **3.** Although biopsy should be done as quickly as possible once the disease is suspected, a short delay after beginning treatment (≈ 7 days) probably does not effect the results.

 Treatment of temporal arteritis should not be delayed to perform a biopsy in a patient in whom temporal arteritis is suspected.

   **4.** Biopsy of a palpably abnormal artery is the most accurate. If the artery is palpably normal, longer and bilateral biopsies are useful.

   **5.** There are cases of biopsy-negative temporal arteritis. One much quoted study gave the following test characteristics for temporal artery biopsy.

     **a.** Sensitivity, 85%; specificity, 100%

     **b.** LR+, ∞ LR–, 0.15

 Even in the setting of a negative temporal artery biopsy, a patient with very high suspicion for temporal arteritis should be monitored closely or treated.

## Treatment

**A.** The treatment of temporal arteritis is corticosteroids.

**B.** Corticosteroids should be started immediately in a patient in whom temporal arteritis is suspected.

**C.** Corticosteroids can be tapered slowly once there has been clinical remission as long as the inflammatory markers (ESR, C-reactive protein) remain depressed.

**D.** Methotrexate might be an option in patients who do not tolerate corticosteroid withdrawal as a steroid-sparing agent.

## MAKING A DIAGNOSIS

Physical exam is notable for vital signs of temperature, 37.1°C; BP, 130/82 mm Hg; pulse, 72 bpm; RR, 10 breaths per minute. Head and neck exam revealed bilateral cataracts with some prominence of the temporal arteries. Heart, lung, and abdominal exams were normal. Breast exam revealed a 2 x 3 cm mass in the left breast that was soft and freely mobile, which seemed unchanged from a description in the patient's chart from 2 years earlier. Extremity exam was notable for bruises over her left elbow and shoulder from a fall. Neurologic exam is fully intact.

Have you crossed a diagnostic threshold for the leading hypothesis, temporal arteritis? Have you ruled out the active alternatives? Do other tests need to be done to exclude the alternative diagnoses?

Temporal arteritis certainly remains high on the differential diagnosis. Her headache and physical exam are both suspicious. Assuming a pretest probability of 40% (the usual percentage of positive biopsies among people in whom temporal arteritis is suspected), the prominence of her temporal arteries (LR+ = 2) increases the likelihood of the diagnosis to 57%.

Both her history of falls and the breast mass (although likely benign) keep subdural hematoma and brain metastasis in the differential diagnosis.

## Alternative Diagnosis: Subdural Hematoma

### Textbook Presentation

Subdural hematoma is usually seen in older patients with a history of falls and neurologic deterioration. The classic triad of symptoms of chronic subdural hematoma is headache, somnolence, and change in mental status.

### Disease Highlights

**A.** Subdural hematomas may be acute (within 24 hours of injury), subacute (1–14 days after injury), or chronic.

**B.** Acute and subacute subdural hematomas generally pose little diagnostic problem. They usually produce evolving, focal neurologic deficits.

**C.** Chronic subdural hematomas can present with subtle symptoms, weeks to months after trauma and can pose a real diagnostic challenge.

**D.** Chronic subdural hematoma is a disease seen in the elderly and others with cerebral atrophy who can accommodate a slowly expanding mass of blood in the subdural space.

**E.** Risk factors for subdural hematomas are frequent falls, alcoholic dependence, and use of anticoagulant medications such as warfarin or aspirin.

### Evidence-Based Diagnosis

**A.** History and physical exam

1. Diagnosis requires a high index of suspicion because the presenting symptoms are often subtle.

2. The mean age at diagnosis is around 70 years in most studies.

3. The most common presenting symptoms are falls and progressive neurologic deficit.

4. Head trauma, transient neurologic deficit, seizure, and headache are also not uncommon modes of presentation.

5. The absence of a trauma history should not be particularly reassuring as this history is often hard to establish.

The most common presenting symptom of chronic subdural hematoma is a history of falls. A high index of suspicion should be present for subdural hematoma in any elderly patient with a history of falls and subacute neurologic deficits.

**B.** Neuroimaging

1. CT scan and MRI are both effective means of diagnosing chronic subdural hematoma.

2. Caution should be used with noncontrast head CT scan because the blood in a chronic subdural hematoma can sometimes be isodense with cortical tissue.

### Treatment

Chronic subdural hematomas are treated with surgical drainage unless they are small and asymptomatic.

## CASE RESOLUTION

Laboratory tests are done, and the patient is sent for a precontrast head CT to look for hemorrhage and a post-contrast study to increase the sensitivity for parenchymal lesions. The patient's test results follow: Hgb, 9.0 g/dL (11.7 g/dL 1 month earlier); Hct, 28.1% (36.6% 1 month earlier); ESR, 125 mm/h. The head CT was normal other than cerebral atrophy expected for the patient's age.

Mrs. T was given 60 mg of prednisone daily and referred for a temporal artery biopsy. This was done 3 days later and was diagnostic for temporal arteritis. Her headache improved after 1 week of therapy. Over the next 2 years, multiple attempts at weaning corticosteroids failed, and the patient continues to take 15 mg of prednisone. While taking prednisone, a spinal compression fracture, acne, diabetes mellitus, and difficult-to-control hypertension develop.

The elevated ESR made the diagnosis of temporal arteritis likely but by no means certain. Taking the pretest probability of 57%, as it stood after the physical exam, an ESR > 100 mm/h raises the probability to 72%. This is probably not high enough to accept the side effects of long-term prednisone therapy without a more definitive diagnosis.

# REVIEW OF OTHER IMPORTANT DISEASES

## Meningitis

### Textbook Presentation

Classically, meningitis presents with the acute onset of the triad of headache, fever, and a stiff neck. Meningitis may occur in the setting of a cluster of cases.

### Disease Highlights

A. The presentation of fever and headache is common and can be worrisome, potentially caused by anything from influenza to meningitis. The differential includes:

1. Viral infections and almost any other febrile illness

2. Meningitis (bacterial, fungal, viral, or parasitic)

3. Encephalitis

4. Sinusitis

5. CNS abscess

6. Septic cavernous sinus thrombosis

B. Although certainly not the most common cause of fever and headache, meningitis is a relatively common, potentially life-threatening illness.

C. Viral causes are 3–4 times more common than bacterial causes and have a generally favorable prognosis.

D. Bacterial meningitis must be treated as a medical emergency.

E. Mortality rates vary by organism but community-acquired bacterial meningitis has a mortality rate of about 25%.

F. Mortality rates are higher for hospital-acquired infections.

G. The most common organisms are listed in Table 18–9.

### Evidence-Based Diagnosis

A. A recent review studied patients in Holland in whom community-acquired bacterial meningitis was diagnosed over a 3 1/2 year time period; the prevalence of various exam features follow:

1. 95% of patients had at least 2 of the findings of headache, fever, stiff neck, or mental status changes

   a. 87% had a headache

   b. 83% had stiff neck

   c. 77% had temperature > 38.0°C

   d. 69% had a change in mental status

2. 33% had focal neurologic findings

3. 34% of those who had imaging done had an abnormal CT scan

B. Patients with suppressed immune systems and the elderly are less likely to have a stiff neck.

1. Two of the most commonly used meningeal signs are Kernig (the inability to extend the knee with a flexed hip) and Brudzinski (the demonstration of flexion of both the knees and hips upon forced flexion of the neck).

2. These signs are present in only about 60% of patients with meningitis.

C. Lumbar puncture

1. Lumbar puncture is the only means of making a definitive diagnosis.

2. The CSF in acute bacterial meningitis will demonstrate WBCs with neutrophil predominance, low glucose, and high protein.

D. Patients with contraindications to lumbar puncture

1. Frequently, the question of contraindication to lumbar puncture is raised.

2. Performing a lumbar puncture in a patient with a CNS mass, elevated intracranial pressure, or a bleeding diathesis places the patient at risk for complications such as herniation, paraspinal hemorrhage, and death.

3. CNS imaging should be performed before lumbar puncture in any patient in whom there is a suspicion of increased intracranial pressure.

4. Findings associated with mass effect on CT scan are

   a. Age > 60 years

   b. Immunocompromise

   c. Preexisting CNS disease

   d. Seizure within the previous week

   e. Abnormal level of consciousness

   f. Inability to answer 2 consecutive questions or follow 2 consecutive commands correctly

   g. Gaze palsy, abnormal visual fields, facial palsy, arm or leg drift, aphasia

 Patients with an abnormal neurologic exam should undergo CNS imaging prior to lumbar puncture.

5. If CNS imaging is required, a patient with suspected meningitis should have blood cultures drawn and then receive empiric antibiotics immediately, undergo a CT scan, and then have the lumbar puncture.

### Treatment

A. As with all infectious diseases, the specific treatment depends on the pathogen.

**Table 18–9.** Common causes of meningitis in adults.

| Organism | Characteristics |
|---|---|
| Viruses | Enteroviruses (echovirus and coxsackievirus) most common<br>More common in children than adults<br>Summer and Fall predominance |
| *Streptococcus pneumoniae* | Most common bacterial meningitis in adults of all ages<br>May occur de novo or by contiguous spread (sinuses, ears)<br>Mortality rates ≈ 30% |
| *Neisseria meningitidis* | Second most common cause overall<br>May occur in epidemics<br>Most commonly seen in young adults<br>Mortality rates ≈ 10% |
| *Listeria monocytogenes* | Disease of older adults (older than 60 years) and immunosuppressed (including patients with diabetes and alcohol abuse) |
| *Haemophilus influenzae* | Previously very common cause of meningitis in children; now rare because of vaccination |

**B.** Because of the severity of meningeal infections, empiric therapy is recommended while waiting for Gram stain and culture results.

**C.** Antibiotic treatment should be ordered when the diagnosis of meningitis is suspected and given immediately after CSF begins to be collected.

**D.** In adult patients with suspected community-acquired meningitis, the current recommendations are to treat empirically with a third-generation cephalosporin and vancomycin.

**E.** If *Listeria monocytogenes* is suspected, ampicillin is also added.

**F.** Corticosteroids should be added to the regimen in patients with a mid-range Glasgow coma scale (8-11).

## Headaches Associated with Head Trauma

### Textbook Presentation

A common presentation of a posttraumatic headache would be a middle-aged person who recently suffered head trauma, usually without detectable cranial or neurologic injury, with a headache similar in quality to tension headaches. The headaches are often associated with symptoms such as irritability or anxiety.

### Disease Highlights

**A.** Head trauma can cause serious cranial or neurologic injury including subdural, epidural or parenchymal hematoma, SAH, cerebral contusion, or depressed skull fracture.

**B.** More commonly, head trauma can cause new headaches or worsen preexisting headache syndromes.

**C.** Trauma-related headaches might occur after minor or major trauma. The IHS requires 2 of the following to qualify as major trauma:

**1.** Loss of consciousness > 30 minutes

**2.** 45 minutes of posttraumatic amnesia

**3.** Objective measures of cranial or neurologic trauma

**D.** There appears to be a significant amount of psychiatric distress and disability associated with posttraumatic headaches.

### Evidence-Based Diagnosis

**A.** Acute evaluation of head trauma

**1.** In a patient with head trauma or a headache seemingly associated with head trauma, the first goal is to identify important and potentially treatable injury.

**2.** The initial test is usually a head CT scan. A difficult question is who can be clinically cleared without a CT scan.

**a.** Two clinical decision rules (The Canadian Head CT Rule and The New Orleans Criteria) are guides to who does and does not need neuroimaging.

**b.** The New Orleans Criteria state that in patients with minor head trauma and a Glasgow Coma Scale of 15 (normal) patients with any of the following should have a head CT: headache, vomiting, age > 60, drug or alcohol intoxication, persistent anterograde amnesia, visible trauma above the clavicle, seizure.

**c.** The Canadian Head CT Rule is referenced at the end of the chapter.

**d.** Both rules have nearly 100% sensitivity for clinically important brain injuries and injuries requiring neurosurgical intervention.

**B.** Diagnosis of posttraumatic headaches

**1.** The next step is to diagnose ongoing headaches as posttraumatic.

**2.** The IHS classifies these headaches into headaches following minor or major trauma (see above) and into acute (occurs within 7 days of the injury and resolves within 3 months) or chronic (occurs within 7 days of the injury and does not resolve within 3 months).

**3.** Headache develops in about 25% of patients following minor trauma.

**a.** These headaches are most likely to be chronic.

**b.** They are also most likely to meet criteria for tension-type headaches.

### Treatment

**A.** The treatment of posttraumatic headaches is generally similar to the treatment of clinically similar headaches.

**B.** It does appear that associated psychological treatment, such as biofeedback and treatment of associated posttraumatic stress syndrome, might be beneficial.

## REFERENCES

Detsky ME, McDonald DR, Baerlocher MO, Tomlinson GA, McCrory DC, Booth CM. Does this patient with headache have a migraine or need neuroimaging? JAMA. 2006;296(10):1274–83.

Edlow JA, Caplan LR. Avoiding pitfalls in the diagnosis of subarachnoid hemorrhage. N Engl J Med. 2000;342(1):29–36.

Forsyth PA, Posner JB. Headaches in patients with brain tumors: a study of 111 patients. Neurology. 1993;43(9):1678–83.

Holroyd KA, O'Donnell FJ, Stensland M, Lipchik GL, Cordingley GE, Carlson BW. Management of chronic tension-type headache with tricyclic antidepressant medication, stress management therapy, and their combination: a randomized controlled trial. JAMA. 2001;285(17):2208–15.

Pascual J, Iglesias F, Oterino A, Vazquez-Barquero A, Berciano J. Cough, exertional, and sexual headaches: an analysis of 72 benign and symptomatic cases. Neurology. 1996;46(6):1520–4.

Raps EC, Rogers JD, Galetta SL et al. The clinical spectrum of unruptured intracranial aneurysms. Arch Neurol. 1993;50(3):265–8.

Smetana GW. The diagnostic value of historical features in primary headache syndromes: a comprehensive review. Arch Intern Med. 2000;160(18):2729–37.

Smetana GW, Shmerling RH. Does this patient have temporal arteritis? JAMA. 2002;287(1):92–101.

Snow V, Weiss K, Wall EM, Mottur-Pilson C. Pharmacologic management of acute attacks of migraine and prevention of migraine headache. Ann Intern Med. 2002;137(10):840–9.

Stiell IG, Clement CM, Rowe BH et al. Comparison of the Canadian CT Head Rule and the New Orleans Criteria in patients with minor head injury. JAMA. 2005;294(12):1511–8.

The International Classification of Headache Disorders: 2nd edition. Cephalalgia. 2004;24 Suppl 1:9–160.

van de Beek D, de Gans J, Spanjaard L, Weisfelt M, Reitsma JB, Vermeulen M. Clinical features and prognostic factors in adults with bacterial meningitis. N Engl J Med. 2004;351(18):1849–59.

van Gijn J, Kerr RS, Rinkel GJ. Subarachnoid haemorrhage. Lancet. 2007;369(9558):306–18.

Weir B. Headaches from aneurysms. Cephalalgia. 1994;14(2):79–87.

Wijdicks EF, Kerkhoff H, van Gijn J. Long-term follow-up of 71 patients with thunderclap headache mimicking subarachnoid haemorrhage. Lancet. 1988;2(8602):68–70.

Younge BR, Cook BE Jr, Bartley GB, Hodge DO, Hunder GG. Initiation of glucocorticoid therapy: before or after temporal artery biopsy? Mayo Clin Proc. 2004;79(4):483–91.

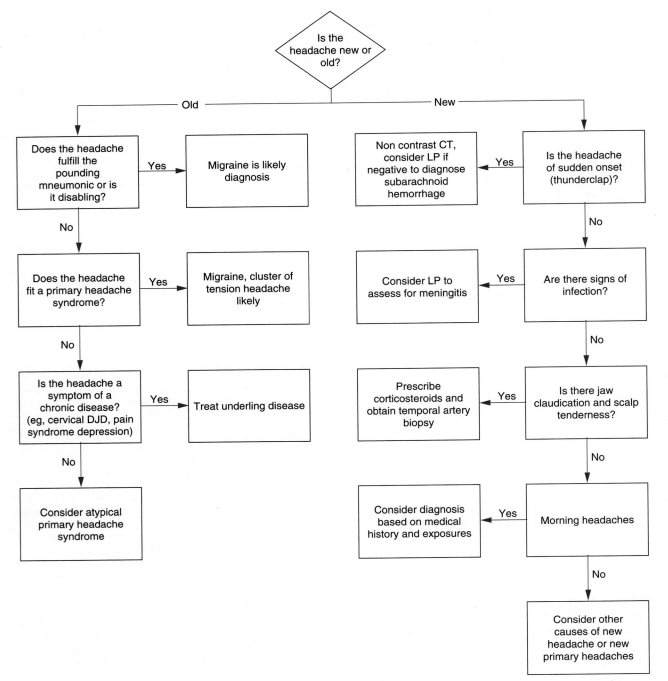

DJD, degenerative joint disease; LP, lumbar puncture; SAH, subarachnoid hemorrhage.

***Figure 18–1.*** Diagnostic approach: headache.

# I have a patient with hypercalcemia.
# How do I determine the cause?

## CHIEF COMPLAINT

PATIENT

Mrs. D is a 60-year-old, African American woman who complains of long-standing constipation. Initial laboratory evaluation reveals a normal TSH, normal electrolytes, and a calcium level of 10.8 mg/dL (nl 8.4–10.2).

**What is the differential diagnosis of hypercalcemia? How would you frame the differential?**

## CONSTRUCTING A DIFFERENTIAL DIAGNOSIS

In general, hypercalcemia is detected in 1 of 3 clinical circumstances. First, hypercalcemia may be discovered during routine laboratory work-ups in patients with no symptoms or in at-risk patients, such as those with malignancy. In fact, most cases of hypercalcemia are diagnosed in asymptomatic persons. Second, hypercalcemia may be found during evaluation of patients with certain symptoms or findings that can be related to hypercalcemia, such as constipation, weakness, fatigue, depression, nephrolithiasis, or osteopenia. Third, severe hypercalcemia may present as altered mental status.

Although most cases of hypercalcemia are due to only a handful of conditions (primary hyperparathyroidism, hypercalcemia of malignancy, renal failure, and the milk-alkali syndrome) the complete differential diagnosis is extensive. What follows is a somewhat abbreviated list organized by etiology.

A. Parathyroid hormone (PTH)–related

  1. Primary hyperparathyroidism

  2. Secondary hyperparathyroidism (due to renal insufficiency and calcium or vitamin D supplementation)

  3. Tertiary hyperparathyroidism

  4. Lithium therapy (causes hypercalcemia in about 10% of patients)

  5. Familial hypocalciuric hypercalcemia

B. Hypercalcemia of malignancy

  1. Secretion of parathyroid hormone–related protein (PTHrP)

    a. Squamous cell carcinomas

    b. Adenocarcinoma of lung, pancreas, kidney, and others

  2. Osteolytic metastasis

    a. Breast cancer

    b. Multiple myeloma

  3. Production of calcitriol (Hodgkin disease)

C. Vitamin D related

  1. Hypervitaminosis D

  2. Granulomatous diseases

D. Other relatively common causes of hypercalcemia

  1. Milk-alkali syndrome (mainly seen in patients with chronic renal failure who are taking calcium carbonate)

  2. Hyperthyroidism

  3. Thiazide diuretics

  4. Falsely elevated serum calcium (secondary to increased serum binding protein)

    a. Hyperalbuminemia

    b. Multiple myeloma

Before returning to the case, it is worthwhile to briefly review the basics of calcium metabolism. Calcium levels are dictated by the actions of PTH and calcitriol (1,25-dihydroxyvitamin D). PTH levels rise and fall in response to serum calcium levels. High levels of PTH stimulate a rise in serum calcium by increasing both renal tubular calcium reabsorption and bone resorption. PTH also stimulates the conversion of calcidiol to calcitriol in the kidneys. Calcitriol leads to a further increase in serum calcium via increased absorption of calcium in the small intestine. Phosphate metabolism is also directed by PTH and calcitriol; PTH generally lowers phosphate levels through its effects on the kidney, while calcitriol generally raises phosphate levels through its effects on the intestine and it inhibitory effects on PTH levels.

1

Mrs. D comes to your office for an initial visit. Her constipation has been long-standing and severe enough to lead to physician visits over the past 5 years. Evaluation with colonoscopy had been normal. Results of laboratory tests, drawn over the last few years by previous physicians, show normal results (including TSH), with the exception of calcium levels in the range of 11 mg/dL. Despite use of stool softeners and high-fiber supplements, she often needs laxatives to move her bowels more than once a week.

In addition to constipation, the patient's other medical problems are hypertension and tobacco use. She feels well. Her medications are atenolol and hydrochlorothiazide. Family history is notable only for hypertension in both parents. She is up-to-date on routine healthcare maintenance (mammography, colonoscopy, Pap smears) and her physical exam is unremarkable.

Following the laboratory results, she was told to stop taking the diuretic and return in 1 week to have her calcium level and BP rechecked.

At this point, what is the leading hypothesis, what are the active alternatives, and is there a must not miss diagnosis? Given this differential diagnosis, what tests should be ordered?

## PRIORITIZING THE DIFFERENTIAL DIAGNOSIS

In healthy ambulatory patients with hypercalcemia, primary hyperparathyroidism is, by far, the leading cause. This disease is common and often asymptomatic or minimally symptomatic. The chronicity of this patient's hypercalcemia, as well as her relatively good health, are pivotal points that make this diagnosis even more likely. Hypercalcemia related to thiazide use is also possible. Although thiazide diuretics generally cause chronic hypercalcemia in patients with other abnormalities in calcium metabolism, they occasionally do cause mild hypercalcemia in patients with no other cause. Familial hypocalciuric hypercalcemia (FHH) is another cause of chronic, usually asymptomatic hypercalcemia. Although it is most usually diagnosed early in life, it can present similarly to primary hyperparathyroidism. Most patients with hypercalcemia due to a malignancy have already been given a diagnosis of cancer when they seek care for hypercalcemia. Sarcoidosis is not a common cause of hypercalcemia but should probably be considered, given the patient's race, if another diagnosis is not made. Table 19–1 lists the differential diagnosis.

 After the thiazide diuretic is discontinued, the calcium level is remeasured and remains unchanged. A PTH level is drawn.

 Is the clinical information sufficient to make a diagnosis? If not, what other information do you need?

## Leading Hypothesis: Primary Hyperparathyroidism

### Textbook Presentation

Primary hyperparathyroidism usually presents with hypercalcemia found during routine laboratory screening. Occasionally, it is detected during the evaluation of nonspecific symptoms, such as fatigue or constipation.

### Disease Highlights

A. Primary hyperparathyroidism most commonly presents with a modestly elevated calcium and few (if any) symptoms rather than the classic presentation of "stones, bones, groans, and psychiatric overtones."

 Primary hyperparathyroidism accounts for more than 90% of cases of hypercalcemia in otherwise healthy ambulatory patients.

**Table 19–1.** Diagnostic hypotheses for Mrs. D.

| Diagnostic Hypotheses | Clinical Clues | Important Tests |
|---|---|---|
| **Leading Hypothesis** | | |
| Primary hyperparathyroidism | Elevated calcium without evident underlying disease | PTH level |
| **Active Alternatives** | | |
| Familial hypocalciuric hypercalcemia | Chronic asymptomatic hypercalcemia | PTH level Family history Urine calcium excretion |
| Thiazide diuretic use | Transient hypercalcemia or exacerbation of hypercalcemia in patient with underlying disease | Resolution with cessation of drug |
| **Active Alternative—Must Not Miss** | | |
| Hypercalcemia of malignancy | Usually presents in patients with known malignancy | Diagnosis of malignancy Demonstration of PTHrP or skeletal metastasis |
| **Other Alternative** | | |
| Sarcoidosis | Pulmonary disease with hilar lymphadenopathy or interstitial lung disease | Demonstration of noncaseating granulomas and exclusion of known causes of granulomatous disease |

B. Etiology of primary hyperparathyroidism
   1. 85% of the cases of primary hyperparathyroidism are due to solitary parathyroid adenomas.
   2. Parathyroid hyperplasia, multiple adenomas, and the rare carcinoma cause the other 15% of cases.
      a. Parathyroid hyperplasia can be sporadic or inherited.
      b. Inherited syndromes of parathyroid hyperplasia include the multiple endocrine neoplasia (MEN) type I and IIA syndromes. Patients with other relevant diagnoses such as pituitary tumors, islet cell tumors, medullary thyroid carcinomas and pheochromocytomas should be evaluated for these syndromes.

C. Clinical manifestations of primary hyperparathyroidism
   1. Nonspecific symptoms such as fatigue, irritability, and weakness are more common among patients with primary hyperparathyroidism.
   2. Decreased bone density is common in patients with primary hyperparathyroidism while classic osteitis fibrosis cystica is exceedingly rare today.
   3. Nephrolithiasis is present in 15–20% of patients with primary hyperparathyroidism.

**4.** Other symptoms of primary hyperparathyroidism probably include increased frequency of hypertension, gout, and calcium pyrophosphate deposition disease.

## Evidence-Based Diagnosis

**A.** Hypercalcemia should be confirmed before evaluating a patient for primary hyperparathyroidism.

   **1.** The calcium level should be remeasured.

   **2.** Albumin or ionized calcium should be measured to account for plasma protein binding. If albumin is measured, then the corrected calcium = calcium (mg/dL) + 0.8(4-albumin (g/dL)).

**B.** Other effects of elevated PTH levels (hypercalciuria, hypophosphatemia, hyperphosphaturia) are seldom useful in differentiating primary hyperparathyroidism from hypercalcemia of malignancy—the second most common cause of hypercalcemia.

**C.** The diagnosis of primary hyperparathyroidism is usually straightforward.

   **1.** The diagnosis is extremely likely in an otherwise healthy patient with chronic hypercalcemia.

   **2.** An elevated PTH level is confirmatory, distinguishing primary hyperparathyroidism from hypercalcemia of malignancy which has low serum PTH levels.

   **3.** About 10% of patients with primary hyperparathyroidism have normal PTH levels (a finding that is in fact inappropriate give the hypercalcemia). In these patients, FHH must be excluded.

## Treatment

**A.** Definitive treatment for primary hyperparathyroidism is surgical parathyroidectomy.

**B.** Who needs surgery?

   **1.** Because of the generally benign course of primary hyperparathyroidism, not everyone needs surgery.

   **2.** Recommendations from consensus panels are based on who is most likely to progress to symptomatic disease and who would benefit most from surgery.

   **3.** Indications for surgery

   **a.** Symptoms of hypercalcemia

   **b.** Elevated serum calcium > 1 mg/dL above normal

   **c.** Creatinine clearance reduction of 30% compared with age-matched controls.

   **d.** 24-hour urine calcium > 400 mg/d (nl < 150 mg/d)

   **e.** Bone density with T score < 2.5 at any site.

   **f.** Age younger than 50

   **g.** Patient preference or patient inability to comply with long-term monitoring

**C.** Monitoring (for patients not undergoing surgery)

   **1.** Assessment of symptoms, calcium level, and renal function every 6–12 months.

   **2.** Bone density screening yearly of the hip, spine, and wrist.

   **3.** Monitoring, possibly radiographically, for development of nephrolithiasis

**D.** This approach to deciding which patients undergo surgery appears to be effective. A recent study observing 52 asymptomatic people for up to 10 years demonstrated the disease is usually not progressive.

   **1.** 38 (73%) had no progression of disease

   **2.** Patients who required surgery did so for the following reasons:

   **a.** Hypercalcemia developed in 2 patients

   **b.** Hypercalciuria developed in 8 patients

   **c.** Low bone density developed in 6 patients

**E.** Parathyroidectomy

   **1.** Parathyroidectomy is markedly effective at inducing normocalcemia (95–98%), improving bone density (100%), and improving symptoms (82%).

   **2.** Preoperative nuclear imaging of the parathyroid glands is very helpful in identifying abnormal glands, thus decreasing the need for detailed neck exploration. The data below is for the identification of abnormal glands.

   **a.** Sensitivity, 69%; specificity, 98%

   **b.** LR+, 34.5; LR−, 0.32

   **3.** Intraoperative PTH assays also serve to improve the surgical success rates.

## MAKING A DIAGNOSIS

Final laboratory test results for Mrs. D follow:

Calcium: 10.9 mg/dL

Inorganic phosphate: 3.3 mg/dL (nl 2.5–4.4)

Ionized calcium: 6.20 mg/dL (nl 4.60–5.40)

PTH: 166 pg/mL (nl < 60 pg/mL)

*A diagnosis of primary hyperparathyroidism was made.*

**Have you crossed a diagnostic threshold for the leading hypothesis, primary hyperparathyroidism? Have you ruled out the active alternatives? Do other tests need to be done to exclude the alternative diagnoses?**

Other than primary hyperparathyroidism, the differential diagnosis of hypercalcemia in a patient with an elevated PTH is lithium use, MEN syndromes, secondary or tertiary hyperparathyroidism, or familial hypocalciuric hypercalcemia. Given the patient's medications, normal renal function, age at presentation, and lack of a family history of hypercalcemia, primary hyperparathyroidism is clearly the most likely diagnosis. FHH would remain a possibility if not for the markedly elevated PTH level. Thiazides diuretics do not cause hypercalcemia via hyperparathyroidism and thus cannot fully explain the patient's hypercalcemia. It could have been a contributing factor in the initial presentation.

## Alternative Diagnosis: Familial Hypocalciuric Hypercalcemia (FHH)

### Textbook Presentation

The diagnosis of FHH is usually made in childhood during evaluation of asymptomatic hypercalcemia or during screening because of a positive family history. The condition may also present during adulthood as hypercalcemia with a normal to slightly elevated PTH.

## Disease Highlights

A. The mutation in FHH makes the calcium sensing receptor, found on various tissues throughout the body, less sensitive to calcium. In the parathyroid glands, this means that higher serum calcium levels are needed to suppress PTH release. The defect leads to:

1. Secretion of PTH inappropriate to calcium levels

2. Renal absorption of calcium inappropriate to calcium levels

B. Most patients with FHH are asymptomatic at the time of presentation.

## Evidence-Based Diagnosis

A. FHH is usually easily distinguished from primary hyperparathyroidism as the former usually has mildly elevated calcium levels and a normal PTH level while the latter has an elevated PTH level.

B. Differentiation can be difficult because patients with FHH sometimes have a mildly elevated PTH, and patients with primary hyperparathyroidism often have mild hypercalcemia and have a normal PTH 10% of the time.

C. Three important distinguishing features are:

1. Patients with FHH usually have family members with FHH. The genetic defect is inherited in an autosomal dominant manner.

2. Urinary calcium excretion is reduced (> 99% reabsorption vs < 99% in primary hyperparathyroidism).

   a. A urinary calcium < 200 mg/day suggests FHH.

   b. A fractional excretion of calcium < 0.01 is nearly diagnostic of FHH. Patients with primary hyperparathyroidism usually have results > 0.02. (Fractional excretion of calcium = (urine calcium × serum creatinine)/(serum calcium × urine creatinine)

3. Serum magnesium is often increased in FHH.

4. Genetic testing is available when the diagnosis is difficult to make.

## Treatment

Treatment for FHH is not necessary because the hypercalcemia is mild and only very rarely leads to complications.

## Alternative Diagnosis: Thiazide-Induced Hypercalcemia

### Textbook Presentation

Thiazide-induced hypercalcemia usually occurs transiently after starting a thiazide diuretic. It is generally mild and is not associated with hyperparathyroidism.

### Disease Highlights

A. Thiazide diuretics have hypocalciuric effects.

1. Sodium depletion causes increased sodium and calcium retention in the proximal tubule.

2. Thiazides probably also augment the effect of PTH.

B. Hypercalcemia is generally mild and should be short lived, because reduced PTH secretion will normalize calcium levels.

C. Some patients may have persistently, although still only mildly, elevated calcium levels.

D. Patients with underlying hyperparathyroidism, or other causes of increased bone turnover, are more likely to have persistent and more pronounced degrees of hypercalcemia.

## Evidence-Based Diagnosis

A. The diagnosis of thiazide-induced hypercalcemia depends on documenting hypercalcemia temporally related to beginning a diuretic.

B. Resolution of the abnormality with cessation of the drug is diagnostic.

C. Patients with more than mild (≅ 0–.5 mg/dL), persistent elevations of calcium while taking a thiazide should be evaluated for other causes of hypercalcemia, as should patients with thiazide-related hypercalcemia who also have an elevated PTH.

## Treatment

A. Because the hypercalcemia is almost always mild and short lived, no treatment is necessary.

B. If the patient has persistent hypercalcemia, evaluate him or her for other causes of hypercalcemia and consider discontinuing the thiazide.

## CASE RESOLUTION

The combination of hypercalcemia and an elevated PTH confirms the diagnosis of primary hyperparathyroidism. Based on the patient's severe constipation, without another cause, the decision was made to treat her hyperparathyroidism. She underwent nuclear scanning of the parathyroid glands and results were normal. Surgical exploration of the neck was performed. A 3 × 3 cm, 4-gram, parathyroid adenoma was found and surgically removed without complication.

On follow-up, the patient had rapid normalization of her calcium levels. Her constipation, however, persisted. In the end, the constipation was considered to be functional and unrelated to the hypercalcemia.

As discussed above, the patient's symptoms are an indication for surgery. However, since the patient's symptoms were nonspecific, they failed to improve after surgery, which is not uncommon. The reported sensitivity of nuclear imaging of the neck for parathyroid adenomas is < 70%, so it is not surprising that the scan was normal.

# CHIEF COMPLAINT

Mrs. W is an 80-year-old woman who is admitted to the hospital from her doctor's office because of lethargy, abdominal pain, and hypercalcemia. She complained to her doctor of 1 year of epigastric pain. The pain had been mild but had become severe and persistent over the last 6 weeks. Her daughter, who found her somewhat confused at their weekly lunch, brought her to the office.

On evaluation in the office, she was found to be lethargic but oriented to person and place. Her vital signs were temperature, 36.9°C; pulse, 94 bpm; BP, 110/90 mm Hg; RR, 14 breaths per minute. She was orthostatic. Her exam was remarkable for cachexia and hepatomegaly.

Initial laboratory test results in the physician's office were:

Sodium: 134 mEq/L

Potassium: 3.9 mEq/L

Chloride: 99 mEq /L

$CO_2$: 26 mEq /L

BUN: 24 mg/dL

Creatinine: 0.8 mg/dL

Glucose: 117 mg/dL

Calcium: 15.0 mg/dL

Albumin: 3.9 g/dL

Total bilirubin: 0.9 g/dL

Conjugated bilirubin: 0.6 g/dL

Alkaline phosphatase: 800 units/L

AST (SGOT): 124 units/L

ALT (SGPT): 86 units/L

Phosphate: 1.4 mg/dL

At this point, what is the leading hypothesis, what are the active alternatives, and is there a must not miss diagnosis? Given this differential diagnosis, what tests should be ordered?

## PRIORITIZING THE DIFFERENTIAL DIAGNOSIS

This is an elderly woman with abdominal pain and significant hypercalcemia. Although primary hyperparathyroidism is a possibility, the degree of hypercalcemia and the abnormalities found on physical exam and laboratory studies are pivotal clues that strongly warrant consideration of other diseases. Hypercalcemia of malignancy needs to be considered given the patient's age and hepatomegaly. Most patients with hypercalcemia of malignancy have a previously diagnosed cancer, but it is possible for symptoms of cancer and hypercalcemia to present simultaneously or for symptoms of hypercalcemia to be the presenting symptoms of the malignancy. Malignancy primarily causes hypercalcemia through the elaboration of PTHrP or through osseous metastasis.

The milk-alkali syndrome should be considered. This syndrome is often caused by ingestion of large amounts of calcium carbonate in an effort to treat dyspepsia. This syndrome typically presents with hypercalcemia, metabolic alkalosis, and renal insufficiency. The presence of only 1 of the syndrome's 3 features makes this diagnosis less likely. The presence of other illnesses or medication use may suggest less common causes of hypercalcemia, such as granulomatous disease. Table 19–2 lists the differential diagnosis.

The patient reports no significant prior medical history but she has not seen a physician in over 5 years. She has been using calcium carbonate (Tums) for her abdominal pain but reports only intermittent use and none for the last few days. She is not taking any other medications. Review of systems is unremarkable other than the previously noted fatigue and abdominal pain.

An abdominal ultrasound done on the day of admission reveals multiple hepatic masses.

Is the clinical information sufficient to make a diagnosis? If not, what other information do you need?

*Table 19–2.* Diagnostic hypotheses for Mrs. W.

| Diagnostic Hypotheses | Clinical Clues | Important Tests |
|---|---|---|
| **Leading Hypothesis** | | |
| Humoral hypercalcemia of malignancy | Presence of malignancy, usually previously diagnosed Squamous cell carcinomas and adenocarcinomas of the lung, pancreas, and kidney most common | PTH-related peptide |
| **Active Alternative** | | |
| Local osteolytic hypercalcemia of malignancy | Presence of malignancy, usually previously diagnosed Multiple myeloma and breast cancer most common | Demonstration of bony metastases |
| **Active Alternative** | | |
| Primary hyperparathyroidism | Elevated calcium without evident underlying disease | PTH level |
| Other Alternative | | |
| Milk-alkali syndrome | Hypercalcemia, metabolic alkalosis, and renal insufficiency | Normal PTH level and history of calcium and absorbable alkali ingestion |

## Leading Hypothesis: Humoral Hypercalcemia of Malignancy

### Textbook Presentation

Hypercalcemia of malignancy is most commonly detected in patients with previously diagnosed cancers. It is uncommon for symptomatic hypercalcemia to be the presenting symptom of a malignancy. Hypercalcemia of malignancy carries a horrendous prognosis with 50% 30-day mortality.

### Disease Highlights

A. Hypercalcemia of malignancy is a heterogeneous process in which malignant cells elevate serum calcium in a number of ways.

   1. The most common cause of hypercalcemia is through elaboration of PTHrP a process called humoral hypercalcemia of malignancy (HHM).

   2. Tumors metastatic to bone may also cause hypercalcemia through local osteolytic effects on the bones, sometimes via local elaboration of PTHrP. This syndrome is discussed below.

   3. It is likely there is a great deal of overlap between these first 2 causes.

   4. Rarely, tumors can cause hypercalcemia by elaborating vitamin D (seen most commonly with lymphoma).

B. The malignancies that commonly cause hypercalcemia are (in approximate order of frequency):

   1. Lung

   2. Breast

   3. Multiple myeloma

   4. Lymphoma

   5. Head and neck

   6. Renal

   7. Prostate

C. PTHrP is a normal, physiologic, protein that is produced by many non-neoplastic tissues.

   1. The protein shares considerable sequence homology to PTH and binds to the same receptor.

   2. PTH and PTHrP affect the bones and kidneys in the same way.

   3. Certain malignancies elaborate the protein in relatively large amounts.

      a. PTHrP is detectable in 80% of patients with hypercalcemia and malignancy.

      b. The most common tumors that produce this protein are squamous cell carcinomas and adenocarcinoma of the lung, pancreas, and kidney.

   4. In hypercalcemia of malignancy secondary to PTHrP, hypercalcemia commonly precedes bony metastasis.

### Evidence-Based Diagnosis

A. Similar to primary hyperparathyroidism, hypercalcemia of malignancy seldom presents significant diagnostic confusion.

B. In patients with a known malignancy, the diagnosis is made by detecting high PTHrP and low PTH levels.

### Treatment

A. All patients with hypercalcemia of malignancy benefit from treatment of the underlying disease.

B. Beyond treatment of the malignancy, treatment aimed directly at hypercalcemia depends on its severity.

C. The mainstays of treatment for moderate and severe elevations of calcium are the bisphosphonates.

   1. Bisphosphonates work by inhibiting osteoclast activity.

   2. Pamidronate and zoledronic acid are both approved for the treatment of hypercalcemia of malignancy in the United States.

D. For patients with severe, symptomatic hypercalcemia, therapy must be more rapidly effective than treatment of the underlying disease or bisphosphonate therapy (which takes about 48 hours to reach full effectiveness).

   1. Saline hydration treats the dehydration that frequently accompanies hypercalcemia and decreases reabsorption of calcium in the proximal tubule of dehydrated, hypercalcemic patients.

   2. Once hydration is attained, a loop diuretic can further assist in achieving calciuresis.

   3. While immediate therapy for hypercalcemia is instituted, a bisphosphonate should be given and long-term treatment of the malignancy should be planned.

E. In all patients being treated for hypercalcemia of malignancy, care should be taken to institute other measures known to decrease serum calcium. Calcium supplements should be stopped, drugs that lead to hypercalcemia (lithium, thiazides) should be held, hypophosphatemia should be treated and weight bearing exercise should be encouraged.

## MAKING A DIAGNOSIS

Given the results of the patient's ultrasound, it is highly likely that she has a malignancy that is causing the hypercalcemia. The next step is to make a definitive diagnosis of the malignancy so that specific treatment can be instituted. Determining how the malignancy is causing hypercalcemia will be part of this evaluation; is the hypercalcemia a result of osseous metastasis or of PTHrP?

The patient was given normal saline for hydration and furosemide for diuresis when mild peripheral edema developed. Her calcium dropped over the first 3 days in the hospital to 11.2 mg/dL, where it remained stable.

As a follow-up to the ultrasound, a chest/abdomen/pelvis CT was ordered. This revealed a large lung mass and multiple liver masses. CT-guided biopsy of the liver was consistent with metastatic squamous cell carcinoma, likely of pulmonary origin.

 Have you crossed a diagnostic threshold for the leading hypothesis, hypercalcemia of malignancy (elaboration of PTHrP)? Have you ruled out the active alternatives? Do other tests need to be done to exclude the alternative diagnoses?

## Alternative Diagnosis: Local Osteolytic Hypercalcemia of Malignancy

### Textbook Presentation

Similar to hypercalcemia of malignancy caused by PTHrP, hypercalcemia due to malignancies metastatic to bone generally presents in patients with previously diagnosed cancer. Breast cancer and multiple myeloma (discussed in detail here) are the most common causes.

Multiple myeloma commonly presents with bone pain (often back pain), anemia, hypercalcemia, or renal insufficiency in patients in their 60s. Plain radiographs commonly demonstrate osteolytic lesions and the diagnosis is made by the demonstration of paraproteinemia and increased plasma cells on bone marrow examination.

## Disease Highlights

A. Breast cancer and multiple myeloma only cause hypercalcemia after metastasizing to bone.

B. The hypercalcemia is due to local osteolytic effects on bone, sometimes related to local PTHrP secretion.

C. Multiple myeloma is caused by a malignant proliferation of plasma cells. The plasma cells usually secrete a single immunoglobulin, called the M component (monoclonal component) that is detected on serum or urine protein electrophoresis.

D. Multiple myeloma most commonly affects patients in the seventh decade of life. Blacks are affected at twice the rate as whites.

E. Symptoms are varied and result from the effect of plasma cell proliferation on multiple systems.

1. Anemia: Secondary to plasma cell infiltration of the bone marrow.

2. Infections: When the M component is excluded, patients with myeloma usually have hypogammaglobulinemia.

3. Bone pain and hypercalcemia: Proliferation of plasma cells in the bone cause osteolytic lesions.

4. Renal insufficiency: Multiple myeloma can cause renal insufficiency in multiple ways:

   a. Light chains may injure the kidney via toxicity to the renal tubules or through obstruction secondary to the heavy burden of filtered protein.

   b. Hypercalcemia

   c. Amyloid deposition in the kidney

   d. Urate nephropathy

5. Serum hyperviscosity may occur from hypergammaglobulinemia; the most common symptoms are headache and visual disturbances.

F. Symptoms at presentation as reported in a recent study

1. Anemia was present in 73% of patients. The anemia was usually mild, normochromic, normocytic.

2. 58% of patients had bone pain at presentation and 67% had lytic bone lesions on radiographs.

3. 19% had renal insufficiency

4. 13% had hypercalcemia > 11 mg/dL

5. M component

   a. 82% of patients had an abnormal serum protein electrophoresis. Of the 18% with a normal serum electrophoresis, 97% had an abnormal urine protein electrophoresis.

   b. The M component most commonly appears in the gamma range and is most commonly IgG.

   c. 16% have only free light chains.

6. A sizable minority (36%) had another plasma cell abnormality present at the time of diagnosis (monoclonal gammopathy of unknown significance, plasmacytoma, amyloidosis).

## Evidence-Based Diagnosis

A. The diagnosis of multiple myeloma is based on the identification of:

1. Marrow plasmacytosis (> 10%)

2. Lytic bone lesions

3. A serum or urine M component or both.

B. Clues to the diagnosis are the presence of normocytic anemia, bone pain, and elevated immunoglobulins.

C. There are a few important issues that may confuse the diagnosis.

1. Filtered light chains are not detected on traditional urine dipsticks. A patient with light chain only myeloma may have normal amounts of serum protein and, apparently, no proteinuria. The presence of a monoclonal gammopathy will be detected with serum and urine protein electrophoresis.

2. The bone lesions of multiple myeloma are almost exclusively osteolytic. They will usually be missed on bone scans but are seen on radiographs.

## Treatment

The treatment of hypercalcemia of malignancy due to local osteolytic metastases is the same as that for HHM discussed above.

# Alternative Diagnosis: Milk-Alkali Syndrome

## Textbook Presentation

There can be many presentations of the milk-alkali syndrome. Acute cases are often seen in women who use calcium carbonate for dyspepsia or osteoporosis who develop hypercalcemia.

## Disease Highlights

A. The milk-alkali syndrome is a syndrome of hypercalcemia, metabolic alkalosis, and renal insufficiency caused by the ingestion of calcium and an absorbable alkali.

B. The syndrome was first described as a result of a proposed ulcer cure that included high doses of magnesium carbonate, sodium bicarbonate, bismuth subcarbonate, and about 1 liter of a milk/cream mixture daily.

C. The pathogenesis likely involves hypercalcemia secondary to the ingestion followed by a resultant decrease in glomerular filtration rate. The combination of renal insufficiency, hypercalcemia, and alkali ingestion then causes the metabolic alkalosis.

D. The modern presentation of the milk-alkali syndrome includes a wide range of calcium values, low to normal phosphate levels, moderate renal insufficiency (average creatinine 4.2 mg/dL in a recent review of published cases), and calcium carbonate as the source of calcium and absorbable alkali.

E. The milk-alkali syndrome is a distant third among the leading causes of hypercalcemia in hospitalized patients, after malignancy and primary hyperparathyroidism.

## Evidence-Based Diagnosis

The diagnosis of milk-alkali syndrome is based on history with supporting laboratory test results (hypercalcemia, metabolic alkalosis, and normal to low PTH).

## Treatment

**A.** Cessation of calcium carbonate intake and hydration is usually sufficient treatment of milk-alkali syndrome.

**B.** Caution should be taken when treating patients with severe milk-alkali syndrome with fluid and loop diuretics. These patients appear to be at particular risk for subsequent, transient, hypocalcemia.

**C.** A subset of patients, possibly those with more prolonged or severe disease complicated by hypovolemia, may never recover normal renal function.

## CASE RESOLUTION

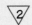

The patient's laboratory test results follow:

PTHrP: 3.3 pmol/L (nl 0–1.9 pmol/L)

PTH: 13 pg/mL (nl < 60)

Mrs. W's hypercalcemia was presumed to be secondary to malignancy with an elevated PTHrP. She was treated with zoledronic acid, while she received hydration. After a long discussion, the patient opted to be treated with palliative chemotherapy. Her condition declined markedly over the next 12 weeks. Chemotherapy was discontinued, and she was transferred to a hospice center where she died 4 weeks later.

Because the patient had metastatic squamous cell lung cancer, her rapid decline was not unexpected. The average life expectancy of patients with squamous cell carcinoma and extensive disease is a little less than 1 year and, as mentioned above, the presence of hypercalcemia worsens the prognosis of a malignancy.

## REVIEW OF OTHER IMPORTANT DISEASES

### Secondary & Tertiary Hyperparathyroidism

#### Disease Highlights

**A.** Secondary and tertiary hyperparathyroidism occur in patients with renal failure.

**B.** Secondary hyperparathyroidism is usually associated with hypocalcemia, since it is the chronic hypocalcemia of renal failure that leads to parathyroid hyperplasia. Therapy for the hyperphosphatemia associated with secondary hyperparathyroidism, however, often leads to hypercalcemia.

  **1.** Hyperphosphatemia develops in patients with renal failure as the renal clearance of phosphate falls.

  **2.** Early in the course of renal failure, hypocalcemia, hypovitaminosis D, and hyperphosphatemia lead to (secondary) hyperparathyroidism. The elevated PTH is adaptive, increasing calcium release from bones and enhancing renal phosphate excretion.

  **3.** As renal failure worsens, hyperparathyroidism becomes counterproductive as the kidneys no longer respond to PTH by excreting phosphate while phosphate continues to be released, with calcium, from the bones.

  **4.** Treatment of hyperphosphatemia in renal failure

    **a.** Calcium carbonate and calcium acetate have been the traditional first-line therapy for hyperphosphatemia in renal failure.

      **(1)** Calcium carbonate and calcium acetate are somewhat effective phosphate binders, decreasing the GI absorption of phosphate.

      **(2)** They do have the downside of frequently failing to lower phosphate levels adequately and of causing hypercalcemia.

      **(3)** The hypercalcemia (and hyperphosphatemia) is often worsened by the effect of calcitriol, also used to treat secondary hyperparathyroidism.

      **(4)** High levels of calcium and phosphate have deleterious cardiovascular effects.

    **b.** Newer therapies may be more effective at treating secondary hyperparathyroidism without raising calcium levels.

      **(1)** Sevelamer is a synthetic phosphate-binding polymer.

      **(2)** The calcium mimetic cinacalcet targets the calcium-sensing receptor in the parathyroid glands, lowering PTH levels.

      **(3)** Newer vitamin D analogues may be able to lower PTH levels with less of a tendency to cause hypercalcemia and hyperphosphatemia.

    **c.** Tertiary hyperparathyroidism occurs when the parathyroid hyperplasia of secondary hyperparathyroidism becomes so severe that PTH production becomes autonomous, causing hypercalcemia beyond that expected by calcium and calcitriol therapy.

#### Evidence-Based Diagnosis

**A.** In patients with renal failure, an elevated calcium level, in the setting of calcium carbonate use and an elevated PTH, is diagnostic of secondary hyperparathyroidism.

**B.** Tertiary hyperparathyroidism is diagnosed when PTH reaches higher levels and does not respond to calcium supplementation and vitamin D.

#### Treatment

**A.** The treatment of secondary hyperparathyroidism is very complicated and is predicated on treating the factors that stimulate PTH secretion in renal failure: hypocalcemia, hypovitaminosis D, and hyperphosphatemia.

**B.** Treatment involves phosphate binders, calcium and/or calcimimetics, and vitamin D analogues all used in an effort to decrease PTH levels without producing hypercalcemia.

**C.** If tertiary hyperparathyroidism occurs and is symptomatic (based on hypercalcemia, bone disease, metastatic calcifications) parathyroidectomy is often required.

## REFERENCES

Beall DP, Scofield RH. Milk-alkali syndrome associated with calcium carbonate consumption. Report of 7 patients with parathyroid hormone levels and an estimate of prevalence among patients hospitalized with hypercalcemia. Medicine (Baltimore). 1995;74:89–96.

Bilezikian JP, Potts JT Jr, Fuleihan Gel H et al. Summary statement from a workshop on asymptomatic primary hyperparathyroidism: a perspective for the 21st century. J Clin Endocrinol Metab. 2002;87:5353–61.

Block GA, Martin KJ, de Francisco AL et al. Cinacalcet for secondary hyperparathyroidism in patients receiving hemodialysis. N Engl J Med. 2004;350:1516–25.

Irvin GL 3rd, Carneiro DM. Management changes in primary hyperparathyroidism. JAMA. 2000;284:934–6.

Kyle RA, Gertz MA, Witzig TE et al. Review of 1027 patients with newly diagnosed multiple myeloma. Mayo Clin Proc. 2003;78:21–33.

Lundgren E, Ljunghall S, Akerstrom G, Hetta J, Mallmin H, Rastad J. Case-control study on symptoms and signs of "asymptomatic" primary hyperparathyroidism. Surgery. 1998;124:980–5.

Marx SJ. Hyperparathyroid and hypoparathyroid disorders. N Engl J Med. 2000;343:1863-75.

Pattou F, Torres G, Mondragon-Sanchez A et al. Correlation of parathyroid scanning and anatomy in 261 unselected patients with sporadic primary hyperparathyroidism. Surgery. 1999;126:1123–31.

Silverberg SJ, Shane E, Jacobs TP, Siris E, Bilezikian JP. A 10-year prospective study of primary hyperparathyroidism with or without parathyroid surgery. N Engl J Med. 1999;341:1249–55.

Sippy B. Gastric and duodenal ulcer: Medical cure by an efficient removal of gastric juice corrosion. JAMA. 1915;64:1625.

Stewart AF. Clinical practice. Hypercalcemia associated with cancer. N Engl J Med. 2005;352:373–9.

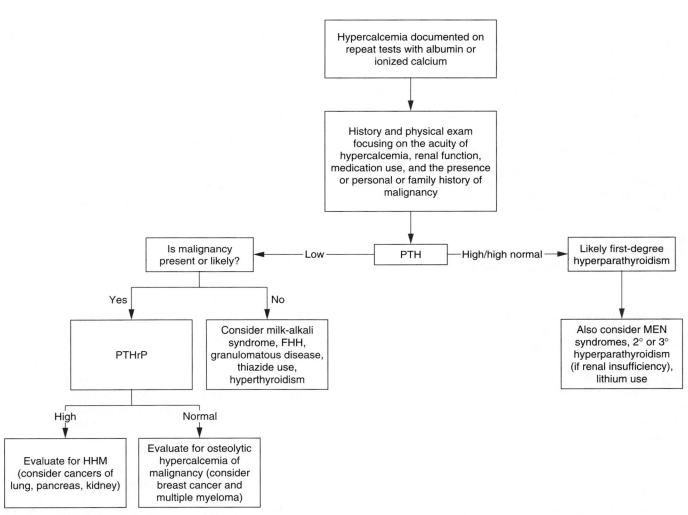

FHH, familial hypocalciuric hypercalcemia; HHM, humoral hypercalcemia of malignancy; MEN, multiple endocrine neoplasia; PTH, parathyroid hormone; PTHrP, parathyroid hormone–related protein.

*Figure 19–1.* Diagnostic approach: hypercalcemia.

# I have a patient with hypertension.
# How do I determine the cause?

## CHIEF COMPLAINT

PATIENT 1

Mr. U is a 48-year-old man with a BP of 165/90 mm Hg.

**What is the differential diagnosis of hypertension? How would you frame the differential?**

## CONSTRUCTING A DIFFERENTIAL DIAGNOSIS

First, what is normal BP, and when is a patient hypertensive? The first step is accurately measuring the BP. Table 20–1 summarizes guidelines for obtaining valid BP measurements.

The most recent Joint National Committee on Prevention, Detection, Evaluation, and Treatment of High BP (JNC 7) classifies BP as follows, based on the mean of 2 seated BP measurements on each of 2 or more office visits:

A. Normal: systolic BP < 120 mm Hg **and** diastolic BP < 80 mm Hg.

B. Prehypertension: systolic BP 120–139 mm Hg **or** diastolic BP 80–89 mm Hg.

C. Stage 1 hypertension: systolic BP 140–159 mm Hg **or** diastolic BP 90–99 mm Hg.

D. Stage 2 hypertension: systolic BP ≥ 160 mm Hg **or** diastolic BP ≥ 100 mm Hg.

Hypertension is either primary (essential) or secondary (resulting from a specific identifiable cause). Causes of secondary hypertension can be organized using an organ/system framework:

A. Primary (essential) hypertension

B. Secondary hypertension

  1. Endocrine

    a. Primary aldosteronism

    b. Pheochromocytoma

    c. Thyroid disease

    d. Hyperparathyroidism

    e. Cushing syndrome

  2. Renal

    a. Chronic kidney disease

    b. Acute renal failure

  3. Vascular

    a. Renovascular disease

    b. Coarctation of the aorta

  4. Pulmonary: sleep apnea

  5. GI: obesity

  6. Drug-induced or drug-related

    a. Prolonged corticosteroid therapy

    b. Nonselective nonsteroidal antiinflammatory drugs (NSAIDs)

    c. Cyclooxygenase (COX)-2 inhibitors

    d. Cocaine

    e. Alcohol

    f. Sympathomimetics (decongestants, anorectics)

    g. Oral contraceptives

    h. Cyclosporine and tacrolimus

    i. Erythropoietin

    j. Stimulants (modafinil, amphetamines)

An algorithm outlining the diagnostic approach to hypertension appears at the end of the chapter.

1

Mr. U's BP is high. He has wanted to avoid taking medication and has been trying to watch his diet and lose weight. Both of his parents and several of his siblings have hypertension. His medical history is notable only for smoking 1 pack/day for 30 years; he does not use alcohol and takes no medications.

**At this point, what is the leading hypothesis, what are the active alternatives, and is there a must not miss diagnosis? Given this differential diagnosis, what tests should be ordered?**

## PRIORITIZING THE DIFFERENTIAL DIAGNOSIS

Ninety-five to 99% of patients with hypertension have essential hypertension. A family history of hypertension increases the pretest probability of essential hypertension and is a pivotal clue in Mr. U's history. Patients between the ages of 20 and 50 have about twice the risk of developing hypertension if they have 1 first-degree relative with hypertension; the relative risk is 3–4 if 2 first-degree relatives have hypertension. Secondary causes are quite rare in *unselected* populations; estimated prevalences are 0.18–4.4% for renovascular hypertension, 0.04–0.2% for pheochromocytoma, 0.01–0.4% for primary hyperaldosteronism, and 0.3% for Cushing syndrome; these conditions may be more prevalent in populations of patients with *resistant* hypertension. More common conditions that can contribute to or cause hypertension include either

***Table 20–1.*** Guidelines for measuring BP.

- The patient should sit for several minutes in a quiet room before BP measurements are taken. Pain, stress, a full urinary bladder, a recent meal, and talking or active listening during measurement affect BP. Having smoked a cigarette within 15–20 minutes can elevate the BP by 5–20 mm Hg.
- Take at least 2 measurements spaced by 1–2 minutes and additional measurements if the first 2 are quite different.
- Using a bladder that is too narrow yields false high readings. Instead of the standard cuff (12–13 cm long, 35 cm wide) use an appropriate larger cuff in patients with increased arm circumference.
- Use phase I (first tapping sound) and V (disappearance) Korotkoff sounds to identify systolic and diastolic BP values, respectively.
- Do not deflate the cuff too rapidly, otherwise individual Korotkoff sounds are missed and too low a value is measured; start with a deflation rate of 2 mm/s.
- Measure the heart rate by palpation and watch out for arrhythmia, which mandates repeated BP measurements.
- At the first visit, measure BP in both arms and take the higher value as the reference; measure BP at 1 minute and 5 minutes after standing upright if the patient has a disorder that frequently causes orthostatic hypotension.

Adapted, with permission, from Messerli FH, Williams B, Ritz E. Essential hypertension. Lancet. 2007;370:591–603.

hyperthyroidism or hypothyroidism, renal insufficiency, excessive alcohol use, sleep apnea, and the use of drugs listed previously. Table 20–2 lists the differential diagnosis.

Mr. U's review of symptoms is negative for chest pain, shortness of breath, claudication, headache, dizziness, palpitations, weight change, constipation, daytime sleepiness, and snoring. On physical exam, BP is 165/90 mm Hg in both arms; pulse, 84 bpm; RR, 16 breaths per minute. He weighs 220 pounds, with a body mass index (BMI) of 30 kg/m². Fundoscopic exam shows some arteriolar narrowing with no hemorrhages or exudates. Jugular venous pressure is normal. Lungs are clear, and cardiac exam shows an $S_4$ but no $S_3$ or murmurs. There are no abdominal bruits; carotid, radial, femoral, posterior tibialis, and dorsalis pedis pulses are normal. There is no peripheral edema. Neurologic exam is normal.

**Is the clinical information sufficient to make a diagnosis? If not, what other information do you need?**

## Leading Hypothesis: Essential Hypertension

### Textbook Presentation

Essential hypertension generally presents as the gradual onset of elevated BP, most often in middle-aged people with positive family histories. Coexisting diabetes or obesity is common but not universal.

### Disease Highlights

A. Patients who are normotensive at age 55 have a 90% lifetime risk of developing hypertension.

B. Across the BP range of 115/75 mm Hg to 185/115 mm Hg, each increment of 20 mm Hg systolic BP or 10 mm Hg diastolic BP doubles the risk of cardiovascular disease.

### Evidence-Based Diagnosis

The evaluation of patients with hypertension focuses primarily on assessing other cardiovascular risk factors and assessing the presence or absence of target organ damage (TOD). Extensive testing for secondary causes is generally not done unless the patient has specific symptoms strongly suggestive of a specific secondary cause or if BP control cannot be achieved. Therefore, there are 3 objectives of testing in patients with hypertension:

A. Objective 1: Assess presence or absence of TOD (Table 20–3).

B. Objective 2: Assess presence or absence of other cardiovascular risk factors.

1. Smoking
2. Obesity (BMI > 30 kg/m²)
3. Physical inactivity
4. Dyslipidemia
5. Diabetes
6. Microalbuminuria or estimated glomerular filtration rate (GFR) < 60 mL/min
7. Age (> 55 for men, > 65 for women)
8. Family history of premature cardiovascular disease (men < 55, women < 65)

C. Objective 3: Identify secondary hypertension.

1. In the absence of any of the clinical clues listed previously, it is unlikely that the patient has renal artery stenosis, hyperaldosteronism, or pheochromocytoma.
2. Testing should focus on screening for more common causes or contributors to hypertension, such as renal or thyroid disease, that are easily diagnosed with simple blood tests.

Initial testing in a patient with hypertension and no clinical clues should include an ECG, electrolytes, BUN, creatinine, calcium, TSH, urine albumin–creatinine ratio, fasting glucose, and fasting lipid panel (total cholesterol, high-density lipoprotein [HDL], triglycerides, low-density lipoprotein [LDL]).

### Treatment

A. Treatment goals

1. Reduce BP.
   a. Target of < 130/80 mm Hg if patient also has diabetes or renal disease
   b. Target of < 140/90 mm Hg for everyone else
2. Modify other cardiovascular risk factors.

**Table 20–2.** Diagnostic hypotheses for Mr. U.

| Diagnostic Hypotheses | Clinical Clues | Important Tests |
|---|---|---|
| **Leading Hypothesis** | | |
| Essential hypertension | Family history Obesity Coexistent diabetes | |
| **Active Alternatives—Most Common** | | |
| Chronic kidney disease | Often none Sometimes edema, malaise | Serum creatinine, estimated GFR |
| Sleep apnea | Obesity (> 120% ideal body weight) Neck circumference > 17 in Frequent snoring Daytime sleepiness Witnessed apnea | Polysomnogram |
| Thyroid disease | *Hyperthyroidism:* Weight loss Loose stools Palpitations Sweating; *Hypothyroidism:* Weight gain Constipation Fatigue | TSH |
| Alcohol | Alcohol history | Alcohol history CAGE questionnaire |
| Drug/medication use | Medication/drug history | Medication/drug history |
| **Other Hypotheses** | | |
| Renal artery stenosis | Abrupt onset or accelerated hypertension Azotemia after use of ACE inhibitor Hypertension refractory to ≥ 3 medications Abdominal or flank bruit Other vascular disease (coronary, carotid, or peripheral) Smoking Severe retinopathy | MRA with gadolinium CT angiography |
| Hyperaldosteronism | Resistant hypertension Hypokalemia | Aldosterone/renin ratio |
| Pheochromocytoma | Labile BP/paroxysmal hypertension Headache Sweating Orthostasis Tachycardia | Plasma metanephrine |

**Table 20–3.** Assessing target organ damage in patients with hypertension.

| Target organ | Clinical manifestations | Important tests |
|---|---|---|
| Heart | Left ventricular hypertrophy | Physical exam ECG Echocardiography in selected patients |
| | Coronary artery disease (angina, myocardial infarction) | History ECG Stress test in selected patients |
| | Heart failure | History Physical exam Echocardiography |
| Brain | Stroke, transient ischemic attack | History Physical exam |
| Kidneys | Proteinuria Chronic kidney disease | Albumin/creatinine ratio Serum creatinine |
| Eyes | Retinopathy | Fundoscopic or ophthalmologic exam |
| Peripheral vasculature | Peripheral vascular disease | History and physical exam ABI measurements in selected patients |

**B.** Nonpharmacologic approaches to treating hypertension (Tables 20–4 and 20–5)

    **1.** 2–6 months is a reasonable length of time for a trial of lifestyle modification

    **2.** Should be discussed with all patients, even if medication also necessary

**C.** Overview of pharmacologic treatment of hypertension

    **1.** In general, can divide patients into those who have other diseases that would guide choice of therapy (called

**Table 20–4.** Nonpharmacologic approaches to managing hypertension.

| Intervention | Approximate reduction in systolic BP |
|---|---|
| Weight reduction | 5–20 mm Hg/10 kg weight loss |
| DASH diet (see Table 20–5) | 8–14 mm Hg |
| Reduced sodium diet (< 2.4 g sodium/day) | 2–8 mm Hg |
| Aerobic exercise, 30 minutes/day, several days/week | 4–9 mm Hg |
| Limitation of alcohol consumption to ≤ 2 drinks/day for men and ≤ 1 drink/day for women | 2–4 mm Hg |

**Table 20–5.** DASH diet.

| Food group | Number of servings |
|---|---|
| Grains/grain products | 7–8/day |
| Vegetables | 4–5/day |
| Fruits | 4–5/day |
| Low-fat dairy products | 2–3/day |
| Meats, poultry, fish | 2–3/day |
| Fats, oils | 2–3/day |
| Sweets | 5/week |
| Nuts, seeds, dried beans | 4–5/week |

See http://www.nhlbi.nih.gov/health/public/heart/hbp/dash/new_dash.pdf for details.

"compelling indications" by JNC 7) and those without such compelling indications

a. No compelling indications
  (1) Start with thiazide diuretic.
  (2) Add ACE inhibitor, β-blocker, angiotensin receptor blocker (ARB), or calcium channel blocker if goal not reached in 1–2 months.
  (3) Optimize dose of second drug until BP goal reached.
  (4) Add third drug from a different class if goal not reached on combination of thiazide diuretic and maximal tolerated dose of second drug; do not combine β-blockers and verapamil because of excessive blockage of atrioventricular (AV) node.

b. Compelling indications
  (1) Heart failure
    (a) Left ventricular (LV) dysfunction without symptoms: use ACE inhibitors and selective β-blockers (carvedilol, metoprolol)
    (b) With symptoms: use loop diuretics, ACE inhibitors, β-blockers, spironolactone
  (2) Ischemic heart disease
    (a) Stable angina: use β-blockers
    (b) Acute coronary syndromes: use β-blockers and ACE inhibitors
    (c) Post-myocardial infarction: use β-blockers, ACE inhibitors
  (3) Diabetes
    (a) Most patients will need at least 2 drugs to achieve BP goal < 130/80 mm Hg.
    (b) Use thiazide diuretic and ACE inhibitor or ARB initially.
    (c) Can add β-blocker or calcium channel blocker in patients who need a third drug.
  (4) Chronic kidney disease
    (a) Use ACE inhibitor or ARB.
    (b) If creatinine > 2.5 mg/dL or estimated GFR < 20 mL/min, use loop diuretic instead of thiazide.

  (5) Cerebrovascular disease
    (a) Use combination of thiazide and ACE inhibitor.
    (b) Beware of rapid reduction of BP in patients with acute stroke.
2. Should also consider cost and dosing frequency: low-cost once-a-day drugs increase compliance
3. If goal is not reached on optimal doses of 3 drugs, consider noncompliance with therapy, excess sodium intake, excess alcohol intake, volume overload from kidney disease, use of medications/drugs that contribute to hypertension, and secondary hypertension.

## MAKING A DIAGNOSIS

Mr. U's initial test results are as follows:

ECG: LV hypertrophy by voltage, otherwise normal

TSH, 1.0 microunit/mL

Urine albumin–creatinine ratio: normal

Na, 145 mEq/L; K, 4.2 mEq/L; Cl, 100 mEq/L; BUN, 11 mg/dL; creatinine, 0.5 mg/dL

Fasting glucose, 90 mg/dL

Fasting lipid panel: total cholesterol, 240 mg/dL; HDL, 40 mg/dL; triglycerides, 100 mg/dL; LDL, 180 mg/dL

 **Have you crossed a diagnostic threshold for the leading hypothesis, essential hypertension? Have you ruled out the active alternatives? Do other tests need to be done to exclude the alternative diagnoses?**

Based on Mr. U's history, physical exam, and initial laboratory test results, it is not necessary to do any further testing for secondary causes of hypertension. He does have other modifiable cardiovascular risk factors (smoking, obesity, and hypercholesterolemia), and some evidence for TOD (early retinopathy and LV hypertrophy).

## CASE RESOLUTION

Mr. U is counseled regarding smoking cessation and referred to a nutritionist for guidance regarding diet and exercise programs. He is started on hydrochlorothiazide, 12.5 mg daily, for his hypertension and atorvastatin, 10 mg daily, for his hypercholesterolemia (Table 20–6). One month later, his BP is 145/85 mm Hg. He has not yet started to exercise and has not quit smoking. You again counsel him regarding the importance of these lifestyle modifications and the possibility of avoiding a second medication if he exercises and loses weight. Six months later, after changing his diet and faithfully exercising 3 times a week, he has lost 5 pounds, and his BP is 135/82 mm Hg; he continues to smoke.

***Table 20–6.*** Guidelines for treatment of hypercholesterolemia.

| Risk category[1] | LDL goal (mg/dL) | LDL levels that should prompt lifestyle changes | LDL levels that should prompt drug therapy |
|---|---|---|---|
| CHD or CHD risk equivalent[2] (10 yr risk > 20%) | < 100[3] | ≥ 100[4] | ≥ 130[3,4] |
| 2+ risk factors[5] (10 yr risk 10–20%) | < 130 | ≥ 130 | ≥ 130 |
| 2+ risk factors (10 year risk < 10%) | < 130 | ≥ 130 | ≥ 160 |
| 0–1 risk factors | < 160 | ≥ 160 | ≥ 190 (drug optional at LDL 160–189) |

[1]10-year risk calculated using Framingham model (see http://hin.nhlbi.nih.gov/ atpiii/calculator.asp)
[2]CHD risk equivalents: Other vascular disease (cerebrovascular, peripheral vascular, abdominal aortic aneurysm), diabetes, Framingham risk > 20%
[3]Some experts recommend an LDL goal of < 70 mg/dL for high-risk patients.
[4]Many experts recommend statin therapy for all patients in this category.
[5]Risk factors: Smoking, hypertension (BP ≥ 140/90 mm Hg, or on antihypertensive therapy), HDL < 40 mg/dL (if HDL > 60 mg/dL, decrease risk factor count by 1), family history of premature CAD (male first-degree relative < 55 years, female first-degree relative < 65 years), age (men ≥ 45 years, women ≥ 55 years)

## CHIEF COMPLAINT

PATIENT 2

Mrs. X is a 66-year-old woman with a long history of hypertension treated with hydrochlorothiazide (25 mg daily), lisinopril (80 mg daily), and amlodipine (10 mg daily). Her BP has generally been in the 140–145/85–95 mm Hg range over the last several years. At her last visit 6 months ago, she weighed 160 pounds and her BP was 140/90 mm Hg. Noting that her BP was above her treatment goal, and that she was on maximal doses of 3 antihypertensive medications, you suggested adding a fourth agent. She declined, preferring to work on lifestyle modifications. Today she weighs 172 pounds, and her BP is 170/95 mm Hg. She feels fine, with no headache, chest pain, shortness of breath, or edema. Other than her antihypertensive medications, she takes only pravastatin. Her medical history is notable for smoking 1 pack/day for 40 years, peripheral vascular disease manifested by stable claudication on walking 6 blocks, and chronic kidney disease, with a serum creatinine of 1.7 mg/dL. Physical exam is notable for clear lungs, an $S_4$ without an $S_3$ or murmurs, and decreased posterior tibial (PT) and dorsalis pedis (DP) pulses. Abdominal exam is normal. There is no peripheral edema, and there are no carotid, femoral, or abdominal bruits.

> At this point, what is the leading hypothesis, what are the active alternatives, and is there a must not miss diagnosis? Given this differential diagnosis, what tests should be ordered?

## PRIORITIZING THE DIFFERENTIAL DIAGNOSIS

Mrs. X's BP has never been very well controlled, and now her control is even worse. Since her hypertension is not controlled on maximal doses of 3 antihypertensive medications, including a diuretic, she meets the definition of resistant hypertension. Although there are patients with essential hypertension who need maximal doses of 4 or even 5 drugs to achieve control, causes of resistant hypertension need to be considered in such patients. These include "pseudoresistance" (inaccurate BP measurements, poor adherence to prescribed medications, white coat hypertension [BP being elevated in the office but normal or lower in other settings]), lifestyle factors (obesity, excessive dietary sodium intake, heavy alcohol intake), drug-related causes (see original differential diagnostic framework), and secondary causes (see original differential diagnostic framework). In patients with resistant hypertension, the estimated prevalence for chronic kidney disease is 1–8%, for renal artery stenosis 3-4%, for hyperaldosteronism 1.5–15%, for thyroid disease 1-3%, and for pheochromocytoma < 0.5%.

The pivotal points in Mrs. X's presentation include her vascular risk factors, suggesting she is at risk for renal artery stenosis. In addition, she does have preexisting renal insufficiency, which could have progressed and caused her BP to increase. Her obesity is a risk factor for obstructive sleep apnea. Another consideration would be hyperaldosteronism, which manifests as resistant hypertension, and often hypokalemia; in recent series, it has been an increasingly common cause of resistant hypertension. She has no symptoms to suggest another cause of secondary hypertension, pheochromocytoma. Table 20–7 lists the differential diagnosis.

She reports that she takes all of her medications every day and never adds salt to her food. She does not drink alcohol and is afraid to use over-the-counter medications. She attributes her weight gain to being somewhat less active due to symptomatic knee osteoarthritis. A recent polysomnogram was normal. Laboratory tests include the following: Na, 140 mEq/L; K, 3.4 mEq/L; Cl, 100 mEq/L; $HCO_2$, 26 mEq/L; BUN, 35 mg/dL; creatinine, 1.8 mg/dL; TSH, 3.2 microunit/mL.

**Table 20–7.** Diagnostic hypotheses for Mrs. X.

| Diagnostic Hypotheses | Clinical Clues | Important Tests |
|---|---|---|
| **Leading Hypothesis** | | |
| Renal artery stenosis | Abrupt onset or accelerated hypertension Azotemia after use of ACE inhibitor Hypertension refractory to ≥ 3 medications Abdominal or flank bruit Other vascular disease (coronary, carotid, or peripheral) Smoking Severe retinopathy | MRA with gadolinium CT angiography |
| **Active Alternatives—Most Common** | | |
| Worsening renal function | None Sometimes edema, malaise | Serum creatinine |
| Adverse lifestyle changes (weight gain, high sodium diet, excess alcohol intake, reduction in exercise, noncompliance with medications) | History | History |
| Use of other medications, especially NSAIDs, decongestants | History | History |
| **Other Hypotheses** | | |
| Hyperaldo-steronism | Resistant hypertension Hypokalemia | Aldosterone/ renin ratio |

 Is the clinical information sufficient to make a diagnosis? If not, what other information do you need?

## Leading Hypothesis: Atherosclerotic Renal Artery Stenosis

### Textbook Presentation

Patients generally have either very abrupt hypertension, hypertension that worsens by > 15% over 6 months, or hypertension refractory to treatment with 3 drugs. The classic patient with atherosclerotic renal artery stenosis has other vascular disease (cerebrovascular disease, coronary artery disease, peripheral arterial disease) or risk factors such as smoking or diabetes.

### Disease Highlights

A. Must distinguish renovascular disease from renovascular hypertension

  1. Renovascular disease means significant stenosis of 1 or both renal arteries.

    a. Can be due to fibromuscular dysplasia (most commonly in young women) or atherosclerosis (90% of cases)

    b. Does not necessarily cause hypertension and can exist in patients with essential hypertension

  2. Renovascular hypertension means hypertension caused by renal hypoperfusion as a result of renal artery stenosis

    a. Stenosis leads to renal ischemia, activating the renin–angiotensin system, which leads to release of renin and production of angiotensin II.

    b. Although plasma renin levels are high initially, they decrease over time.

    c. Aldosterone secretion and vasoconstriction then occur, leading to hypertension.

    d. Aldosterone secretion also causes salt and water retention and hypokalemia.

    e. Ischemic nephropathy occurs when renal blood flow is so reduced that GFR decreases and there is loss of renal function.

    f. Some patients with bilateral renal artery stenosis present with episodic, unexplained pulmonary edema ("flash pulmonary edema"); echocardiograms in such patients show normal systolic function.

B. About 50% of patients with renal artery stenosis have renovascular hypertension.

### Evidence-Based Diagnosis

A. Clinical characteristics

  1. Abdominal bruits, moderate to severe retinopathy, and peripheral vascular disease are often present.

  2. Predictive value of abdominal bruits

    a. Should listen over all 4 abdominal quadrants and also spine and flanks between T12 and L2

    b. Should be systolic and diastolic

    c. Prevalence of 6.5–31% in a healthy population; prevalence of 28% in patients with hypertension

    d. Prevalence of 78–87% in patients with proven renal artery stenosis

    e. Sensitivity 39–63%, specificity 90–99%

  3. Family history of hypertension often absent

  4. Hypokalemia often seen as a result of stimulation of aldosterone release; metabolic alkalosis also often seen.

  5. A clinical predication model has been developed (Table 20–8); it should not be considered totally accurate but does give an estimate of pretest probability.

  6. Response to ACE inhibition

    a. A reversible increase in serum creatinine can develop in some patients with bilateral renal artery stenosis (or unilateral stenosis in patients with only 1 functioning kidney) when starting ACE inhibitor therapy.

***Table 20–8.*** Clinical predication rule for estimating pretest probability of renal artery stenosis.

| Predictor | Points (no history of smoking) | Points (former or current smoker) |
|---|---|---|
| Age | | |
| 20 | 0 | 3 |
| 30 | 1 | 4 |
| 40 | 2 | 4 |
| 50 | 3 | 5 |
| 60 | 4 | 5 |
| 70 | 5 | 6 |
| Female | 2 | 2 |
| Signs and symptoms of vascular disease | 1 | 1 |
| Onset of hypertension within 2 years | 1 | 1 |
| BMI < 25 kg/m² | 2 | 2 |
| Presence of abdominal bruit | 3 | 3 |
| Serum creatinine | | |
| 0.4 | 0 | 0 |
| 0.7 | 1 | 1 |
| 0.9 | 2 | 2 |
| 1.1 | 3 | 3 |
| 1.7 | 6 | 6 |
| 2.3 | 9 | 9 |
| Lipid-lowering therapy | 1 | 1 |

Score of 9 = pretest probability of 10%
Score of 10 = pretest probability 15–20%
Score of 12 = pretest probability over 30%
(Reproduced, with permission, from Krijnen P, van Jaarsveld BC, Steyerberg EW, Man't Veld AJ et al. A clinical predication rule for renal artery stenosis. Ann Intern Med. 1998;129:705–11.)

      **(1)** The peak creatinine occurs somewhere between 4 days and 2 months.

      **(2)** Creatinine returns to baseline within 1 week of stopping the ACE inhibitor.

    **b.** One study reported that, in a population of high-risk patients, a 20% increase in creatinine had 100% sensitivity and 70% specificity for the diagnosis of renal artery stenosis (defined as > 50% bilateral stenosis).

**B.** Imaging studies

    **1.** Intra-arterial digital subtraction angiography (DSA) is the gold standard.

      **a.** Can also be therapeutic through performance of angioplasty or placement of stent

      **b.** Complications include bleeding, dissection, embolization, and contrast nephropathy

    **2.** Duplex ultrasonography (two-dimensional ultrasound imaging combined with Doppler flow measurements)

      **a.** Sensitivity 90–95%, specificity 60–90%; LR+ = 2.4–9; LR– = 0.11–0.17

      **b.** Test characteristics not as good with less experienced technicians, and it is extremely difficult to obtain images in obese patients.

      **c.** Renal artery/aortic peak systolic velocity ratio > 3.5 *and* a renal artery peak velocity > 2 m/sec correspond well to a stenosis of > 60%.

    **3.** Magnetic resonance angiography (MRA) with gadolinium

      **a.** Reported sensitivity ranges from 88% to 95% with a specificity of 94% (corresponding to LR+ of ~15 and LR– of 0.03–0.05)

      **b.** The largest single study found that for atherosclerotic renal artery stenosis, the sensitivity was 78% and specificity 88% (LR+ = 6.5, LR– = 0.25); for fibromuscular dysplasia, the sensitivity was only 22% but the specificity was 96%.

    **4.** CT angiography

      **a.** The range of reported sensitivity/specificity is similar to MRA with gadolinium, but nephrotoxic contrast is required.

      **b.** In the study noted above, for atherosclerotic renal artery stenosis, the sensitivity was 77% and specificity 94% (LR+ = 12.8, LR– = 0.24); for fibromuscular dysplasia, the sensitivity was 28% and specificity was 99%.

**C.** Blood tests

    **1.** Plasma renin level

      **a.** Sensitivity 57%, specificity 66%

      **b.** LR+ = 1.7, LR– = 0.65

    **2.** Captopril augmented plasma renin level

      **a.** Diuretics and ACE inhibitors held for 2 weeks; renin measured before and 30 minutes after captopril dose

      **b.** A positive test is plasma renin > 21 ng/mL/h, an absolute increase of at least 10 ng/mL/h, or an increase of 150%

      **c.** 96% sensitivity, 55% specificity; LR+ = 2.1, LR– = 0.07

## Treatment

**A.** Not clear which patients benefit from revascularization

**B.** Asymmetric renal blood flow on nuclear studies and ultrasonographic renal resistance index might identify responders.

**C.** Cure of hypertension is unusual, but number of medications necessary to achieve control often reduced

**D.** Revascularization might preserve renal function.

**E.** Risk factor management (eg, cholesterol, smoking, diabetes mellitus) is important.

## MAKING A DIAGNOSIS

Mrs. X suffers from claustrophobia and does not want to have an MRI scan. Consequently, you order a duplex ultrasound to evaluate her renal arteries. The report reads "technically difficult study; no evidence for renal artery stenosis."

Have you crossed a diagnostic threshold for the leading hypothesis, renovascular hypertension? Have you ruled out the active alternatives? Do other tests need to be done to exclude the alternative diagnoses?

Worsening renal insufficiency and "adverse lifestyle changes" have been ruled out by the history and unchanged serum creatinine. Primary aldosteronism needs to be considered in patients with resistant hypertension, especially those with hypokalemia.

## Alternative Diagnosis: Primary Hyperaldosteronism

### Textbook Presentation

Primary hyperaldosteronism is usually diagnosed when a patient with hypertension has unexplained hypokalemia.

### Disease Highlights

A. Etiology

1. Results from a unilateral aldosterone-producing adenoma in 30–60% of cases (Conn syndrome)

2. Results from idiopathic bilateral adrenal hyperplasia in most other patients

3. Rarer causes include microadenomas, unilateral adrenal hyperplasia, and adrenal carcinoma.

B. True prevalence unknown but could be as high as 12–15% in selected populations of patients with resistant hypertension.

C. Pathophysiology

1. High aldosterone levels lead to salt and water retention and potassium wasting.

2. Because aldosterone is being produced autonomously, it is not suppressed by volume expansion, as it is normally.

3. Volume expansion suppresses plasma renin levels.

D. Most patients (50–60%) have a normal potassium level.

 A normal potassium level does not rule out hyperaldosteronism.

### Evidence-Based Diagnosis

A. Evaluation for hyperaldosteronism should be considered in hypertensive patients with potassium levels < 3.5 mEq/L, those with severe diuretic induce hypokalemia (K < 3.0 mEq/L), those with resistant hypertension, and those with hypertension and an incidental adrenal adenoma.

B. The testing is complicated and may be best done in consultation with an endocrinologist.

C. The plasma aldosterone concentration/plasma renin activity ratio (ARR) is the most commonly used screening test; it is elevated in patients with primary hyperaldosteronism.

1. Hypokalemia must be corrected before testing.

2. All antihypertensive agents should be stopped for 2 weeks, if possible.

   a. Calcium channel blockers, α-blockers, and hydralazine do not significantly affect the test results.

   b. Aldosterone antagonists and β-blockers must be stopped.

   c. ACE inhibitors, ARBs, and diuretics can cause false-negative results.

3. Measure the plasma aldosterone concentration (ng/dL) and the plasma renin activity (ng/mL/h) simultaneously in the morning after the patient has been ambulatory for 2 hours; because of sampling variability, 3 separate specimens should be obtained.

4. The optimal cutoff value and the test characteristics are not totally clear, but the following parameters are commonly used:

   a. An ARR < 23.6 rules out primary hyperaldosteronism.

   b. An ARR > 30 has a sensitivity of 90% and a specificity of 75% (LR+ = 3.6; LR− = 0.13).

   c. An ARR > 67 rules in primary hyperaldosteronism.

D. After a positive ARR, confirmatory testing should be done.

1. Saline loading, sometimes with captopril or fludrocortisone, is done to demonstrate lack of suppression of aldosterone.

2. Adrenal imaging, usually with MRI, is done to look for adenomas.

### Treatment

A. Surgery for macroadenomas after demonstration of activity with adrenal venous sampling for aldosterone

B. Otherwise, treat with the aldosterone antagonist spironolactone.

## CASE RESOLUTION

2

Because Mrs. X is somewhat overweight, and the duplex ultrasound was technically difficult, the normal study does not rule out renovascular hypertension. Options at this point include performing an imaging study with a better sensitivity, such as MRA, and testing for the alternative diagnosis of primary hyperaldosteronism. Considering her risk factors, renovascular hypertension is much more likely than primary hyperaldosteronism and should be investigated more thoroughly.

You explain why getting the MRA is important and offer Mrs. X a short-acting benzodiazepine to be taken 1 hour before the scan. She is able to complete the test without incident; it shows a 90% stenosis of her right renal artery. Nuclear imaging studies demonstrate decreased blood flow to the right kidney, and Mrs. X's BP fails to improve with the addition of a fourth agent. She then undergoes right renal artery stenting, and her BP becomes well controlled on 3 medications.

## CHIEF COMPLAINT

PATIENT

Mr. J is 45-year-old man with a 10-year history of hypertension. When you last saw him 1 year ago, his BP was 160/95 mm Hg. He ran out of his medications 6 months ago and was unable to obtain refills because of financial problems. Today, he has stopped by to see your nurse for new prescriptions. Because he is complaining of a headache, she checked his BP and then runs to find you because it is 220/112 mm Hg.

 At this point, what is the leading hypothesis, what are the active alternatives, and is there a must not miss diagnosis? Given this differential diagnosis, what tests should be ordered?

## PRIORITIZING THE DIFFERENTIAL DIAGNOSIS

Mr. J's BP clearly needs to be lowered, and the primary question is how quickly this needs to be accomplished. In other words, is this a **hypertensive emergency** or **hypertensive urgency**? These syndromes are defined by the degree of BP elevation and whether there is acute end organ damage. A hypertensive emergency exists when there is severe BP elevation and acute target organ involvement: acute neurologic syndromes (encephalopathy, cerebrovascular accident, intracerebral or subarachnoid hemorrhage), acute aortic dissection, acute myocardial infarction/acute coronary syndrome, acute pulmonary edema, acute renal failure, severe preeclampsia/eclampsia, microangiopathic hemolytic anemia, or acute postoperative hypertension. In hypertensive urgency, there is severe BP elevation without any acute TOD. The exact definition of "severe BP elevation" has not been established, but many experts use a cutoff of > 180/100 mm Hg.

 A hypertensive emergency is defined by the presence of clinical symptoms, not by the degree of BP elevation.

To some extent, the degree of the acute TOD in patients with very elevated BP depends on the time course of the BP elevation. For example, normotensive women in whom acute hypertension develops from eclampsia can have significant TOD at pressures of 160/100 mm Hg, whereas patients with chronic hypertension can be asymptomatic at much higher pressures. So, despite his very elevated BP, it is quite likely that Mr. J falls into the "hypertensive urgency" rather than the "hypertensive emergency" category. Nevertheless, hypertensive emergency is always the "must not miss" diagnosis in such patients (Table 20-9).

 You tell the nurse to put Mr. J in an exam room. On further history, he has no shortness of breath, chest pain, edema, abdominal pain, feelings of confusion, vomiting, or focal weakness or numbness. He generally appears well and is clearly happy to have a new job with insurance.

**Table 20–9.** Diagnostic hypotheses for Mr. J.

| Diagnostic Hypotheses | Clinical Clues | Important Tests |
|---|---|---|
| **Leading Hypothesis** | | |
| Hypertensive urgency | Absence of hypertensive emergency syndromes | |
| **Active Alternative—Must Not Miss** | | |
| Hypertensive emergencies | | |
| Myocardial infarction | Chest pain | ECG Cardiac enzymes |
| Aortic dissection | Chest, back pain Diastolic murmur Absent pulses | Chest radiograph Transesophageal echocardiogram Chest CT |
| Pulmonary edema | Dyspnea Crackles $S_3$ | Chest radiograph |
| Hypertensive encephalopathy | Headache Nausea/vomiting Delirium Seizures Coma Papilledema | MRI |
| Acute renal failure | Nausea Fatigue | Serum creatinine |

Physical exam confirms BP of 220/112 mm Hg, pulse of 84 bpm, and RR of 16 breaths per minute. It is difficult to see his disks on fundoscopic exam, but you do not think there is papilledema. Lungs are clear, jugular venous pressure is not elevated, there is an $S_4$ and a 2/6 systolic ejection murmur without an $S_3$, abdomen is nontender, there is no peripheral edema, and neurologic exam is normal.

 Is the clinical information sufficient to make a diagnosis? If not, what other information do you need?

## Leading Hypothesis: Hypertensive Urgency

### Textbook Presentation

A patient with chronic hypertension has extremely high BP; by definition, patients have no symptoms or signs of acute TOD.

### Evidence-Based Diagnosis

A. Must rule out acute TOD through history, physical, and selected laboratory tests.

B. All patients should have a serum creatinine and urinalysis performed.

C. Patients with symptoms suggestive of myocardial ischemia or pulmonary edema should have an ECG, chest radiograph, and cardiac enzymes.

D. Patients with neurologic signs or symptoms need a head CT scan and sometimes a brain MRI.

## Treatment

A. In stable outpatients with chronically elevated BP, there is NOT an urgent need to reduce the BP, and it is fine if it takes several days for the BP to be reduced.

1. In patients who have stopped their medications, it is usually sufficient just to restart them.

2. Can also just choose 2 agents, such as a diuretic and either a calcium channel blocker or ACE inhibitor, and start them

3. Oral agents that are short acting, such as captopril, felodipine, furosemide, and clonidine, lower BP more quickly than long-acting and sustained-released preparations.

4. Whether or not such patients need to be observed depends on their reliability and comorbid conditions.

B. Too rapid reduction of BP can lead to hypotension and cerebral hypoperfusion.

C. IV and sublingual medications can have unpredictable effects on BP and should be avoided in asymptomatic patients.

1. IV hydralazine causes a progressive and sometimes precipitous fall in BP 5–15 minutes after administration.

2. Although the circulating half-life of hydralazine is only 3 hours, the half time of its effect on BP is 10 hours.

3. Sublingual nifedipine causes completely unpredictable lowering of BP and should never be used.

Do not be in a hurry to normalize BP in patients without acute TOD!

## MAKING A DIAGNOSIS

Mr. J's serum creatinine is 1.4 mg/dL, unchanged from 1 year ago. His urinalysis is normal. Mr. J wants to know if he can have a couple of acetaminophen tablets for his headache, get his prescriptions, and leave; he has to pick up his son at school.

Have you crossed a diagnostic threshold for the leading hypothesis, hypertensive urgency? Have you ruled out the active alternatives? Do other tests need to be done to exclude the alternative diagnoses?

## Alternative Diagnosis: Hypertensive Emergencies

Acute coronary syndromes, aortic dissection, subarachnoid hemorrhage, and pulmonary edema are discussed in other chapters. This section focuses on hypertensive encephalopathy.

### Textbook Presentation

Patients present with the acute or subacute development of lethargy, confusion, headache, and visual disturbances, sometimes followed by seizures (focal or generalized) and coma. The syndrome can occur with or without proteinuria and retinopathy.

### Disease Highlights

A. Cerebral blood flow is autoregulated within specific limits.

1. In normotensive people, cerebral blood flow is unchanged between mean arterial pressures (MAP) of 60–120 mm Hg (mean arterial pressure = [(2 × diastolic) + systolic]/3)

   a. Cerebral vasoconstriction limits hyperperfusion up to a MAP of 180 mm Hg.

   b. Above a MAP of 180 mm Hg, autoregulation is overwhelmed.

2. In hypertensive patients, cerebral blood flow can be maintained at MAPs of up to 200 mm Hg.

   a. Thought to be due to arteriolar thickening

   b. Such patients also need higher MAPs to maintain adequate cerebral blood flow (ie, abrupt lowering of the BP to a MAP of < 100–110 mm Hg can potentially lead to cerebral ischemia).

B. Failure of autoregulation leads to cerebral vasodilation, endothelial dysfunction, and cerebral edema.

C. The classic MRI finding in hypertensive encephalopathy is subcortical vasogenic edema.

1. Also called reversible posterior leukoencephalopathy syndrome (RPLS)

2. Generally in the posterior regions of the brain due to relatively sparse sympathetic innervation of the vertebrobasilar territory leading to more disruption of autoregulatory mechanisms, increased perfusion, and edema

3. Can also see changes in the brainstem and anterior brain

4. In one series, 92% of patients with RPLS presented with encephalopathy, 39% with visual symptoms, and 53% with headache; 87% of patients had seizures.

5. Also seen with eclampsia and use of some immunosuppressive agents and cytotoxic drugs; in one series, 68% of patients with RPLS had hypertension, 11% eclampsia, 11% immunosuppressive use, and 11% other causes

6. Reversible with treatment of hypertension or removal of inciting agent, with MRI findings resolving in days to weeks; long-term antiepileptic therapy is not necessary.

### Evidence-Based Diagnosis

A. Hypertensive encephalopathy is primarily a clinical diagnosis.

B. A head CT should be done to exclude intracranial hemorrhage (intracerebral or subarachnoid bleeding).

C. An MRI should be done to exclude acute ischemic stroke and to look for RPLS.

MRI is much more sensitive than CT (83% vs 16% sensitivity; specificity of both > 95%) for the diagnosis of acute ischemic stroke.

### Treatment (Table 20–10)

A. Treating hypertension in the setting of hypertensive encephalopathy

***Table 20–10.*** Summary of treatment of hypertensive emergencies.

| Target organ involved | Preferred agents | Comments |
|---|---|---|
| Aortic dissection: Must use vasodilator AND β-blocker | Labetalol OR Nicardipine + esmolol OR Nitroprusside + esmolol or IV metoprolol | *Labetalol:* combined selective α-adrenergic and nonselective β-adrenergic blocker; maintains cardiac output, renal, cerebral, coronary blood flow<br>*Nicardipine:* dihydropyridine calcium channel blocker; strong cerebral and coronary vasodilator; reduces coronary and cerebral ischemia<br>*Esmolol:* ultrashort-acting cardioselective β-adrenergic blocker; suitable when cardiac output, BP and HR are increased<br>*Nitroprusside:* arterial and venous vasodilator; decreases cerebral blood flow; contains cyanide |
| Hypertensive encephalopathy | Nicardipine OR Labetalol OR Fenoldopam | *Fenoldopam:* vasodilates by acting on peripheral dopamine-1 receptors; improves creatinine clearance + sodium excretion |
| Cerebral infarction or hemorrhage | Nicardipine OR Labetalol OR Fenoldopam | |
| Myocardial ischemia/ infarction | Labetalol OR esmolol PLUS nitroglycerin | *Nitroglycerin:* potent venodilator; reduces preload and cardiac output; causes reflex tachycardia |
| Acute pulmonary edema/systolic dysfunction | Nicardipine OR fenoldopam OR nitroprusside PLUS nitroglycerin PLUS loop diuretic | |
| Renal insufficiency | Nicardipine OR fenoldopam | |
| Eclampsia | Labetalol OR nicardipine | Nitroprusside and ACE inhibitors should not be used in pregnant patients |
| Acute postoperative hypertension | Esmolol OR nicardipine OR labetalol | |

1. All patients should be admitted to the hospital; many will need to be treated in the ICU with IV medications.

2. Little or no evidence to guide choice of specific drugs or rate of BP lowering in hypertensive encephalopathy

3. Guidelines recommend lowering the MAP by no more than 25% in the first 2 hours and achieving a BP of 160/100 mm Hg (MAP = 120 mm Hg) within 6 hours.

4. Agents commonly used include labetalol, nicardipine, or fenoldopam, all of which are thought to maintain cerebral blood flow.

B. Treating hypertension in the setting of acute ischemic stroke

1. Most patients have acutely elevated BP regardless of pre-existing hypertension as the body attempts to maintain cerebral blood flow to the ischemic territory.

2. Autoregulation is impaired in ischemic areas, so lowering the BP can lead to a significant reduction in cerebral blood flow, potentially exacerbating cerebral ischemia.

3. The BP elevation generally decreases spontaneously with time.

4. Guidelines recommend treating hypertension in acute ischemic stroke *only if:*

a. The diastolic BP is > 120 mm Hg and/or the systolic BP is > 220 mm Hg

b. The patient has noncerebral acute TOD

c. Thrombolysis is planned, in which case the target BP is 180/105 mm Hg

5. IV labetalol is the drug of choice for acute treatment because it can be easily titrated and does not reduce cerebral blood flow.

6. BP should be reduced by no more than 10-15% in the first 24 hours.

7. Oral agents should be started 10 days after the acute event.

C. Treating hypertension in the setting of subarachnoid or intracerebral hemorrhage

1. There is no evidence that hypertension causes further bleeding, and elevated BP might be necessary to maintain cerebral perfusion.

2. BP should be lowered in a controlled manner when the systolic BP is > 200 mm Hg, the diastolic > 110 mm Hg, or the MAP > 130 mm Hg.

3. Nicardipine has been shown to be effective in intracerebral hemorrhage.

# CASE RESOLUTION

▽3

Mr. J has no signs or symptoms of stroke, intracranial hemorrhage, pulmonary edema, myocardial ischemia, or aortic dissection. He has a headache, but he does not have other symptoms, such as lethargy or confusion, to suggest hypertensive encephalopathy. His renal function is stable and his urinalysis is normal. Although his fundi were not optimally visualized, it is unlikely that he has acute end organ damage considering his overall presentation. There is no need to perform any further testing at this point.

Mr. J's previous regimen was hydrochlorothiazide, 25 mg; metoprolol ER, 50 mg; and amlodipine, 10 mg. You instruct him to fill his prescriptions after he picks up his son at school, to take the amlodipine tonight, and then to take all 3 medications in the morning. When he returns in 2 days, his BP is 160/100 mm Hg; 3 weeks later it is 145/90 mm Hg.

# REVIEW OF OTHER IMPORTANT DISEASES

## Pheochromocytoma

### Textbook Presentation

The classic presentation is a patient with attacks of paroxysmal hypertension, headache, palpitations, and sweating occurring several times daily, weekly, or every few months. Patients generally have orthostatic hypotension on physical exam.

### Diseases Highlights

A. 95% of patients have headache, sweating, OR palpitations.

B. 10% of pheochromocytomas are malignant and tend to have a less typical presentation.

C. 10–15% are familial (multiple endocrine neoplasia type 2, von Hippel-Lindau disease, neurofibromatosis); these are more often asymptomatic (and normotensive) than sporadic cases.

D. See Table 20–11 for distribution of symptoms, taken from a series of patients with pheochromocytoma, about half of whom presented with paroxysmal hypertension and about half of whom had persistent hypertension.

### Evidence-Based Diagnosis

A. Pretest probability of 0.5% in hypertensive patients who have suggestive symptoms

B. Pretest probability of 4% in patients with incidentally discovered adrenal masses

C. Plasma metanephrine is the single best test to rule out pheochromocytoma (Table 20–12).

1. Patients should fast overnight and be supine for 20 minutes prior to the blood draw.

2. Because caffeine and acetaminophen interfere with the assay, patients should avoid caffeine for 12 hours and acetaminophen for 5 days prior to testing.

3. The standard upper limit of normal for plasma metanephrines is 61 ng/L.

**Table 20–11.** Signs and symptoms in pheochromocytoma.

| Symptom | Patients with pheochromocytoma and paroxysmal hypertension | Patients with pheochromocytoma and persistent hypertension |
|---|---|---|
| Severe headaches | 92% | 72% |
| Sweating | 65% | 69% |
| Palpitations and/or tachycardia | 73% | 51% |
| Anxiety/panic | 60% | 28% |
| Tremulousness | 51% | 26% |
| Chest or abdominal pain | 48% | 28% |
| Nausea ± vomiting | 43% | 26% |

a. The overall (sporadic and hereditary cases) sensitivity at this cut off is 99% with a specificity of 89%.

b. A plasma metanephrine > 236 ng/L is 100% specific for the diagnosis of pheochromocytoma.

D. Patients with positive biochemical testing should undergo adrenal imaging.

1. CT: sensitivity of 93–100% for detecting adrenal pheochromocytomas, 90% for extra-adrenal tumors; specificity 50–70%

**Table 20–12.** Diagnostic tests for sporadic pheochromocytoma.[1]

| Test | Sensitivity (%) | Specificity (%) | LR+ | LR– |
|---|---|---|---|---|
| Plasma free metanephrines | 99 | 82 | 5.5 | 0.012 |
| Plasma catecholamines | 92 | 72 | 2.9 | 0.11 |
| 24-hour urine fractionated metanephrines | 97 | 45 | 1.76 | 0.06 |
| 24-hour urine catecholamines | 91 | 75 | 3.64 | 0.12 |
| 24-hour urine total metanephrines | 88 | 89 | 8 | 0.13 |
| 24-hour urine vanillylmandelic acid level (VMA) | 77 | 86 | 5.5 | 0.26 |

[1]Test characteristics for the diagnosis in patients with hereditary pheochromocytoma are different and can be found in (Data from Lenders JWM. JAMA. 2002;287:1427–34.)

**2.** MRI: sensitivity 90%; specificity also 50–70%; better than CT for identifying vascular invasion

**3.** [131]I-MIBG or positron emission tomography scanning is sometimes used when the biochemistry is positive and both CT and MRI are negative.

## Treatment

**A.** Surgery is the definitive treatment.

**B.** Must give both α- and β-blocking agents preoperatively

  **1.** The α-blocker opposes catecholamine-induced vasoconstriction.

  **2.** The β-blocker opposes the reflex tachycardia that occurs with α-blockade.

  **3.** Unopposed β-blockade will cause inhibition of epinephrine induced vasodilation, leading to increased BP, left heart strain, and possibly HF.

  **4.** Should be done in consultation with an endocrinologist because of the complexities of ensuring adequate α-blockade

 Never give a patient with a pheochromocytoma a β-blocker without first giving an α-blocker.

**C.** 27–38% of patients have residual hypertension.

**D.** Patients with familial pheochromocytoma often have multiple, bilateral tumors; the optimal approach to therapy is not clear.

## REFERENCES

Calhoun DA, Jones D, Textor S et al. Resistant hypertension: diagnosis, evaluation, and treatment: a scientific statement from the American Heart Association Professional Education Committee of the Council for High Blood Pressure Research. Circulation. 2008;117:e510–26.

Chobanian AV, Bakris GL, Black HR et al. The Seventh Report of the Joint National Committee on Prevention, Detection, Evaluation, and Treatment of High Blood Pressure. JAMA. 2003;289:2560–72.

Doi SAR, Abalkhail S, Al-Qudhaiby et al. Optimal use and interpretation of the aldosterone renin ratio to detect aldosterone excess in hypertension. J Human Hypertension. 2006;20:482–89.

Krijnen P, van Jaarsveld BC, Steyerberg EW, Man't Veld, AJ et al. A clinical predication rule for renal artery stenosis. Ann Intern Med. 1998;129:705–11.

Lee VH, Wijdicks EFM, Manno EM, Rabinstein AA. Clinical spectrum of reversible posterior leukoencephalopathy syndrome. Arch Neurol. 2008;65:205–10.

Lenders JWM, Pacak K, Walther MM et al. Biochemical diagnosis of pheochromocytoma. Which test is best? JAMA. 2002;287:1427–34.

Manger WM, Gifford RW. Pheochromocytoma. J Clin Hypertension. 2002;4:62–72.

Marik PE, Varon J. Hypertensive crises. Chest. 2007;131:1949–62.

Mittendorf EA, Evans DB, Lee JE, Perrier ND. Pheochromocytoma: advances in genetics, diagnosis, localization, and treatment. Hematol Oncol Clin N Am. 2007;21:509–25.

Turnbull JM. Is listening for abdominal bruits useful in the evaluation of hypertension? JAMA. 1995;274:1299–1301.

Van de Ven PJG, Beutler JJ, Kaatee R et al. Angiotensin converting enzyme inhibitor induced renal dysfunction in atherosclerotic renovascular disease. Kidney Int. 1998;53:986–93.

Vasbinder G, Nelemans PJ, Kessels A et al. Accuracy of computed tomographic angiography and magnetic resonance angiography for diagnosing renal artery stenosis. Ann Intern Med. 2004;141:674–82.

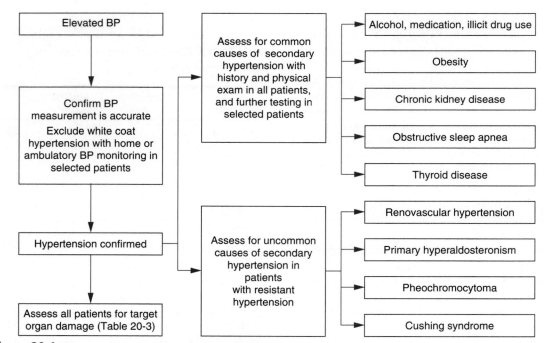

***Figure 20-1.*** Diagnostic approach: evaluation of hypertension.

# I have a patient with hyponatremia. I have a patient with hypernatremia. How do I determine the cause?

## HYPONATREMIA

## CHIEF COMPLAINT

PATIENT 1

Mr. D is a 42-year-old man who is brought to the emergency department by the police department. He is disoriented and confused. Initial labs reveal a serum sodium concentration of 118 mEq/L.

**What is the differential diagnosis of hyponatremia? How would you frame the differential?**

## CONSTRUCTING A DIFFERENTIAL DIAGNOSIS

Hyponatremia develops when the body is unable to excrete free water. Hyponatremia is defined as serum sodium concentration <134 mEq/L and is significant when the concentration is <130 mEq/L. The first step in evaluating the hyponatremic patient is to review the history and laboratory results for a few diagnostic fingerprints that may be present (ie, a history of thiazide ingestion suggests diuretic-induced hyponatremia, hyperkalemia suggests primary adrenal insufficiency, a urine osmolality ≈100 mOsm/L suggests psychogenic polydipsia, and marked hyperglycemia suggests hyperglycemia-induced hyponatremia.) For most patients, these tests will not be diagnostic and the key **pivotal** point in the differential diagnosis is to determine the patient's volume status and identify who is clinically hypervolemic, euvolemic, or hypovolemic. This step narrows the differential diagnosis and is necessary to properly interpret test results. Correct classification of the patient's volume status requires a review of the history, physical exam findings, and laboratory results (Figure 21–1). After the patient's volume status has been determined, the different etiologies can be considered (Figure 21–2).

## Differential Diagnosis of Hyponatremia

A. Hypervolemia
   1. Heart failure (HF)
   2. Cirrhosis
   3. Nephrotic syndrome
   4. Renal failure (glomerular filtration rate [GFR] <5 mL/min)

B. Euvolemia
   1. Syndrome of inappropriate antidiuretic hormone (SIADH)

      a. Cancers (eg, pancreas, lung)

      b. CNS disease (eg, cerebrovascular accident, trauma, infection, hemorrhage, mass)

      c. Pulmonary diseases (eg, infections, respiratory failure)

      d. Drugs

         (1) Thiazides

         (2) Antidiuretic hormone (ADH) analogues (vasopressin, desmopressin acetate [DDAVP], oxytocin)

         (3) Chlorpropamide (6–7% of treated patients)

         (4) Carbamazepine

         (5) Antidepressants (tricyclics and selective serotonin reuptake inhibitors) and antipsychotics

         (6) Nonsteroidal antiinflammatory drugs (NSAIDs)

         (7) Ecstasy (MDMA)

         (8) Others (cyclophosphamide, vincristine, nicotine, opioids, clofibrate)

   2. Hypothyroidism
   3. Psychogenic polydipsia
   4. Secondary adrenal insufficiency
   5. Exercise-associated hyponatremia

C. Hypovolemia
   1. Salt and water loss with free water replacement

      a. Severe diarrhea with free water ingestion

      b. Large burns with free water replacement

      c. Third-spacing with free water replacement

   2. Primary adrenal insufficiency
   3. Renal disease

      a. Diuretics

      b. Salt-wasting nephropathy

Before proceeding, it is useful to briefly review the pathophysiology of hyponatremia. Hyponatremia develops when patients do not excrete their daily ingested excess (or free) water. Free water excretion requires 3 distinct mechanisms (Figure 21–3):

1. Glomerular filtration

2. Separation of water from solute so that free water can be excreted. This occurs in the thick ascending loop of Henle. This section of the tubule is impermeable to water. Therefore, sodium pumped out of the lumen leaves free water within the tubule.

3. Excretion of free water. Finally, water must travel through the tubules without being reabsorbed into the kidney. This requires absent or low levels of ADH. (ADH increases the permeability of the tubules [via aquaporin channels] allowing water within the tubules to leak back into the interstitium.)

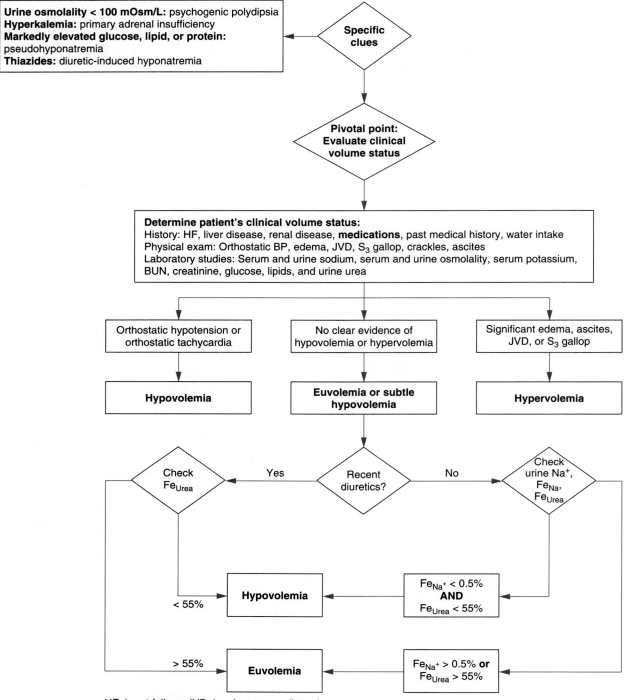

**Urine osmolality < 100 mOsm/L:** psychogenic polydipsia
**Hyperkalemia:** primary adrenal insufficiency
**Markedly elevated glucose, lipid, or protein:**
pseudohyponatremia
**Thiazides:** diuretic-induced hyponatremia

Specific clues

Pivotal point: Evaluate clinical volume status

**Determine patient's clinical volume status:**
History: HF, liver disease, renal disease, **medications**, past medical history, water intake
Physical exam: Orthostatic BP, edema, JVD, $S_3$ gallop, crackles, ascites
Laboratory studies: Serum and urine sodium, serum and urine osmolality, serum potassium,
BUN, creatinine, glucose, lipids, and urine urea

Orthostatic hypotension or orthostatic tachycardia

No clear evidence of hypovolemia or hypervolemia

Significant edema, ascites, JVD, or $S_3$ gallop

**Hypovolemia**

**Euvolemia or subtle hypovolemia**

**Hypervolemia**

Check $Fe_{Urea}$

Yes

Recent diuretics?

No

Check urine $Na^+$, $Fe_{Na}$, $Fe_{Urea}$

< 55%

**Hypovolemia**

$Fe_{Na^+} < 0.5\%$
**AND**
$Fe_{Urea} < 55\%$

> 55%

**Euvolemia**

$Fe_{Na^+} > 0.5\%$ **or**
$Fe_{Urea} > 55\%$

HF, heart failure; JVD, jugular venous distention.

***Figure 21–1.*** Determination of volume status in true (hypo-osmolar) hyponatremia.

In short, free water excretion requires glomerular filtration, a functioning thick ascending loop of Henle, and low levels of ADH. Interference with these 3 mechanisms contributes to hyponatremia.

## Symptoms of Hyponatremia

The adverse effects and manifestations of hyponatremia depend on its severity and rapidity of development. Acute hyponatremia

leaves the brain hypertonic relative to the serum. This osmotic gradient drives water into the brain, resulting in cerebral edema and CNS symptoms. Typically, patients with serum sodium levels >130 mEq/L are asymptomatic; those with levels from 125 mEq/L to 130 mEq/L may have nausea, vomiting, or abdominal symptoms. Headache, agitation, and confusion may develop in patients with levels < 125 mEq/L. Levels below 120 mEq/L have been associated with seizures and coma. Severe acute hyponatremia may

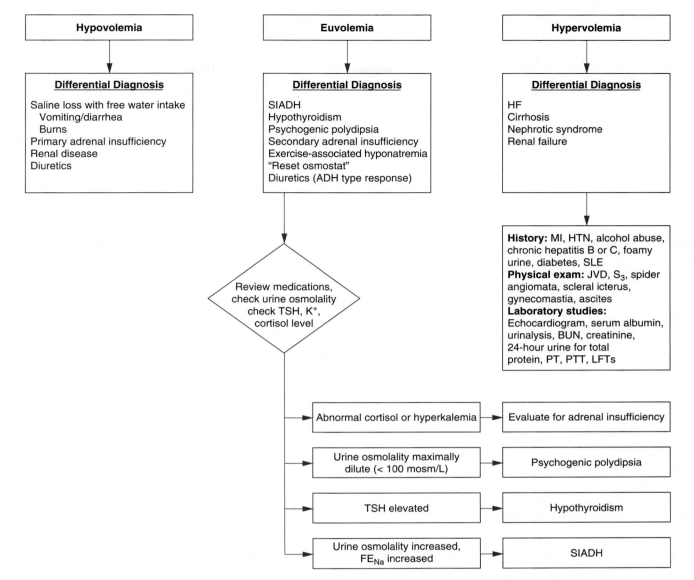

ADH, antidiuretic hormone; HF, heart failure; HTN, hypertension; JVD, jugular venous distention; LFTs, liver function tests; MI, myocardiial infarction; PT, Prothrombin time; PTT, partial thromboplastin time; SIADH, syndrome inappropriate antidiuretic hormone; SLE, systemic lupus erythematosus.

***Figure 21–2.*** Differential diagnosis of true (hypo-osmolar) hyponatremia by volume status.

cause brain damage, brainstem herniation, respiratory arrest, and death. Rhabdomyolysis may occur. On the other hand, chronic hyponatremia allows neurons to decrease their intracellular osmolality and thereby causes less cerebral edema. Although minor symptoms are common, seizures and herniation are much less frequent in chronic hyponatremia.

Because the classification scheme of hyponatremia relies on the correct determination of the patient's volume status, it is important to ask, "How reliable is the physical exam for classifying the patient's volume status?"

A. In patients with hypervolemic hyponatremia, the hypervolemia is easily detected because the hyponatremia only develops in advanced disease (ie, HF, cirrhosis, or nephrotic syndrome).

1. There is often a known history of HF, cirrhosis, or nephrosis.

2. Physical findings of volume overload (eg, edema, jugular venous distention [JVD], $S_3$, and ascites) are usually present.

B. In contrast, separating euvolemic patients from hypovolemic patients is more difficult.

1. Hypovolemic patients may have a history of volume loss (ie, diarrhea, intense prolonged sweating) or physical findings of hypotension, tachycardia, or orthostatic hypotension.

2. However, many hypovolemic patients with hyponatremia appear euvolemic, and the history and physical findings

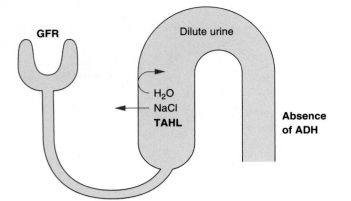

**Figure 21–3.** Pathophysiology of free water excretion. Free water diuresis requires (1) GFR, (2) functioning TAHL, and (3) absence of ADH. (ADH, antidiuretic hormone; GFR, glomerular filtration rate; TAHL, thick ascending loop of Henle.)

are neither sensitive nor specific for hypovolemia with LRs around 1.0 (Table 21–1).

C. Given the limitations of the history and physical exam, certain laboratory tests are critical to distinguish euvolemic patients from hypovolemic patients. The 3 most accurate biochemical parameters are the spot urine sodium, the fractional excretion of sodium ($FE_{Na}$), and the fractional excretion of urea ($FE_{urea}$). All parameters were studied in patients who were either euvolemic or hypovolemia. *Hypervolemic* patients

**Table 21–1.** Sensitivity and specificity of the clinical and lab exam to detect hypovolemia in hyponatremic patients.[1]

| Criteria | Sensitivity (%) | Specificity (%) | LR+ | LR– |
|---|---|---|---|---|
| Clinical evaluation[2,3] | 25–47 | 48–78 | 0.9–1.3 | 1.1– 0.9 |
| Urine sodium concentration < 30 mEq/L | 71–80 | 88–100 | 5.9– ∞ | 0.2– 0.3 |
| Urine sodium concentration < 20 mEq/L | 47 | 94 | 7.8 | 0.6 |
| $FE_{Na+}$ < 0.5% | 100 | 58–80 | 2.4– 5.0 | 0 |
| $FE_{Na+}$ < 0.5% and $FE_{urea}$ < 55% | 94 | 100 | ∞ | 0.06 |

[1]These studies included euvolemic and hypovolemic patients. Hypervolemic patients and those taking diuretics were excluded.
[2]Criteria included ≥ 2 of the following: (compatible history, decreased skin turgor or dry axilla or thirst, ≥ 0.5-kg weight loss, > 10% decreased systolic pressure, 10% increase in standing pulse rate, BUN/Cr > 20 mg/dL).
[3]Required 3 of the following: dry mouth mucosa, decreased skin turgor, absent jugular venous distention, orthostatic fall in systolic BP > 10%, orthostatic increase pulse > 10%.

(with ascites or edema) were excluded because hyponatremia in these patients is usually due to *ineffective circulating volume,* and thus such patients usually avidly reabsorb sodium. Obtaining urine sodium measurements in them may mislead clinicians into thinking these patients are hypovolemic. The accuracy of these tests in euvolemic and hypovolemic patients is summarized in Table 21–1. These results are for patients not taking diuretics, since diuretics promote sodium loss and interfere with the ability to interpret the urine sodium concentration and $FE_{Na+}$.

1. Spot urine sodium
   a. Most hypovolemic patients avidly reabsorb sodium resulting in decreased urine sodium concentration.
   b. Average urinary sodium in hypovolemic patients: 18.4 mEq/L, compared with 72 mEq/L in euvolemic patients
   c. False-negative results (elevated urine sodium in hypovolemic patients) may be seen in hypovolemia secondary to:
      (1) Primary adrenal insufficiency in which the hypoaldosteronism directly leads to sodium wasting.
      (2) Vomiting with accompanying metabolic alkalosis. The metabolic alkalosis causes an obligatory urinary $HCO_3^-$ loss, which is accompanied by sodium. Urine chloride may be low in such cases.
   d. False-positive results (low urine sodium in euvolemic patients) may be seen in certain euvolemic patients.
      (1) Psychogenic polydipsia. These patients are euvolemic but usually have low urine sodium *concentration* due to dilution of the excreted sodium in vast quantities of water.
      (2) Some patients with SIADH *ingest* little sodium causing decreased urinary sodium output.

2. Fractional excretion of sodium
   a. $FE_{Na} = (U_{Na}^+ \times P_{Cr})/(P_{Na}^+ \times U_{Cr})$
   b. Compares fraction of sodium excreted to fraction of sodium filtered. In hypovolemic states, the fraction excreted should be low (< 0.5%).
   c. $FE_{Na}^+$ is an exceptionally sensitive measure of hypovolemia (sensitivity 100%). An elevated $FE_{Na}$ > 0.5% rules out hypovolemia except in patients taking diuretics.
   d. Patients taking diuretics have obligatory sodium losses, raising the $FE_{Na}$ even in the face of hypovolemia. In such patients, the $FE_{urea}$ can be helpful (see below).
   e. Specificity is imperfect. Certain euvolemic patients may have a low $FE_{Na}$.
      (1) SIADH patients with a low salt intake; eg, the $FE_{Na}^+$ of a patient with a low sodium intake (1.6 g/d) (and normal renal function) would be 0.4%.
      (2) Some patients with psychogenic polydipsia (one-third of such patients have a low $FE_{Na}^+$).

3. Fractional excretion of urea
   a. $(FE_{urea}) = (U_{urea} \times P_{Cr})/(P_{urea} \times U_{Cr})$
   b. Compares fraction of urea excreted to urea filtered. In euvolemic states, urea is rapidly excreted ($FE_{urea}$ > 55%)
   c. Two studies suggest a combination of both low $FE_{Na}$ (< 0.5%) and low $FE_{urea}$ (< 55%) was highly sensitive and specific for hypovolemia.

**d.** FE$_{urea}$ in hypovolemic patients taking diuretics is usually low and may be more useful than FE$_{Na}$ in such patients.

**4.** In summary, a high Fe$_{Na+}$ rules out hypovolemia (except for patients taking diuretics) and a low Fe$_{Na}^+$ combined with a low FE$_{urea}$ rules in hypovolemia.

Urine sodium and FENa help properly classify patients as euvolemic or hypovolemic.

**5.** Although not routinely used, renin and aldosterone levels are higher on average in hypovolemic patients than euvolemic patients (renin 63 pg/mL vs 24 pg/mL, respectively; aldosterone 274 ng/mL vs 98 ng/mL, respectively). Elevated levels suggest hypovolemia but low levels are not diagnostic of euvolemia.

Due to his confusion, Mr. D is unable to relate his past medical history. His chart is requested. Physical exam reveals a disheveled man appearing older than his stated age. He is unshaven and smells of alcohol. His vital signs are BP, 90/50 mm Hg; pulse, 90 bpm; temperature, 36.0°C; RR, 18 breaths per minute. He has no orthostatic change in BP. Neck veins are flat. His lungs are clear to auscultation. Cardiac exam reveals a regular rate and rhythm. There is no JVD, S$_3$ gallop, or murmur. His abdomen is distended, and his flanks are bulging. Extremity exam reveals 3+ pitting edema extending all the way up his thighs.

Laboratory studies reveal a glucose of 100 mg/dL, K+ 3.8, a BUN of 28 mg/dL, creatinine 1.0 mg/dL, and a serum osmolality of 252 mOsm/L. Urine osmolality is 480 mOsm/L.

At this point, what is the leading hypothesis, what are the active alternatives, and is there a must not miss diagnosis? Given this differential diagnosis, what tests should be ordered?

## PRIORITIZING THE DIFFERENTIAL DIAGNOSIS

The first step in evaluating the patient with hyponatremia is to determine whether there is a history of thiazide use and to review the laboratory results to determine whether there are any highly specific results that point to a particular diagnosis (ie, hyperglycemia, hyperkalemia, or a maximally dilute urine) (see Figure 21–1). Mr. D's serum glucose is normal, ruling out marked hyperglycemic hyponatremia, and the absence of hyperkalemia makes primary adrenal insufficiency less likely. The urine osmolality is high enough to effectively rule out psychogenic polydipsia (see below). The second and **key pivotal point** in the evaluation of hyponatremia is to ascertain whether Mr. D is hypervolemic, euvolemic, or hypovolemic. Mr. D's marked peripheral edema clearly indicates that he is *hypervolemic*. The 4 causes of hypervolemic hyponatremia include HF, nephrotic syndrome, cirrhosis, and renal failure. Of these, cirrhosis seems most likely. The smell of alcohol raises the suspicion of alcohol abuse and liver disease, and the bulging flanks suggest ascites, which in turn suggests cirrhosis.

***Table 21–2.*** Diagnostic hypotheses for Mr. D.

| Diagnostic Hypothesis | Clinical Clues | Important Tests |
|---|---|---|
| **Leading Hypothesis** | | |
| Cirrhosis | *History:* Heavy alcohol use, hepatitis C or chronic hepatitis B, esophageal varices *Physical exam:* Scleral icterus, spider angiomata, gynecomastia, ascites (bulging flanks, shifting dullness) | Serum albumin, ALT, AST, bilirubin, PT, PTT, hepatitis B surface antigen, hepatitis C antibody, liver ultrasound and Doppler |
| **Active Alternatives—Most Common** | | |
| Nephrotic syndrome | History of foamy urine, diabetes, SLE | Serum albumin, urinalysis, 24-hour urine total protein, BUN, creatinine |
| **Active Alternatives—Must Not Miss** | | |
| Heart failure | History of myocardial infarction or poorly controlled hypertension S$_3$ gallop, JVD, crackles on lung exam, peripheral edema | Echocardiogram, ECG |

HF is also possible although Mr. D has neither an S$_3$ gallop nor JVD. Nonetheless, HF should still be considered since neither finding is sensitive for HF. Renal failure is effectively ruled out by his normal creatinine, but we do not have any information yet about proteinuria. Table 21–2 lists the differential diagnosis.

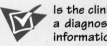

Review of Mr. D's past medical record reveals that he has a long history of alcohol-related complications. Six months ago he was hospitalized for bleeding esophageal varices.

Is the clinical information sufficient to make a diagnosis of cirrhosis? If not, what other information do you need?

## Leading Hypothesis: Cirrhosis

### Textbook Presentation

See Chapter 15, Edema for a full discussion. Patients with cirrhosis may have ascites, variceal hemorrhage, encephalopathy, jaundice, hypoalbuminemia, coagulopathy, and elevated transaminases.

### Disease Highlights

**A.** Hyponatremia is a marker of severe cirrhosis found in 3% of patients with Child-Pugh class A, 16% in class B, and 31% of class C.

**Table 21–3.** Comparison of findings in patients who have cirrhosis with and without hyponatremia.

| | Patients without Hyponatremia | Patients with Hyponatremia |
|---|---|---|
| Small liver size | 25% | 85% |
| Child-Pugh class C | 31% | 60% |
| BP | 112/59 mm Hg | 99/54 mm Hg |
| Hepatorenal syndrome | 5% | 17–85%[1] |
| Hepatic encephalopathy | 15% | 38% |

[1]The wide variation between the incidence of hepatorenal syndrome in patients with hyponatremia and cirrhosis reflects the incidence in different patient populations. The rate of 85% was reported in patients hospitalized for an acute complication.

B. Hyponatremia is associated with a higher frequency of adverse outcomes (including hepatorenal syndrome, hepatic encephalopathy, spontaneous bacterial peritonitis, and death), especially if there is no clear precipitant (Table 21–3). One study of hospitalized patients reported a 25% mortality among cirrhotic patients without hyponatremia compared with 93% among those with hyponatremia. Another study of patients awaiting liver transplant reported a 4% mortality among those without hyponatremia compared with 35% among patients with hyponatremia.

C. Among patients with cirrhosis and ascites, 22% have sodium ≤ 130 mEq/L.

D. Pathogenesis of hyponatremia in cirrhosis

1. Hypoalbuminemia and splanchnic dilatation (possibly secondary to elevated nitric oxide) cause decreased effective circulating volume and decreased systemic vascular resistance respectively, which leads to decreased mean arterial pressure, resulting in

   a. Elevated ADH (particularly important)

   b. Decreased GFR

   c. Increased proximal reabsorption of solute causing decreased solute delivery to loop of Henle

2. Renal arteriolar vasoconstriction further decreases GFR and increases proximal sodium reabsorption.

3. NSAIDs may worsen edema by reducing GFR and worsen hyponatremia. NSAIDs also lower renal $PGE_2$, which normally antagonizes ADH.

E. Hyponatremia may worsen hepatic encephalopathy.

### Evidence-Based Diagnosis

A. No clinical finding is terribly sensitive for cirrhosis.

1. Jaundice, 14%

2. Variceal bleeding, 50%

3. Ascites, 30%

4. Encephalopathy, 50–70%

5. Splenomegaly, 36–92%

B. However, certain physical exam findings are common in cirrhotic patients *with* hyponatremia.

1. Ascites present in 100%

2. Peripheral edema seen in 59%

C. Laboratory studies: Mean urine sodium 4 mEq/L (measurements made after diuretics have been stopped for 5 days). (Decreased effective circulating volume causes increased renal reabsorption of sodium.)

### Treatment

A. Since the hyponatremia develops gradually, symptoms due to the hyponatremia are uncommon. Fluid restriction is recommended particularly in symptomatic patients.

B. Short-term, preliminary studies, suggest tolvaptan, an ADH V2 receptor antagonist, can help correct hyponatremia in patients with cirrhosis, HF, and SIADH. Combined ADH receptor antagonists V1a-V2 (conivaptan) should not be used in patients with cirrhosis as they may induce hypotension.

## MAKING A DIAGNOSIS

Lab studies reveal an albumin of 2.1 g/dL, bilirubin 6.2 mg/dL, AST (SGOT) 85 units/L, ALT (SGPT) 45 units/L, INR of 1.8. An abdominal ultrasound reveals moderate ascites and a small liver with coarse architecture suggestive of cirrhosis.

Have you crossed a diagnostic threshold for the leading hypothesis, cirrhosis? Have you ruled out the active alternatives? Do other tests need to be done to exclude the alternative diagnoses?

Mr. D's findings point fairly conclusively to hypervolemic hyponatremia secondary to cirrhosis. The prior history of varices and ascites point to portal hypertension while the jaundice, hypoalbuminemia, and increased INR suggest synthetic failure by the liver. HF secondary to an alcoholic cardiomyopathy is still possible. Other causes of hypervolemia hyponatremia, such as nephrotic syndrome, are less likely but possible. Finally, there is no history of thiazide use to suggest diuretic-induced hyponatremia.

## Alternative Diagnosis: HF & Hyponatremia

### Textbook Presentation

Typically, patients with HF complain of shortness of breath, dyspnea on exertion, fatigue, and orthopnea. (See Chapter 14, Dyspnea for a complete discussion of HF.)

### Disease Highlights

A. Patients with HF and hyponatremia have marked *increases* in total body sodium retention and content.

B. In patients with hyponatremia, free water clearance is impaired and water retention *exceeds* sodium retention.

C. Free water clearance is impaired in large part secondary to elevated ADH levels. The fall in cardiac output triggers carotid baroreceptors which in turn stimulate ADH release. A decreased GFR (due to decreased renal perfusion) and an increase in proximal sodium reabsorption also impair free water excretion.

**D.** Hyponatremia is observed in patients with severe HF and is associated with an increased risk of death.

**E.** Diuretic therapy (particularly thiazides) can worsen the hyponatremia.

### Evidence-Based Diagnosis

See HF discussion in Chapter 14, Dyspnea.

### Treatment

**A.** Treatment of underlying HF

   **1.** Similar to other patients with HF (see Chapter 14, Dyspnea).

   **2.** ACE inhibitors: Hyponatremia suggests activation of the renin angiotensin system and such patients are susceptible to hypotension when ACE inhibitors are used. Therefore, therapy with ACE inhibitors should be initiated at *low* doses. ACE inhibitors can help restore sodium levels to normal.

   **3.** Avoid NSAID use, which can decrease prostaglandin-dependent renal blood flow and worsen renal function.

**B.** Treatment of hyponatremia

   **1.** Exclude overdiuresis with free water replacement

   **2.** Restrict water intake < 1000 mL/d

   **3.** Discontinue thiazide diuretics

   **4.** Furosemide in symptomatic, volume-overloaded patients

   **5.** The selective ADH V2 receptor antagonist tolvaptan may prove useful (see above).

## Alternative Diagnosis: Nephrotic Syndrome

### Textbook Presentation

See Chapter 15, Edema for full discussion. Patients typically complain of edema.

### Disease Highlights

**A.** Lesions may be primary and idiopathic (eg, minimal change lesion) or secondary to systemic disease (eg, diabetes mellitus, malignancy).

**B.** Glomerular lesion leads to albuminuria and hypoalbuminemia. Patients with nephrotic syndrome are total body sodium *overloaded.* The effective *intravascular* volume may be decreased or increased.

   **1.** In some patients, hypoalbuminemia and decreased oncotic pressures lead to both edema and ineffective circulating volume. This in turn elevates ADH, reduces free water clearance, and promotes hyponatremia.

   **2.** In other patients, renal insufficiency impairs sodium and free water clearance. Patients are hypervolemic and some patients are hyponatremic.

   **3.** Pseudohyponatremia may be seen secondary to marked hypertriglyceridemia.

### Evidence-Based Diagnosis

**A.** Nephrotic syndrome is characterized by urine protein excretion ≥ 3.5 g/d, edema, hypoalbuminemia, and hyperlipidemia.

**B.** Renal biopsy can help identify certain underlying disease states.

### Treatment

Free water restriction.

## CASE RESOLUTION

> An echocardiogram reveals normal left ventricular function and a urinalysis reveals only 1+ proteinuria not suggestive of nephrotic syndrome. A paracentesis is performed to rule out spontaneous bacterial peritonitis and is normal.

Mr. D's history, physical exam, and laboratory findings clearly point to severe cirrhosis. HF and nephrotic syndrome are effectively ruled out by the echocardiogram and urinalysis. An important aspect of his care is to ensure a safe and gradual return of his serum sodium to normal.

### Treatment of Hyponatremia Associated with Hypervolemia

Correction of hyponatremia must be done carefully. Rapid correction may cause permanent brain damage.

**A.** In chronic hyponatremia, physiologic adaptations protect the brain from cerebral edema by lowering intraneuronal osmolality.

**B.** Rapid *correction* of hyponatremia leaves the brain hypotonic relative to plasma, which can result in catastrophic demyelinization and the dreaded complication of central pontine myelinolysis (see below).

**C.** Asymptomatic or mildly symptomatic patients

   **1.** Free water restriction is the therapy of choice.

   **2.** The goal of therapy is to correct the serum sodium by ≤ 0.5 mEq/L/h. Some authorities suggest a maximum correction of ≤ 8 mEq/L/d.

**D.** Patients with **severe** neurologic symptoms from hyponatremia (seizures, coma)

   **1.** Renal consultation is advised.

   **2.** ICU monitoring is usually appropriate.

   **3.** Hypertonic saline (3%) can be given to such patients.

   **4.** For patients with severe symptoms, the goal is an initial correction rate of 1–2 mEq/L/h for 3–4 hours or until symptoms (ie, seizures or coma) abate.

   **5.** A maximum of 8–12 mEq/L/d (0.33 mEq/L/h) correction is still recommended.

   **6.** Formulas can help estimate the initial rate of infusion. However, actual responses may vary, and patients must have frequent sodium measurements to ensure an appropriate rate of correction.

   **7.** The impact of 1 L of fluid can be calculated as follows:

     **a.** $\{(\text{Infusate Na} - \text{Plasma } [\text{Na}^+])/(\text{TBW} + 1)\}$

       **(1)** Total body water (TBW) = 0.6 × weight (kg) men

       **(2)** TBW = 0.5 × weight (kg) women

       **(3)** Infusate Na = 154 mEq/L for normal saline

       **(4)** Infusate Na = 513 mEq/L for 3% normal saline

**b.** Example: Assume an asymptomatic 70 kg male. Initial [Na] = 110 mEq/L

**(1)** TBW = 0.6 × 70 (kg) = 42 L

**(2)** Using *normal saline* [Na⁺] = 154 mEq/L

   **(a)** Increase in [Na⁺] = {(154 − 110)/(42 + 1)} = 1 mEq per liter infused

   **(b)** If the desired correction rate is 0.33 mEq/L/h, then the 1 L would be administered over 3 hours.

**(3)** If the patient was seizing, more rapid correction would be advised using *3% normal saline* [Na⁺] = 513 mEq/L

   **(a)** Increase in [Na⁺] = {(513 − 110)/(42 + 1)} = 9.3 mEq per liter infused

   **(b)** If the desired rate of correction for the first 3 hours was 2 mEq/L/h, then 2/9.3 × 1000 (= 215 mL/h) would be administered per hour for the first 3 hours

**c.** Electrolytes should be monitored every 2 hours.

**d.** Furosemide is often administered to prevent intravascular volume overload. Furosemide may also increase free water loss.

**e.** Hypertonic saline should be stopped if *any* of the following criteria are met:

**(1)** Life-threatening symptoms abate (regardless of the persistence of hyponatremia)

**(2)** Serum sodium > 120 mEq/L

**(3)** Total magnitude of correction > 25 mEq/L

**(4)** Additionally, the rate of change should be < 12 mEq/L/d

**E.** Complications: Central pontine myelinolysis

**1.** Typically, patients have severe chronic hyponatremia that is rapidly corrected; 2–6 days later spastic quadriparesis and pseudobulbar palsy develop. Death may occur.

**2.** May occur when hyponatremia is corrected too rapidly (> 12 mEq/L/d or > 0.5 mEq/L/h).

**3.** Pons is most commonly affected but other areas of white matter may be affected.

**4.** Premenopausal women appear to be at substantially higher risk for this complication than men.

> ▽1
>
> Mr. D. has mild, not severe, symptoms from hyponatremia. Rapid correction of hyponatremia must be avoided. Hypertonic saline is not indicated. He is begun on free water restriction and his sodium gradually improves to 128 mEq/L. His mental status returns to normal.

## CHIEF COMPLAINT

> PATIENT ▽2
>
> Mrs. L is a 60-year-old woman who comes to see you for a follow-up of her hypertension. She reports no specific complaints except perhaps some mild fatigue. On physical exam, her BP is well controlled at 126/84 mm Hg. Routine chemistries reveal a serum sodium of 128 mEq/L. Her potassium and other electrolytes and creatinine are normal. Her glucose is 108 mg/dL and BUN 28 mg/dL. Urine specific gravity is 1.025.

**At this point, what is the leading hypothesis, what are the active alternatives, and is there a must not miss diagnosis? Given this differential diagnosis, what tests should be ordered?**

## PRIORITIZING THE DIFFERENTIAL DIAGNOSIS

The first step is to review her medications to determine whether she is taking a thiazide diuretic and to look for hyperkalemia, marked hyperglycemia, or a maximally dilute urine. Her hypertension is treated with amlodipine (a calcium channel blocker) and her potassium and blood glucose are normal. Although her urine osmolality is not reported, her urine specific gravity is *not* highly dilute, and does not suggest psychogenic polydipsia. The next pivotal step is to classify Mrs. L's volume status as hypervolemic,

euvolemic, or hypovolemic. A careful exam should search for signs of hypervolemia (edema, JVD, ascites, S₃ gallop, or crackles) and for signs of hypovolemia (hypotension, tachycardia, or orthostatic hypotension). If Mrs. L is not hypervolemic, urine sodium and FE_Na can further help distinguish euvolemia from hypovolemia.

> ▽2
>
> Mrs. L denies any history that suggests volume loss (vomiting, diarrhea, or excessive perspiration). Furthermore, she has no history of any diseases associated with hypervolemic states (HF, cirrhosis, renal failure, or nephrotic syndrome). She denies any dyspnea on exertion or orthopnea. On physical exam, BP is normal with no significant change going from lying to standing. There is no pretibial or pedal edema. Cardiovascular exam reveals no JVD, S₃ gallop, or crackles. There are no signs of ascites (bulging flanks, shifting dullness).
>
> Mrs. L's urine studies reveal a urine sodium concentration of 60 mEq/L, urine osmolality 480 mOsm/L, and a FE_Na of 5%.

Mrs. L's history and exam do not suggest hypervolemia. Her exam does not suggest hypovolemia. Furthermore, neither her urine sodium nor her FE_Na are low (as would be expected if she were hypovolemic). Therefore, Mrs. L has euvolemic hyponatremia. The differential diagnosis of euvolemic hyponatremia includes SIADH, adverse effect of medication, glucocorticoid insufficiency, hypothyroidism, and psychogenic polydipsia. At this point the leading

**Table 21–4.** Diagnostic hypotheses for Mrs. L.

| Diagnostic Hypotheses | Clinical Clues | Important Tests |
|---|---|---|
| **Leading Hypothesis** | | |
| SIADH | History of cancer (or cancer risks) Unusual cough Hemoptysis or lymphadenopathy Neurologic or pulmonary disease HIV | Urine Na+ > 40 mEq/L $FE_{Na}$ > 1% Urine osmolality > 300 mOsm/L Exclusion of hypothyroidism and adrenal insufficiency |
| **Active Alternative—Most Common** | | |
| Medication | Medication history | Response to discontinuation of medication |
| Hypothyroidism | Fatigue, cold intolerance | TSH |
| **Active Alternative—Must Not Miss** | | |
| Adrenal insufficiency | Long-term corticosteroid therapy, pituitary disease, HIV, sarcoid | Corticotropin stimulation test |

hypothesis is uncertain. Table 21–4 lists the differential diagnosis. Further history may help prioritize the differential diagnosis.

> Past medical history: Hypertension treated with amlodipine. Social history: 40-pack-year history of smoking. Alcohol use is minimal. Review of systems positive only for a cough that has been present over the last 1–2 months.

Mrs. L's history is not particularly diagnostic. As noted above, she is not taking a thiazide diuretic, one of the most common medications causing hyponatremia. Her recent cough and tobacco history raises the possibility of SIADH from a lung cancer. Adrenal insufficiency is a potentially life-threatening cause of hyponatremia and should be considered a "must not miss" diagnosis. Although hyperkalemia suggests adrenal insufficiency, a normal potassium does not rule it out.

**Is the clinical information sufficient to make a diagnosis? If not, what other information do you need?**

## Leading Hypothesis: SIADH

### Textbook Presentation

Patients are often (although not always) elderly, with a chief complaint of confusion or weakness. Alternatively, mild hyponatremia may be discovered incidentally on serum chemistries.

### Disease Highlights

A. Most common cause of hyponatremia

B. Secondary to inappropriate ADH release despite hypotonicity and euvolemia.

C. Patients are clinically euvolemic. Clinically inapparent volume expansion due to water retention leads to urinary sodium loss.

D. Etiologies

  1. Cancer, 15%

    **a.** Ectopic production by small cell carcinoma of the lung is the most common malignancy.

    **b.** Pancreatic cancer, lymphoma, endometrial cancer, leukemia, and other tumors may cause SIADH.

  2. Neurologic disease (eg, meningitis, tumors, trauma, cerebrovascular accidents)

  3. Intrathoracic disease (eg, pneumonia, tuberculosis, HIV)

  4. Drugs: Carbamazepine (20–30% of patients), MDMA, ADH analogues (vasopressin, DDAVP, oxytocin [5% of patients]), thiazides, chlorpropamide, NSAIDs, antidepressants (tricyclics and selective serotonin reuptake inhibitors), antipsychotics, cyclophosphamide, vincristine, nicotine, opioids, clofibrate

  5. AIDS

    **a.** SIADH may be secondary to *Pneumocystis* pneumonia, CNS infections, or cancer.

    **b.** Hyponatremia may also be due to HIV-related adrenal insufficiency or diarrhea (with free water ingestion).

  6. Hypothyroidism

    **a.** Hyponatremia may occur in 10% of patients with hypothyroidism but is rarely symptomatic.

    **b.** In part secondary to ADH release

    **c.** Elevated ADH levels may be secondary to decreased cardiac output.

  7. Idiopathic

E. Reset osmostat

  1. A variant of SIADH in which ADH control is modulated to maintain serum sodium levels at a lower range than normal. Patients retain ability to excrete water load at new equilibrium point.

  2. Therefore, hyponatremia is not progressive.

  3. Patients typically have serum sodium levels between 125 mEq/L and 135 mEq/L.

  4. Very dilute urine osmolality may be seen following water load (< 100 mOsm/L).

  5. Etiology is similar to SIADH.

  6. Treatment is directed at the underlying disorder.

### Evidence-Based Diagnosis

A. Standard criteria

  1. Effective plasma osmolality < 275 mOsm/L; can be calculated using the following equation: Effective osmolarity = $(2 \times Na^+) + (Glucose/18)$

  2. Urine sodium is typically > 40 mEq/L.

  3. $FE_{Na}$ is usually > 1%.

   4. Urine osmolality not maximally dilute due to active ADH (urine osmolality > 100 mOsm/L, usually > 300 mOsm/L)

   5. Patient clinically euvolemic and other causes of euvolemic hyponatremia excluded (hypothyroidism, psychogenic polydipsia, adrenal insufficiency, diuretic use)

B. 13–42% of patients have low urine sodium and low $FE_{Na}$ due to low sodium intake.

C. All patients had elevated $FE_{urea}$ (> 55%).

## Treatment

A. Determine and treat underlying etiology.

   1. Review medications; consider CT scan of the chest and head.

   2. SIADH often resolves with treatment of the underlying disorder (ie, cancer). Recurrent SIADH suggests cancer recurrence.

   3. Water restriction is the cornerstone of therapy.

B. **Determine acuity and symptomatology**

   1. As noted above, the correction of hyponatremia must be done carefully. Rapid correction of chronic hyponatremia may result in permanent brain damage.

   2. Therefore, the approach must be individualized based on the acuity and severity of the hyponatremia.

C. Asymptomatic, chronic hyponatremia

   1. Fluid restriction < 1 L/d

   2. Discontinue any medication that may cause SIADH.

D. Symptomatic or documented acute hyponatremia < 48 hours

   1. In patients with moderate symptoms, normal saline with furosemide (20 mg once or twice daily) to correct sodium at a rate < 0.5 mEq/L/h. (Normal saline without furosemide may worsen hyponatremia. Since sodium handling is intact [but water is not], the administered sodium may be excreted but the accompanied water is retained, causing decreased serum sodium.)

   2. In patients with severe symptoms (eg, seizures or coma) 3% normal saline to correct sodium at a rate of 1–2 mEq/L/h can be used until life-threatening symptoms abate (usually a few hours). Authorities recommend limiting sodium correction to 8–12 mEq/L/d.

Do not increase serum sodium concentration by > 8–12 mEq/L/d.

   3. ADH receptor antagonists. A variety of both selective (tolvaptan) and nonselective (conivaptan) ADH receptor antagonists have been developed and demonstrated to increase serum sodium levels faster than placebo. Their precise role needs to be defined.

   4. Demeclocycline

      a. Has also been used if fluid restriction is inadequate to restore normal sodium levels.

      b. Blocks intracellular effect of ADH by interfering with the generation and action of cyclic adenosine monophosphate (cAMP)

      c. Can cause photosensitivity and nephrotoxicity

## MAKING A DIAGNOSIS

The urine osmolality is 480 mOsm/L. The serum osmolality is 266 mOsm/L. Her TSH is normal at 2.3 milliunits/L.

Have you crossed a diagnostic threshold for the leading hypothesis, SIADH? Have you ruled out the other active alternatives that cause euvolemic hyponatremia? Do other tests need to be done to exclude the alternative diagnoses?

Mrs. L's elevated $FE_{Na}$ (5%) and urine osmolality are consistent with SIADH. It is important to consider the alternative diagnosis before concluding that she in fact has SIADH. If SIADH is confirmed, a search for the underlying cause is appropriate.

## Alternative Diagnosis: Diuretic-Induced Hyponatremia

### Textbook Presentation

The most common clinical situation is a small elderly woman taking a thiazide diuretic for hypertension. Patients may be asymptomatic or complain of weakness, lethargy or occasionally confusion due to hyponatremia.

### Disease Highlights

A. One of the most common causes of hyponatremia

B. Often associated with more severe hyponatremia than frequently seen due to other etiologies (mean serum sodium, 116 mEq/L)

C. Most commonly seen with thiazide diuretics; rarely seen with loop diuretics

D. More common in patients over 70 (OR 3.9)

E. 70% of patients are women

F. Hyponatremia can be multifactorial; pathogenesis may vary in different patients.

   1. Most patients are hypovolemic (although this may not be clinically evident).

      a. Thiazide diuretics interfere with NaCl transport in cortical diluting segments. This limits NaCl transport out of the tubule, reducing formation of free water within the tubule, which leads to decreased free water excretion.

      b. Decreased GFR causes increased proximal sodium reabsorbtion leading to reduced distal sodium delivery and free water clearance.

      c. Volume depletion may elevate ADH levels.

      d. Sodium losses are occasionally marked.

      e. One study suggested that hypovolemic patients often presented after prolonged use of diuretics (mean duration, 103 days) and were often asymptomatic.

   2. Some patients are hypervolemic or euvolemic.

      a. Thiazides can increase ADH without volume depletion (ie, SIADH).

      b. Increased water intake coupled with impaired free water excretion leads to hyponatremia.

**c.** In patients with thiazide-induced SIADH, hyponatremia often develops within days of initiating a thiazide diuretic; it can be severe and symptomatic.

**F.** NSAID use may increase the risk of thiazide-induced hyponatremia.

**G.** Hyponatremia may persist for 1 month after discontinuation of thiazide.

## Evidence-Based Diagnosis

**A.** Clinical dehydration evident in only 24% of patients

**B.** Symptoms included lethargy 49%, dizziness 47%, vomiting 35%, confusion 17%, and seizures 0.9%.

**C.** Despite volume depletion, urine sodium concentration and $FE_{Na}$ may be elevated if diuretic action is still present.

Urine sodium > 30 mEq/L and $FE_{Na+}$ > 0.5% in 55% of diuretic-treated hyponatremic patients.

**D.** $FE_{urea}$ is usually low due to true volume depletion.

**E.** Several features help distinguish thiazide-induced hypovolemia and hyponatremia from thiazide-induced SIADH. Features that suggest a thiazide-induced SIADH-like process include the rapid development of hyponatremia, clinical euvolemia, as well as a high $FE_{Na}$ and high $FE_{urea}$ as well as a serum uric acid level < 4.0 mg/dL. Sensitivity, 90%; specificity, 75%; LR+, 6.0; LR−, 0.13.

## Treatment

**A.** Stopping the diuretic is usually adequate.

**B.** Hypovolemic patients

**1.** Consider careful volume resuscitation with normal saline.

**2.** Correct sodium concentration at rate < 0.5 mEq/L/h (see formulas above to calculate correct rate).

**3.** Unlike hypervolemic patients, fluid resuscitation in a hypovolemic patient may lead to a drop in ADH levels. This may result in rapid water losses and an overly rapid and dangerous correction of the serum sodium concentration. Serum sodium levels should be monitored closely and electrolyte replacement may need to be terminated if serum sodium levels or urinary output rise abruptly.

**4.** Hypertonic saline can be used if severe neurologic symptoms are present (see calculations above; common estimate is 2 mL/kg/h of 3% normal saline for 3–4 hours).

**C.** Euvolemic patients and SIADH likely: restrict free water.

**D.** Some authorities recommend checking serum sodium in elderly women 1–3 days after initiating thiazide diuretic, particularly if they take NSAIDs.

## Alternative Diagnosis: Adrenal Insufficiency

### Textbook Presentation

Patients may have chronic symptoms of fatigue, weight loss, nausea, vomiting, orthostasis, and abdominal pain or acute symptoms, such as a clinical constellation that suggests septic shock (hypotension and fever). Adrenal insufficiency may also cause hypoglycemia. Both primary and secondary adrenal insufficiency may cause hyponatremia.

### Disease Highlights

**A.** Etiology

**1.** Adrenal insufficiency may be primary or secondary.

**a.** Primary adrenal insufficiency occurs when damage to the adrenal gland results in inadequate cortisol production. ACTH increases because the hypothalamic pituitary axis attempts to compensate for the hypocortisolism.

**b.** Secondary adrenal insufficiency develops when damage to the hypothalamic pituitary system results in inadequate corticotropin (ACTH) production thereby producing inadequate adrenal stimulation and hypocortisolism.

**2.** Both primary and secondary adrenal insufficiency cause hypocortisolism. Cortisol normally suppresses ADH release. Decreased cortisol causes increased ADH levels and hyponatremia.

**3.** Primary adrenal insufficiency

**a.** May decrease the synthesis of other adrenal hormones

**(1)** Aldosterone, DHEA, and catecholamine synthesis may be impaired.

**(2)** Aldosterone deficiency results in salt losses and clinical hypovolemia. The hypovolemia may further stimulate ADH release. Finally, the aldosterone deficiency may also cause hyperkalemia.

Suspect primary adrenal insufficiency in hyponatremic patients with hyperkalemia.

**(3)** DHEA deficiency affects women (but not men due to testicular androgen synthesis). Findings may include decreased libido, decreased axillary and pubic hair, and amenorrhea.

**(4)** Catecholamine synthesis is also usually impaired (except in autoimmune adrenal disease).

**b.** Etiologies of primary adrenal insufficiency

**(1)** Autoimmune adrenalitis (80–90% of cases in developed nations)

**(2)** HIV infection: Up to 20% of patients with HIV have adrenal insufficiency.

**(3)** Tuberculosis (most common cause in developing nations)

**(4)** Less common etiologies: Fungal or cytomegalovirus infections, bilateral adrenal hemorrhage (seen in septic shock, postoperative patients, and in patients taking anticoagulants), infiltration (cancer), inherited disorders and certain drugs (ketoconazole, rifampin, phenytoin, and others)

**4.** Secondary adrenal insufficiency (hypothalamic-pituitary insufficiency)

**a.** Results in *isolated* cortisol deficiency which, in turn, causes elevated ADH levels and hyponatremia.

**b.** Aldosterone is primarily under control of the renin-angiotensin system and is unaffected so that patients are often euvolemic and do not suffer from hyperkalemia.

**c.** Etiologies

**(1)** Iatrogenic due to corticosteroid therapy

**(a)** Up to 50% of patients taking long-term corticosteroid therapy (ie, > 7.5 mg/d prednisone for > 3 weeks) have adrenal insufficiency

**(b)** Recovery of hypothalamic-pituitary-adrenal axis may take 9–12 months.

**(2)** Sepsis

**(3)** Pituitary tumors (30% of patients with a pituitary macroadenoma exhibit adrenal insufficiency)

**(4)** Less common etiologies: Pituitary infarction, irradiation, autoimmune hypophysitis, traumatic brain injury, HIV, sarcoidosis, hemorrhage, hemochromatosis, empty sella syndrome

 Suspect hypopituitarism as the cause of hyponatremia in any patient with a history of pituitary disease (eg, macroadenoma, infarction, empty sella syndrome).

**d.** Hyponatremia may be precipitated by intercurrent illness, leading to inadequate cortisol response; 43% of patients with secondary adrenal insufficiency had superimposed infection when presenting with hyponatremia.

**B.** Adrenal crisis

**1.** 3% of patients per year

**2.** Often secondary to insufficient increases in glucocorticoid during times of stress

## Evidence-Based Diagnosis

**A.** History and physical exam

**1.** Acute adrenal insufficiency (adrenal crisis) presents similarly to septic shock with hypotension, abdominal pain, vomiting, and fever. This is rare in patients with secondary adrenal insufficiency because aldosterone secretion is preserved in such patients.

**2.** Chronic adrenal insufficiency

**a.** May present with a variety of nonspecific symptoms (eg, fatigue, weakness, weight loss).

**b.** The frequency of presenting symptoms may be overestimated in the literature dominated by very old case series that discovered advanced disease.

**c.** Hypotension and hyperpigmentation are seen only in primary adrenal insufficiency

**(1)** Hypotension occurs due to concomitant aldosterone deficiency and occurs in ≅ 90% of patients with primary adrenal insufficiency.

**(2)** Hyperpigmentation

**(a)** Develops secondary to an increased release of proopiomelanocortin (POMC), the precursor hormone that contains both ACTH and melanocyte-stimulating hormone.

**(b)** Typically develops in exposed areas such as the face, dorsum of hands and knuckles, as well as the palmer creases of interphalangeal joints. There may also be a blue black hyperpigmentation of the buccal mucosa.

**(c)** Older reports suggest hyperpigmentation was invariable in primary adrenal insufficiency. A more recent report found hyperpigmentation in only 18% of such patients.

**d.** Other findings in chronic adrenal insufficiency

**(1)** Weakness, tiredness, fatigue: 100%

**(2)** Weight loss and anorexia: 100%

**(3)** Gastrointestinal symptoms

**(a)** Nausea: 86%

**(b)** Vomiting: 75%

**(c)** Diarrhea: 16%

**(4)** Postural dizziness: 12%

**(5)** Psychiatric manifestations (memory impairment, delirium, depression, and psychosis): 5–50%

**(6)** Vitiligo: 10–20%

**(7)** Salt craving: 16%

**B.** Laboratory tests (Figure 21–4)

**1.** Morning cortisol levels

**a.** Cortisol secretion demonstrates a marked diurnal variation.

**b.** Early morning cortisol levels can help establish or refute adrenal insufficiency.

**(1)** Morning levels > 15 mcg/dL (415 nmol/L) rule out adrenal insufficiency.

**(2)** Morning levels between 3 mcg/dL and 15 mcg/dL are nondiagnostic.

**(3)** Morning levels < 3 mcg/dL (80 nmol/L) establishes adrenal insufficiency.

**2.** In patients with adrenal insufficiency, ACTH measurements (8 AM) differentiate primary from secondary adrenal insufficiency.

**a.** ACTH is elevated in primary adrenal insufficiency.

**b.** ACTH is low in adrenal insufficiency secondary to hypothalamic-pituitary dysfunction.

**3.** Diagnostic testing in patients with low or borderline cortisol and elevated ACTH (suspected primary adrenal insufficiency)

**a.** ACTH stimulation test is the test of choice. (Cosyntropin is the synthetic agent used.)

**(1)** Can be performed any time of day

**(2)** 250 mcg cosyntropin given IM or IV

**(3)** Serum cortisol measured 30–60 minutes later

**(4)** Level < 18 mcg/dL (500 nmol/L) rules in adrenal insufficiency

**(5)** Sensitivity, 97.5%; specificity, 95%; LR+, 19.5; LR–, 0.026

**b.** Adrenal imaging with CT scanning is appropriate in patients with an abnormal cosyntropin stimulation test.

**c.** HIV testing should be considered.

**d.** Antibodies against 21-hydroxylase are accurate in the diagnosis of autoimmune adrenalitis.

**4.** Diagnostic testing in patients with low or borderline cortisol and low ACTH: suspected secondary or tertiary (pituitary-hypothalamic) based adrenal insufficiency

**a.** ACTH stimulation

**(1)** *Chronic* (> 1 month) secondary or tertiary adrenal insufficiency results in adrenal atrophy and such patients may not respond to exogenous ACTH. They are likely to have low cortisol levels and an abnormal cosyntropin stimulation test.

**(2)** On the other hand, patients with acute secondary adrenal insufficiency (ie, recent pituitary infarction or pituitary surgery) will not yet have adrenal gland atrophy.

**(a)** In such patients, *exogenous* ACTH will result in an appropriate bump in cortisol. Thus, such

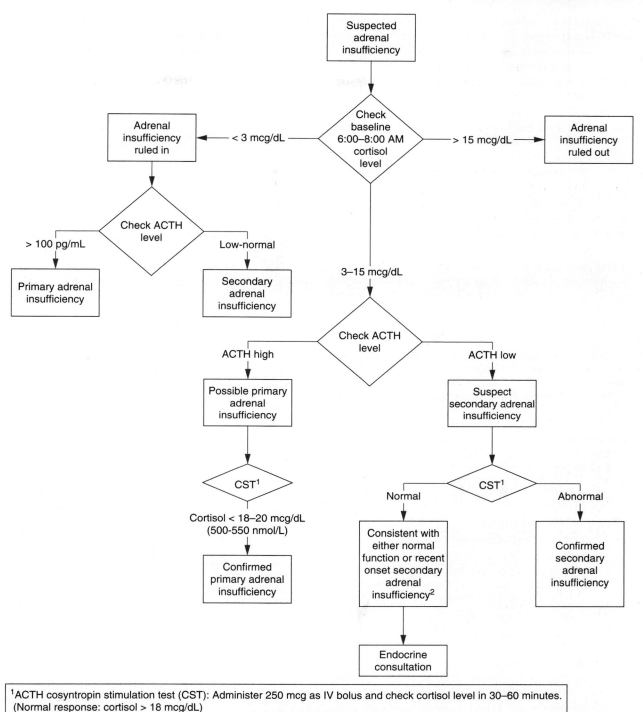

**Figure 21–4.** Evaluation of suspected adrenal insufficiency.

[1]ACTH cosyntropin stimulation test (CST): Administer 250 mcg as IV bolus and check cortisol level in 30–60 minutes.
 (Normal response: cortisol > 18 mcg/dL)
[2]Recent secondary adrenal insufficiency should be suspected in patients with recent pituitary surgery.

patients can have a normal cortisol response in spite of disease (false-negative).

**(b)** Such patients require tests that challenge the entire hypothalamic-pituitary axis, such as the insulin tolerance test.

**(c)** However, this is a complex test that requires experience to avoid complications of hypoglycemia. Endocrine consultation is advised.

**b.** Pituitary MRI is indicated in patients with secondary adrenal insufficiency.

5. Evaluation of adrenal insufficiency in acutely ill patients in the ICU is complex.

   a. Severe stressors normally elevate cortisol levels so that cosyntropin stimulation tests are unnecessary.

   b. Hypoalbuminemia complicates the interpretation of cortisol results in ICU patients.

     (1) Many ICU patients have normal free (active) cortisol levels but low *total* cortisol levels due to low levels of binding proteins.

     (2) Free cortisol levels are not widely available, and the low total levels give the misimpression of adrenal insufficiency.

6. Serum electrolytes are abnormal in many but not all patients with adrenal insufficiency.

   a. Hyponatremia: 88% of patients

   b. Hyperkalemia: 18–64% of patients

7. Urine electrolytes in hyponatremic patients with adrenal insufficiency: Decreased cortisol causes lack of suppression of ADH, leading to increased ADH and laboratory values similar to SIADH: Average urinary sodium, 110 mmol/L; average urine osmolality, 399 mOsm/L

8. Eosinophilia has been reported in 17% of patients.

9. As noted above, hyponatremia may occur in primary or secondary adrenal insufficiency due to increased ADH hormone levels. Hyperkalemia occurs only in primary adrenal insufficiency due to aldosterone deficiency.

## Treatment

A. Long-term therapy

  1. In both primary and secondary insufficiency, therapy must replace normal corticosteroid output *and the dosage must be automatically increased at times of stress to prevent life-threatening adrenal crisis.*

  2. Primary adrenal insufficiency

   a. Prednisone or dexamethasone

     (1) Daily dose: 5 mg (prednisone) or 0.5 mg (dexamethasone) once daily at bedtime. Additional medications may affect glucocorticoid metabolism. Drug interactions need to be carefully considered

     (2) Prevention of adrenal crisis

       (a) Strenuous physical activity: Add 5–10 mg hydrocortisone

       (b) Pregnancy: Doses may need to be increased in the third trimester and in the peripartum period. Endocrine consultation is advised.

       (c) Hyperthyroidism: Double or triple daily dose

       (d) Febrile illness or invasive diagnostic procedures: Double or triple daily dose

       (e) Major surgery or trauma: 50 mg every 8 hours of IV hydrocortisone

       (f) A medical alert bracelet should be worn to alert caretakers of adrenal insufficiency and the need for stress dosing in emergencies. In addition, patients in remote areas should have injectable glucocorticoids for emergency situations.

   b. Mineralcorticoid

     (1) 0.05–0.2 mg/d of fludrocortisone

     (2) Monitor potassium levels as well as BP

   c. DHEA (50 mg/d) can be considered for women with impaired sense of well being despite glucocorticoid and mineralcorticoid replacement.

  3. Secondary adrenal insufficiency

   Glucocorticoids as for primary adrenal insufficiency

B. Treatment of adrenal crisis

  1. Hydrocortisone 100 mg IV and then 100 mg IV every 6–8 hours. For patients who are still being evaluated for adrenal insufficiency, dexamethasone is substituted for hydrocortisone because it is not detected by the cortisol assays.

  2. Normal saline (often up to 1 L/h)

When adrenal crisis is suspected, blood tests should be drawn for cortisol and ACTH. Treatment should commence immediately and not await laboratory results.

## CASE RESOLUTION

The serum cortisol level following 250 mcg of corticotropin is 800 nmol/L. Her glucose is 100 mg/dL.

Mrs. L's urine osmolality is not dilute, effectively ruling out psychogenic polydipsia. Her TSH and corticotropin stimulation tests are also normal, ruling out hypothyroidism and adrenal insufficiency. (Secondary adrenal insufficiency of recent onset is still theoretically possible, but nothing in the history suggests the patient is at risk for pituitary disease.) Therefore, Mrs. L has SIADH. The final step will be to determine the etiology of the SIADH. As noted above, SIADH can result from a variety of pulmonary, neurologic, or malignant causes. Following clinical clues is important. Her recent cough and long history of tobacco use suggests an underlying pulmonary etiology.

A chest film reveals a 5-cm pulmonary mass adjacent to the right hilum. Bronchoscopy and biopsy confirms small cell carcinoma of the lung. Mrs. L is referred to medical oncology. Her hyponatremia is controlled with free water restriction.

## REVIEW OF OTHER IMPORTANT DISEASES

## Hypovolemic Hyponatremic Syndromes

### Textbook Presentation

Hyponatremia may develop in volume-depleted patients if sodium losses (resulting from vomiting, diarrhea, or excessive perspiration) are replaced with free water. Patients may have orthostatic hypotension or dry mucous membranes.

## Disease Highlights

**A.** The primary controller of ADH release is serum osmolality. Hypo-osmolality normally inhibits ADH release leading to free water diuresis.

**B.** *Significant* hypovolemia can stimulate ADH release independent of serum osmolality.

**C.** Free water ingestion in face of elevated ADH levels causes hyponatremia.

**D.** Typical urine findings include

    **1.** Decreased urine sodium concentration (< 30 mEq/L)

    **2.** Decreased $FE_{Na}$ (< 0.5%)

    **3.** Increased urine osmolality (> 450 mOsm/L)

    **4.** Prerenal azotemia (BUN/Cr > 20)

    **5.** Elevated uric acid

## Treatment

**A.** For mildly symptomatic patients, normal saline can be used (see calculations above).

**B.** For severely symptomatic patients, 3% normal saline can be used.

**C.** Serum sodium corrections may occur faster than predicted by formulas because volume resuscitation suppresses ADH release.

**D.** Frequent monitoring of serum sodium is mandatory.

# Exercise-Associated Hyponatremia

## Textbook Presentation

Patients with exercise-associated hyponatremia (EAH) usually present during or within hours of completing an endurance event (marathon). Symptoms range from weakness and nausea to coma, seizures, and death.

## Disease Highlights

**A.** Typically follows prolonged workout

    **1.** Hyponatremia (Na < 135 mEq/L) developed in 13-29% of endurance athletes completing marathons or ironman competitions.

    **2.** Severe hyponatremia (< 130 mEq/L) developed in 2% of runners in the Boston Marathon and critical hyponatremia (< 120 mEq/L) developed in 0.6%.

**B.** Etiology is secondary to an increase in total body water, in turn secondary to a combination of both excessive fluid intake combined in some patients with inappropriate ADH release.

    **1.** Hyponatremia developed in 17% of runners who gained > 2 kg during the race, compared with 1.2% of runners who gained < 2 kg.

    **2.** Hyponatremia should suppress ADH. The finding that 44% of runners with exercise-associated hyponatremia have non-suppressed ADH levels suggests that SIADH contributes to hyponatremia in some patients. This is supported by the absence of urination during treatment for exercise-associated hyponatremia (despite apparent normovolemia).

**C.** As noted above, the leading risk factor is weight gain during the event. Some studies have also reported an increased risk in women and NSAID users.

**D.** Rapid onset of hyponatremia renders the plasma hypotonic relative to the brain, leading to cerebral edema.

**E.** Hyponatremia and cerebral edema cause neurologic symptoms including confusion, headaches, seizures, coma, and death.

**F.** Pulmonary edema has been reported in patients with exercise-associated hyponatremia.

## Treatment

**A.** Prevention

    **1.** Athletes should be advised to weigh themselves before and after exercise, and counseled to avoid excessive weight gain (> 2 kg).

    **2.** Thirst should be used as a guide to drinking during marathon events rather than fixed, regular, fluid intake.

    **3.** Sporadic weight checks during endurance events could also detect athletes with significant weight gain at risk for exercise-associated hyponatremia.

**B.** Treatment

    **1.** Individuals who collapse or have neurologic symptoms during or following endurance events should be immediately evaluated for exercise-associated hyponatremia (as well as hyperthermia, hypoglycemia, and myocardial infarction).

    **2.** Unlike chronic hyponatremia, exercise-associated hyponatremia develops rapidly and does not allow the brain time to adapt to the hypo-osmolarity.

    **3.** Therefore, a more aggressive treatment approach is safer and recommended to correct the acute hyponatremia in patients with symptomatic exercise-associated hyponatremia.

    **4.** 3% normal saline is recommended. For patients with significant neurologic symptoms (confusion, coma, seizures), 100 mL (of 3% normal saline) over the first 10 minute is recommended followed 3% normal saline at rates of 1 mL/kg/h for the first few hours.

    **5.** Central pontine myelinolysis from over-rapid correction of chronic hyponatremia has not been reported in patients treated for acute symptomatic exercise-associated hyponatremia.

# Psychogenic Polydipsia

## Textbook Presentation

Psychogenic polydipsia typically occurs in patients with a psychiatric history and unexplained hyponatremia. Patients are unaware of or do not usually admit to excessive water intake. SIADH may also be seen in psychiatric patients.

## Disease Highlights

**A.** Increased water intake suppresses ADH, which increases free water excretion and the formation of a dilute urine.

**B.** Hyponatremia develops only when massive water ingestion is sufficient to overcome maximal urinary free water excretion (usually requires > 8–10 L/d fluid intake).

**C.** Urine osmolality maximally dilute ($\cong$ 100 mOsm/L)

**D.** Reported in 6–20% of chronically ill, hospitalized psychiatric patients

**E.** Since volume status is normal, renal excretion of sodium is usually normal, and $FE_{Na}$ is usually > 1%. However, spot urine sodium *concentration* is low due to dilution by massive water intake.

**F.** Complications are secondary to both hyponatremia and marked polyuria (incontinence, hypocalcemia, hydronephrosis (from massive urinary output), and HF.

**G.** Although a maximally dilute urine is expected to be found in psychogenic polydipsia, this is not always the case. Several problems can aggravate the hyponatremia in psychogenic polydipsia and complicate the diagnosis.

    **1.** Psychotic episodes may cause a transient release of ADH or an increased renal responsiveness to ADH.

    **2.** In addition, psychiatric medications can induce concomitant SIADH. This accentuates the hyponatremia and can produce a higher than expected urine osmolality.

    **3.** Finally, medications with anticholinergic activity can lead to dry mouth and increase water intake.

### Evidence-Based Diagnosis

**A.** Water restriction test can prove the diagnosis by demonstrating rapid resolution of hyponatremia.

**B.** Mean urine sodium concentration is 18 mEq/L.

**C.** $FE_{Na} > 0.5\%$ in 66%

**D.** $FE_{urea} > 55\%$ in 100%

**E.** Mean urine osmolality $144 \pm 23$ mOsm/L vs. 500 mOsm/L in SIADH and 539 mOsm/L in hypovolemic patients.

### Treatment

**A.** Careful free water restriction allows gradual restoration of serum sodium concentration.

**B.** For severe neurologic symptoms (eg, seizures, coma), hypertonic saline can be used.

## Ecstasy (MDMA) Intoxication

### Textbook Presentation

Patients are typically college students, attending clubs (raves), who may have delirium, agitation, or seizures.

### Disease Highlights

**A.** MDMA is a synthetic sympathomimetic amphetamine that stimulates the release of norepinephrine, dopamine, and serotonin, and blocks their reuptake.

**B.** Frequent drug of abuse (up to 5–10% of high school seniors in 1 study)

**C.** Symptoms and signs include those of sympathetic overload (agitation, tachycardia, hyperthermia, hypertension) as well as delirium, seizures, and death. Other common symptoms include muscle tension (trismus), diaphoresis, blurred vision, and ataxia.

**D.** Complications include malignant hypertension, stroke, arrhythmias, myocardial infarction, pneumothorax, hyperpyrexia, rhabdomyolysis, organ system failure, and hyponatremia.

**E.** Hyponatremia develops in some patients due to ADH release and a consequent SIADH-like syndrome. Hyperthermia and diaphoresis may promote drinking large volumes, which is aggravated by "recommendations" to drink large amounts of water.

**F.** Hyponatremia may be severe and cause cerebral edema, seizures, coma, and death.

### Evidence-Based Diagnosis

**A.** MDMA is excreted in the urine and can be detected by specific tests.

**B.** Numerous congeners of MDMA exist.

**C.** Urine studies may not detect various congeners and the diagnosis is often made clinically.

### Treatment

**A.** The treatment of MDMA intoxication is beyond the scope of this text. Treatment will focus on the hyponatremia.

**B.** Fluid restriction is recommended and normally results in normalization of the serum sodium within 24 hours.

**C.** For symptomatic severe hyponatremia (ie, persistent seizures in a patient with serum sodium < 115 mEq/L), hypertonic saline is recommended. Benzodiazepines are recommended for the seizures.

## Pseudohyponatremia

### Textbook Presentation

Certain rare conditions interfere with the accurate measurement of sodium and cause the sodium concentration to appear *spuriously* low. These conditions are referred to as **pseudohyponatremia.** Causes include *marked* hyperlipidemia and *marked* hyperproteinemia. In these conditions, the serum sodium in the plasma phase is actually normal and the measured serum osmolality is normal. However, the measured serum sodium is low because the plasma phase within any aliquot is smaller than normal due to the marked increase in lipid or proteins causing the instrument to calculate a low serum sodium level. These conditions may be suspected in patients with marked hyperproteinemia (ie, patients with multiple myeloma or following immunoglobulin infusions), or marked hyperlipidemia or when there is a significant difference between the measured and calculated serum osmolality. Since the *calculated* osmolality uses the measured serum sodium level (which is spuriously low), the calculated osmolality is also spuriously low whereas the measured serum osmolality is correct. The difference between the two (the *osmolar gap)* is elevated. The osmolar gap can be calculated by the following equations:

Osmolar gap = Measured serum osmolality – calculated serum osmolality
(normal < 10)

Calculated serum osmolality = 2 × sodium + glucose/18 + BUN/2.8

    Marked hyperglycemia works somewhat differently. Marked hyperglycemia draws water into the intravascular space and thereby produces hyponatremia. In this situation, the hyperglycemia makes the serum hyper-osmolar. This discussion will be limited to patients with hyponatremia secondary to marked hyperglycemia.

### Disease Highlights

**A.** In poorly controlled diabetes, intravascular glucose acts as an osmotic agent drawing water from the cells into the plasma resulting in hyponatremia.

**B.** Serum osmolality is elevated (due to the marked hyperglycemia).

**C.** The elevated serum osmolality stimulates ADH release further accentuating hyponatremia.

**D.** Correction factors can help predict the serum sodium concentration after the hyperglycemia is treated (and the intravascular water relocates to the intracellular space). The optimal correction factor is controversial.

**E.** Experiments suggest that the sodium concentration will increase by 2.4 mEq/L for every 100 mg/dL that glucose falls with treatment. A sodium of 129 mEq/L in a patient with a serum glucose of 1000 mg/dL would correct as follows:

1. Serum glucose will fall 900 mg/dL with treatment (to about 100 mg/dL).
2. Correct sodium concentration by 2.4 per 100 mg/dL fall in glucose.

3. $9 \times 2.4 = 21.6$
4. Corrected sodium = $129 + 21.6 = 150.6$

---

## HYPERNATREMIA

### CHIEF COMPLAINT

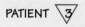

PATIENT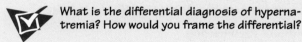

Mr. R is an 80-year-old nursing home resident with a history of severe dementia brought to the emergency department with lethargy and confusion. Serum chemistries reveal a sodium level of 168 mEq/L.

 What is the differential diagnosis of hypernatremia? How would you frame the differential?

### CONSTRUCTING A DIFFERENTIAL DIAGNOSIS

Hypernatremia is almost always secondary to a free water deficit. The differential diagnosis of hypernatremia is markedly simpler than that of hyponatremia.

Hypernatremia and hyperosmolality are potent stimulators of thirst, which acts to stimulate water ingestion and protects against hypernatremia. Therefore, hypernatremia occurs almost exclusively in patients who are either unaware of their thirst or physically unable to get to water. The most common clinical scenarios involve infants or debilitated elderly patients with severe dementia. In such patients, normal insensible water losses or increased water loss (ie, from diarrhea) are not matched by oral intake and hypernatremia develops. The urine osmolality in such patients is typically high (> 700 mOsm/L). In over 50% of elderly patients, a superimposed process (ie, pneumonia, urinary tract infection or cerebrovascular accident) is present. The 30-day mortality in elderly hypernatremic patients has been reported at 41.5%.

Clinicians should search for an underlying cause in patients discovered to have hypernatremia.

Hypernatremia may also develop in patients with marked hyperglycemia. The osmotic diuresis results in a free water loss and may result in hypernatremia if free water intake is impaired due to an altered sensorium. This may not be obvious on initial laboratory results because the hyperglycemia draws water from the intracellular compartment into the intravascular compartment diluting the sodium concentration. With treatment of the hyperglycemia, the hypernatremia worsens as water moves back to the intracellular space.

Other causes of hypernatremia are rare and will be touched upon here only briefly. Hypernatremia may develop in patients who have an impairment in renal *water conservation* (ie, diabetes insipidus [DI]). Even in these patients, increased thirst normally prompts increased water intake and allows such patients to compensate and maintain normonatremia. (These patients complain of polydipsia and polyuria.) Hypernatremia may develop when a superimposed process limits water intake. The urine osmolality in such patients is inappropriately low (< 700 mOsm/L). DI can result from pituitary processes which decrease ADH production, or renal processes, which cause resistance to ADH. Finally, very rare causes of hypernatremia include hypothalamic lesions, which render patients unaware of thirst despite a normal sensorium, or increased salt intake (ie, infusion of hypertonic saline or salt water ingestion). See Figure 21–5, Evaluation of hypernatremia.

### Differential Diagnosis of Hypernatremia

A. Impaired water intake: urine osmolality > 700 mOsm/L
   1. Neurologic disease (eg, dementia, delirium, coma, stroke)
   2. Water unavailable (ie, desert conditions)
B. Osmotic diuresis with impaired water intake
   1. Hyperosmolar hyperglycemia
   2. Postobstructive diuresis
C. Rare etiologies
   1. DI (if associated with decreased water intake)
      a. Neurogenic DI (decreased ADH production)
      b. Nephrogenic DI (ADH resistance)
         (1) Long-term lithium ingestion
         (2) Hypercalcemia
   2. Hypothalamic lesions causing decreased thirst
   3. Increased salt intake
      a. Salt water ingestion
      b. Hypertonic saline

 How reliable is the history and physical exam for detecting hypernatremia?

Signs and symptoms develop due to dehydration (tachycardia, orthostatic hypotension, dry mucous membranes and axilla) and due to the hypernatremia (depressed sensorium, coma, focal deficits, and seizures). Hypernatremia-induced brain shrinkage can also result in rupture of cerebral veins and subarachnoid hemorrhage. Symptoms are more severe with rapidly developing hypernatremia. The clinical findings in patients with hypernatremia are summarized in Table 21–5. No finding was highly sensitive for hypernatremia.

### PRIORITIZING THE DIFFERENTIAL DIAGNOSIS

The most common cause of hypernatremia is inadequate water intake, which develops in patients with severe neurologic dysfunction

**Table 21–5.** Findings in patients with hypernatremia.

| Finding | Sensitivity (%) | Specificity (%) | LR+ | LR− |
|---|---|---|---|---|
| Tachycardia | 17.8 | 94 | 2.97 | 0.87 |
| Orthostatic BP | 61.5 | 50.6 | 1.24 | 0.76 |
| Abnormal subclavicular skin turgor[1] | 73.3 | 79 | 3.49 | 0.34 |
| Dry oral mucosa[2] | 49 | 87.8 | 4.02 | 0.58 |

[1]Defined as lasting ≥ 3 seconds after 3 seconds of pinching.
[2]Defined as placing the finger inside the cheek and assessing whether it is wet or dry.

(ie, dementia). Often, some other illness has supervened to further compromise the patient's state of alertness and oral intake. Marked hyperglycemia should always be considered a "must not miss" alternative. Inadequate water conservation due to DI is possible but far less common. Table 21–6 lists the differential diagnosis.

> ▽3
>
> The nursing home reports that Mr. R has had a cough for the last 3 days with low-grade fever. Over the last 48 hours, he has become progressively less responsive

**Table 21–6.** Diagnostic hypotheses for Mr. R.

| Diagnostic Hypotheses | Clinical Clues | Important Tests |
|---|---|---|
| **Leading Hypothesis** | | |
| Inadequate water consumption | Altered sensorium History of neurologic or physical disability limiting access/ ingestion of water Concomitant illness | Urine osmolarity > 700-800 mOsm/L Chest radiograph Urinalysis and culture |
| **Active Alternative—Most Common** | | |
| Diabetes insipidus | Complaints of polydipsia, polyuria | Urine osmolality < 700 mOsm/L |
| Central | History of CNS trauma, surgery, CVA, sarcoidosis | ADH levels low; Administration of exogenous ADH markedly increases urine osmolality |
| Nephrogenic | Lithium ingestion | ADH levels elevated; Exogenous ADH minimally elevates urine osmolarity |
| **Active Alternative—Must Not Miss** | | |
| Hyperglycemia | Diabetes mellitus, concurrent illness | Markedly elevated serum glucose |

and his oral intake and urinary output have dropped dramatically.

Mr. R is minimally responsive to stimuli. Vital signs are BP, 110/70 mm Hg; pulse, 110 bpm; temperature, 38.1°C; RR, 20 breaths per minute. His oral mucosa is parched and his axilla dry. Lung exam is difficult to evaluate due to poor effort. Cardiac exam reveals tachycardia; neck veins are flat. There is no $S_3$ or $S_4$. Chest radiograph reveals a right lower lobe infiltrate. Laboratory findings: Na, 168 mEq/L; K, 4.2 mEq/L; $HCO_3^-$, 24 mEq/L; chloride, 134 mEq/L; BUN, 45 mg/dL; creatinine, 1 mg/dL. Serum glucose is 150 mg/dL.

> ☑ Is the clinical information sufficient to make a diagnosis? If not, what other information do you need?

## Leading Hypothesis: Hypernatremia Secondary to Inadequate Water Intake

### Textbook Presentation

Patients with hypernatremia due to inadequate water ingestion usually have an altered neurologic status or physical disability. A superimposed illness may worsen cognitive function, worsening oral intake and promote hypernatremia. Mental status is almost always impaired and may vary from confusion to frank coma.

### Evidence-Based Diagnosis

The diagnosis is easily confirmed by the presence of hypernatremia, increased urine osmolality, and absence of hyperglycemia.

### Treatment

A. The brain adapts to hypernatremia by increasing intracellular osmolality to minimize cellular dehydration.

B. Rapid correction of hypernatremia leaves the brain hypertonic relative to the plasma. This promotes osmotic movement of water into the brain and cerebral edema. Seizures and death can occur.

C. Hypernatremia should be corrected slowly ≅ 0.5 mEq/L/h (≤12 mEq/L/d).

D. Calculating infusion rates

1. In hypernatremic patients, total body water (TBW) = 0.5 × weight (kg) (men); TBW = 0.4 × weight (kg) (women)

2. Example: Suppose a 70-kg man has a serum sodium of 165 mEq/L

   a. TBW = 0.5 × 70 = 35 L

   b. Change in serum $Na^+$ per liter of IV fluid infused =

      (1) (infusate $Na^+$ − serum $Na^+$)/(TBW + 1)

      (2) Give D5W (infusate $Na^+$ = 0) →

      (3) (0 − 165)/(35 + 1) = 4.6 mEq fall *per liter* of D5W infused

      (4) Since the target decrease is 0.5 mEq/h and each liter will drop the sodium by 4.6 mEq, the liter must be given over 9.2 hours → infusion rate of 1000 mL/9.2 h = 108 mL/h

**(5)** If 0.45% normal saline (which has an infusate concentration of 77 mEq/L) is used, the rate would be 204 mL/h.

**c.** Ongoing losses must be added.

**3.** Many such patients are markedly hypovolemic on presentation. Patients who are hypotensive should initially receive normal saline to restore adequate perfusion and then be switched to D5W at the appropriate rate.

## MAKING A DIAGNOSIS

An elevated urine osmolality can confirm urinary concentrating ability and establish inadequate fluid intake (versus inadequate conservation) as the etiology. An evaluation of the underlying precipitant is also important.

Mr. R's urine osmolality is 850 mOsm/L. Blood cultures grow Streptococcus pneumoniae.

As in the overwhelming majority of cases of hypernatremia, the diagnosis is straightforward. The history, exam, and elevated urine osmolality all confirm hypernatremia due to decreased intake. Urine concentrating ability is intact. Serum glucose is normal. Further diagnostic testing is not required.

## CASE RESOLUTION

Mr. R is given D5W. His body weight is measured at 140 lbs (63 kg). The rate of free water administration must be determined. He is given piperacillin-tazobactam to treat his aspiration pneumonia.

Three days after D5W is started, his electrolytes are normal. He gradually returns to his baseline neurologic function and is discharged after 6 days of therapy to continue his oral antibiotics at the nursing home.

## REFERENCES

Almond CS, Shin AY, Fortescue EB et al. Hyponatremia among runners in the Boston Marathon. N Engl J Med. 2005;352(15):1550–6.

Angeli P, Wong F, Watson H, Gines P, Investigators C. Hyponatremia in cirrhosis: Results of a patient population survey. Hepatology. 2006;44(6):1535–42.

Chassagne P, Druesne L, Capet C, Menard JF, Bercoff E. Clinical presentation of hypernatremia in elderly patients: a case control study. J Am Geriatr Soc. 2006;54(8):1225–30.

Chow KM, Kwan BC, Szeto CC. Clinical studies of thiazide-induced hyponatremia. J Ntl Med Assoc. 2004;96(10):1305–8.

Chung HM, Kluge R, Schrier RW, Anderson RJ. Clinical assessment of extracellular fluid volume in hyponatremia. Am J Med. 1987;83(5):905–8.

Dunlop D. Eighty-Six Cases of Addison's Disease. BMJ. 1963;2(5362):887–91.

Musch W, Decaux G. Utility and limitations of biochemical parameters in the evaluation of hyponatremia in the elderly. Int Urol Nephrol. 2001;32(3):475–93.

Musch W, Thimpont J, Vandervelde D, Verhaeverbeke I, Berghmans T, Decaux G. Combined fractional excretion of sodium and urea better predicts response to saline in hyponatremia than do usual clinical and biochemical parameters. Am J Med. 1995;99(4):348–55.

Nerup J. Addison's disease--clinical studies. A report of 108 cases. Acta Endocrinologica. 1974;76(1):127–41.

Porcel A, Diaz F, Rendon P, Macias M, Martin-Herrera L, Giron-Gonzalez JA. Dilutional hyponatremia in patients with cirrhosis and ascites. Arch Intern Med. 2002;162(3):323–8.

Ruf AE, Kremers WK, Chavez LL, Descalzi VI, Podesta LG, Villamil FG. Addition of serum sodium into the MELD score predicts waiting list mortality better than MELD alone. Liver Transplant. 2005;11(3):336–43.

Siegel AJ, Verbalis JG, Clement S et al. Hyponatremia in marathon runners due to inappropriate arginine vasopressin secretion. Am J Med. 2007;120(5):461 e11–7.

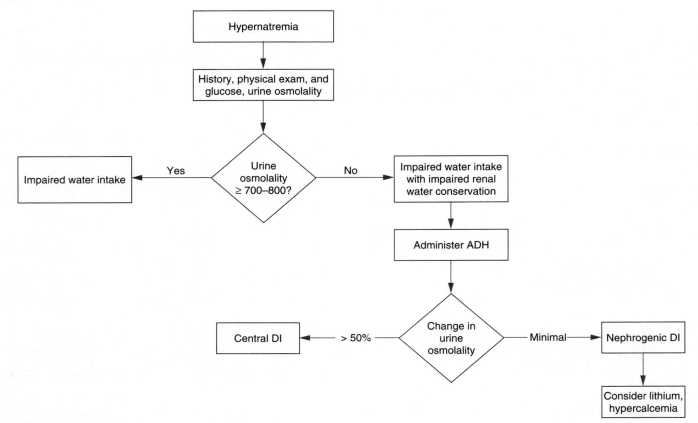

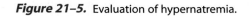

DI, diabetes insipidus.

***Figure 21–5.*** Evaluation of hypernatremia.

# I have a patient with jaundice or abnormal liver enzymes. How do I determine the cause?

## CHIEF COMPLAINT

**PATIENT** ▽1

Ms. B is a 56-year-old woman who comes to your office because her skin and eyes have been yellow for the past 2 weeks.

**What is the differential diagnosis of jaundice? How would you frame the differential?**

## CONSTRUCTING A DIFFERENTIAL DIAGNOSIS

The differential diagnosis of jaundice, or hyperbilirubinemia, is often organized pathophysiologically. It is helpful to review some basic physiology first.

**A.** Oxidation of the heme moiety of Hgb generates biliverdin, which is metabolized into **unconjugated bilirubin,** and then bound to albumin.

**B.** There are 3 steps in bilirubin metabolism in the liver:

  **1. Uptake:** The unconjugated bilirubin-albumin complex reaches the liver cell, bilirubin dissociates, and then enters the hepatocyte.

  **2. Conjugation:** Unconjugated bilirubin and glucuronic acid combine to make **conjugated bilirubin.**

  **3. Excretion:** The hepatocyte excretes conjugated bilirubin into the bile.

    **a.** The rate-limiting step of bilirubin metabolism in the liver

    **b.** If excretion is impaired, conjugated bilirubin travels back through the sinusoidal membrane of the hepatocyte into the bloodstream.

**C.** Conjugated bilirubin in the bile is transported through the biliary ducts into the duodenum; it is not reabsorbed by the intestine.

  **1.** Can be excreted unchanged in the stool

  **2.** Can be converted to **urobilinogen** by colonic bacteria

    **a.** Urobilinogen can be reabsorbed, entering the portal circulation.

    **b.** Some is taken up by the liver and re-excreted into the bile.

    **c.** Some bypasses the liver and is excreted by the kidney, thus appearing in the urine in small amounts.

**D. Unconjugated bilirubin is not found in the urine** because it is bound to albumin and cannot be filtered by the glomeruli.

**E. Conjugated bilirubin is filtered and excreted in the urine** when there is hyperbilirubinemia.

The first key point in the differential diagnosis of hyperbilirubinemia is determining which kind of bilirubin is elevated.

Dark, tea-colored urine means the patient has conjugated hyperbilirubinemia.

Light stools, often described as "clay colored," occur when extrahepatic obstruction prevents bilirubin from entering the intestine.

If there is unconjugated hyperbilirubinemia (when > 80% of the bilirubin is unconjugated), use a pathophysiologic framework:

**A.** Increased bilirubin production

  **1.** Hemolysis

  **2.** Dyserythropoiesis

  **3.** Extravasation of blood into tissues

**B.** Impaired hepatic bilirubin uptake

  **1.** Heart failure

  **2.** Sepsis

  **3.** Drugs (rifampin, probenecid, chloramphenicol)

  **4.** Fasting

  **5.** Portosystemic shunts

**C.** Impaired bilirubin conjugation (decreased hepatic glucuronosyltransferase activity)

  **1.** Hereditary

    **a.** Gilbert syndrome

    **b.** Crigler-Najjar syndrome

  **2.** Acquired

    **a.** Neonates

    **b.** Hyperthyroidism

    **c.** Ethinyl estradiol

    **d.** Liver disease (causes mixed hyperbilirubinemia; usually predominantly conjugated)

    **e.** Sepsis

Most patients with unconjugated hyperbilirubinemia have hemolysis, Gilbert syndrome, heart failure, or sepsis.

Although many sources organize the differential diagnosis for conjugated hyperbilirubinemia (when > 50% is conjugated) using a pathophysiologic framework, a more practical, clinical approach uses the results of other liver function tests:

**A.** Normal liver enzymes (ALT [SGPT], AST [SGOT])

    **1.** Sepsis or systemic infection

    **2.** Rotor syndrome

    **3.** Dubin-Johnson syndrome

**B.** Elevated liver enzymes

    **1.** Transaminases more elevated than alkaline phosphatase: **hepatocellular** pattern

        **a.** Acute viral or alcoholic hepatitis

        **b.** Alcoholic or nonalcoholic steatohepatitis

        **c.** Chronic hepatitis (viral, alcoholic, autoimmune)

        **d.** Cirrhosis of any cause

        **e.** Drugs

    **2.** History suggestive of obstruction or alkaline phosphatase more elevated than transaminases, or both: **cholestatic** pattern

        **a.** Extrahepatic cholestasis (biliary obstruction)

        **b.** Intrahepatic cholestasis (primarily due to impaired excretion)

            **(1)** Viral hepatitis

            **(2)** Alcoholic hepatitis

            **(3)** Cirrhosis

            **(4)** Drugs and toxins

            **(5)** Sepsis

            **(6)** Total parenteral nutrition

            **(7)** Postoperative jaundice

            **(8)** Infiltrative diseases (amyloidosis, lymphoma, sarcoidosis, tuberculosis)

            **(9)** Primary sclerosing cholangitis

            **(10)** Primary biliary cirrhosis

So regardless of how you organize this differential, the first step is to determine whether the hyperbilirubinemia is primarily unconjugated or conjugated. The differential of unconjugated hyperbilirubinemia is relatively limited. If the hyperbilirubinemia is conjugated, the second step is to determine whether there is extrahepatic obstruction or intrinsic liver dysfunction due to 1 of many possible etiologies. Although other liver function tests can serve as a guide, it is clear from the way the above differentials overlap that these tests are not very specific. Table 22–1 summarizes the commonly used liver tests. An algorithm showing the diagnostic approach to hyperbilirubinemia is at the end of this chapter.

> ▽ ①
>
> Ms. B also tells you she has dark urine, light-colored stools, anorexia, and fatigue. She has no nausea, vomiting, abdominal pain, or fever. Ms. B's physical exam shows scleral icterus and jaundice as well as marked hepatomegaly, with her liver edge palpable 6–7 cm below the costal margin. The liver extends across the midline. There is a palpable organ in the left upper quadrant that is either the liver or the spleen. There is no abdominal tenderness or distention. There is no peripheral edema, and the rest of her exam is normal.

**Table 22–1.** Biochemical markers used to evaluate the liver.

| Test | Aspect of Liver Assessed | Origins |
| --- | --- | --- |
| Aspartate aminotransferase (AST [SGOT]) | Hepatocyte integrity | Liver Heart Skeletal muscle Kidney Brain RBC |
| Alanine aminotransferase (ALT [SGPT]) | Hepatocyte integrity | Liver |
| Alkaline phosphatase (AP) | Cholestasis | Liver Bone Intestine Placenta |
| Gamma-glutamyl transpeptidase (GGTP) | When elevated with AP, indicates liver origin of AP | Liver |
| Bilirubin (conjugated) | Cholestasis | Liver |
| Serum albumin | Reflects synthetic capacity of liver | Liver or diet |
| Prothrombin time | Reflects synthetic capacity of liver | Vitamin K dependent clotting factors synthesized by liver |

 **How reliable is the physical exam for detecting hyperbilirubinemia?**

**A.** Jaundice

    **1.** Detectable on physical exam when total bilirubin is > 2.5–3.0 mg/dL

 Scleral icterus is detectable before jaundice of the skin.

    **2.** For bilirubin > 3.0 mg/dL, sensitivity of physical exam is 78.4% and specificity is 68.8% (LR+ = 2.5, LR– = 0.31).

    **3.** For bilirubin > 15.0 mg/dL, sensitivity of physical exam is 96.4%.

**B.** Hepatomegaly: The test characteristics of the physical exam for finding hepatomegaly are not well established.

**C.** Splenomegaly

    **1.** Percussion looks for loss of tympany as the enlarged spleen impinges on the air-filled lung, stomach, and colon.

        **a.** Dullness instead of tympany in Traube space (sixth rib superiorly, midaxillary line laterally, and left costal margin inferiorly); **in nonobese patients who have not eaten recently,** has an LR+ of 4.3 and an LR– of 0.26.

b. Dullness by the Castell method (percussing at the lowest intercostal space in the left anterior axillary line in both expiration and inspiration) has an LR+ of 4.8 and an LR– of 0.21.

2. Palpation (combining studies with a variety of palpation methods) has LR+ of 7.25–13.5 and an LR– of 0.45–0.74.

D. Ascites

1. The best 2 historical findings are

a. Increased abdominal girth (LR+ = 4.16, LR– = 0.17)

b. Ankle swelling (LR+ = 2.80, LR– = 0.10)

2. The best physical exam findings are

a. Fluid wave (LR+ = 6.0, LR– = 0.4)

b. Shifting dullness (LR+ = 2.7, LR– = 0.3)

c. Proper physical exam technique must be used to obtain these LRs.

3. Ultrasound can detect 100 mL of ascites

Given the pivotal historical points (dark urine and light colored stools) and the pivotal physical exam findings of jaundice, massive hepatomegaly, and possible splenomegaly, you are confident that Ms. B has hyperbilirubinemia and suspect that it will be primarily conjugated. You obtain the following initial tests: total bilirubin, 13 mg/dL; direct bilirubin, 9.6 mg/dL; AST, 250 units/L; ALT, 113 units/L; alkaline phosphatase, 503 units/L; albumin, 2.8 g/dL; prothrombin time (PT), 15.4 s (control 11.1 s). WBC = 22,000 cells/mcL with 80% PMNs, 16% lymphocytes, and 4% monocytes.

At this point, what is the leading hypothesis, what are the active alternatives, and is there a must not miss diagnosis? Given this differential diagnosis, what tests should be ordered?

## PRIORITIZING THE DIFFERENTIAL DIAGNOSIS

The first pivotal point to consider is the marked hepatomegaly, which suggests chronic liver disease, most likely due to the common etiologies of alcohol abuse or chronic hepatitis C, or both. The next pivotal point is the pattern of the biochemical abnormalities. The combination of a substantially elevated alkaline phosphatase and moderately elevated transaminases is consistent with a cholestatic pattern, due either to disease causing intrahepatic cholestasis or to extrahepatic obstruction. Viral or alcoholic hepatitis, with or without cirrhosis, would be the most common diseases that cause both hepatocellular and cholestatic abnormalities; the AST being greater than the ALT is a pivotal finding that points toward alcoholic liver disease. Extrahepatic obstruction must be considered also, since she could have an obstruction in addition to chronic liver disease. Cancer and stricture are more likely causes of painless jaundice than common bile duct stones. Pancreatic cancer is the most common malignancy that causes extrahepatic obstruction; cholangiocarcinoma and ampullary carcinoma are 2 other possibilities. Occasionally, obstruction is due to benign polyps in the biliary tree. Table 22–2 lists the differential diagnosis.

**Table 22–2.** Diagnostic hypotheses for Ms. B.

| Diagnostic Hypotheses | Clinical Clues | Important Tests |
|---|---|---|
| **Leading Hypothesis** | | |
| Alcoholic hepatitis | Alcohol history Hepatomegaly Signs of cirrhosis (palmar erythema, angiomata) AST > ALT | CT scan Liver biopsy |
| **Active Alternative—Most Common** | | |
| Viral hepatitis | Exposure to body fluids, needles, or contaminated food Signs of cirrhosis if chronic hepatitis B or C | Hepatitis A antibody Hepatitis B antigen and antibodies Hepatitis C antibody |
| **Active Alternative—Must Not Miss** | | |
| Pancreatic cancer | Jaundice (with or without pain) Weight loss Alkaline phosphatase elevation > transaminase elevation | CT scan MRCP ERCP, Endoscopic ultrasound |
| **Other Hypotheses** | | |
| Common bile duct (CBD) stones | Lack of pain makes gallstones unlikely, although multiple CBD stones can present painlessly | CT scan MRCP Endoscopic ultrasound ERCP |
| Strictures or polyps | Painless jaundice | CT scan MRCP Endoscopic ultrasound ERCP |
| Ampullary carcinoma or cholangiocarcinoma | Painless jaundice Endoscopic | CT scan MRCP ultrasound ERCP |

Ms. B had a blood transfusion in Latvia in 1996. She has no history of injection drug use or smoking, but she has consumed between 2 glasses and 1 bottle of wine daily for years. Her past medical history is notable only for *Helicobacter pylori*–positive gastric and duodenal ulcers 6 years ago, treated with eradication therapy. She is taking no medications.

Is the clinical information sufficient to make a diagnosis? If not, what other information do you need?

# Leading Hypothesis: Alcoholic Liver Disease

## Textbook Presentation

Alcoholic liver disease encompasses a broad spectrum of abnormalities, beginning with steatosis, progressing to steatohepatitis and sometimes cirrhosis. The amount of alcohol necessary to develop advanced alcoholic liver disease varies among individuals, but in general, is about 40–80 g (4–8 drinks) daily for several years. The risk is higher for women at any given level of alcohol consumption.

## 1. Steatosis

### Textbook Presentation

Steatosis is usually asymptomatic, with normal or mildly elevated transaminases. Hepatomegaly is present in 70% of patients with biopsy proven steatosis.

### Disease Highlights

A. Potentiates liver damage from other insults, such as viral hepatitis or acetaminophen toxicity, and promotes obesity-related liver disease.

B. Found in 50% of patients who consume > 6 drinks (60 g) per day.

C. Usually completely reversible with abstinence from alcohol, although 1 study found that 18% of patients who became abstinent still progressed to cirrhosis.

D. Cirrhosis develops in 37% of those who continue to drink.

### Treatment

Abstain from alcohol.

## 2. Alcoholic Steatohepatitis

### Textbook Presentation

The classic manifestations of alcoholic steatohepatitis (also called alcoholic hepatitis) are fever, malaise, jaundice, and tender hepatomegaly.

### Disease Highlights

A. In reality, there is a broad range of presentations, including asymptomatic or isolated hepatomegaly; malnutrition is seen in 90% of patients.

B. Since cirrhosis can coexist, alcoholic hepatitis can also present with complications of portal hypertension, such as ascites, varices, and encephalopathy.

C. Found in 10–35% of heavy drinkers, and 38–56% of those who continue to drink progress to cirrhosis

D. 3-month mortality between 15% (mild alcoholic hepatitis) and 55% (severe alcoholic hepatitis)

E. Several tools have been developed to risk stratify patients with alcoholic hepatitis

  1. The Modified Discriminant Function (mDF)

    a. mDF = 4.6 × (patient PT – control PT) + serum bilirubin level

    b. If the mDF is > 32, the short-term mortality rate is > 50%; if the MDF is < 32, the mortality rate is 17%

    c. For predicting mortality, the sensitivity is 67–86% and the specificity is 48–62%.

  2. The Mayo End-stage Liver Disease (MELD) score

    a. This score incorporates the total bilirubin, INR, and serum creatinine.

    b. An online calculator is available at http://www.mayoclinic.org/meld/mayomodel7.html

    c. A MELD score > 11 was found to have a sensitivity of 86% and a specificity of 82% for 30-day mortality.

    d. A MELD score > 18 was found to have similar sensitivity and specificity; a score > 20 1 week after admission had a sensitivity of 91% and specificity 85%.

  3. Glasgow Alcoholic Hepatitis Score (GAHS)

    a. Includes age, WBC count, BUN, PT/INR, and total bilirubin

    b. A score ≥ 9 is associated with a poor prognosis and has an accuracy of 81% in predicting 28-day mortality

### Evidence-Based Diagnosis

A. Transaminases are elevated but generally < 6–7 times the upper limit of normal.

B. GGTP (gamma-glutamyl transpeptidase) is often elevated, and the GGTP/alkaline phosphatase ratio is often > 2.5.

C. AST:ALT ratio often, but not always, > 2

  1. 70–80% of patients in various studies.

  2. Another study showed mean ratio of 2.6 for patients with alcoholic liver disease, compared with mean of 0.9 for patients with nonalcoholic steatohepatitis; however, there was some overlap.

D. Imaging (with ultrasound or CT) is most helpful for ruling out other diagnoses; can variably see fatty infiltration, hepatomegaly, ascites, or cirrhosis.

E. Liver biopsy is the gold standard for diagnosis but is not always necessary.

### Treatment

A. Abstain from alcohol.

B. Consider selected medications in severe, acute steatohepatitis.

  1. In 1 study, pentoxifylline was shown to reduce mortality and development of hepatorenal syndrome in hospitalized patients with mDF > 32.

  2. There are conflicting data on corticosteroids, but there is some evidence of mortality benefit in selected patients: specifically, those with mDF > 32 or spontaneous encephalopathy (or both), in the absence of infection, GI bleeding, and renal failure.

## 3. Cirrhosis

A. See Chapter 15, Edema for a discussion of cirrhosis.

B. The prognosis of alcoholic cirrhosis varies, depending on whether the patient stops consuming alcohol.

  1. 5-year survival of 90% if patient becomes abstinent

  2. 5-year survival of 70% if patient continues to consume alcohol

  3. 5-year survival of 30–50% once complications of cirrhosis appear

## MAKING A DIAGNOSIS

Ms. B's transaminases are consistent with, but not diagnostic of, alcoholic liver disease. An imaging study is necessary not to rule in alcoholic liver disease, but rather to exclude alternative diagnoses. As discussed in Chapter 3, Abdominal Pain, ultrasound is the best first test to look for stones. However, in this patient, pancreatic or other malignancies are more likely causes of extrabiliary obstruction than stones; therefore, an abdominal CT scan is the best first test. Tests for hepatitis are necessary in all patients with liver disease and are especially important in Ms. B because of her history of a blood transfusion.

Ms. B has an abdominal CT scan, which shows an enlarged, nodular liver, moderate ascites, and a normal pancreas. Her hepatitis A IgM antibody, HBsAg and hepatitis B IgM core antibody, and hepatitis C antibody are all negative.

 Have you crossed the diagnostic threshold for the leading hypothesis, alcoholic hepatitis? Have you ruled out the active alternatives? Do other tests need to be done to exclude the alternative diagnoses?

## Alternative Diagnosis: Pancreatic Cancer

### Textbook Presentation

Patients with pancreatic cancer often have vague abdominal pain for weeks or months, followed by weight loss and perhaps the abrupt onset of painless jaundice.

### Disease Highlights

A. > 90% of cases are ductal carcinomas; 70–80% are in pancreas head and 20–25% in pancreas body or tail

B. Clinical presentation
   1. Symptoms are insidious and often present for more than 2 months.
   2. Abdominal pain is the most common presenting complaint, occurring in up to 80% of patients.
      a. Often described as gnawing, visceral pain, sometimes radiating from the epigastrium to the sides or back
      b. Sometimes improves with bending forward; worse at night or after eating
      c. Back pain is prominent if splanchnic nerve or celiac plexus infiltration occurs
   3. Weight loss is common.
   4. Jaundice
      a. In 80% of patients with cancers in the head; more if mass is > 2 cm
      b. Can occur when the cancer is in the body or tail but is then due to liver metastases
      c. Can be painless or associated with abdominal pain
   5. Rare presentations include acute pancreatitis, malabsorption, migratory thrombophlebitis, and GI bleeding.

### Evidence-Based Diagnosis

A. Multidetector CT scan ("pancreas protocol CT")
   1. Sensitivity = 86%; specificity = 90%
   2. Sensitivity lower for cancers < 2 cm (71%) versus those > 2 cm (89%)

B. Magnetic resonance cholangiopancreatography (MRCP): sensitivity = 84%, specificity = 97%

C. Endoscopic ultrasound
   1. Sensitivity = 95–98%; specificity = 75–100%
   2. Specificity = 100% if fine-needle aspiration (FNA) also performed

D. Endoscopic retrograde cholangiopancreatography (ERCP)
   1. Sensitivity 70%, specificity 94%
   2. No longer used to diagnose pancreatic cancer at many centers due to complications of pancreatitis and hemorrhage
   3. Still used for biliary stent placement in patients with unresectable biliary obstruction and for removal of common bile duct stones

E. CA 19–9
   1. For levels above 37–40 units/mL: sensitivity = 76–90%, specificity = 68–98%
   2. For levels above 100–120 units/mL, specificity = 87–100%
   3. For levels > 1000 units/mL, specificity = 94–100%

F. There is no universally accepted standard algorithm to diagnose pancreatic cancer
   1. The choice of imaging studies depends on the expertise available, with endoscopic ultrasound being the most operator-dependent.
   2. Most clinicians would start the evaluation with a CT scan, followed by either CT or endoscopic ultrasound–guided FNA if a mass is found on CT.
   3. Endoscopic ultrasound is better than CT for detecting small lesions, and should be done in patients with suggestive symptoms and normal CT scans.
   4. While CA 19-9 is not sensitive enough to rule out pancreatic cancer, very high levels are highly specific.

### Treatment

A. Complete resection is possible in ~15% of patients; 5-year survival is still only 10–25%.

B. Palliative approach for patients with nonresectable cancer
   1. Biliary diversion, either percutaneous or surgical
   2. Radiation therapy for pain relief
   3. Gemcitabine for improved quality of life, but not increased survival
   4. Median survival is 6 months.

## CASE RESOLUTION

1

With an LR- of 0.16, a normal CT scan does not always rule out pancreatic cancer. However, in this patient, given that her CT scan shows evidence of advanced liver disease (a more likely diagnosis for her), it is not necessary to do further imaging studies. The other active alternative, chronic hepatitis, is ruled out by her negative serologies. These test results, combined with her alcohol intake history, makes alcoholic liver disease the most likely diagnosis. At this point, some clinicians would proceed with treatment for alcoholic hepatitis, while others would confirm the diagnosis and, for prognostic purposes, establish the presence or absence of cirrhosis with a liver biopsy.

Her liver biopsy showed acute alcoholic hepatitis with cirrhosis. Because her mDF was > 32, she was treated with prednisolone. She was also advised to abstain from alcohol. She completed the course of prednisolone and has remained abstinent. Several weeks later, her bilirubin was normal and she felt well.

## CHIEF COMPLAINT

PATIENT

Mr. R is a 24-year-old graduate student with no past medical history who comes to see you because his girlfriend thought his eyes looked yellow yesterday. He has felt tired and a bit queasy for the last couple of weeks but thought he was just overworked and anxious. He has had some aching pain in the right upper quadrant and epigastrium, not related to eating or bowel movements. He has had no fevers, chills, or sweats. He has noticed dark urine for 1 or 2 days but attributed it to not drinking enough.

On physical exam, he appears tired. He has scleral icterus, and his liver is palpable 2 cm below the costal margin and is mildly tender. The spleen is not palpable, and the rest of his abdomen is nontender and nondistended. He has no edema, and the rest of his exam is normal.

At this point, what is the leading hypothesis, what are the active alternatives, and is there a must not miss diagnosis? Given this differential diagnosis, what tests should be ordered?

## PRIORITIZING THE DIFFERENTIAL DIAGNOSIS

The differential diagnosis for fatigue, nausea, and vague abdominal pain is broad, but the pivotal findings of scleral icterus and tender hepatomegaly point toward a hepatic source.

Mr. R's clinical picture is consistent with that of 90% of patients with viral hepatitis: a history of anorexia, malaise, and nausea, and a physical exam showing hepatomegaly, hepatic tenderness, or both. Hepatitis A is the most frequent cause of acute viral hepatitis; hepatitis C is the second most frequent but is usually asymptomatic acutely. Hepatitis B can also present acutely. By virtue of being common, alcoholic hepatitis is another active alternative diagnosis, and the presentation can mimic that of viral hepatitis. Biliary obstruction is always a consideration in patients with jaundice, but the prodrome and type of abdominal pain are not typical. Table 22–3 lists the differential diagnosis.

Hepatitis is unlikely in the absence of nausea, anorexia, malaise, hepatomegaly, or hepatic tenderness.

2

He has no past medical history and takes no medicines; he does not smoke or use illicit drugs. He drinks 1–2 beers most weeks, and occasionally shares a bottle of wine with friends. He has never had a blood transfusion or a tattoo. He enjoys trying different restaurants, and frequently eats sushi and ceviche. Initial laboratory tests include the following: total bilirubin, 6.5 mg/dL; conjugated bilirubin, 4 mg/dL; ALT, 1835 units/L; AST, 1522 units/L; alkaline phosphatase, 175 units/L; WBC, 9800 cells/mcL (normal differential); Hgb, 14.5 g/dL; Hct, 44%.

**Table 22–3.** Diagnostic hypotheses for Mr. R.

| Diagnostic Hypotheses | Clinical Clues | Important Tests |
|---|---|---|
| **Leading Hypothesis** | | |
| Acute hepatitis A | Exposure to potentially contaminated food Travel Right upper quadrant (RUQ) pain Nausea ± vomiting Malaise | IgM anti-HAV |
| **Active Alternative—Most Common** | | |
| Acute alcoholic steatohepatitis | History of binge drinking Hepatomegaly Signs of cirrhosis (palmar erythema, angiomata) AST > ALT | CT scan Liver biopsy Ultrasound |
| **Active Alternative—Must Not Miss** | | |
| Hepatitis B or C | Exposure to needles/body fluids RUQ pain Nausea ± vomiting Malaise | Hepatitis B: HBsAg IgM anti-HBc Hepatitis C: Anti-HCV HCV RNA |
| **Other Hypotheses** | | |
| Epstein Barr virus (EBV) or cytomegalovirus (CMV) hepatitis | Adenopathy Pharyngitis | EBV, CMV antibodies |
| Biliary obstruction | Biliary colic | Ultrasound |

Is the clinical information sufficient to make a diagnosis? If not, what other information do you need?

## Leading Hypothesis: Hepatitis A

### Textbook Presentation

The classic presentation is the gradual onset of malaise, nausea, anorexia, and right upper quadrant pain, followed by jaundice.

### Disease Highlights

A. Prevalence: Accounts for 20–40% of cases of viral hepatitis in the United States.

B. Clinical manifestations

1. Symptoms develop in 70% of adults, compared with < 30% of children under the age of 6.

2. Average incubation period is 25–30 days (range 15–49 days), followed by prodromal symptoms of fatigue, malaise, nausea, vomiting, anorexia, fever, and right upper pain; about 1 week later, jaundice appears.

3. 70% of patients have jaundice, and 80% have hepatomegaly.

4. Other physical findings include splenomegaly, cervical lymphadenopathy, rash, arthritis, and leukocytoclastic vasculitis.

5. Uncommon extrahepatic manifestations include vasculitis, arthritis, optic neuritis, transverse myelitis, thrombocytopenia, and aplastic anemia.

C. Transmission

1. Fecal-oral transmission, either sporadically or in an epidemic form

    a. Contaminated water, shellfish, frozen strawberries, etc.

    b. Contamination from infected restaurant worker

    c. Exposure history not always clear

2. No maternal-fetal transmission

D. Clinical course

1. Generally self-limited, with rare cases of fulminant hepatic failure (< 1% of patients with hepatitis A)

    a. Fulminant course is more common in patients with underlying hepatitis C.

    b. 1.1% fatality rate in adults > age 40

2. 85% fully recover in 3 months, and nearly all by 6 months

3. Transaminases normalize more rapidly than serum bilirubin

E. Prevention

1. Vaccination is available for preexposure prophylaxis.

    a. Immunity develops within 4 weeks in 90% of patients and within 26 weeks in 100% of patients.

    b. A second dose given 6–12 months later provides persistent immunity.

2. Can use immune serum globulin with or without vaccination for postexposure prophylaxis.

    a. Immune globulin provides 3–5 months of protection against hepatitis A and can be used for preexposure prophylaxis in patients who need immediate coverage.

    b. Immune globulin is 69–89% effective in preventing symptomatic illness when used postexposure.

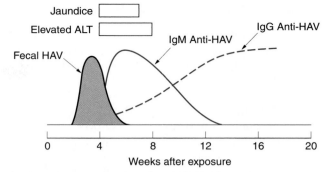

**Figure 22–1.** Natural history of hepatitis A symptoms and antibodies. ALT, alanine aminotransferase; HAV, hepatitis A virus.

### Evidence-Based Diagnosis

A. Liver function tests

1. ALT and AST are generally over 1000 units/L, and may be as high as 10,000 units/L; ALT is generally > AST.

2. Bilirubin commonly > 10 mg/dL

3. Alkaline phosphatase is usually modestly elevated.

B. Antibody tests (Figure 22–1)

1. Serum IgM anti-HAV detects acute illness, being positive even before the onset of symptoms and remaining positive for 4–6 months

2. LR+ = 99, LR− = 0.01

3. Serum IgG anti-HAV appears in the convalescent phase of the disease and remains positive for decades.

### Treatment

A. Supportive therapy: rest, oral hydration, and antiemetic medications as needed

B. Admit if INR is elevated or patient is unable to hydrate orally.

C. Liver transplant if fulminant hepatitis and liver failure occur

## MAKING A DIAGNOSIS

Considering the hepatocellular pattern of Mr. R's liver test abnormalities, the acute onset of his symptoms, and his lack of signs of chronic liver disease, the pretest probability for some form of viral hepatitis is so high that it is not necessary to consider other diagnoses at this point. Although Mr. R's history of food exposure suggests hepatitis A, it is generally necessary to test for all 3 of the primary hepatitis viruses since the exposure history for both hepatitis B and C is often unclear.

His hepatitis A IgM antibody is positive, with negative HBsAg, IgM anti-HBc, and anti-HCV.

Have you crossed a diagnostic threshold for the leading hypothesis, acute hepatitis A? Have you ruled out the active alternatives? Do other tests need to be done to exclude the alternative diagnoses?

## Alternative Diagnosis: Acute Hepatitis B

### Textbook Presentation

The classic presentation is the gradual onset of malaise, nausea, anorexia, right upper quadrant pain, followed by jaundice. Hepatitis B is often subclinical.

### Disease Highlights

A. Prevalence of hepatitis B virus (HBV) carriers

   1. 0.1–2% (low prevalence) in the United States, Canada, and Western Europe

   2. 3–5% (medium prevalence) in Mediterranean countries, Japan, central Asia, the Middle East, and Latin and South America

   3. 10–20% (high prevalence) in Southeast Asia, China, and sub-Saharan Africa

B. Clinical manifestations

   1. 70% of patients have subclinical infection or are anicteric; 30% of patients have icteric hepatitis.

   2. Incubation period is 1–4 months.

   3. Symptoms are similar to those of hepatitis A, but serum sickness-like syndrome can be part of the prodrome (fever, rash, arthralgias).

C. Transmission

   1. In high prevalence areas, transmission is primarily perinatal, occurring in 90% of babies born to HBeAg-positive mothers; it can be prevented by neonatal vaccination.

   2. In medium prevalence areas, childhood infection occurs from contaminated household objects, via minor breaks in the skin or mucous membranes.

   3. In low prevalence areas, transmission is most often sexual, via percutaneous inoculation (eg, injection drug use, accidental needlestick, tattooing, body piercing, acupuncture), or from contaminated blood transfusion.

D. Clinical course

   1. Fulminant hepatic failure occurs in 0.1–0.5% of patients.

   2. Transaminases normalize in 1–4 months if acute infection resolves.

   3. Elevation of ALT for > 6 months indicates progression to chronic hepatitis.

E. Prevention of hepatitis B

   1. Vaccination for preexposure prophylaxis

   2. Vaccination and HB immune globulin within 12 hours for perinatal exposure and within 1 week for postexposure prophylaxis

   3. Vaccinated individuals will have positive HBsAb tests

### Evidence-Based Diagnosis

A. Liver function tests: similar to hepatitis A

B. **Hepatitis B surface antigen (HBsAg)** appears 1–10 weeks after acute exposure, prior to symptoms or elevations of transaminases (Figure 22–2).

   1. Should be present in patients with acute symptoms

   2. Should clear in 4–6 months

   3. LR+ = 27, LR− = 0.2

C. **Hepatitis B surface antibody (HBsAb)** appears after disappearance of HBsAg; there can be a "window period" of several

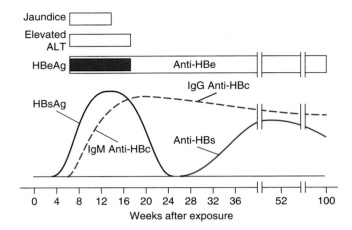

**Figure 22–2.** Natural history of acute hepatitis B infections.

weeks to months between the disappearance of HBsAg and the appearance of HBsAb.

D. **IgM hepatitis B core antibody (IgM anti-HBc)** appears shortly after HBsAg and is the only marker of acute infection detectable during the "window period."

   1. LR+ = 45, LR− = 0.1

   2. However, IgM anti-HBc can remain detectable for 2 years, and titer can increase during exacerbations of chronic hepatitis B.

### Treatment

A. Supportive therapy: rest, oral hydration, and antiemetic medications as needed

B. Admit if INR is elevated or patient is unable to hydrate orally.

C. Liver transplant if fulminant hepatitis occurs

## Alternative Diagnosis: Chronic Hepatitis B

### Textbook Presentation

Manifestations can range from asymptomatic, to isolated fatigue, to cirrhosis with portal hypertension. There is often no history of acute hepatitis B.

### Disease Highlights

A. Defined as presence of HBsAg for more than 6 months

B. After acute infection, HBV persists in the liver and serum at very low levels; patients in whom chronic hepatitis B develops have an impaired immune response to HBV.

C. Risk of progression from acute to chronic hepatitis B varies, depending on the host

   1. < 1% when the acute infection is acquired by an immunocompetent adult

   2. 90% when the infection is acquired perinatally

   3. 20% when the infection is acquired during childhood

D. 10–20% have extrahepatic findings (eg, polyarteritis nodosa, glomerular disease)

E. HBsAg is generally detectable for life (0.5–2%/year become HBsAg negative)

***Table 22–4.*** Chronic hepatitis B virus (HBV) infection.

| Phase | Laboratory Findings | Histology | Highlights | Natural History |
|---|---|---|---|---|
| Immune tolerance | HBeAg positive<br>HBV DNA level very high<br>ALT normal | Minimal or no inflammation | Occurs in perinatally acquired HBV<br>Short or absent when infection acquired later<br>An immune response to HBeAg does not occur | Lasts 1-4 decades and then transitions to HBeAg positive chronic hepatitis |
| HBeAg positive chronic hepatitis (Immune Clearance) | HBeAg positive<br>HBV DNA moderately high; can fluctuate<br>Elevated ALT | Active inflammation and fibrosis | Recurrent "flares" of liver enzymes that may result in loss of HBeAg, transient decrease in HBV with persistence of HBeAg, or hepatic decompensation<br>Frequency and severity of flares correlates with risk of cirrhosis and HCC | Spontaneous conversion to HBeAg negative state occurs in 10–20% of patients annually<br>Seroconversion more likely in older patients, those with higher ALT levels, and those with genotype B<br>Annual incidence of cirrhosis 2–5% |
| Inactive HBsAg carrier state | HBeAg negative<br>HBeAb positive<br>HBV DNA low to undetectable<br>ALT normal | Minimal inflammation and fibrosis; inactive cirrhosis sometimes seen | Can remain in this phase for years or even indefinitely | In one study, 67% stayed inactive carriers, 4% reverted to HBeAg positive, 24% developed HBeAg negative chronic hepatitis, and 8% cirrhosis |
| HBeAg negative chronic hepatitis (reactivation of HBV replication) | HBeAg negative<br>HBeAb positive<br>HBV DNA detectable<br>Elevated ALT | Continued inflammation<br>Variable fibrosis<br>Sometimes cirrhosis | Can progress to this state from either inactive carrier state or HBeAg positive chronic hepatitis state<br>Disease activity fluctuates, with periods of normal ALT levels | Can progress silently for years<br>Annual incidence of cirrhosis 8–10%<br>0.5–1%/year spontaneous clearance of HBsAg |

**F.** There are 4 phases of chronic HBV (Table 22–4); not all patients experience all 4 phases.

**G.** Risk factors for progression from chronic hepatitis to cirrhosis include frequent alcohol intake, concurrent hepatitis C or HIV infection, high levels of HBV replication, and HBV genotype C.

**H.** Chronic hepatitis B is a risk factor for hepatocellular carcinoma (HCC)

  **1.** Annual incidence < 1% for non-cirrhotic chronic carriers and 2–3% for those with cirrhosis.

  **2.** Additional risk factors include frequent alcohol intake, concurrent hepatitis C infection, high levels of HBV replication, and HBV genotype C.

  **3.** Screening with ultrasound and alpha-fetoprotein levels is recommended every 6–12 months.

## Evidence-Based Diagnosis

**A.** HBsAg is always positive.

**B.** See Table 22–4 for patterns of HBeAg, HBV DNA, and ALT in different phases.

## Treatment

**A.** HBeAg-positive patients have high rates of early progression to chronic active hepatitis and cirrhosis and should be treated.

**B.** Asymptomatic HBeAg-negative patients with viral loads below $10^5$ genomes/mL and normal transaminases are usually not treated; those with higher viral loads and abnormal transaminases are sometimes treated.

**C.** Markers of successful therapy include loss of HBeAg, with seroconversion to anti-HBe antibodies (in HBeAg-positive patients), and reduction of the viral load.

**D.** True cure is rare (1–5% of patients).

**E.** Current treatment options include interferon alfa, lamivudine, and adefovir.

## Alternative Diagnosis: Hepatitis C

### Textbook Presentation

Most patients are asymptomatic, with jaundice developing in less than 25%. When present, symptoms are similar to those of other viral hepatitis and last 2–12 weeks.

### Disease Highlights

**A.** Prevalence

  **1.** 20% of cases of acute hepatitis

  **2.** Prevalence of HCV infection in the United States is 1.6%

**B.** Transmission

  **1.** Currently, 1 per 2 million blood transfusions transmit hepatitis C; up to 10% of transfusion recipients prior to 1990 were infected.

**2.** Now, hepatitis C is primarily transmitted through injection drug use, with occasional cases due to ear or body piercing, sex with an injection drug user, or accidental needlesticks.

**3.** Household contacts are rarely infected.

**4.** Transmission between monogamous partners is about 1%/year; risk of sexual transmission is higher if index carrier also has HIV or multiple partners.

**5.** Perinatal transmission occurs in 4.6-10% of cases.

**C.** Clinical course

**1.** Most patients are asymptomatic during the acute infection.

**2.** Average incubation period is 7–8 weeks.

**3.** Fulminant hepatitis is rare.

**4.** Extrahepatic manifestations are common, being found in about 75% of patients.

   **a.** Fatigue, arthralgias, paresthesias, myalgias, pruritus, and sicca syndrome are found in > 10% of patients.

   **b.** Vasculitis secondary to cryoglobulinemia is found in 1% of patients, although cryoglobulinemia is present in about 40%.

   **c.** Depression and anxiety are more common than in uninfected persons.

**5.** 15–40% of patients clear the infection within 6 months.

**6.** 60–85% of patients have detectable HCV RNA at 6 months and therefore have chronic hepatitis C.

**D.** Chronic hepatitis C

**1.** There are 5 stages of liver disease:

   **a.** Stage 0: No fibrosis

   **b.** Stage 1: Fibrous expansion of portal tracts

   **c.** Stage 2: Periportal fibrosis

   **d.** Stage 3: Bridging fibrosis

   **e.** Stage 4: Cirrhosis

**2.** There is no correlation between ALT levels and liver histology.

**3.** Although there are noninvasive techniques that can predict the degree of fibrosis (see Chapter 15, Edema), it is necessary to do a liver biopsy to accurately determine the activity and severity of the disease.

**4.** 27–41% of patients progress at least 1 stage over 5 years.

**5.** Cirrhosis develops in 4–24% of patients after 20 years of infection.

   **a.** Rates are low in community cohorts and cohorts of blood donors (4–7%).

   **b.** Rates are higher in other populations (24%).

   **c.** Liver histology is the best predictor of progression to cirrhosis.

   **d.** Other predictors of progression to cirrhosis include age at infection (> 40 years of age → more progression), duration of infection, consumption of alcohol > 50 g/d, HIV or HBV coinfection, male sex, higher ALT, baseline fibrosis, and possibly steatosis.

   **e.** 5-year survival for compensated cirrhosis is 80% but drops to 50% once decompensation occurs.

   **f.** HCC develops in 1–7% of patients per year.

**E.** Prevention: no vaccine available; no role for immunoglobulin

**Evidence-Based Diagnosis**

**A.** Anti-HCV antibody tests

**1.** Main screening assay is an **enzyme immunoassay (EIA)**

   **a.** Sensitivity of 92–95% for second-generation test (EIA-2) and 97% for third-generation test (EIA-3)

   **b.** Positive predictive value (true positive EIAs/all positive EIAs) is 50–61% in low prevalence populations, such as blood donors, and 88–95% in high prevalence populations.

   **c.** Can be negative in immunocompromised patients, such as organ transplant recipients, HIV-infected patients, or hemodialysis patients, even in presence of active viral infection

   **d.** Positive in 50% of patients with acute hepatitis C at time of presentation; mean time to seroconversion is 10 weeks but can occur within 4 weeks

**2.** Patients with high pretest probability of infection and a negative antibody test should have an HCV RNA assay performed

**B.** HCV RNA tests (Figure 22–3)

**1.** Qualitative HCV RNA tests

   **a.** Highly sensitive (96–98%) and specific (> 99%)

   **b.** Very low limits of detection (< 50 international units/mL)

   **c.** Qualitative tests are used to confirm viremia, particularly in blood and organ donation screening

**2.** Quantitative HCV RNA tests

   **a.** Specificity 96–98.9%

   **b.** Lower limit of detection generally higher than that of qualitative tests (~600 international units/mL), but some newer assays have limits of detection as low as 10 international units/mL

   **c.** Quantitative tests are used to monitor response to treatment

**C.** Genotype testing

**1.** Used for prediction of response to treatment and choice of treatment duration

**2.** Genotypes do not change, so this test needs to be done only once.

**3.** In the United States, 71.5% of cases are from genotype 1, 13.5% from genotype 2, 5.5% from genotype 3, and 1.15 from genotype 4.

**D.** When should you order the different antibody and RNA tests? (see Algorithm, Testing in Hepatitis C, at end of chapter)

**1.** In a patient with **acute hepatitis,** order the anti-HCV EIA first; if it is negative, order a qualitative HCV RNA, which is detectable before the antibody.

**2.** In a patient with **chronic liver disease or an elevated ALT,** order the anti-HCV EIA.

   **a.** Nearly all results are true-positives, so confirmatory testing is not required.

   **b.** If you choose to do a confirmatory test, the best is a quantitative HCV RNA, since the results will be used to monitor the response to treatment; if the quantitative HCV RNA is negative, order the more sensitive qualitative HCV RNA.

**3.** When a positive anti-HCV EIA is found in blood donors, or in patients with normal ALT levels, confirmatory testing with a highly sensitive assay is necessary.

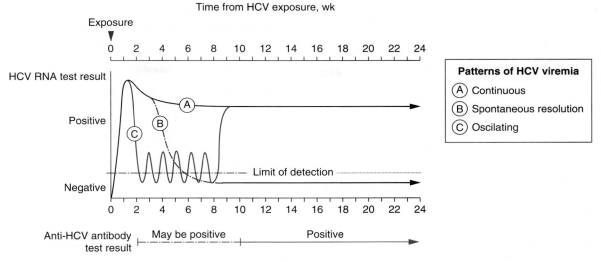

Time from HCV exposure, wk

**Patterns of HCV viremia**
Ⓐ Continuous
Ⓑ Spontaneous resolution
Ⓒ Oscilating

JAMA, February 21, 2007—Vol 297, No. 7

**Figure 22-3.** Patterns of HCV RNA test results. (Reproduced, with permission, from Scott JD et al. Molecular diagnostics of hepatitis C virus infection: a systematic review. JAMA. 2007;297:724–32.)

**4.** Immunocompromised patients with suspected hepatitis C who are EIA antibody negative should have a qualitative test.

## Treatment

**A.** Goals of treatment: Prevention of cirrhosis and its complications, reduction of extrahepatic manifestations, and reduction of transmission

**B.** A sustained virologic response is defined as non-detectable HCV RNA 6 months after completion of therapy.

**C.** Testing negative for HCV RNA at 4 and 12 weeks predicts the likelihood of a sustained virologic response

**D.** Patients with higher viral loads (> 800,000 international units/mL, equivalent to 2 million copies/mL) have higher relapse rates and are often treated longer than those with lower viral loads.

**E.** Currently, the best results are seen with a combination of pegylated interferon and ribavirin.

## CASE RESOLUTION

Mr. R clearly has acute hepatitis A, presumably from contaminated food. Although he is nauseated, he is able to drink adequate fluid. His INR is normal at 1.1. You recommend rest and oral hydration for Mr. R, and serum immune globulin and vaccination for his girlfriend. He feels much better when he returns 1 month later.

The best test of the liver's synthetic function is the PT. It is important to check the INR in all patients with hepatitis to look for signs of liver failure.

## CHIEF COMPLAINT

PATIENT ▽3

Mr. H is a 55-year-old man with unexpected transaminase abnormalities.

What is the differential diagnosis of asymptomatic transaminase elevations? How would you frame the differential?

## CONSTRUCTING A DIFFERENTIAL DIAGNOSIS

The basic framework is to separate hepatic from nonhepatic causes.

**A.** Hepatic causes
  **1.** Alcohol abuse
  **2.** Medication
  **3.** Chronic hepatitis B or C
  **4.** Nonalcoholic fatty liver disease (NAFLD)
  **5.** Autoimmune hepatitis
  **6.** Hemochromatosis

7. Wilson disease (in patients < 40 years old)

8. $\alpha_1$-Antitrypsin deficiency

B. Nonhepatic causes

1. Celiac sprue

2. Inherited disorders of muscle metabolism (AST elevation only)

3. Acquired muscle disease (AST elevation only)

4. Strenuous exercise (AST elevation only)

Mr. H comes in for a routine appointment. He feels fine. His past medical history is notable for type 2 diabetes and hypertension. His medications include metformin, atorvastatin, hydrochlorothiazide, and lisinopril. He does not smoke, and he has a beer with dinner occasionally. His physical exam shows a BP of 125/80 mm Hg, pulse of 80 bpm, RR of 16 breaths per minute, weight 230 lbs, and height 5 ft 9 in (BMI = 34.0). Pulmonary, cardiac, and abdominal exams are all normal.

Laboratory test results from his last visit include a creatinine of 0.9 mg/dL, a HgbA$_{1C}$ of 6.8%, an LDL of 95 mg/dL, a bilirubin of 0.8 mg/dL, an AST of 85 units/L, an ALT of 92 units/L, and a normal alkaline phosphatase. You then note that his transaminases were 45 units/L and 53 units/L, respectively, when last checked a year earlier.

At this point, what is the leading hypothesis, what are the active alternatives, and is there a must not miss diagnosis? Given this differential diagnosis, what tests should be ordered?

## PRIORITIZING THE DIFFERENTIAL DIAGNOSIS

In the absence of an obvious nonhepatic cause of liver enzyme elevations, the initial approach is to focus on the hepatic causes. The prevalence of the liver diseases in the differential diagnosis varies widely, depending on the population studied. For example, in a study of over 19,000 young, healthy military recruits, of whom 99 had enzyme elevations, only 11 were found to have any liver disease (4 had hepatitis B, 4 had hepatitis C, 2 had autoimmune hepatitis, 1 had cholelithiasis). A study of 100 blood donors with elevated enzymes found that 48% had alcoholic liver disease, 22% had NAFLD, and 17% had hepatitis C. In another study, patients with elevated enzymes in whom a diagnosis could not be made by history or blood tests underwent liver biopsy; NAFLD was found in over 50% of them.

The pivotal points in the history and physical exam are the patient's diabetes and elevated BMI. NAFLD is extremely common in obese, diabetic patients, so Mr. H is at high risk for this disease. He has no specific risk factors for chronic hepatitis, but often the exposure history is unclear and these diagnoses cannot be ruled out without further testing. His alcohol intake is minimal, but sometimes even small amounts of alcohol can cause liver enzyme elevations. He is also taking 2 medications, metformin and atorvastatin, that can cause elevation of liver enzymes. (Although statins cause transaminase elevation in 0.5–2.0% of patients, the clinical significance is unclear, and progression to liver failure is rare. The American College of Cardiology recommends measuring transaminases at baseline, at 12 weeks, and then annually.) The final possibility to consider at this point is

**Table 22–5.** Diagnostic hypotheses for Mr. H.

| Diagnostic Hypotheses | Clinical Clues | Important Tests |
|---|---|---|
| **Leading Hypothesis** | | |
| Nonalcoholic fatty liver disease | Obesity (BMI > 30) Diabetes | Ultrasound Liver biopsy |
| **Active Alternatives—Most Common** | | |
| Hemochromatosis | Family history Diabetes | Serum iron/TIBC Ferritin |
| Alcohol | Intake history AST > ALT | Abstinence |
| Medication | Medication history (prescriptions and nonprescription) | Stopping the medication |
| **Active Alternatives—Must Not Miss** | | |
| Hepatitis B or C | Exposure to body fluids, needles | HBsAg Anti-HBc Anti-HBs Anti-HCV |
| **Other Hypotheses** | | |
| Autoimmune hepatitis | Other autoimmune disease | Serum protein electrophoresis Antinuclear antibody Anti-smooth muscle antibody Liver biopsy |
| Wilson disease | Age < 40 Neuropsychiatric symptoms | Ceruloplasmin |
| $\alpha_1$-Antitrypsin deficiency | Emphysema | $\alpha_1$-Antitrypsin level and phenotype |

hemochromatosis, a fairly common gene mutation that can present with liver enzyme abnormalities and diabetes. Table 22–5 lists the differential diagnosis.

Mr. H first abstains from alcohol for 2 weeks; his repeat liver enzymes show AST = 90 units/L and ALT = 95 units/L. He then stops his atorvastatin and metformin for 1 week, with no change in his transaminases. PT, albumin, and CBC are all normal.

Is the clinical information sufficient to make a diagnosis? If not, what other information do you need?

## Leading Hypothesis: NAFLD

### Textbook Presentation

Patients are often asymptomatic but sometimes complain of vague right upper quadrant discomfort. It is common to identify patients

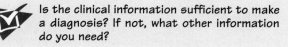

by finding hepatomegaly on exam or asymptomatic transaminase elevations.

## Disease Highlights

**A.** Definition

   **1.** A spectrum of liver abnormalities all of which include hepatic steatosis in the absence of significant alcohol use

   **2.** Stages

     **a.** Steatosis (also called fatty liver [FL])

     **b.** Non-alcoholic steatohepatitis (NASH)

     **c.** Cirrhosis

**B.** Epidemiology and etiology

   **1.** Risk factors include the metabolic syndrome, obesity, type 2 diabetes, insulin resistance, and hyperlipidemia.

   **2.** Prevalence varies based on population studied

     **a.** 20–30% in Western adults, with only 2–3% being NASH

     **b.** 70% in diabetics

     **c.** 91% in obese patients (BMI > 35 kg/m²) undergoing bariatric surgery, with 37% being NASH

   **3.** Most common cause of abnormal liver test results in the United States.

   **4.** Other causes of NAFLD

     **a.** Nutritional (eg, total parenteral nutrition, starvation, rapid weight loss, malnutrition, bariatric surgery)

     **b.** Drugs (eg, methotrexate, amiodarone, estrogens, glucocorticoids, aspirin, cocaine, antiretroviral agents)

     **c.** Metabolic or genetic

     **d.** Other (eg, inflammatory bowel disease, HIV, environmental hepatotoxins)

**C.** Clinical course

   **1.** Most patients with pure steatosis are stable and do not develop progressive liver disease; about 12–40% develop NASH with early fibrosis after 8–13 years.

   **2.** Progressive liver disease can develop in patients with NASH, with about 15% progressing to cirrhosis over 8–13 years.

   **3.** Risk factors for progression include weight gain and presence of portal tract fibrosis on initial biopsy.

   **4.** HCC develops in about 7% of cirrhotic patients over 10 years.

## Evidence-Based Diagnosis

**A.** Blood tests

   **1.** Transaminase elevation is usually < 4 times normal; AST:ALT ratio is usually less than 1, but not if there is advanced disease

   **2.** Serum ferritin is elevated in 50% of patients.

   **3.** Alkaline phosphatase and GGT are often mildly elevated.

**B.** Imaging

   **1.** Ultrasound for the diagnosis of steatosis

     **a.** Sensitivity, 89%; specificity, 93%, although the sensitivity may be lower for mild degrees of steatosis

     **b.** LR+, 12.7; LR−, 0.12

   **2.** The test characteristics of CT scan are similar to those of ultrasound.

   **3.** No imaging study can reliably distinguish steatosis from more advanced NAFLD.

**C.** Liver biopsy is the gold standard for diagnosis and staging.

It is necessary to rule out other causes of liver disease listed in the above differential before diagnosing NAFLD.

## Treatment

**A.** Weight loss

**B.** Exercise

**C.** Control of diabetes

**D.** Control of hyperlipidemia

# MAKING A DIAGNOSIS

You should take somewhat of a stepwise approach to evaluating asymptomatic liver enzyme abnormalities. As was done with Mr. H, the first step is to stop alcohol and, if possible, potentially hepatotoxic medications, and then remeasure the liver enzymes. Although aspects of the history can increase the likelihood of a specific diagnosis, the history is not sensitive or specific enough to make a diagnosis, and it is necessary to test somewhat broadly. If liver enzyme abnormalities persist after stopping alcohol and potentially hepatotoxic medications, the American Gastroenterological Association recommends beginning with a prothrombin times; serum albumin; CBC; hepatitis A, B, and C serologies; and iron studies (serum iron, total iron-binding capacity [TIBC], ferritin).

IgM and IgG anti-HAV are both negative. HBsAg and IgM anti-HBc are negative; IgG anti-HBc and anti-HBs are positive. Anti-HCV is negative. The transferrin saturation is 35%, and the serum ferritin is 190 ng/mL.

**Have you crossed a diagnostic threshold for the leading hypothesis, NAFLD? Have you ruled out the active alternatives? Do other tests need to be done to exclude the alternative diagnoses?**

## Alternative Diagnosis: Hereditary Hemochromatosis

### Textbook Presentation

Most patients are asymptomatic, but a few have extrahepatic manifestations of iron overload (see below). Some patients are identified by screening the family members of affected individuals.

### Disease Highlights

**A.** Iron deposition occurs throughout the reticuloendothelial system, leading to a broad range of potential manifestations.

   **1.** In the liver leads to cirrhosis and then to HCC

   **2.** In the heart leads to dilated cardiomyopathy

   **3.** In the pituitary leads to secondary hypogonadism

   **4.** In the pancreas leads to diabetes

   **5.** In the joints leads to arthropathy

   **6.** In the thyroid leads to hypothyroidism

**B.** > 90% of patients are homozygous for the autosomal recessive *HFE* C282Y mutation.

C. The gene expression is quite variable, with a high penetrance of iron overload (ie, increased ferritin levels) but a low penetrance of clinical disease.

D. In a recent study, nearly 100,000 primary care patients were screened for iron overload and *HFE* mutations.

1. 299 patients were homozygous for the C282Y mutation.

   a. The prevalence of homozygosity was 0.44% in whites, 0.11% in Native Americans, 0.027% in Hispanics, 0.014% in blacks, 0.012% in Pacific Islanders, and 0.000039% in Asians.

   b. The prevalence of heterozygosity for the mutation was 10% in whites, 5.7% in Native Americans, 2.9% in Hispanics, 2.3% in blacks, 2% in Pacific Islanders, and 0.12% in Asians.

2. The transferrin saturation (see definition below) was > 50% in 84% of male homozygotes and > 45% in 73% of females.

3. The serum ferritin was > 300 mcg/L in 88% of male homozygotes and was > 200 mcg/L in 57% of females.

E. 72% of patients with serum ferritin levels > 1000 mcg/L have cirrhosis, compared with 7.4% of those with ferritin levels < 1000 mcg/L.

F. Screening primary care populations for hemochromatosis is not recommended by the United States Preventive Services Task Force (USPSTF) or the American College of Physicians.

### Evidence-Based Diagnosis

A. Liver biopsy with measurement of hepatic iron index is the gold standard.

B. Initial testing should be done with a transferrin saturation (serum iron/TIBC [TIBC = serum iron + unsaturated iron-binding capacity]) or the unsaturated iron-binding capacity, and a serum ferritin (the test characteristics are for identifying homozygous patients).

1. Transferrin saturation ≥ 50% in men

   a. Sensitivity = 82.4%; specificity = 92.5%

   b. LR+ = 10.9, LR− = 0.19

2. Transferrin saturation ≥ 45% in women

   a. Sensitivity = 73.8%; specificity = 93.1%

   b. LR+ = 10.8, LR− = 0.28

3. Unsaturated iron-binding capacity (UIBC) < 24 mcmol/L in men

   a. Sensitivity = 87.9%, specificity = 92.5%

   b. LR+ = 11.8, LR− = 0.13

4. UIBC < 29 mcmol/L in women

   a. Sensitivity = 81.4%, specificity = 92.5%

   b. LR+ = 10.8, LR− = 0.2

5. Ferritin ≥ 200 ng/mL

   a. Men

      (1) Sensitivity, 78%; specificity, 76%

      (2) LR+ = 3.25, LR− = 0.23

   b. Women

      (1) Sensitivity, 54%; specificity, 95%

      (2) LR+ = 20, LR− = 0.48

C. Patients who have a transferrin saturation ≥ 45% and an elevated ferritin should undergo *HFE* gene testing, looking for the hereditary hemochromatosis mutations.

All first-degree relatives of patients with hereditary hemochromatosis should undergo gene testing, regardless of the results of the iron studies.

1. If C282Y/C282Y homozygous mutation is found

   a. If age is < 40 years, ferritin < 1000 ng/mL, and transaminases are normal, proceed to treatment

   b. Otherwise, perform liver biopsy to determine severity

2. If other mutations or no mutations are found, look for other causes of iron overload or perform liver biopsy for diagnosis.

### Treatment

Periodic phlebotomy to reduce the iron overload has been shown to reduce the risk of progression to cirrhosis.

## CASE RESOLUTION

Mr. H's transaminase levels remained elevated after abstaining from alcohol and discontinuing medications, making those diagnoses unlikely. His hepatitis A and C serologies are negative; his hepatitis B serologies are consistent with a previous infection and not chronic hepatitis B. His transferrin saturation is normal, and the slightly elevated ferritin is not specific for any particular disease.

At this point, you could order an antinuclear antibody (ANA), smooth muscle antibody (SMA), ceruloplasmin, and $\alpha_1$-antitrypsin levels and phenotype. However, considering his age, gender, and lack of other symptoms or illnesses, autoimmune hepatitis, Wilson disease, and $\alpha_1$-antitrypsin deficiency are all very unlikely. At this point, NAFLD is by far the most likely diagnosis. An ultrasound is not absolutely necessary, but it could confirm the diagnosis of NAFLD.

Mr. H has an ultrasound, which shows an enlarged liver with diffuse fatty infiltration. He begins to walk 20 minutes 4 times/week, and reduces his portion sizes. His transaminases remain stable for the next several months. One year later, he has lost 20 pounds, and his transaminases have decreased to around 40.

## REFERENCES

Adams PC, Barton JC. Hemochromatosis. Lancet. 2007;370:1855–60.

Adams PC, Reboussin DM, Barton JC et al. Hemochromatosis and iron overload screening in a racially diverse population (HEIRS study). N Engl J Med. 2005;352:1769–78.

Adams PC, Reboussin DM, Leiendecker-Foster C et al. Comparison of the unsaturated iron-binding capacity with transferring saturation as a screening test to detect C282Y homozygotes for hemochromatosis in 101,168 participants in the HEIRS study. Clin Chem. 2005;51:1048–52.

American Gastroenterological Association. Evaluation of liver chemistry tests. Gastroenterology. 2002;123:1364–66.

Bialek SR, Terrault NA. The changing epidemiology and natural history of hepatitis C virus infection. Clin Liver Dis. 2006;10:697–715.

Brundage SC, Fitzpatrick AN. Hepatitis A. Am Fam Physician. 2006;73:2162–68.

DeWitt J, Devereaux B, Chriswell M et al. Comparison of endoscopic ultrasonography and multidetector computed tomography for detecting and staging pancreatic cancer. Ann Intern Med. 2004;141:753–63.

Giannini EG, Testa R, Savarino V. Liver enzyme alteration: a guide for clinicians. CMAJ. 2005;172:367–79.

Grover SA, Barkun AN, Sackett DL. Does this patient have splenomegaly? JAMA. 1993;270:2218–21.

Hung OL, Kwon NS, Cole AE et al. Evaluation of the physician's ability to recognize the presence or absence of anemia , fever, and jaundice. Acad Emerg Med. 2000;7:146–56.

Katz MH, Savides TJ, Moossa AR, Bouvet M. An evidence based approach to the diagnosis and staging of pancreatic cancer. Pancreatology. 2005;5:576–90.

Mills SJ, Harrison SA. Comparison of the natural history of alcoholic and nonalcoholic fatty liver disease. Curr Gastroenterol Rep. 2005;7:32–6.

Naylor CD. Physical examination of the liver. JAMA. 1994;271:1859–64.

Sass DA, Shaikh OS. Alcoholic hepatitis. Clin Liver Dis. 2006;10:219–37.

Scott JD, Gretch Dr. Molecular diagnostics of hepatitis C virus infection: a systematic review. JAMA. 2007;297:724–32.

Srikureja W, Kyulo NL, Runyon BA, Hu KQ. MELD score is a better prognostic model than Child-Turcotte-Pugh score or Discriminant Function score in patients with alcoholic hepatitis. J Hepatol. 2005;700–6.

Williams JW, Simel DL. Does this patient have ascites? JAMA. 1992;267:2645–48.

Yim JH, Lok AS. Natural history of chronic hepatitis B infection: what we knew in 1981 and what we know in 2005. Hepatology. 2006;43:S173–S181.

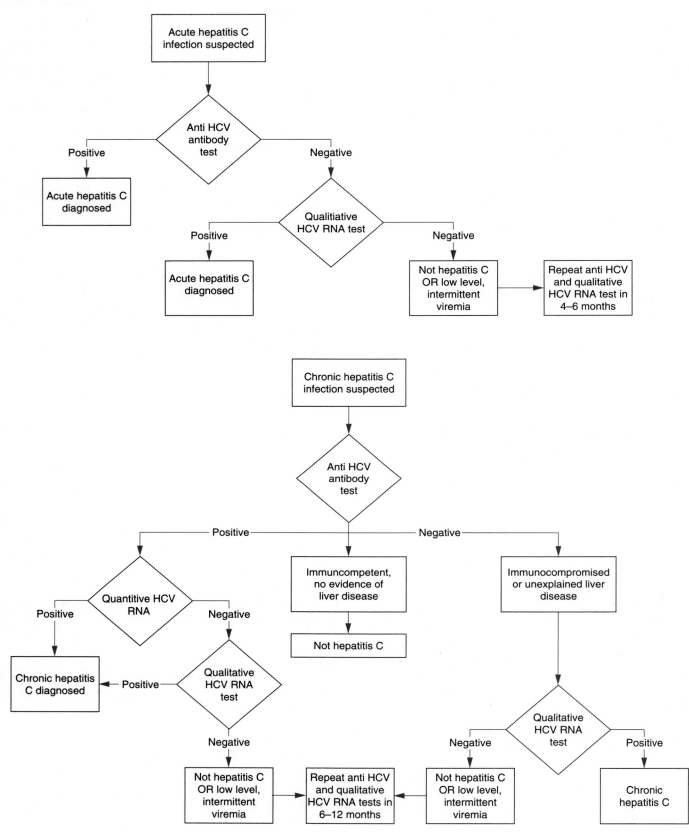

**Testing in Hepatitis C Infection**

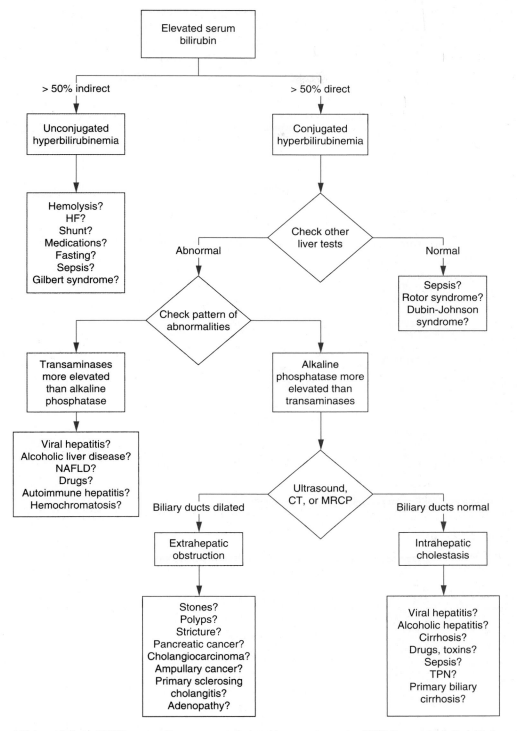

HF, heart failure; MRCP, magnetic resonance cholangiopancreatography; NAFLD, nonalcoholic fatty liver disease; TPN; total parenteral nutrition.

**Diagnostic Approach to Hyperbilirubinemia**

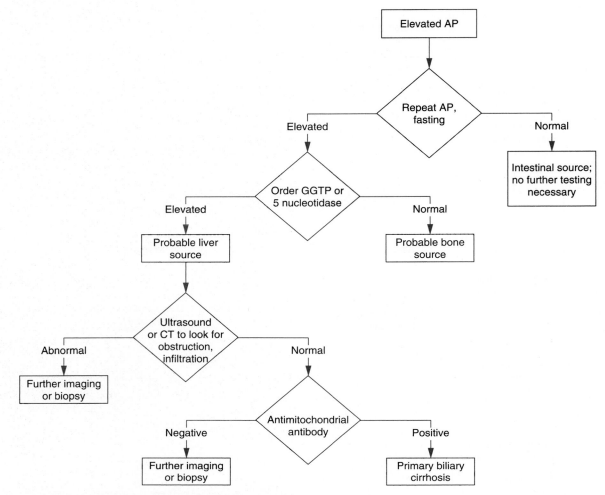

AP, alkaline phosphatase; GGTP, gamma-glutamyl transpeptidase.

**Diagnostic Approach to Elevated Alkaline Phosphatase**

# I have a patient with joint pain. How do I determine the cause?

## CHIEF COMPLAINT

PATIENT ▽1

Mrs. K is a 75-year-old woman who complains of a painful left knee.

What is the differential diagnosis of joint pain? How would you frame the differential?

## CONSTRUCTING A DIFFERENTIAL DIAGNOSIS

The causes of joint pain range from common to rare and from not particularly dangerous to joint- and life-threatening. Even the most benign causes of joint pain can lead to serious disability. The evaluation of a patient with joint pain calls for a detailed history and physical exam (often focusing on extra-articular findings) and occasionally the sampling of joint fluid and possibly analyzing serologic tests.

There are three pivotal features in organizing the approach to joint pain. First, is the pain articular or extra-articular? Although this distinction may seem obvious, abnormalities of periarticular structures can mimic articular disease. Second, is a single joint or are multiple joints involved? Finally, are the involved joints inflamed or not?

The first pivotal point in making a diagnosis in a patient with joint pain is to determine whether the patient's pain is truly articular, real joint pain, or periarticular.

The differential diagnosis below is organized by these pivotal points: the number of joints involved (monoarticular vs polyarticular) and by whether or not the joint is inflamed (judged by physical exam, joint fluid analysis, or both). Recognize that all of the monoarticular arthritides can present in a polyarticular distribution, and classically polyarticular diseases may occasionally only affect a single joint.

The joint distribution of diseases that cause joint pain is variable; monoarticular arthritides may present with polyarticular findings and vice versa.

A. Monoarticular arthritis
  1. Inflammatory
    a. Infectious
      (1) Gonococcal arthritis
      (2) Nongonococcal septic arthritis
      (3) Lyme disease

    b. Crystalline
      (1) Monosodium urate (gout)
      (2) Calcium pyrophosphate dihydrate deposition disease (CPPD or pseudogout)
  2. Noninflammatory
    a. Osteoarthritis (OA)
    b. Traumatic
    c. Avascular necrosis
B. Polyarticular arthritis
  1. Inflammatory
    a. Rheumatologic
      (1) Rheumatoid arthritis (RA)
      (2) Systemic lupus erythematosus (SLE)
      (3) Psoriatic arthritis
      (4) Other rheumatic diseases
    b. Infectious
      (1) Bacterial
        (a) Bacterial endocarditis
        (b) Lyme disease
      (2) Viral
        (a) Rubella
        (b) Hepatitis B
        (c) HIV
        (d) Parvovirus
      (3) Postinfectious
        (a) Enteric
        (b) Urogenital
        (c) Rheumatic fever
  2. Noninflammatory: OA

▽1

Mrs. K's symptoms started after she stepped down from a bus with unusual force. The pain became intolerable within about 6 hours of onset and has been present for 3 days now. She otherwise feels well. She reports no fevers, chills, dietary changes, or sick contacts.

On physical exam she is in obvious pain, limping into the exam room on a cane. Her vital signs are temperature, 37.0°C; RR, 12 breaths per minute; BP, 110/70 mm Hg; pulse, 80 bpm. The only abnormality on exam is the

(continued)

right knee. It is red, warm to the touch, and tender to palpation. The range of motion is limited to only about 20 degrees.

> At this point, what is the leading hypothesis, what are the active alternatives, and is there a must not miss diagnosis? Given this differential diagnosis, what tests should be ordered?

## PRIORITIZING THE DIFFERENTIAL DIAGNOSIS

Pivotal points in this case are that the patient's symptoms clearly localize to articular, rather than periarticular structures since the exam reveals an inflamed joint with limited range of motion. Therefore, the differential diagnosis focuses primarily on the causes of inflammatory monoarticular arthritis, such as septic arthritis, gout, pseudogout, and trauma.

Salient points of the patient's presentation are the rapid onset of the pain; the mild, antecedent trauma; and the lack of systemic symptoms, such as fever, fatigue, or weight loss.

Given the patient's age, the single inflamed joint, and high incidence of gout, this diagnosis is the leading hypothesis. CPPD (also called pseudogout) is common in the knee of elderly patients, so this must also be high in the differential diagnosis. Traumatic injury to the knee, such as a meniscal injury or intra-articular fracture, are probably less likely given the mild nature of the injury and the inflammation of the joint.

An infectious arthritis is probably less likely, given the sudden onset and lack of systemic symptoms, but are must not miss hypotheses since they are potentially disastrous if left untreated. Gonococcal and nongonococcal septic arthritis are possibilities. Lyme disease can affect multiple joints but most commonly causes a monoarticular arthritis of the knee. Table 23–1 lists the differential diagnosis.

Mrs. K has never had a similar episode before. Her other medical problems include diabetes with diabetic nephropathy, hypertension, and hypercholesterolemia. Her medications are insulin, enalapril, atorvastatin, and hydrochlorothiazide. There is no history of alcohol or drug abuse.

> Is the clinical information sufficient to make a diagnosis? If not, what other information do you need?

## Leading Hypothesis: Gout

### Textbook Presentation

Gout classically presents in older patients with acute and severe pain of the great toe. The pain generally begins acutely and becomes unbearable within hours of onset. Patients often say that they are not even able to place a bed sheet over the toe. On physical exam, the first metatarsophalangeal (MTP) joint is warm, swollen, and red.

***Table 23–1.*** Diagnostic hypotheses for Mrs. K.

| Diagnostic Hypotheses | Clinical Clues | Important Tests |
|---|---|---|
| **Leading Hypothesis** | | |
| Gout | Previous episodes Rapid onset Involvement of first MTP joint | Classic presentation or demonstration of sodium urate crystals in synovial fluid |
| **Active Alternative** | | |
| CPPD (pseudogout) | May present as chronic or acute arthritis | Demonstration of crystals in synovial fluid or classic radiographic findings |
| **Active Alternative—Must Not Miss** | | |
| Bacterial arthritis (gonococcal or nongonococcal) | Fever with monoarticular or polyarticular arthritis | Positive synovial (or other body) fluid cultures |
| Lyme disease | Exposure to endemic area History of tick bite Rash | Clinical history Serologies Response to treatment |
| **Other Alternative** | | |
| Traumatic injury | Usually history of severe trauma | Appropriate imaging (radiograph for fracture, MRI for cartilaginous injury) |

### Disease Highlights

**A.** Gout is the most common crystal-induced arthropathy.

**B.** Gouty attacks occur when sodium urate crystallizes in synovial fluid inducing an inflammatory response and causing an abrupt, remarkably painful arthritis.

**C.** The primary risk factor for gout is hyperuricemia.

**D.** Location

    **1.** The classic location for gout is the first MTP joint (podagra).

    **2.** The joints of the lower extremities and the elbows are also common sites.

**E.** Gouty attacks often occur after abrupt changes in uric acid levels. Common causes are:

    **1.** Large protein meals

    **2.** Alcohol binges

    **3.** Initiation of thiazide or loop diuretics

    **4.** New renal failure

**F.** Gouty attacks can also be induced by trauma, hospitalization, or surgery.

**G.** The initial attack nearly always involves a single joint, while later attacks may be polyarticular.

**H.** Forms of gout

    **1.** Acute gouty arthritis is by far the most common type of gout.

    **2.** Chronic arthritis can develop in patients who have untreated hyperuricemia.

***Table 23–2.*** Characteristics of synovial fluid.

| Characteristic | Normal | RA or Similar OA | Acute Crystal or Arthritides | Septic Arthritis |
|---|---|---|---|---|
| Color and clarity | Yellow and clear | Yellow and clear | Yellow green and cloudy | Yellow green and opaque |
| Volume | 0–4 mL | 1–10 mL | 5–50 mL | 15–50 mL |
| WBC/mcL | < 500 | < 2000 | 1000–50,000 | 10,000–100,000 |
| %PMN | < 25 | < 50 | > 50 | > 75 |

OA, osteoarthritis; PMN, polymorphonuclear; RA, rheumatoid arthritis.

**3.** Tophaceous gout occurs when there is macroscopic deposition of sodium urate crystals in and around joints.

**4.** The kidney can also be affected by gout. Patients can develop sodium urate stones or a urate nephropathy.

**I.** Evaluation of a patient with gout

**1.** Patients with a new diagnosis of gout should be evaluated for alcoholism, renal insufficiency, myeloproliferative disorders, and hypertension.

**2.** Patients in whom gout first occurs in their teens and twenties should be evaluated for disorders of purine metabolism.

## Evidence-Based Diagnosis

**A.** Acute, inflammatory, monoarticular arthritis is an absolute indication for arthrocentesis.

**B.** Sampling synovial fluid will not only rule out potentially joint destroying septic arthritis but will also usually make a diagnosis.

 Every acute, inflammatory joint effusion should be tapped.

**C.** Arthrocentesis

**1.** Joint fluid is routinely sent for cell count, Gram stain, culture, and crystal analysis.

**2.** Normal joint fluid is small in volume and clear with a very low cell count.

**3.** Characteristics of abnormal synovial fluid are shown in Table 23–2. These numbers should be used as estimates.

**4.** Joint fluid obtained during an acute flare of a crystal arthritis will be highly inflammatory in nature.

**5.** The only setting in which it is reasonable not to tap a monoarticular effusion is when a septic joint is extremely unlikely and there is truly no diagnostic question. This may be the case

**a.** When a patient has recurrent inflammatory flares secondary to documented process (gout).

**b.** When the diagnosis is clear (podagra for gout or joint trauma in a patient with a bleeding diathesis for hemarthrosis).

**D.** Clinical diagnosis

**1.** Despite the crucial role of arthrocentesis in the diagnosis of acute monoarticular arthritis, the diagnosis of gout can occasionally be made with some certainty without joint aspiration.

**2.** The following clinical points make a diagnosis of gout probable:

**a.** More than 1 attack of acute arthritis

**b.** Maximal inflammation in < 1 day

**c.** Monoarthritis

**d.** Joint erythema

**e.** First MTP involvement

**f.** Unilateral MTP arthritis

**g.** Unilateral tarsal acute arthritis

**h.** Tophus

**i.** Asymmetric joint swelling

**j.** Hyperuricemia

**k.** Bone cysts without erosion on radiograph

**l.** Negative joint fluid culture

**3.** The test characteristics of a combination of these findings are provided in Table 23–3.

**4.** The presence of six findings highly consistent with gout rules in the diagnosis even without arthrocentesis.

**5.** Fever may accompany acute attacks.

**a.** Present in 44% of patients

**b.** 10% of patients have fevers > 39.0°C

**6.** Other findings that make gout more probable are

**a.** Hypertension

**b.** Use of thiazide or loop diuretics

**c.** Obesity

**d.** Alcohol use

***Table 23–3.*** Test characteristics of combined findings for the diagnosis of gout.

| Criteria | Sensitivity | Specificity | LR+ | LR– |
|---|---|---|---|---|
| 6 or more of the clinical points[1] | 87% | 96% | 22 | 0.13 |
| 5 or more of the clinical points[1] | 95% | 89% | 8.6 | 0.05 |
| Serum uric acid > 7 mg/dL | 90% | 54% | 1.9 | 0.19 |

[1]See text for list of clinical points.
Modified from Black ER. Diagnostic strategies for common medical problems. Philadelphia: American College of Physicians, 1999: p. 396.

**Table 23–4.** Immediate therapies for gout with potential adverse effects.

| Therapy | Potential Adverse Effects |
|---|---|
| Nonsteroidal anti inflammatory drugs | Nephrotoxicity<br>GI toxicity |
| Colchicine | GI toxicity (diarrhea) |
| Oral corticosteroids | GI toxicity<br>Hyperglycemia |
| Intra-articular corticosteroids | Complications of joint injection<br>Hyperglycemia |

### Treatment

A. Therapy for gout is classified as either abortive (to treat an acute flare) or prophylactic (to prevent flares and the destructive effects on the joints and kidneys).

B. Abortive therapy is outlined in Table 23–4.

   1. All of the therapies are effective, and the choice is usually made by the potential adverse effects.

   2. Most frequently, patients will be treated with a combination of a potent nonsteroidal anti-inflammatory drug (NSAID) and colchicine.

C. Prophylactic therapy

   1. There are 5 basic indications for prophylactic therapy:

      a. Frequent attacks

      b. Disabling attacks

      c. Urate nephrolithiasis

      d. Urate nephropathy

      e. Tophaceous gout

   2. Prophylactic therapy should begin with nonpharmacologic interventions to decrease uric acid levels and decrease the risk of gouty flares.

      a. Abstinence from alcohol use

      b. Weight loss

      c. Discontinuation of medications that impair urate excretion (eg, aspirin, thiazide diuretics).

   3. Potential prophylactic treatments are listed below.

      a. NSAIDs

      b. Colchicine

      c. Allopurinol

      d. Probenecid

      e. Sulfinpyrazone

      f. Febuxostat

   4. Colchicine should be used during the initiation of urate-lowering therapy to prevent recurrent gouty flares.

      a. NSAIDs may be added if necessary.

      b. Colchicine is usually continued for the first 6 months of urate-lowering therapy.

   5. Allopurinol is usually the first antihyperuricemic drug used, although it is relatively contraindicated in patients with renal or hepatic insufficiency.

   6. If allopurinol is ineffective, uric acid excretion should be measured. Patients with low uric acid excretion (present in 80% of patients with gout) should be given a uricosuric agent, such as probenecid.

## MAKING A DIAGNOSIS

The evaluation of this patient clearly requires joint aspiration. Septic arthritis is in the differential of any acutely inflamed joint. Although Mrs. K has only 4 criteria for gout (maximal inflammation in < 1 day, monoarthritis, joint erythema, and asymmetric joint swelling), gout remains likely, especially given the presence of hypertension and her use of a thiazide.

Radiographs of the knee demonstrate evidence of mild OA but no evidence of fracture. Joint fluid is aspirated from the patient's knee.

Have you crossed a diagnostic threshold for the leading hypothesis, gout? Have you ruled out the active alternatives? Do other tests need to be done to exclude the alternative diagnoses?

## Alternative Diagnosis: CPPD

### Textbook Presentation

CPPD generally presents in older patients. It may present with an acute flare (pseudogout) or, more commonly, as a degenerative arthritis with suspicious radiographic findings that distinguish it from OA. Patients often have other diseases associated with CPPD, such as hyperparathyroidism.

### Disease Highlights

A. CPPD is a crystal-induced arthropathy that can be clinically indistinguishable from gout, except for the presence of calcium pyrophosphate dihydrate crystals in the joint fluid.

B. Like gout, it is caused by the inflammatory response to crystals in the synovial space.

C. There are many other similarities between pseudogout and gout.

   1. Both cause acute painful monoarticular attacks.

   2. Both can cause polyarticular flares.

   3. Flares can be induced by trauma or illness.

   4. Both can potentially cause destructive arthropathy.

   5. Incidence increases with age.

D. There are some aspects of the disease quite distinct from gout.

   1. Episodic "gout-like" flares only occur in a small percentage of patients.

   2. CPPD commonly manifests as a degenerative arthritis (in about 50% of patients).

   3. It has highly specific radiologic features.

   4. It most commonly affects the knee.

Although CPPD is commonly thought of as pseudogout, it more commonly presents as a chronic degenerative arthritis.

E. Pseudogout has been associated with a number of diseases, the most common of which are:

1. Hyperparathyroidism

2. Hypocalciuric hypercalcemia

3. Hemochromatosis

4. Hypothyroidism

5. Gout

6. Hypomagnesemia

7. Hypophosphatasia

## Evidence-Based Diagnosis

A. Definite diagnosis of CPPD arthritis requires demonstration of the calcium pyrophosphate crystals in synovial fluid.

B. Certain radiographic findings are quite suggestive. The classic findings are punctate and linear calcific densities, most commonly seen in the cartilage of the knees, hip, pelvis, and wrist.

C. Proposed criteria offer findings that should alert the physician to the possibility of CPPD:

1. Acute arthritis of a large joint, especially the knees, in the absence of hyperuricemia.

2. Chronic arthritis with acute flares.

3. Chronic arthritis that involves joints that would be atypical for OA such as the wrists, metacarpophalangeal (MCP) joints, and shoulders.

D. Evaluation of a patient with pseudogout should include testing for related diseases. The evaluation generally includes measuring the levels of the following:

1. Calcium

2. Magnesium

3. Phosphorus

4. Alkaline phosphatase

5. Iron, ferritin, and total iron-binding capacity (TIBC)

6. TSH

7. Uric acid

## Treatment

A. Treat an associated underlying disease, when present.

B. Acute attacks can be managed with

1. NSAIDs

2. Joint aspiration with corticosteroid injection

3. Colchicine

C. Chronic degenerative arthritis is difficult to treat. NSAIDs are usually used.

## Alternative Diagnosis: Septic Arthritis

### Textbook Presentation

Septic arthritis usually presents as subacute joint pain, the knee being most common, associated with low-grade fever and progressive pain and disability. Because the infection usually begins with hematogenous spread, a risk factor for bacteremia (such as injection drug use) is sometimes present.

### Disease Highlights

A. Septic arthritis usually occurs via hematogenous spread of bacteria.

B. Joint distribution

1. The knee is the most commonly affected joint.

2. Monoarticular arthritis is the rule, with multiple joints involved in < 15% of patients.

3. Infection is most common in previously abnormal joints, such as those affected by OA or RA.

C. *Staphylococcus aureus* is the most common organism followed by species of streptococcus.

### Evidence-Based Diagnosis

A. Clinical findings

1. Fever is common, present in most patients.

   a. A recent meta-analysis found that 57% of patients with septic arthritis had fever.

   b. Recognize that this means that over 40% of patients with septic arthritis are afebrile.

   c. Fever > 39.0°C is rare.

2. Findings predictive of a septic arthritis causing joint pain are recent joint surgery (LR+ 6.9) and the presence of a prosthetic knee or hip in the presence of a skin infection (LR+ 15.0).

 Fever cannot distinguish septic arthritis from other forms of monoarticular arthritis. Patients with gout may be febrile while those with septic joints may not.

B. Laboratory findings

1. WBC > 10,000/mcL is seen in only 50% of patients.

2. Definitive diagnosis is made by Gram stain and culture.

   a. Gram stain of synovial fluid is positive in about 75% of patients with septic arthritis.

   b. The yield is highest with *S aureus*.

3. Elevated synovial fluid WBC count can be predictive in making the diagnosis.

   a. Synovial fluid WBC count > 100,000/mcL: LR+ 28, LR+ 0.71.

   b. Lower WBC cut offs are not predictive.

4. Joint fluid culture is positive in about 90% of cases.

5. Blood (and sputum, when appropriate) should also be cultured as this may help identify an organism if one is not isolated from the synovium. About 50% of patients will have positive blood cultures.

 Because of the potential for septic arthritis to cause joint destruction, a single, acutely inflamed joint should be assumed infected until proved otherwise.

### Treatment

A. Antibiotic therapy is directed by Gram stain findings.

B. Empiric therapy should cover *S aureus*.

C. The affected joint should also be drained, either with a needle, arthroscope, or arthrotomy (opening the joint in the operating room).

1. Small joints can usually be drained and lavaged with serial arthrocentesis.
2. Large joints usually require surgical drainage.
3. The knee is an exception, a large joint that, in many cases can be treated with serial arthrocentesis.

E. Patients who receive treatment within 5 days of symptom onset have the best prognosis.

## Alternative Diagnosis: Disseminated Gonorrhea

### Textbook Presentation

Disseminated gonorrhea is classically seen in young, sexually active women who have fever and joint pain. The most common presentation is severe pain of the wrists, hands, and knees with warmth and erythema diffusely over the backs of the hands. A rash may sometimes be present.

### Disease Highlights

A. Disseminated gonorrhea is a disease with rheumatologic manifestations that is seen in young, sexually active persons.

B. Women are 3 times more likely to have the disease than men.

 Disseminated gonorrhea usually occurs in patients without a history of a recent sexually transmitted disease.

C. Disseminated gonorrhea seems to present in 1 of 2 ways (with a good deal of overlap): a classic septic arthritis or a triad of tenosynovitis, dermatitis, and arthralgia.

1. The triad presentation seems to reflect a high-grade bacteremia with reactive features.
2. The tenosynovitis presents predominantly as a polyarthralgia of the hands and wrists.
3. The rash is a scattered, papular, or vesicular rash.
4. The more classic, monoarticular septic joint presentation occurs in about 40% of patients.
5. Table 23–5 gives the frequency of various findings in these 2 types of presentation.

**Table 23–5.** Physical signs and culture results in patients with disseminated gonorrhea.

| Characteristic | Septic Arthritis | Triad |
|---|---|---|
| % Female | 63% | 77% |
| Tenosynovitis | 21% | 87% |
| Fever | 32% | 50% |
| Skin lesions | 42% | 90% |
| Positive blood cultures | 0% | 43% |
| "Tapable" joint effusion[1] | 100% | 0% |

[1]Note that this is how the groups were distinguished.
Modified from O'Brien JP, Goldenberg DL, Rice PA. Disseminated gonococcal infection: a prospective analysis of 49 patients and a review of pathophysiology and immune mechanisms. *Medicine (Baltimore)*. 1983;62:395–406.

### Evidence-Based Diagnosis

A. Diagnosis is based on isolating the organism.

B. Besides synovial fluid cultures, blood, pharyngeal, and genital cultures should also be sent.

C. If all cultures are negative, the disease can still be diagnosed if there is a high clinical suspicion and a rapid response to appropriate antibiotics.

 Negative cultures do not necessarily exclude the diagnosis of disseminated gonorrhea.

### Treatment

A. Ceftriaxone 1 g IV or IM every 24 hours or cefotaxime 1 g IV every 8 hour.

B. IV therapy is generally recommended for 24–48 hours after improvement.

## Alternative Diagnosis: Lyme Disease

### Textbook Presentation

Lyme disease presents in different ways at different stages of the disease. A classic presentation of the joint symptoms is a patient with acute, inflammatory knee pain who has been in an area where the disease is endemic. There may be a history of a previous tick bite, rash, or nonspecific febrile illness.

### Disease Highlights

A. Lyme disease is caused by the spirochete *Borrelia burgdorferi*, transmitted by a number of species of *Ixodes* ticks.

B. The tick most commonly transmits the disease during its nymphal stage.

C. The disease is endemic in certain places.

1. In the United States: along the northern Atlantic Coast; in Wisconsin and Minnesota; in California and Oregon
2. In Europe: Germany; Austria; Slovenia; Sweden

D. The clinical picture differs somewhat between that in the United States and that in Europe and Asia. The presentation in the United States is discussed below.

E. Peak incidence is in June and July, with disease occurring from March through October.

F. The disease is generally divided into 3 stages.

1. Early localized disease
   a. Skin findings are most common, usually a large area of localized erythema.
      (1) 80% of patients have an acute rash.
      (2) 50% of the rashes occur below the waist.
      (3) The mean diameter of the rash is 10 cm.
      (4) About 60% of the rashes are an area of homogeneous erythema.
      (5) About 30% of rashes are the more classic target lesion.
      (6) About 10% of the patients have multiple lesions.

 Only about 30% of patients with Lyme disease have the classic target rash on presentation.

**b.** Other symptoms include

    **(1)** Myalgias and arthralgias (59%)

    **(2)** Fever (31%)

    **(3)** Headache (28%)

**2.** Early disseminated disease can involve the heart and the CNS.

  **a.** Atrioventricular (AV) node block is the most common cardiac manifestation.

  **b.** Headache is the most common CNS finding, while meningitis and cranial nerve palsies (especially CN7) also occur.

**3.** Joint symptoms predominate late in the disease.

  **a.** Occurs in about 60% of patients months after infection.

  **b.** Monoarticular knee arthritis is the most common.

  **c.** Intermittent attacks or an oligoarticular arthritis may also occur.

  **d.** Arthritis can become chronic, even in treated patients, in about 10% of cases.

### Evidence-Based Diagnosis

**A.** Definitive diagnosis of Lyme disease is based on clinical characteristics, exposure history, and antibody titers.

**B.** Antibodies may be negative early in the disease and are thus not helpful in the setting of acute infection.

**C.** Antibodies are nearly 100% sensitive in the setting of arthritis.

### Treatment

**A.** There are multiple antibiotic regimens effective in the treatment of localized and disseminated Lyme disease.

**B.** Prophylactic treatment with a single dose of doxycycline given after a tick bite is effective at preventing Lyme disease but is generally not recommended given the low likelihood of being infected with Lyme disease after a tick bite, even in endemic areas.

**C.** Treatment of arthritis caused by Lyme disease is either 4 weeks of oral antibiotics or 2–4 weeks of intravenous antibiotics.

**D.** Chronic and debilitating symptoms from Lyme disease rarely develop after appropriate treatment and, when they do occur, the etiology of these symptoms is not clear.

## CASE RESOLUTION

Mrs. K's synovial fluid aspiration yielded 25 mL of translucent, yellow fluid. The WBC was about 55,000/mcL with 56% PMNs. The Gram stain was negative, and crystal exam with polarized light microscopy demonstrates negatively birefringent crystals consistent with monosodium urate crystals, thus making the diagnosis of gout.

The inflammatory joint fluid could have been predicted by the exam. Acute gout is commonly associated with very inflamed joints, often with very high WBC counts. The positive crystal exam makes the diagnosis of gout.

The patient was treated with NSAIDs and colchicine with a good response. Because this was Mrs. K's first attack, prophylactic therapy was not instituted.

---

## CHIEF COMPLAINT

PATIENT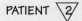

Mrs. C is a 50-year-old woman who comes to your office complaining of joint pain. She reports the pain has been present for about 2 years. The pain affects her hands and her wrists. She describes the pain as "a dull aching" and "a stiffness." It is worst in the morning and improves over 2 to 3 hours. She says that on particularly bad days she uses NSAIDs with moderate relief.

At this point, what is the leading hypothesis, what are the active alternatives, and is there a must not miss diagnosis? Given this differential diagnosis, what tests should be ordered?

## PRIORITIZING THE DIFFERENTIAL DIAGNOSIS

Although morning stiffness is common with most types of arthritis, Mrs. C's prolonged symptoms are suggestive of an inflammatory arthritis. She does not seem to have other systemic symptoms, and she has no history of a recent infection. Considering these pivotal features in this case, those of a polyarticular, inflammatory arthritis, the differential diagnosis is broad.

RA has to lead the differential diagnosis for a middle-aged woman with a symmetric, inflammatory arthritis. The chronicity, age at onset, and joint distribution all support this diagnosis. Psoriatic arthritis can be indistinguishable from RA, especially early in its course, and needs to be considered. SLE can also present as a chronic, inflammatory arthritis. The patient is older than the average age of onset for SLE, and we have not heard about other organ system involvement.

Degenerative arthropathies, such as OA and CPPD, should be considered, but the joint distribution and inflammatory nature of the arthritis makes these less likely. Table 23–6 lists the differential diagnosis.

Mrs. C is otherwise well, except for a history of mild hypertension managed with an angiotensin-receptor blocker. She reports no other joint pains. She does not have a history of psoriasis.

Her vitals signs are temperature, 37.1°C; BP, 128/84 mm Hg; pulse, 84 bpm; RR, 14 breaths per minute. Her

(continued)

***Table 23–6.*** Diagnostic hypotheses for Mrs. C.

| Diagnostic Hypotheses | Clinical Clues | Important Tests |
|---|---|---|
| **Leading Hypothesis** | | |
| Rheumatoid arthritis | Morning stiffness Symmetric polyarthritis Commonly involves the MCP joints | Clinical diagnosis Rheumatoid factor |
| **Active Alternative** | | |
| Psoriatic arthritis | Psoriasis Dactylitis Spinal arthritis Often asymmetric Often involves the DIP joints | Clinical diagnosis |
| Systemic lupus erythematosus | Multisystem disease Most common in young, African American women | Clinical diagnosis aided by serologies and diagnostic criteria |
| **Other Alternative** | | |
| Osteoarthritis | Chronic arthritis in weight-bearing joints In the hands, DIP and PIP involvement more common than MCP involvement | Radiograph of affected joints |

general physical exam is essentially normal. There is a 2/6 systolic ejection murmur. Joint exam reveals limited range of motion of the MCPs and wrists bilaterally. There is swelling of the third and fourth MCP on the right and the third on the left. There is pain at the extremes of motion and a boggy quality to the joints. A detailed skin exam is normal. The patient is wearing nail polish on the day of the visit.

 **Is the clinical information sufficient to make a diagnosis? If not, what other information do you need?**

## Leading Hypothesis: RA

### Textbook Presentation

RA is most commonly seen in middle-aged patients with a symmetric polyarthritis manifesting itself with painful, stiff, and swollen hands. Morning stiffness is often a predominant symptom. Swollen and tender wrists, MCP, and proximal interphalangeal (PIP) joints are usually seen on exam. Laboratory evaluation may reveal an anemia of chronic inflammation and a positive rheumatoid factor (RF) and positive anti-cyclic citrullinated peptide (anti-CCP).

### Disease Highlights

**A.** RA is the paradigm for idiopathic inflammatory arthritides.

**B.** The sine qua non of RA is the presence of an inflammatory synovitis, most commonly involving the hands. This synovitis eventually forms a destructive pannus that injures articular and periarticular tissue.

**C.** RA is fairly common, present in about 1% of the population, so the diagnosis should be considered in any adult patient presenting with joint symptoms and true findings of arthritis on exam.

 RA should be considered in any adult with a chronic, symmetric polyarthritis.

**D.** Common findings in RA, all included in The American College of Rheumatology (ACR) diagnostic criteria for RA are:

  **1.** Symmetric arthritis of the hands

  **2.** Presence of serum RF

  **3.** Presence of radiographic changes typical of RA on hand and wrist radiographs.

**E.** Morning stiffness is a classic finding.

  **1.** Although many people are stiff upon awakening, those with inflammatory arthritis can experience stiffness for an hour or more.

  **2.** Morning stiffness improves with therapy.

 Prolonged morning stiffness is a good clue to an inflammatory arthritis.

**F.** The joints most commonly involved are

  **1.** Hand

    **a.** Wrists, MCP, and PIP joints are most commonly affected.

    **b.** Distal interphalangeal (DIP) joints are often spared.

    **c.** Ulnar deviation of the MCPs as well as swan neck and boutonnière deformities are classic findings.

  **2.** Elbow

  **3.** Knee

  **4.** Ankle

  **5.** Cervical spine

    **a.** Usually presents as neck pain and stiffness.

    **b.** C1–C2 instability can occur secondary to associated tenosynovitis.

      **(1)** This can produce cervical myelopathy.

      **(2)** Advisable to radiographically image the cervical spines of patients with RA prior to elective endotracheal intubation.

**G.** Once RA is established, joint destruction begins to occur and can be seen on radiographs. The chronic synovitis causes erosions of bone and cartilage.

**H.** Long-standing RA can cause severe joint deformity through destruction of the joint and injury to the periarticular structures.

**I.** Nonarticular findings in RA

  **1.** Rheumatoid nodules, when present, are usually over extensor surfaces.

**2.** Dry eyes are common.

**3.** Pulmonary disease (eg, pulmonary nodules or interstitial lung disease) is more common in RA than in most other rheumatologic diseases.

**4.** Pericardial disease

   **a.** Asymptomatic pericardial effusion is most common.

   **b.** Restrictive pericarditis can occur.

**5.** Anemia

   **a.** RA is the textbook cause of anemia of inflammation.

   **b.** See Chapter 6, Anemia for a more complete discussion.

## Evidence-Based Diagnosis

**A.** The diagnosis of RA can be difficult because it may resemble other causes of inflammatory arthritis around the time of onset.

**B.** Serologies

**1.** RF is a nonspecific test.

   **a.** It is occasionally positive in healthy people and in a number of inflammatory states such as infections, sarcoidosis, and periodontal disease.

   **b.** The test characteristics of RF vary in different studies but a recent meta-analysis found the following: sensitivity, 69%; specificity, 85%; LR+, 4.86; LR– 0.38.

**2.** Anti-CCP is a newer test that is more predictive of RA than RF. The same meta-analysis found the following: sensitivity, 62%; specificity, 95%; LR+, 12.46; LR– 0.36.

A positive anti-CCP is very predictive of a diagnosis of RA.

**3.** In practice, RF and anti-CCP are used together. In the right clinical situation, patients with both tests positive are at high risk for RA.

**C.** The ACR has developed diagnostic criteria for RA.

**1.** A patient must have 4 of the following to make a diagnosis. If present, any 1 of the first 4 must have been present for at least 6 weeks.

   **a.** Morning stiffness (lasting at least 1 hour before maximal improvement)

   **b.** Simultaneous arthritis of more than 2 joint areas

   **c.** Arthritis of hand joints

   **d.** Symmetric arthritis

   **e.** Rheumatoid nodules

   **f.** Serum RF

   **g.** Typical radiographic changes on hand and wrists

**2.** Although meant to standardize research and not to be used as diagnostic criteria, they are helpful in highlighting the clinical characteristics of RA.

**D.** The ACR criteria can be used to help guide diagnosis.

**1.** The test characteristics for the criteria are shown in the first 2 lines of Table 23–7. They demonstrate that the criteria are only moderately helpful in making a diagnosis.

**2.** As demonstrated in the bottom 4 rows of the table, the criteria can be helpful at the extremes.

**3.** The most specific individual criteria are rheumatoid nodules (LR+ > 30) and consistent radiographic changes (LR+ 11).

## Treatment

**A.** The treatment for RA has changed rapidly in recent years and is now really the purview of the rheumatologist.

**B.** The treatments are often divided into those that treat the symptoms of the disease and those that modify the course of the disease.

**C.** The drugs used to treat the symptoms of the disease are:

**1.** NSAIDs

   **a.** Generally used early in the course of the disease for symptom relief while a diagnosis is being made.

   **b.** Rarely, patients with very mild disease can remain on these medications alone.

**2.** Corticosteroids

   **a.** Generally provide excellent symptom control

   **b.** Their effect on slowing joint destruction from RA is very controversial.

**D.** Disease-modifying antirheumatic drugs (DMARDs) include sulfasalazine, hydroxychloroquine, methotrexate, leflunomide, etanercept, and infliximab.

**1.** Methotrexate is the most commonly used drug in this class.

**2.** Patients with more severe disease also commonly receive the TNF-α inhibitors etanercept or infliximab or leflunomide, a drug that impairs T-cell function.

**Table 23–7.** Test characteristics for the ACR criteria for the diagnosis of RA.

| No. of Criteria | Time Frame | Sensitivity | Specificity | LR+ | LR– |
|---|---|---|---|---|---|
| ≥ 4 (ACR criteria) | Within 1 year of symptoms | 66% | 82% | 3.67 | 0.41 |
| ≥ 4 (ACR criteria) | After 2 years of follow-up | 91% | 75% | 3.64 | 0.12 |
| 0–1 | Within 1 year | 91% | 50% | 1.82 | 0.18 |
| 0–1 | After 2 years | 98% | 42% | 1.69 | 0.05 |
| 6–7 | Within 1 year | 9% | 100% | ∞ | 0.91 |
| 6–7 | After 2 years | 37% | 100% | ∞ | 0.63 |

ACR, American College of Rheumatology; RA, rheumatoid arthritis.

**3.** New therapies include rituximab, which depletes B-lymphocytes, and abatacept, which blocks costimulation of T-lymphocytes.

## MAKING A DIAGNOSIS

The presentation of Mrs. C's symptoms is typical for RA. She already fulfills 4 of the ACR criteria for RA. Further evaluation should be directed toward gathering other information that might suggest RA and make other diagnoses less likely.

A CBC with iron studies, RF, anti-CCP, and antinuclear antibodies (ANA) are done. Radiographs are ordered with fine details of the hands.

Have you crossed a diagnostic threshold for the leading hypothesis, RA? Have you ruled out the active alternatives? Do other tests need to be done to exclude the alternative diagnoses?

## Alternative Diagnosis: Psoriatic Arthritis

### Textbook Presentation

Psoriatic arthritis most commonly presents as joint pain in middle-aged patients with a history of psoriasis. There are signs and symptoms of an inflammatory arthritis often involving the wrists, MCP, PIP, and DIP joints symmetrically. Exam of the skin reveals psoriasis and psoriatic nail changes.

### Disease Highlights

**A.** Psoriasis is a very common skin disease that can be complicated by arthritis.

**B.** Psoriatic arthritis is one of the seronegative spondyloarthropathies.

   **1.** The ACR defines the seronegative spondyloarthropathies as diseases characterized by inflammatory axial spine involvement, asymmetric peripheral arthritis, enthesopathy, and inflammatory eye diseases.

   **2.** Patients with these diseases classically have a negative ANA and RF, giving the group the "seronegative" moniker.

   **3.** Other seronegative spondyloarthropathies are ankylosing spondylitis, reactive arthritis, and the arthritis associated with inflammatory bowel disease.

**C.** The distribution of the arthritis in psoriatic arthritis is quite variable but follows 3 general presentations:

   **1.** Oligoarthritis often involving large joints and the hands. Dactylitis, a swelling of the entire finger causing a "sausage digit" secondary to both arthritis and tenosynovitis, is a classic finding.

   **2.** A polyarthritis similar to RA

   **3.** A spinal arthritis

**D.** Psoriatic arthritis can be indistinguishable from RA, especially early in the course of both diseases.

   **1.** Radiographs of the hands can show erosions.

**2.** About 10% of patients with psoriatic arthritis have a positive RF.

**E.** Distinguishing features include:

   **1.** Common involvement of DIP joints

   **2.** Spine involvement that is uncommon in RA

   **3.** Arthritis mutilans, a syndrome in which there is marked boney destruction around joints causing "telescoping digits."

### Evidence-Based Diagnosis

**A.** The most diagnostic feature of psoriatic arthritis is the presence of psoriasis.

   **1.** Psoriasis precedes the development of arthritis in about 70% of cases.

   **2.** Arthritis and psoriasis begin contemporaneously in about 15% of patients.

   **3.** In about 15% of patients, there is no psoriasis at the onset of disease, although there maybe a family history of the skin disease.

**B.** A very careful skin exam should be done in all patients in whom the diagnosis is suspected.

**C.** Nail findings

   **1.** Psoriasis can cause recognizable changes in the nails (eg, pitting, an oil stained appearance).

   **2.** Nail changes occur in only about 20% of people with psoriasis but in about 80% of people with psoriasis and arthritis.

   **3.** Nail changes are especially common in people with DIP arthritis.

 A detailed skin and nail exam is important when considering the diagnosis of psoriatic arthritis. Nail polish should be removed for the visit.

### Treatment

The treatment of psoriatic arthritis is similar to the treatment of RA.

## Alternative Diagnosis: SLE

### Textbook Presentation

SLE would classically present in a young woman with fatigue and arthritis, commonly of the hands. There are often suspicious findings in the history such as an episode of pleuritis or undiagnosed anemia.

### Disease Highlights

**A.** SLE is a truly systemic autoimmune disease primarily affecting women of childbearing age.

**B.** Various groups are more prone to disease.

   **1.** Female:male ratio is about 9:1.

   **2.** There is a genetic component with about 5% of patients reporting a first-degree relative with the disease.

   **3.** Women of color are most commonly affected.

**C.** Almost every organ can be involved, although the joints, skin, serosa, and kidneys are most commonly affected.

**Table 23–8.** Clinical manifestations of SLE at onset and during disease.

| Signs and Symptoms | Prevalence at Onset | Prevalence at any Time |
|---|---|---|
| Arthralgia | 77% | 85% |
| Rashes | 53% | 78% |
| Constitutional | 53% | 77% |
| Renal involvement | 38% | 74% |
| Arthritis | 44% | 63% |
| Raynaud phenomenon | 33% | 60% |
| CNS involvement (most commonly headache) | 24% | 54% |
| GI (most commonly abdominal pain) | 18% | 45% |
| Lymphadenopathy | 16% | 32% |
| Pleurisy | 16% | 30% |
| Pericarditis | 13% | 23% |

SLE, systemic lupus erythematosus.

**Table 23–9.** Test characteristics for the ACR criteria (4 or more criteria) and individual criteria in the diagnosis of SLE.

| Finding | Sensitivity | Specificity | LR+ | LR− |
|---|---|---|---|---|
| ACR criteria | 80% | 98% | 40 | 0.2 |
| Malar rash | 57% | 96% | 14 | 0.45 |
| Discoid rash | 18% | 99% | 18 | 0.83 |
| Photosensitivity | 43% | 96% | 11 | 0.59 |
| Oral ulcers | 27% | 96% | 6.8 | 0.76 |
| Arthritis | 86% | 37% | 1.4 | 0.38 |
| Serositis | 56% | 86% | 4.0 | 0.51 |
| Renal disorder | 51% | 94% | 8.5 | 0.52 |
| Hematologic disorder | 20% | 98% | 10 | 0.80 |
| Neurologic disorder | 59% | 89% | 5.4 | 0.46 |

ACR, American College of Rheumatology; SLE, systemic lupus erythematosus. Adapted from Black ER. *Diagnostic strategies for common medical problems.* Philadelphia: American College of Physicians, 1999:421.

**D.** The pathogenesis of the disease is related to the formation of autoantibodies to a number of nuclear antigens. The ANA is the most common.

**E.** The most common features of SLE, both at presentation and later in follow-up, are listed in Table 23–8.

### Evidence-Based Diagnosis

**A.** The diagnosis of SLE, especially in people with mild disease, can be difficult.

**B.** The ACR has developed criteria to standardize the diagnosis for research purposes.

   **1.** The criteria are:

      **a.** Malar rash

      **b.** Discoid rash

      **c.** Photosensitivity

      **d.** Oral ulcers

      **e.** Arthritis (nonerosive arthritis)

      **f.** Serositis (pleuritis or pericarditis)

      **g.** Renal disorder (proteinuria or cellular casts)

      **h.** Neurologic disorder (headache, seizures, or psychosis without other cause)

      **i.** Hematologic disorder (hemolytic anemia or any cytopenia)

      **j.** Immunologic disorder (anti-DNA, anti-SM, or antiphospholipid antibodies)

      **k.** ANA

   **2.** The diagnosis of SLE requires the presence of 4 or more of these criteria.

   **3.** Although the same reservations about using diagnostic criteria clinically that were discussed above in the section of RA apply here, the SLE criteria are frequently used.

   **4.** The test characteristics of these criteria are given in Table 23–9. Also included in this table are the test characteristics for the various individual criteria.

   **5.** The presence of a malar rash or satisfaction of the ACR criteria are highly supportive of the diagnosis of SLE.

**C.** Autoantibodies

   **1.** Measuring autoantibodies is very important in SLE because they provide important diagnostic information.

   **2.** ANA and anti-DsDNA

      **a.** ANA is the most sensitive test for SLE. It is very nonspecific.

      **b.** Anti-DsDNA is highly specific. It is also associated with the presence of lupus nephritis.

      **c.** ANA does not vary with disease activity while anti-DsDNA does.

      **d.** The test characteristics of ANA and Anti-DsDNA are given in Table 23–10.

 A negative ANA essentially rules out SLE. A positive anti-DsDNA essentially rules in SLE.

      **e.** Staining patterns are often reported with the ANA.

         **(1)** These patterns correlate, to some extent, with the other specific antibodies discussed below and their use has, to a great extent, been supplanted by these tests.

**Table 23–10.** Test characteristics for ANA and DsDNA in the diagnosis of SLE.

| Test | Sensitivity | Specificity | LR+ | LR− |
|------|-------------|-------------|-----|-----|
| ANA | 99% | 80% | 4.95 | 0.01 |
| DsDNA | 73% | 98% | 36.5 | 0.28 |

ANA, antinuclear antibodies; SLE, systemic lupus erythematosus.
Adapted from Black ER. *Diagnostic strategies for common medical problems.* Philadelphia: American College of Physicians, 1999:423.

(2) In general, the meaning of the staining patterns are as follows:

(a) Homogeneous: Seen in SLE, RA, and drug-induced lupus

(b) Peripheral: Most specific pattern for SLE

(c) Speckled: Least specific pattern. Commonly seen with low titer ANAs in people without rheumatic disease

(d) Nucleolar: Common in patients with scleroderma and Raynaud phenomenon.

3. Other serologies are helpful because they tend to be associated with various subsets of disease.

a. Anti-RNP: Associated with Raynaud phenomenon and myositis

b. Anti-SSA/Ro and anti-SSB/La: Associated with Sjögren syndrome and photosensitivity

c. Anti-RNP: Associated with CNS manifestations of SLE

4. Table 23–11 outlines a variety of serologies that may be obtained in persons in whom rheumatologic disease is suspected.

D. Complement

1. Complement levels are helpful in tracking the activity of SLE.

2. C3, C4, and CH50 levels tend to decline during episodes of lupus activity.

**Treatment**

A. Similar to RA, the treatment of SLE is complicated and to a great extent the purview of the rheumatologist.

B. In general, NSAIDs, corticosteroids, and immunosuppressants are the mainstay of therapy.

C. NSAIDs are generally used for symptomatic relief of inflammatory symptoms with careful monitoring because of their potential nephrotoxic effects.

D. Corticosteroids and hydroxychloroquine are commonly used in long-term therapy and high-dose corticosteroids are used for disease exacerbations.

E. Cyclophosphamide, mycophenolate mofetil, and azathioprine are the most commonly used immunosuppressants in SLE. They are used most widely for the treatment of lupus nephritis.

**Table 23–11.** Common serologies in rheumatologic diseases.

| Antibody | Clinical Association |
|----------|---------------------|
| Anti-DsDNA | Nephritis in SLE |
| Anti–Smith | SLE |
| Anti-RNP | Raynaud phenomenon and myositis in SLE |
| Anti Ribosomal P | CNS disease in SLE |
| Anti SSA/Ro, Anti SSB/La | Sjögren syndrome and skin disease in SLE and Sjögren syndrome |
| Anti-histone antibodies | Drug-induced lupus |
| Anti-jo-1 | Polymyositis/dermatomyositis |
| Anti-DNA topoisomerase I (Scl-70), anti-RNA polymerase I and III | Systemic sclerosis (scleroderma) |
| ANCA | Many vasculitic diseases including Wegener granulomatosis, microscopic polyangiitis, and Churg-Strauss syndrome |
| Anti-U1 RNP antibodies | Mixed connective tissue disease |
| Anti-GBM | Anti-GBM antibody (Goodpasture disease) |

## CASE RESOLUTION

Mrs. C's laboratory and radiology test results are as follows: Hgb, 10.5 g/dL; Hct, 31.0%; serum ferritin, 95 ng/mL (nl > 45 ng/mL); serum iron, 36 mcg/dL (nl 40–160 mcg/dL); TIBC, 200 mcg/dL (nl 230–430); RF, 253 international units/mL (nl < 10 international units/mL); anti-CCP 1000 units/mL (nl < 100 units/mL) ANA, 2560 titer (nl < 80); anti- DsDNA, < 10 titer (nl < 10); radiographs of hand, periarticular erosions of the 3 clinically involved MCP joints.

The diagnosis of RA is now fairly certain. The clinical picture, as well as the laboratory test showing an anemia of chronic inflammation, elevated RF and anti-CCP, and positive ANA all support the diagnosis. (About 40% of patients with RA have positive ANAs.) The first step in management is to control Mrs. C's symptoms. NSAIDs and prednisone are likely to accomplish this. There are already signs of joint destruction on the radiographs, so aggressive therapy with disease-modifying drugs is indicated.

# CHIEF COMPLAINT

PATIENT

Ms. T is a 21-year-old woman who comes to see you complaining of rash and joint pain for the past 2 days. She reports being well until 2 days ago when she awoke with severe pain in both knees and mild pain in both wrists. No other joints were involved. She also noted a nonpruritic rash on her distal arms and legs. She describes the rash as "splotchy." The joint pain has worsened over the last 2 days, and she reports that both her knees are swollen.

 At this point, what is the leading hypothesis, what are the active alternatives, and is there a must not miss diagnosis? Given this differential diagnosis, what tests should be ordered?

## PRIORITIZING THE DIFFERENTIAL DIAGNOSIS

Ms. T has acute onset polyarticular joint symptoms. From her history of knee swelling, it is likely that she has arthritis rather than arthralgias. The pivotal points of acute onset and polyarticular involvement combined with the patient's demographics and associated symptoms help narrow the differential diagnosis.

In a young woman with arthritis and a rash, SLE needs to be considered. As discussed above, rash, arthralgias, and arthritis are among the most common presenting symptoms in patients with SLE. The acuity of the onset and lack of other organ system involvement would be a little unusual for patients with SLE. RA would be less likely given the patient's age; however, Still disease, a variant of RA, may present acutely in young patients.

Various infectious arthritides need to be considered. Many viral illnesses can cause arthritis. Parvovirus is probably the most common. Bacterial illnesses can cause polyarthritis in many different ways. Septic arthritides, discussed above, can be polyarticular as can disseminated gonorrhea. Bacterial endocarditis can cause aseptic polyarthritis and often causes arthralgia of multiple joints. Acute rheumatic fever classically causes a migratory polyarthritis and rash. Lyme disease, discussed above, is most commonly monoarticular. Reactive arthritis, occurring after enteric or urogenital infections, is also a possibility.

Given that the viral arthritides are more common than bacterial ones and, as far as we know, the patient has been previously well, viral arthritis is probably more likely than bacterial disease. Table 23–12 lists the differential diagnosis.

On further history, Ms. T reports that 10 days before she came to see you she experienced 2 days of fatigue, myalgias, and fever to 39.4°C. There were no other symptoms. These symptoms resolved uneventfully.

She reports no travel outside Chicago, where she is in school, for the last year. She does not use recreational drugs. She is not sexually active.

On physical exam, she appears healthy. Her vital signs are temperature, 36.9°C; BP, 106/68 mm Hg; pulse, 84 bpm; RR, 14 breaths per minute. On extremity exam,

**Table 23–12.** Diagnostic hypotheses for Ms. T.

| Diagnostic Hypotheses | Clinical Clues | Important Tests |
|---|---|---|
| **Leading Hypothesis** | | |
| Systemic lupus erythematosus | Multisystem disease Most common in young, African American women | Clinical diagnosis aided by serologies and diagnostic criteria |
| **Active Alternative** | | |
| Viral arthritis, parvovirus most common | Usually a history of preceding illness | Antibody titers and serology |
| **Active Alternative—Must Not Miss** | | |
| Rheumatic fever | Migratory polyarthritis Carditis Erythema marginatum | Jones criteria |
| Bacterial arthritis (gonococcal or nongonococcal) | Fever with monoarticular or polyarticular arthritis | Positive synovial (or other body) fluid cultures |
| **Other Alternative** | | |
| Reactive arthritis | History of recent colonic or urogenital infection Presence of arthritis, urethritis, and iritis | Clinical diagnosis |

her wrists have normal range of motion. There is pain with extremes of flexion and extension in the wrists and MCPs. There is mildly decreased range of motion and warmth in the knees as well as small effusions.

Skin exam reveals a diffuse erythematous rash with macules on the hands, feet, and distal extremities. Palms and soles are spared. The remainder of the exam was normal. There is no heart murmur.

The patient's history forces us to reorder our differential. The history of a recent febrile illness has to make a viral arthritis or postinfectious arthritis most likely. Lyme disease and bacterial endocarditis are very unlikely given her lack of suspicious exposure and the fact that she is presently well. SLE remains on the differential but is less likely.

 In a patient with acute polyarthritis, a detailed history of recent illnesses must be taken.

 Is the clinical information sufficient to make a diagnosis? If not, what other information do you need?

## Leading Hypothesis: Parvovirus

### Textbook Presentation

Parvovirus is commonly seen in young people who are in contact with children (mothers, teachers, daycare workers, and pediatricians). Parvovirus often presents 10 days after a flu-like illness with a macular rash and moderately severe arthralgias of the joints of the upper extremities. There is no fever and symptoms improve over the course of weeks.

### Disease Highlights

**A.** There are 5 major manifestations of the parvovirus infection in humans.

  **1.** Erythema infectiosum (fifth disease) in children

  **2.** Acute arthropathy in adults

  **3.** Transient aplastic crises in patients with chronic hemolytic diseases

  **4.** Chronic anemia in immunocompromised persons

  **5.** Fetal death complicating maternal infection prior to 20 weeks gestation.

**B.** In adults, the acute disease often proceeds in 2 phases with the arthritis following a systemic febrile infection.

  **1.** Initial phase

    **a.** Nonspecific symptoms such as fever, malaise, headache, myalgia, diarrhea, and pruritus

    **b.** Generally resembles a nonspecific viral infection

  **2.** Second phase

    **a.** Follows initial phase by 10 days with joint symptoms and rash dominating the clinical picture.

    **b.** Arthropathy accompanies about 50% of adult infections.

    **c.** The arthritis is a symmetric polyarthritis commonly involving the following joints:

      **(1)** Elbows

      **(2)** Wrists

      **(3)** Hands

      **(4)** Knees

      **(5)** Ankles

      **(6)** Feet

    **d.** The rash lasts 2–3 days.

      **(1)** It is usually a peripheral macular rash that occasionally spreads to the trunk.

      **(2)** Many different rashes have been described.

**C.** The incidence of parvovirus infection peaks between January and June.

**D.** Attack rates of 50–60%.

**E.** Contact with children is common among patients.

**F.** Other viruses cause arthritis less commonly. These are listed in Table 23–13.

### Evidence-Based Diagnosis

**A.** The diagnosis of parvovirus can be difficult because it can mimic other diseases.

**B.** Distinguishing the disease from SLE can be challenging.

**Table 23–13.** Common viral causes of arthritis.

| Virus | Disease Characteristics |
|---|---|
| Rubella | Seen in about 50% of infections<br>Occurs occasionally with vaccination<br>Associated with rash |
| Hepatitis B | Arthritis usually precedes jaundice but is associated with transaminitis<br>Rash may be present |
| HIV | May be symptom of seroconversion or occur at other times during illness |
| Mumps, arboviruses, adenoviruses, coxsackieviruses, and echoviruses all associated with arthritis | |

  **1.** Both may present with arthritis, arthralgias, and rash.

  **2.** Both are more common in women than men.

  **3.** ANA can be transiently elevated in patients with parvovirus.

**C.** Diagnosis is made by identifying IgM to parvovirus in the serum of patients with a suspicious symptom complex.

### Treatment

**A.** The treatment of parvovirus is symptomatic.

**B.** NSAIDs generally provide good relief of symptoms.

**C.** Symptoms usually resolve within a couple of weeks, but as many as 10% of patients have symptoms that last longer.

## MAKING A DIAGNOSIS

Ms. T was treated with NSAIDs and given a return appointment in 1 week. Laboratory tests were sent and revealed the following: Chem-7, normal; liver function tests, normal; WBC, 6800/mcL; Hgb, 12.9 g/dL; Hct, 37.9%; platelet, 182,000/mcL; ESR, 68 mm/h; rapid strep test, negative. ANA, streptococcal antibody titers, blood cultures, stool cultures, and parvovirus titer were pending at the time of discharge from her first appointment.

**Have you crossed a diagnostic threshold for the leading hypothesis, parvovirus? Have you ruled out the active alternatives? Do other tests need to be done to exclude the alternative diagnoses?**

Parvovirus, or another viral arthritis, is high on the differential. Laboratory testing to rule in the most likely disease and rule out other possible diseases is reasonable. The normal liver function tests rule out hepatitis B as the cause of the patient's symptoms. Negative blood cultures will make endocarditis even less likely than it is based on the history alone. Lyme disease was thought so unlikely that serologies were not even sent. Stool cultures were sent to evaluate the possibility of a reactive arthritis.

# Alternative Diagnosis: Reactive Arthritis

## Textbook Presentation

Reactive arthritis classically presents as a subacute arthritis, often involving the knees, ankles, and back. Physical exam reveals arthritis. There may be a history of an antecedent infection and symptoms of urethritis and conjunctivitis.

## Disease Highlights

A. Reactive arthritis is an acute arthritis complicating enteric and urogenital infections. This was formerly called Reiter syndrome.

B. Reactive arthritis is often accompanied by other extra-articular manifestations such as urethritis or conjunctivitis.

C. Reactive arthritis is 1 of the seronegative spondyloarthropathies.

D. The bacteria implicated in reactive arthritis are:

   1. *Shigella*
   2. *Salmonella*
   3. *Yersinia*
   4. *Campylobacter*
   5. *Chlamydia*

E. GI infections are equally likely to be the inciting event in men and women. Arthritis complicating chlamydial infection is rare in women.

F. The mean age at diagnosis is 26 years.

G. More often than not, the inciting infection is asymptomatic.

 Reactive arthritis often presents without an apparent antecedent infection.

H. Manifestations of the disease begin 2–4 weeks after the inciting infection.

   1. Urethritis is frequently the first finding followed by eye findings and then arthritis.

   2. The asymmetric arthritis has a predilection for the lower extremities.

      a. Knees, ankles, and joints in the feet are the most common locations.

      b. Dactylitis, heel pain, and back pain also occur in 50–60% of patients.

   3. Other associated findings include rash, nail changes, and oral ulcers.

   4. Table 23–14 shows the prevalence of various findings.

## Evidence-Based Diagnosis

A. The diagnosis is a clinical one.

B. A high clinical suspicion is warranted in a young patient with an asymmetric oligoarthritis.

## Treatment

A. In most patients, symptoms resolve within 1 year.

B. NSAIDs are useful in treating the acute symptoms.

C. Culture positive enteric or chlamydial infections should be treated.

**Table 23–14.** Features of reactive arthritis.

| Feature | Prevalence |
| --- | --- |
| History of diarrhea | 6% |
| Urethritis | 46% |
| Conjunctivitis | 31% |
| **Location of arthritis** | |
| Knees | 68% |
| Ankles | 49% |
| Feet | 64% |
| Fever > 38.3 °C | 32% |
| HLA-B27 | 81% |

From Arnett FC. Incomplete Reiter's syndrome: Clinical comparisons with classical triad. Ann Rheum Dis 1979;38(Suppl 1):suppl 73–78. Adapted and reproduced with permission from the BMJ Publishing Group.

D. A subset of patients experience relapse, development of a chronic arthritis, or development of ankylosing spondylitis.

# Alternative Diagnosis: Rheumatic Fever

## Textbook Presentation

Rheumatic fever classically presents in a child in the weeks following streptococcal pharyngitis. The 5 cardinal manifestations are arthritis, carditis, rash, subcutaneous nodules, and chorea. The arthritis is typically migratory, involving the knees, ankles, and hands.

## Disease Highlights

A. Rheumatic fever is an inflammatory disease that follows streptococcal pharyngitis by 2–4 weeks.

B. Unlike in children, clinical documentation of a previous streptococcal infection is rare in adults and the most pronounced symptoms are joint pain and stiffness.

C. The arthritis is generally described as a migratory polyarthritis.

   1. Individual joints are usually affected for less than a week.

   2. The joints in the legs are usually affected first.

   3. Subjective complaints are often more prominent than objective findings.

D. Carditis

   1. May involve any, or all, parts of the heart—pericarditis, myocarditis, endocarditis, or pancarditis.

   2. Endocarditis commonly causes valvular lesions that may progress over years to symptomatic valve disease, especially mitral stenosis.

## Evidence-Based Diagnosis

A. The diagnosis of rheumatic fever is based on the Jones Criteria.

B. The criteria require evidence of an antecedent group A streptococcal infection (culture, antibody titer) with either 2 major criteria or 1 major and 2 minor criteria given in Table 23–15.

**Table 23–15.** Jones criteria for the rheumatic fever.

| Major Criteria | Minor Criteria |
|---|---|
| Polyarthritis | Fever |
| Carditis (pericarditis, myocarditis, endocarditis) | Arthralgia |
| Chorea | Inflammatory markers (eg, CRP, ESR) |
| Rash—Erythema marginatum Subcutaneous nodules | PR segment prolongation |

CRP, C-reactive protein; ESR, erythrocyte sedimentation rate.

## Treatment

**A.** Anti-inflammatories

    **1.** Aspirin is the mainstay of therapy.

    **2.** Corticosteroids are given to patients with severe carditis.

**B.** Antibiotics

    **1.** Penicillin for treatment of pharyngitis.

    **2.** Lifelong prophylactic therapy with penicillin is usually recommended after the initial therapy.

## CASE RESOLUTION

Parvovirus clearly fits this patient's presentation. Reactive arthritis is possible although the patient's recent illness was not GI. Rheumatic fever seems less likely. Although she does have multiple Jones criteria (polyarthritis, arthralgia, elevated erythrocyte sedimentation rate [ESR]) and although the lack of a sore throat during the recent illness is not terribly helpful, the patient does not have a migratory arthritis or evidence of present streptococcal carriage.

> **3**
>
> Ms. T's blood work came back negative except for a positive ANA (titer 1:80) and a positive parvovirus IgM. She was treated with NSAIDs with good relief of her symptoms. Her rash resolved over 3–4 days, and joint pain was gone at a follow-up visit 2 weeks later.

## CHIEF COMPLAINT

> **PATIENT**  **4**
>
> Mr. L is a 55-year-old man who comes to see you complaining of right hip pain. He reports suffering with the pain for about 2 years. The pain is worst in the morning and evening. In the morning, it is associated with stiffness of his hip. The stiffness lasts about 5 minutes and then improves. At the end of the day he routinely feels a dull ache that is worse if he has had a very active day. He recently noticed that he is unable to cross his legs (right over left) without significant discomfort.

 At this point, what is the leading hypothesis, what are the active alternatives, and is there a must not miss diagnosis? Given this differential diagnosis, what tests should be ordered?

## PRIORITIZING THE DIFFERENTIAL DIAGNOSIS

Mr. L is a middle-aged man with chronic, monoarticular symptoms. The time course, single joint involvement and noninflammatory nature of the process (we have not heard about warmth, erythema, or prolonged morning stiffness) are the pivotal points in this case.

Reviewing the initial differential diagnosis, the articular process that best fits the history is OA, a chronic, noninflammatory, often monoarticular, arthritis. OA is so common in older adults that it becomes the diagnosis to disprove in all patients who have pain consistent with OA. The disease most commonly affects the

fingers, knee, hip, and spine. CPPD is another chronic degenerative arthritis that could produce similar symptoms and should be considered.

In patients with noninflammatory monoarticular symptoms, consider the specific periarticular symptoms that can affect the particular joint.

When considering the periarticular syndromes that cause hip pain, it is important to identify where exactly the patient feels the pain. Lumbar spine disease with radicular symptoms can cause pain in the buttocks or lateral hip. Trochanteric bursitis is a common cause of lateral hip pain. Inguinal hernias may cause groin pain. Femoral stress fractures may cause groin or lateral hip pain. Although such stress fractures are rare and are most commonly seen in young women, they should not be missed. Table 23–16 lists the differential diagnosis.

 "Hip pain" is a nonspecific complaint. It is important to identify the exact location of the pain.

> **4**
>
> When asked to pinpoint the location of his pain, Mr. L reports that he primarily feels it in the groin. Rest, acetaminophen, and heat all seem to help the pain. He comes in today because he is in more constant pain, and he has begun to limp on bad days. His past history is remarkable only for mild asthma. He denies any previous injury to the hip. He has never been hospitalized or taken corticosteroids. His only medication is albuterol.
>
> Vital signs are temperature, 37.0°C; RR, 12 breaths per minute; BP, 132/70 mm Hg; pulse, 72 bpm. On physical

**Table 23–16.** Diagnostic hypotheses for Mr. L.

| Diagnostic Hypotheses | Clinical Clues | Important Tests |
|---|---|---|
| **Leading Hypothesis** | | |
| Osteoarthritis | Chronic pain in weight-bearing joints | Radiograph of affected joints |
| **Active Alternative** | | |
| CPPD | May present as chronic or acute arthritis | Demonstration of crystals in synovial fluid or classic radiographic findings |
| **Active Alternatives—Nonarticular** | | |
| Inguinal hernia | Pain worse with straining | Physical exam |
| Trochanteric bursitis | Lateral hip pain Tenderness over the bursa | Physical exam Response to injection therapy |
| Lumbar nerve root compression | Positive straight leg raise | Physical exam MRI |
| **Active Alternative—Must Not Miss** | | |
| Femoral stress fractures | Most common in young women involved in weight-bearing exercise | MRI Bone scan |

exam, there is no warmth, erythema, or tenderness around the hip or over the trochanteric bursa. Testicular exam and hernia exam are normal. Flexion and extension of the right hip are nearly normal. There is decreased range of motion in hip rotation with about 10 degrees in internal rotation and 20 degrees in external rotation.

 **Is the clinical information sufficient to make a diagnosis? If not, what other information do you need?**

## Leading Hypothesis: OA

### Textbook Presentation

OA most commonly presents in older patients as chronic joint pain and stiffness. Pain is usually worse with activity and improves with rest. Knees, hips, and hands are most commonly affected. On exam of joints, there is bony enlargement without significant effusions but with mild tenderness along the joint lines and limited range of motion. Radiographs are diagnostic.

### Disease Highlights

A. OA is a disease of aging, with peak prevalence in the eighth decade. However, as obesity is risk factor, it may be seen in much younger people with severe obesity.

B. More common in women than men.

C. Although often referred to as "wear and tear" arthritis, the pathophysiology is actually quite complicated.

D. Joint destruction manifests as loss of cartilage with change to the underlying bone manifesting as bony sclerosis and osteophyte formation.

E. Joint distribution
   1. OA is most common in the knees, hips, hands, and spine.
   2. Nearly any joint can be affected.
   3. Non–weight-bearing joints other than the hand, such as the elbow, wrist, and shoulder, are rarely affected by primary OA. The ankle is also not a common location.

F. Classic symptoms include
   1. Pain with activity
   2. Relief with rest
   3. Periarticular tenderness
   4. Occasional mildly inflammatory flares
   5. Gelling: Joint stiffness brought on by rest and rapidly resolving with activity.
   6. Late in the disease, constant pain with joint deformation and severe disability is common.

G. Physical exam findings
   1. Generally there is bony enlargement, crepitus, and decreased range of motion without signs of inflammation or synovial thickening.
   2. Knee
      a. Crepitus
      b. Tenderness on joint line
      c. Varus or valgus displacement of the lower leg related to asymmetric loss of the articular cartilage.
   3. Hip
      a. Marked decrease first in internal and then external rotation
      b. Groin pain with rotation of the hip
   4. Hand
      a. Tenderness and bony enlargement of the first carpometacarpal joint
      b. Joint involvement in decreasing order of prevalence is DIP, PIP, MCP.
      c. Heberden nodes (prominent osteophytes of the DIP joints)
      d. Bouchard nodes (prominent osteophytes of the PIP joints)
   5. Spine
      a. Signs of spinal OA vary depending on location.
      b. Pain and limited range of motion are common.
      c. Radicular symptoms resulting from osteophyte impingement on nerve roots is seen.
      d. Spinal stenosis with associated symptoms (radiculopathy and pseudoclaudication) can result from bony hypertrophy.

### Evidence-Based Diagnosis

A. The diagnosis of OA is clinical, based on a combination of compatible history, physical exam, and radiologic findings.

B. Because of the high prevalence of OA, the diagnosis should lead the differential in any patient with suspicious symptoms.

**C.** Diagnostic criteria have been established.

    **1.** Hand

        **a.** Pain, aching, or stiffness

        **b.** 3 of the following

            **(1)** Hard tissue enlargement of at least 2 of the following joints:

                **(a)** Second and third DIP joints

                **(b)** Second and third PIP joints

                **(c)** First MCP joint

            **(2)** Hard tissue enlargement of 2 or more DIP joints

            **(3)** Fewer than 3 swollen MCP joints

            **(4)** Deformity of at least 1 of the joints listed in above entries a through c.

    **2.** Hip

        **a.** Hip pain

        **b.** 2 of the following:

            **(1)** ESR < 20 mm/h

            **(2)** Osteophytes on radiograph

            **(3)** Joint space narrowing on radiograph

    **3.** Knee: There are multiple criteria, the easiest to remember is

        **a.** Knee pain

        **b.** Osteophytes on radiograph, and

        **c.** 1 of the following

            **(1)** Age older than 50 years

            **(2)** Stiffness < 30 minutes

            **(3)** Crepitus

**D.** The test characteristics for these criteria are shown in Table 23–17.

## Treatment

**A.** Nonpharmacologic

    **1.** Patient education and improved social support have been shown to improve pain and improve the efficacy of pharmacologic interventions.

    **2.** Weight loss is key in decreasing symptoms of lower extremity OA.

    **3.** Physical and occupational therapy can help patients with functional impairment due to OA.

**B.** Pharmacologic

    **1.** Acetaminophen

        **a.** Standard initial therapy given its effectiveness and low side-effect profile.

        **b.** Equally effective to NSAIDs for mild to moderate OA.

    **2.** NSAIDS are probably more effective than acetaminophen for severe OA.

    **3.** Oral combinations of glucosamine and chondroitan sulfate probably are modestly effective in some patients and have a very favorable side-effect profile.

    **4.** Intra-articular medications

        **a.** Intra-articular corticosteroids are very effective for acute flares of OA.

        **b.** Hyaluronic acid given by intra-articular injection may provide a small benefit to some patients.

    **5.** Tramadol and opioid analgesics are reasonable choices for patients with severe symptoms.

**C.** Surgical

    **1.** Arthroscopic surgery for OA is probably ineffective.

    **2.** Hip and knee replacement can have remarkable effects on decreasing pain and improving function in patients in whom conservative therapy has failed.

## MAKING A DIAGNOSIS

Mr. L's history and physical exam are very suggestive of OA, but CPPD remains a possibility. Most of the periarticular syndromes that were considered initially have been made unlikely by the exam. Lumbar spine disease with radicular symptoms would not cause the limited range of motion that is seen on the patient's exam. Patients with trochanteric bursitis usually have more acute symptoms than did this patient, and there is tenderness over the bursa. Mr. L does not have a hernia on exam. Femoral stress fractures may cause groin pain but should not really cause limited range of motion. That said, this is a diagnosis that must not be missed, so further consideration should be given.

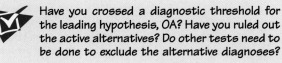

The working diagnosis of OA was made and the patient was given 1000 mg of acetaminophen twice daily. A radiograph was ordered.

Have you crossed a diagnostic threshold for the leading hypothesis, OA? Have you ruled out the active alternatives? Do other tests need to be done to exclude the alternative diagnoses?

## Alternative Diagnosis: Femoral Stress Fractures

### Textbook Presentation

Femoral stress fractures are most commonly seen in young female athletes. Symptoms begin acutely with persistent groin pain that worsens as the day progresses. On physical exam, there is often mild tenderness over the proximal one-third of the femur. Range of motion of the hip is normal. Radiographs are usually normal.

### Disease Highlights

**A.** Like other types of stress fractures, femoral stress fractures are most common

    **1.** In athletes who have recently increased their level of training

**Table 23–17.** Test characteristics for the diagnosis of OA.

| Joint | Sensitivity | Specificity | LR+ | LR− |
|-------|-------------|-------------|-----|-----|
| Hand | 94% | 87% | 7.2 | 0.07 |
| Hip | 89% | 91% | 9.9 | 0.12 |
| Knee | 91% | 86% | 6.5 | 0.1 |

OA, osteoarthritis.

***Table 23–18.*** Some common periarticular pain syndromes.

| Area of Pain | Diagnosis | History | Physical and Diagnostic Evaluation |
|---|---|---|---|
| Neck and shoulder | Acute cervical sprain | Pain and stiffness over neck and upper thoracic vertebrae<br>Often first noticed when rising in the morning | Pain with tilting head<br>Muscle spasm often palpable |
| | Cervical radiculopathy | Pain and stiffness of cervical spine, usually with radiation to upper back and arm<br>Occasionally manifests solely as pain between spine and scapula | Radicular symptoms can be reproduced with manipulation of cervical spine<br>MRI diagnostic |
| | Rotator cuff/Impingement syndrome | Pain inferior to acromioclavicular joint | Tenderness inferior to acromioclavicular joint<br>Pain with passively raising shoulder while preventing "shrugging" |
| | Rotator cuff tear | Pain similar to above<br>Occurs after injury in younger patients<br>Often spontaneous in older patients | Weakness in abduction<br>Positive Job test (patient resists downward force to an internally rotated, anteriorly stretched arm) |
| Elbow | Lateral and medial epicondylitis | Pain over tendon insertion on medial and lateral epicondyle | Tenderness at site of pain<br>Exacerbated with wrist flexion (medial) or extension (lateral) |
| | Olecranon bursitis | Pain over olecranon bursa | Tenderness and swelling over the olecranon bursa |
| Hand | DeQuervain tenosynovitis | Pain at the lateral base of the thumb | Worse with pincer grasp<br>Positive Finkelstein maneuver (ulnar deviation of wrist with fingers curled over thumb) |
| Hip | Trochanteric bursitis | Pain over bursa<br>Patient often notes pain when lying on area at night | Tenderness over bursa<br>Sometimes visualized on radiograph |
| | Meralgia paresthetica | Pain or numbness over lateral thigh<br>Often after weight gain or loss | Neuropathic-type pain<br>Abnormal sensation over lateral femoral cutaneous nerve distribution |
| Knee | Patellofemoral syndrome | Anterior knee pain, often worse climbing or descending stairs | Crepitus beneath patella |
| | Meniscal and ligamentous injuries | Ligament injuries tend to be traumatic<br>Classically associated with the knee giving way<br>Meniscal injuries may be traumatic or degenerative<br>Knee locking is classic | Ligament injuries will manifest as laxity on exam<br>Meniscal injuries as a click<br>MRI is diagnostic |
| Foot and ankle | Achilles tendinitis | Pain over distal tendon<br>Pain and stiffness worse after inactivity | Tenderness over insertion of tendon |
| | Plantar fasciitis | Pain anterior to heel<br>Worse with first standing | History usually diagnostic<br>Radiograph may show heel spur |
| | Morton neuroma | Pain between the second and third or third and fourth metatarsal heads | Tenderness at the area of pain |
| Polyperiarticular | Fibromyalgia | Diffuse pain syndrome<br>Often nonrestorative sleep | Diagnosis depends on tenderness at 11 or more specific locations |
| | Polymyalgia rheumatica | Pain and disability of large muscles of shoulder and hips | Disease is often associated with signs of inflammatory disease (anemia, elevated CRP and ESR) |

CRP, C-reactive protein; ESR, erythrocyte sedimentation rate.

**2.** In women

**3.** In persons with decreased bone density

**B.** The most common stress fractures are tibial and metatarsal.

**C.** Femoral stress fractures usually present with hip or groin pain with preserved range of motion of the hip.

### Evidence-Based Diagnosis

**A.** Stress fractures in general and femoral stress fractures in particular are often not apparent on initial radiographs.

**B.** MRI and bone scans are considered the diagnostic test of choice.

### Treatment

**A.** Many stress fractures heal with reduced physical activity and short-term immobilization.

**B.** Femoral stress fractures may resolve with decreased weight bearing (crutches) or may require casting or internal fixation.

## CASE RESOLUTION

4

The patient's hip radiograph showed changes consistent with OA.

The combination of a high clinical suspicion, pain, and consistent findings on a radiograph confirms the diagnosis.

## REVIEW OF OTHER IMPORTANT DISEASES

### Periarticular Syndromes

There are textbooks written about the numerous periarticular syndromes that commonly present to primary care physicians, orthopedists, and rheumatologists. Table 23–18 briefly outlines some of the most common.

## REFERENCES

Arnett FC. Incomplete Reiter's syndrome: clinical comparisons with classical triad. Ann Rheum Dis. 1979;38 Suppl 1:suppl 73–8.

Black ER. *Diagnostic strategies for common medical problems.* 2nd ed. Philadelphia: American College of Physicians; 1999.

Margaretten ME, Kohlwes J, Moore D, Bent S. Does this adult patient have septic arthritis? JAMA. 2007;297(13):1478–88.

Nishimura K, Sugiyama D, Kogata Y et al. Meta-analysis: diagnostic accuracy of anti-cyclic citrullinated peptide antibody and rheumatoid factor for rheumatoid arthritis. Ann Intern Med. 2007;146(11):797–808.

O'Brien JP, Goldenberg DL, Rice PA. Disseminated gonococcal infection: a prospective analysis of 49 patients and a review of pathophysiology and immune mechanisms. Medicine (Baltimore). 1983;62(6):395–406.

*Primer on the rheumatic diseases.* 12th ed. Atlanta, GA: Arthritis Foundation; 2001.

Shmerling RH. Origin and utility of measurement of rheumatoid factors. In: Rose B, ed. UpToDate, 2007.

Steere AC. Lyme disease. N Engl J Med. 2001;345(2):115–25.

Terkeltaub RA. Clinical practice. Gout. N Engl J Med. 2003;349(17):1647–55.

**Diagnostic Approach: Joint Pain**

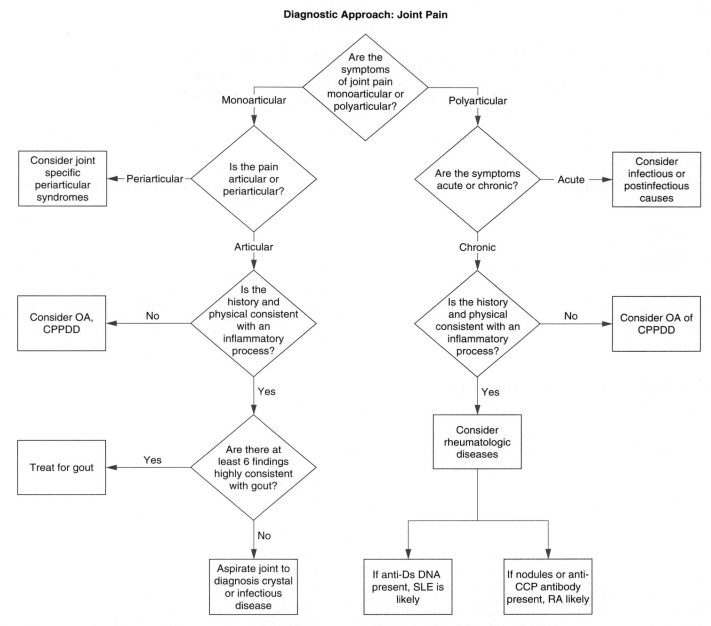

Anti-cyclic citrullinated peptide; CPPDD, calcium pyrophosphate dihydrate deposition disease; OA, osteoarthritis; SLE, systemic lupus erythematosus.

# I have a patient with a rash.
# How do I determine the cause?

## CHIEF COMPLAINT

PATIENT 1

Ms. N is a 23-year-old woman who comes to see you complaining of a rash.

☑ What is the differential diagnosis of a rash? How would you frame the differential?

## CONSTRUCTING A DIFFERENTIAL DIAGNOSIS

In clinical practice, rashes are diagnosed through pattern recognition probably more than with any other complaint. This is an effective way of making a diagnosis when the diagnosis is obvious or when the observer is very experienced. The risk with pattern recognition is that diagnostic hypotheses are heavily influenced by recent experience, rare diagnoses tend not to be considered, and physicians often reach premature closure on an incorrect diagnosis.

The most useful way of organizing the differential diagnosis of a rash is to base it on the morphology of the lesion. To correctly categorize a lesion's morphology, the physician must first identify the primary lesion, the typical element of the eruption. Once the primary lesion is identified, the eruption can be categorized based on morphology and then the specific diagnosis identified. This process can be difficult. The primary lesion is often affected by secondary changes such as excoriation, erosion, crusting, and even coalescence. The differential diagnosis of one lesion can also be extensive. After determining the morphology of the primary lesion, the next step in making the diagnosis is often to observe the distribution of lesion. Some eruptions will have characteristic distributions. What follows are some important definitions, followed by a differential diagnosis of some of the most common primary lesions.

1. Macule: lesion without elevation or depression, < 1 cm
2. Patch: lesion without elevation or depression, > 1 cm
3. Papule: any solid, elevated "bump" < 1 cm
4. Plaque: raised plateau-like lesion of variable size, no depth, often a confluence of papules
5. Nodule: solid lesion with palpable elevation, 1–5 cm
6. Tumor: solid growth, > 5 cm
7. Cyst: encapsulated lesion, filled with soft material
8. Vesicle: elevated, fluid-filled blister, < 1 cm
9. Bulla: elevated, fluid-filled blister, > 1 cm
10. Pustule: elevated, pus-filled blister, any size
11. Wheal: inflamed papule or plaque formed by transient and superficial local edema
12. Comedone: a plug of keratinous material and skin oils retained in a follicle; open is black, closed is white

Papulosquamous eruptions present with papules and plaques associated with superficial scaling. Folliculopapular eruptions begin as papules arising in a perifollicular distribution. Dermal reaction patterns result from infiltrative and inflammatory processes involving the dermal and subcutaneous tissues. Petechia and purpura occur when there is leakage of blood products into surrounding tissues from inflamed or damaged blood vessels. Blistering disorders present with vesicles and bullae.

A. Papulosquamous eruptions (papules and plaques)
  1. Eczematous dermatitis
    a. Atopic dermatitis
    b. Allergic contact dermatitis
    c. Irritant contact dermatitis
  2. Pityriasis rosea
  3. Tinea infections
  4. Psoriasis
  5. Seborrheic dermatitis
B. Folliculopapular eruptions (perifollicular papules)
  1. Acne vulgaris
  2. Rosacea
  3. Folliculitis
  4. Perioral dermatitis
C. Dermal reaction patterns
  1. Urticaria
  2. Sarcoidosis
  3. Granuloma annulare
  4. Erythema nodosum
D. Purpura and petechiae
  1. Palpable purpura
    a. Leukocytoclastic vasculitis
     (1) Henoch-Schönlein purpura
     (2) Allergic vasculitis
    b. Infectious
     (1) Bacteremia
     (2) Rocky Mountain spotted fever
  2. Nonpalpable purpura
    a. Thrombocytopenia
    b. Medication related

c. Benign pigmented purpura

d. Bacteremia

e. Disseminated intravascular coagulation

f. Actinic/senile purpura

g. Corticosteroid associated

h. Amyloidosis

E. Blistering disorders (vesicles, pustules, and bullae)

   1. Autoimmune

     a. Bullous pemphigoid

     b. Pemphigus vulgaris

     c. Epidermolysis bullosa acquisita

   2. Congenital

     a. Epidermolysis bullosa

     b. Epidermolytic hyperkeratosis

   3. Infectious

     a. Varicella zoster

     b. Herpes simplex

     c. Impetigo

     d. Staphylococcal scalded skin

   4. Hypersensitivity syndromes

     a. Stevens-Johnson syndrome

     b. Toxic epidermal necrolysis

*Ms. N complains of frequent "breakouts" on her face for the last several years. She reports the use of many topical over-the-counter agents over the years. She complains of feeling greasy and the need to "squeeze pus" out of lesions on a regular basis.*

*On examination, over the forehead, cheeks, and chin there are many erythematous papules, occasional pustules, and open and closed comedones. There is a predominance of larger nodules along the jaw line. Similar erythematous papules involve the upper back and chest. There is neither significant background erythema nor scaling in the scalp, eyebrows, or nasolabial folds. Figure 24–1 shows her on her initial visit.*

**At this point, what is the leading hypothesis, what are the active alternatives, and is there a must not miss diagnosis? Given this differential diagnosis, what tests should be ordered?**

## PRIORITIZING THE DIFFERENTIAL DIAGNOSIS

The pivotal clues in this case are the morphology of the lesion and its distribution. This patient has a folliculopapular eruption that predominantly affects the face, chest, and upper back. Primary lesions of inflammatory papules, pustules, and comedones place acne at the top of the differential. The history is typical for acne: a chronic course with intermittent flares.

Other folliculopapular conditions must be considered. The lack of background erythema and telangiectasias makes a diagnosis of rosacea less likely. Perioral dermatitis typically presents as monomorphic small papules. It is closely associated with the use

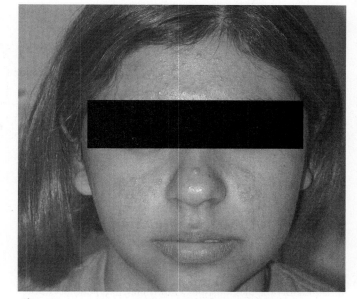

***Figure 24–1.*** Ms. N on initial presentation. (See Plate 1.)

of topical corticosteroids and cosmetics. Treatment usually requires cessation of these agents and the administration of antibiotics with cutaneous antiinflammatory activity. The mixture of lesion type, with comedones as well as papules and nodules, and the more diffuse distribution makes acne more likely than perioral dermatitis. An infectious folliculitis is possible, but the course of the disease makes this extremely unlikely (Table 24–1).

***Table 24–1.*** Diagnostic hypotheses for Ms. N.

| Diagnostic Hypotheses | Clinical Clues | Important Tests |
|---|---|---|
| **Leading Hypothesis** | | |
| Acne vulgaris | Presence of comedones, papules, pustules, nodules Flares with menses Distribution over the face, chest and back | Clinical diagnosis |
| **Active Alternative** | | |
| Rosacea | History of flushing Presence of telangiectasias and possibly inflammatory papules | Clinical diagnosis |
| **Other Alternative** | | |
| Perioral dermatitis | Monomorphic eruption of fine erythematous papules clustered around mouth | Clinical diagnosis |

The patient is in good health and is not overweight. She is not taking any oral medications. She reports regular menstrual cycles and notes that the breakouts are worse around the time of her period. She does not report easy flushing or any increased hair growth on the face or chest. She has one healthy child.

**Is the clinical information sufficient to make a diagnosis? If not, what other information do you need?**

## Leading Hypothesis: Acne Vulgaris

### Textbook Presentation

Typically, acne vulgaris presents in adolescence with chronic, waxing and waning lesions. A variety of lesions are present, including inflammatory papules, pustules, comedones, and nodulocysts over the face, chest, and back.

### Disease Highlights

**A.** Description of lesion: inflammatory papules, pustules, comedones, and nodulocysts over the face, chest, and back. (See Figure 24–1.)

**B.** Acne is a highly prevalent condition, most common during mid-to-late adolescence.

**C.** Acne may persist beyond adolescence, especially in women.

**D.** Acne is caused by the obstruction of sebaceous follicles on the face and trunk. Three factors are involved in the development of the lesions:

    **1.** Increased sebum production (androgen dependent) obstructs follicles.

    **2.** Excessive desquamation of epithelial cells and keratin into follicles causes obstruction.

    **3.** Inflammation secondary to proliferation of the anaerobe *Propionibacterium acnes.*

**E.** Although the 3 factors discussed above are responsible for the overwhelming majority of acne, it is important to keep in mind other factors that may be contribute to the disease.

    **1.** Hyperandrogen states (eg, polycystic ovary syndrome [PCOS] or androgenic progestins in oral contraception).

    **2.** Exposure to topical comedogens (cocoa butter, mineral oil, lanolin, fatty acids).

    **3.** Numerous factors that lead to follicular obstruction (eg, habits or clothing that cause skin trauma or obstruct pores, and hot humid environments or heavy sweating leading to keratin over-hydration).

    **4.** Medications known to trigger or exacerbate acne (eg, corticosteroids, isoniazid, lithium, androgens)

Evidence-Based Diagnosis

**A.** The diagnosis is typically clinical.

**B.** Histopathology will vary depending on the lesion. Comedones have a distinctive histologic appearance.

**C.** Work-up for hyperandrogenism is appropriate when there are signs of polycystic ovary disease, virilization, or an atypical presentation (such as later in life).

## Treatment

**A.** Establish that there are none of the acne precipitants discussed above.

**B.** Review general skin care techniques for acne-prone skin.

    **1.** Vigorous scrubbing can aggravate acne by promoting development of inflammatory lesions.

    **2.** Abrasive cleaners and mechanical devices also aggravate acne by promoting inflammation.

    **3.** Use of a mild cleanser with lukewarm water and one's hands is best.

    **4.** Use of moisturizers should be minimized and all cosmetics and lotions should be oil-free.

    **5.** Minimize contact of facial skin with hair gels and other styling products (pomade acne).

**C.** Medical therapy is aimed at the 3 factors involved in acne development.

    **1.** Decreasing sebum production

        **a.** No topical therapies are effective

        **b.** Estrogen

            **(1)** Most effective at doses of > 50 mcg of ethinyl estradiol

            **(2)** Common oral contraceptive pills containing ≤ 35 mcg ethinyl estradiol are still helpful.

        **c.** Antiandrogens (spironolactone)

        **d.** Isotretinoin (see later discussion)

    **2.** Alteration of epithelial turnover and cohesiveness

        **a.** Topical retinoids: tretinoin, tazarotene

        **b.** Adapalene: a naphthoic acid with retinoid activity

    **3.** *P acnes* proliferation and accompanying inflammation

        **a.** Topical antibiotics

            **(1)** Erythromycin

            **(2)** Clindamycin

            **(3)** Metronidazole

            **(4)** Benzoyl peroxide

        **b.** Systemic antibiotics

            **(1)** Tetracycline class

            **(2)** Erythromycin

            **(3)** Clindamycin

**D.** Guidelines for the use of these medications are as follows:

    **1.** Predominantly comedonal acne: retinoid or adapalene

    **2.** Mild inflammatory acne: topical antibiotic with or without retinoid or adapalene

    **3.** Moderate to severe but noncystic inflammatory acne: systemic antibiotic in combination with a topical regimen

    **4.** Nodular cystic acne: isotretinoin

        **a.** Because of potential adverse effects with isotretinoin, it should only be prescribed by clinicians experienced in its use.

        **b.** Isotretinoin has the potential to cause hypertriglyceridemia and depression.

        **c.** Isotretinoin is a potent teratogen and effective contraception must be assured.

**E.** Additional considerations

    **1.** Oral contraceptives are useful in women with a strong hormonal component.

**2.** Spironolactone can be useful in adult women with recalcitrant acne.

## MAKING A DIAGNOSIS

A clinical diagnosis of acne is most likely. Although PCOS might by considered based on the older age of the patient and the distribution of lesions along the jaw line, the patient lacks the oligomenorrhea that, along with evidence of hyperandrogenism, is necessary for making the diagnosis.

A clinical diagnosis of acne is made, and discussion begins as to the most appropriate therapy.

 Have you crossed a diagnostic threshold for the leading hypothesis, acne vulgaris? Have you ruled out the active alternatives? Do other tests need to be done to exclude the alternative diagnoses?

## Alternative Diagnosis: Rosacea

### Textbook Presentation

Commonly presents in adults with a facial rash. There is gradual development of telangiectasias and persistent centrofacial erythema occasionally with inflammatory red papules and papulopustules. Comedones are absent. There is often a history of easy flushing. The rash may worsen with sun exposure, ingestion of spicy food and hot liquids, emotional stress, and exercise.

### Disease Highlights

**A.** Description of lesion: centrofacial persistent facial erythema, telangiectasias, and, occasionally, inflammatory papules and papulopustules (Figure 24–2).

**B.** Rosacea is most common in fair-skinned individuals of northern European descent but can be seen in people with darker skin as well.

**C.** Women are more commonly affected than men.

**D.** However, complicated disease with sebaceous gland hyperplasia and rhinophyma (sebaceous overgrowth causing deformity of the nose) develops more often in men.

**E.** Although rosacea typically begins later than acne and reaches a peak in middle age, the two can overlap.

**F.** Although sun exposure is thought to be a trigger of rosacea, and sun-damaged skin is frequently observed, self-reported sun sensitivity is infrequent.

### Evidence-Based Diagnosis

**A.** Diagnosis is by clinical presentation.

**B.** Histopathology varies according to the stage and variant of the disease and is often nonspecific.

### Treatment

**A.** Sun protection

**B.** Avoidance of triggers of flushing

    **1.** Sun exposure

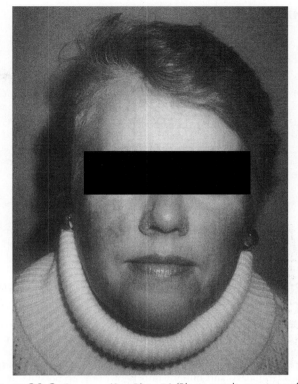

**Figure 24–2.** Rosacea. (See Plate 2.) (Photograph courtesy of Dr. Anne E. Laumann.)

    **2.** Ingestion of spicy foods and hot liquids

    **3.** Emotional stressors

    **4.** Physical exertion: encourage frequent cool-downs

**C.** Topical agents: metronidazole decreases erythema and prevents papules and papulopustules.

**D.** Systemic agents: oral antibiotics of the tetracycline class control severe eruptions of inflammatory lesions.

**E.** Laser treatment

    **1.** Used to ablate telangiectasias and improve background erythema.

    **2.** May be helpful to reduce rhinophyma.

## CASE RESOLUTION

A management plan was discussed with the patient, including an appropriate skin care regimen, appropriate product selection, and use of systemic and topical medications. At follow-up in 3 months, the patient had significantly fewer active lesions with evidence of dyspigmentation associated with resolving lesions.

## CHIEF COMPLAINT

PATIENT 2

Mr. B is a 13-year-old boy who was in good health until 1 week ago, when he noted that the left side of his chest was painful. One day before his visit, he noticed a rash on the left side of his chest, just lateral to his sternum. He describes the rash as small bumps, blisters, and red patches. He says that the skin is extremely sensitive to light touch. He otherwise feels well, without fever or constitutional symptoms.

At this point, what is the leading hypothesis, what are the active alternatives, and is there a must not miss diagnosis? Given this differential diagnosis, what tests should be ordered?

## PRIORITIZING THE DIFFERENTIAL DIAGNOSIS

Several general etiologic categories need to be considered when presented with a patient with new-onset blisters or vesicles. Blisters can be a symptom of infection, autoimmune disease, or a reaction to an external stimulus. Infectious causes include varicella zoster virus (VZV), presenting either as chickenpox or herpes zoster (shingles), and bullous impetigo. Both are possible in this patient. The prodromal pain suggests VZV. Bullous impetigo can cause blisters in a young, healthy person, but these blisters often begin in intertriginous areas. Bullous impetigo is most common in children. Grouped blisters suggest VZV or herpes simplex virus (HSV), whereas other blistering diseases may demonstrate large distinct blisters or erosions.

Bullous arthropod bites can affect patients of any age. A history of exposure should be elicited. The numerous, small, clustered lesions in this case make arthropod bites a less likely diagnosis. Bullous pemphigoid and other autoimmune blistering disorders are rare but possible. Stevens-Johnson syndrome is unlikely given the subacute onset but is certainly a "must not miss" diagnosis (Table 24–2).

2

The patient reports no significant medical history. He recently finished a course of amoxicillin for pharyngitis. He does also frequently help his mother with gardening. The patient is afebrile with normal vital signs. The physical exam demonstrates clusters of small vesicles, filled with clear fluid, overlying erythematous skin. There is no lymphadenopathy. The rest of the skin exam is unremarkable (Figure 24–3).

Is the clinical information sufficient to make a diagnosis? If not, what other information do you need?

## Leading Hypothesis: Varicella Zoster Virus (Herpes Zoster/Shingles)

### Textbook Presentation

This condition usually presents as a rash over a single, unilateral dermatome. The lesions begin as closely grouped vesicles on an

**Table 24–2.** Diagnostic hypotheses for Mr. B.

| Diagnostic Hypotheses | Clinical Clues | Important Tests |
|---|---|---|
| **Leading Hypothesis** | | |
| Varicella zoster virus | Prodromal pain symptoms Localized lesions in a dermatomal distribution | Usually diagnosed clinically Tzanck smear, direct fluorescent antibody test of skin scraping, culture |
| **Active Alternatives** | | |
| Bullous impetigo | Acute onset, related to skin trauma | Bacterial culture of lesion |
| Bullous arthropod bites | Pruritus Lack of constitutional symptoms Exposure history | Clinical |
| Bullous pemphigoid | May present with early urticarial lesions and pruritus Later intact blisters | Skin biopsy and direct immunofluorescence of skin |
| **Active Alternative—Must Not Miss** | | |
| Stevens-Johnson syndrome | Rapidly progressive rash with associated mucosal lesions | Skin biopsy |

erythematous base. Over 2–3 days, the lesions become pustular and then crust over after 7–10 days. Pain and paresthesias along the involved dermatome often precede the rash by a few days.

### Disease Highlights

A. Description of the lesion: small, tightly grouped vesicles on an erythematous base occurring in one dermatome.

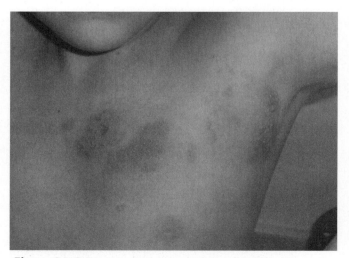

**Figure 24–3.** Mr. B. on initial presentation. (See Plate 3.)

(See Figure 24–3.) Very early in the presentation, the lesions are large papules that then become vesicular, then pustular, and ultimately crusted.

**B.** Characteristics of the lesion

   **1.** The rash tends to occur in the region where the rash of primary VZV infection (chickenpox) was most severe.

      **a.** The most common dermatomes are trigeminal and T3-L2.

      **b.** It is not uncommon to have a few vesicles in contiguous dermatomes.

   **2.** New lesions may appear for several days, occasionally for up to 7 days.

**C.** Shingles is caused by reactivation of VZV in a dorsal root ganglion.

**D.** Complications

   **1.** Herpes zoster ophthalmicus

      **a.** Can occur when there is involvement of the first division trigeminal nerve.

      **b.** Herpes zoster ophthalmicus carries high risk of corneal damage.

   **2.** Ramsay Hunt syndrome

      **a.** Reactivation of VZV within the geniculate ganglion

      **b.** Causes a Bell palsy (facial paralysis) and ear pain

      **c.** Vesicles can often be seen in the ear canal.

      **d.** Vestibular and hearing disturbances (vertigo and hearing loss or tinnitus) are frequently reported.

**E.** Disseminated varicella zoster may occur, most often in immunocompromised patients.

**F.** Shingles in the elderly

   **1.** Shingles can be associated with significant morbidity in elderly patients.

   **2.** The rash is more severe and generally lasts longer in the elderly.

   **3.** Postherpetic neuralgia, a potentially debilitating, long-term pain syndrome, is also most common in the elderly.

### Evidence-Based Diagnosis

**A.** The diagnosis of shingles is usually made clinically without additional tests.

**B.** Detection of virus by immunofluorescent techniques is rapid and sensitive.

**C.** The bedside Tzanck smear of material scraped from a fresh vesicle can be supportive evidence but cannot distinguish between VZV and HSV.

**D.** Viral culture is the gold standard for diagnosis.

### Treatment

**A.** In the immunocompetent, the eruption is self-limited; supportive care with pain relievers may be all that is necessary.

**B.** Patients with any involvement of the eye should be evaluated by an ophthalmologist.

**C.** Antiviral agents

   **1.** When the rash is diagnosed within the first 72 hours, systemic antiviral medications are useful.

   **2.** They decrease the duration and severity of the disease.

   **3.** They prevent dissemination.

   **4.** Early treatment with antiviral agents may also prevent the development of postherpetic neuralgia.

 The use of antiviral drugs is not beneficial if the rash of herpes zoster has been present for more than 72 hours.

**D.** Symptomatic care: soaks and topical antipruritics might be useful.

**E.** Corticosteroids

   **1.** There are data that the use of corticosteroids in conjunction with antiviral agents reduces the duration of the rash and the acute pain syndrome.

   **2.** The use of corticosteroids remains somewhat controversial because the studies have shown higher rates of adverse events in patients treated with corticosteroids.

**F.** Infection control

   **1.** The vesicle fluid is infectious to individuals who have not had chickenpox or been vaccinated.

   **2.** Infection risk can, therefore, be reduced by preventing direct contact with the vesicle fluid.

**G.** Postherpetic neuralgia

   **1.** Most commonly complicates disease in the elderly

   **2.** Potentially severe neuropathic pain syndrome

   **3.** Can be treated with tricyclic antidepressants, gabapentin, or opioids

   **4.** Intrathecal methylprednisolone and lidocaine are effective for refractory disease.

**H.** Prevention

   **1.** A vaccine is now available for the prevention of herpes zoster.

   **2.** The original trial of this vaccine was conducted in a population over 60 years of age and demonstrated a 48.5% reduction in episodes of zoster (NNT = 63) and a 45% reduction in cases of postherpetic neuralgia (NNT = 434).

   **3.** The vaccine is recommended for patients over 60.

   **4.** Because this is a live-virus vaccine, it is contraindicated in patients who are immunosuppressed, pregnant, or planning pregnancy.

## MAKING A DIAGNOSIS

Given the patient's prodromal symptoms, VZV is the leading diagnosis. Because the rash was believed to be somewhat atypical, a fresh vesicle was unroofed with a scalpel tip and the base of the vesicle was scraped and smeared onto a microscope slide. The slide was transported to the laboratory for a direct fluorescent antibody assay.

The diagnosis of varicella zoster is often clinical. The distribution and clinical appearance of lesions, as well as the associated prodromal symptoms, can make the diagnosis obvious. Impetigo, bullous arthropod bites, and autoimmune blistering diseases will typically demonstrate larger distinct blisters or erosions. Stevens-Johnson syndrome and other drug reactions must always be considered when medications are in use. This patient was taking amoxicillin. The clinical appearance of the lesions, their localized distribution, and the overall time course of the symptoms is not consistent with this eruption, so VZV must still lead the list.

Have you crossed a diagnostic threshold for the leading hypothesis, varicella zoster? Have you ruled out the active alternatives? Do other tests need to be done to exclude the alternative diagnoses?

## Alternative Diagnosis: Bullous Impetigo

### Textbook Presentation

Most commonly seen in children, bullous impetigo presents as flaccid, transparent bullae in the intertriginous areas. The blisters rupture easily and leave a rim of scale and a shallow moist erosion.

### Disease Highlights

A. Description of the lesion: flaccid bullae on normal skin (Figure 24–4)

B. Location of the lesion

1. Develops on grossly intact skin as a result of local toxin production.

2. This is in contrast to nonbullous impetigo, shown in Figure 24–5, resulting from *Staphylococcus* or *Streptococcus* infection, which tends to affect previously traumatized skin.

3. Lesions most commonly develop on moist, intertriginous skin.

C. Superficial skin infection that most commonly affects infants and young children

D. The causative agent is *Staphylococcus aureus.*

E. The blistering is caused by the production of exfoliatin or epidermolytic toxins.

### Evidence-Based Diagnosis

A. Diagnosis is by clinical presentation.

B. Culture of blister fluid or the moist edge of a crusted plaque may be diagnostic.

### Treatment

A. Oral antibiotics active against *S aureus* should be prescribed for bullous impetigo. The possibility of methicillin-resistant *S aureus* (MRSA) must be considered.

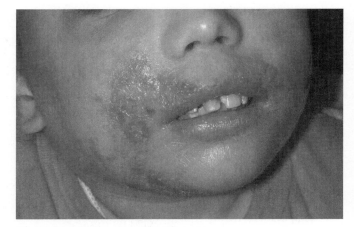

***Figure 24–5.*** Impetigo. (See Plate 5.)

B. Localized nonbullous impetigo may be adequately treated with topical antibiotics effective against gram-positive cocci such as:

1. Bacitracin

2. Polymyxin

3. Mupirocin

C. Recurrent infections may indicate staphylococcal carriage. Eradication measures including daily washing with chlorhexidine gluconate, intranasal mupirocin ointment, and oral rifampin and doxycycline have been modestly successful.

D. Family members and close contacts may also be colonized and warrant investigation and treatment when appropriate.

## Alternative Diagnosis: Bullous Arthropod Bites

### Textbook Presentation

This condition commonly presents as a cluster of tense blisters on exposed skin. The blisters tend to be large (≥ 1 cm) and surrounding skin is normal.

### Disease Highlights

A. Description of the lesion: large, often tense blisters on normal skin (Figure 24–6).

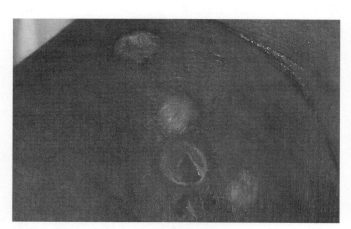

***Figure 24–4.*** Bullous impetigo. (See Plate 4.)

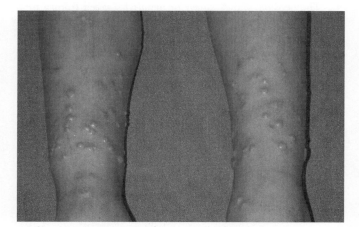

***Figure 24–6.*** Bullous arthropod bites. (See Plate 6.)

B. Character and location of the lesion

1. The lesions tend to develop in exposed areas of the skin, such as the extremities.

2. The patient will otherwise appear well.

3. The lesions are typically extraordinarily pruritic.

4. Although the blisters arise from otherwise normal skin, surrounding inflammatory changes from rubbing and scratching are often present.

C. Arthropod bite reactions are dermal hypersensitivity reactions to antigens in the saliva of insects.

D. Fleas and bedbugs are common culprits.

### Evidence-Based Diagnosis

A. Diagnosis is made by clinical presentation.

B. Histopathology can be supportive, demonstrating edema, a subepidermal blister, and a dermal inflammatory infiltrate with numerous eosinophils.

### Treatment

A. Avoidance of future bites with use of protective clothing and insect repellants.

B. Attention to eradicating the source of the biting insects, such as on pets, nests, etc.

C. Supportive local care to prevent secondary infection and relieve pruritus.

## Alternative Diagnosis: Bullous Pemphigoid

### Textbook Presentation

Bullous pemphigoid is usually seen in elderly patients with the sudden onset of 1–2 cm tense blisters and bright red, urticarial plaques. Lesions often begin on the lower extremities and progress upward.

### Disease Highlights

A. Description of the lesion: tense bullae arising on skin that may be normal, erythematous, or urticarial (Figure 24–7).

B. Bullous pemphigoid is an autoimmune disease primarily affecting the elderly.

C. Autoantibodies are targeted against components of the epidermal basement membrane zone, thus triggering separation and blistering.

D. The lesions heal without scarring.

E. Most cases occur sporadically without obvious precipitating factors.

F. Character and location of the lesion

1. Predilection of blisters for the extremities

2. Lesions range from asymptomatic to intensely pruritic.

3. Mucosal surfaces are rarely involved.

G. Antibodies to several elements of the basements membrane zone have been isolated. These distinct antibodies cause other blistering syndromes, such as pemphigus vulgaris and epidermolysis bullosa acquisita.

### Evidence-Based Diagnosis

A. Histopathology provides supportive information, demonstrating a subepidermal blister plane and accumulation of eosinophils.

B. Immunopathology confirms the diagnosis by demonstrating linear deposits of IgG and C3 at the dermal–epidermal junction.

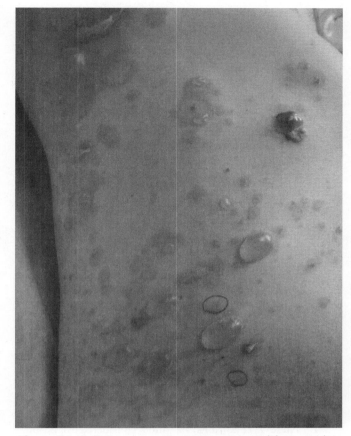

***Figure 24–7.*** Bullous pemphigoid. (See Plate 7.) (Photograph courtesy of Dr. Keith Duffy.)

C. In 70–80% of patients, circulating IgG that recognizes the identified antigens of the basement membrane zone can be found.

### Treatment

A. Topical, potent corticosteroids can be effective.

B. Extensive disease can be treated with systemic corticosteroids.

C. Steroid-sparing immunosuppressives are used to limit the toxicities of systemic corticosteroids in chronic disease.

D. Alternative antiinflammatory regimens such as tetracycline and nicotinamide may be effective.

E. Remission is usually obtained within a few weeks; however, some degree of long-term therapy may be necessary.

F. Refractory cases may respond to plasmapheresis or intravenous gammaglobulin.

## Alternative Diagnosis: Stevens-Johnson Syndrome

### Textbook Presentation

Stevens-Johnson syndrome typically presents in a patient with fever, malaise, headache, and myalgias who is taking a potentially causative medication. After about 1 week of symptoms, a macular rash develops on the chest and face. These lesions subsequently blister and then rapidly erode. The skin is usually excruciatingly tender.

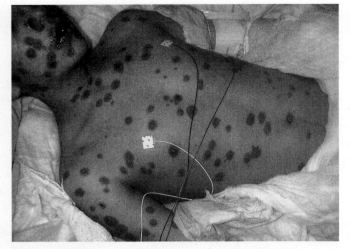

**Figure 24–8.** Stevens-Johnson syndrome. (See Plate 8.)

**Table 24–3.** Medications most commonly implicated in Stevens-Johnson syndrome or toxic epidermal necrolysis.

| Medications | OR |
| --- | --- |
| **Short-term** | |
| Sulfonamide antibiotics | 172 |
| Aminopenicillins | 6.7 |
| Quinolones | 10 |
| Cephalosporins | 14 |
| **Long-term** | |
| Carbamazepine | 90 |
| Phenobarbital | 45 |
| Phenytoin | 53 |
| Valproic acid | 25 |
| Piroxicam | 12 |
| Allopurinol | 52 |
| Corticosteroids | 54 |

Data from Roujeau JC, Kelly JP, Naldi L et al. Medication use and the risk of Stevens-Johnson syndrome or toxic epidermal necrolysis. N Engl J Med. 1995; 333:1600–7. Copyright © 1995 Massachusetts Medical Society. All rights reserved.

## Disease Highlights

**A.** Description of the lesion: flaccid bullae and vesicles that develop centrally within preexisting target lesion. The bullae rapidly erode, leaving red and raw skin (Figure 24–8).

**B.** Stevens-Johnson syndrome and toxic epidermal necrolysis are hypersensitivity reaction patterns involving the skin.

  **1.** These 2 conditions are often considered to be on a spectrum of severity. Stevens-Johnson syndrome involves less body surface area, whereas toxic epidermal necrolysis leads to considerable areas of full-thickness skin sloughing.

  **2.** Although the precise cause has not been found, drugs are involved in most cases.

**C.** More than 200 drugs have been implicated as causes of Stevens-Johnson syndrome and toxic epidermal necrolysis.

**D.** A well-done case-control trial identified the most likely culprits. These are listed in Table 24–3 with their associated ORs.

**E.** Disease course

  **1.** Prodromal symptoms, characterized by fever, malaise, headache, myalgias, as well as GI and respiratory complaints, occur over 1–2 weeks.

  **2.** The rash occurs initially on the face and central trunk as pink to red macules and papules.

  **3.** The rash may spread and evolve rapidly, with individual lesions becoming targetoid with dusky centers and ultimately coalescing into larger plaques.

  **4.** Flaccid bullae and vesicles may develop centrally within targets as the skin necroses.

  **5.** Blisters form and rapidly erode, leaving red and raw skin that becomes coated by a gray-white pseudomembrane.

  **6.** Mucous membranes

    **a.** Lesions on mucous membranes may accompany or precede the skin rash.

    **b.** The mucosal surfaces may be tender and burning.

    **c.** The lips are often swollen, cracked, bleeding, and crusted.

  **7.** The skin is extremely tender.

 A hallmark of Stevens-Johnson syndrome and toxic epidermal necrolysis is the presence of exquisite skin tenderness.

## Evidence-Based Diagnosis

**A.** Histopathology supports the clinical impression.

**B.** Pathology demonstrates epidermal necrosis with minimal evidence of epidermal and dermal inflammation.

## Treatment

**A.** If an offending drug is present, it must be discontinued.

**B.** Studies support the use of intravenous immunoglobulin in the early stages of the disease to abort progression.

**C.** Use of systemic corticosteroids is controversial. Studies have not proven that the benefit outweighs risk of immunosuppression.

**D.** Supportive care in a burn unit is recommended.

## CASE RESOLUTION

Within the hour the laboratory reported fluorescent antibody labeling of VZV, thus confirming the diagnosis of varicella zoster. The patient was prescribed valacyclovir for 7 days. He was instructed to keep the skin lesions covered to prevent contacts from being exposed to the infective vesicle fluid. He was counseled to avoid close contact with young infants and immunosuppressed individuals until all skin lesions are crusted.

## CHIEF COMPLAINT

PATIENT  ③

Ms. M is a 16-year-old developing girl who has many small red flaky patches, first on her trunk and now spreading to her extremities over the last 2 weeks (Figure 24–9). She denies any history of similar eruptions. She states she is otherwise feeling well. This eruption is not particularly itchy. On examination, there are many 1–2 cm discrete, brightly erythematous plaques and papules with adherent white scale. The lesions are predominantly on the trunk but extend onto the extremities. Some lesions appear somewhat linear in configuration, whereas most are round to oval in shape. The scale is confluent over the surface of the lesions. The nails are normal and the palms and soles are clear. The oropharynx is injected with some tonsillar enlargement but without exudates. The tongue appears geographic. The rest of the physical exam is unremarkable.

At this point, what is the leading hypothesis, what are the active alternatives, and is there a must not miss diagnosis? Given this differential diagnosis, what tests should be ordered?

## PRIORITIZING THE DIFFERENTIAL DIAGNOSIS

The appearance of the eruption suggests that this condition is papulosquamous in morphology (ie, it is composed primarily of papules and plaques with scale). Common causes of papulosquamous eruptions are psoriasis, pityriasis rosea, fungal infections, and nummular dermatitis.

The patient's age, acute onset of the rash, and the pattern of small papules and plaques are pivotal points suggesting either guttate psoriasis or pityriasis rosea. In addition, the finding of pharyngeal injection suggests that there may be an infectious component (as is common with guttate psoriasis). The configuration of the lesions and the scale can be very helpful in narrowing the differential diagnosis. This patient's scale is confluent over the surface of

the lesions, consistent with guttate psoriasis, whereas tinea and pityriasis rosea typically have an annular scale. Nummular dermatitis is usually found on the extremities and is associated with significant pruritus, making it an unlikely diagnosis in this case. Secondary syphilis needs to be considered as a "must not miss" diagnosis. Syphilis can present with plaques, but they often involve the palms and soles and lack an adherent scale (Table 24–4).

On further questioning, the patient does recall a sore throat several weeks ago. Her medical history is unremarkable. Her family history is remarkable only for a father with psoriasis.

Is the clinical information sufficient to make a diagnosis? If not, what other information do you need?

## Leading Hypothesis: Guttate Psoriasis

### Textbook Presentation

Guttate psoriasis generally presents with small, round, and slightly oval lesions on the back and trunk. The lesions have somewhat silvery, adherent scales.

**Table 24–4.** Diagnostic hypotheses for Ms. M.

| Diagnostic Hypotheses | Clinical Clues | Important Tests |
|---|---|---|
| **Leading Hypothesis** | | |
| Guttate psoriasis | Presents after acute pharyngitis Discrete small red plaques with adherent silvery scale | Morphology and pattern of lesions and positive throat culture |
| **Active Alternatives** | | |
| Pityriasis rosea | Classically starts with a single "herald patch" 1-2 weeks prior to disseminated eruption | Clinical diagnosis |
| Tinea corporis | Solitary or few lesions Annular lesions with a leading edge of scale Pruritic | Identification of fungus with KOH or culture. |
| Nummular dermatitis | Well-defined plaques with crust and papulovesicles Pruritic Symmetric distribution on extremities | Clinical diagnosis |
| Secondary syphilis | Palms and soles involved Thinner plaques without adherent scale | RPR, FTA |

*Figure 24–9.* Ms. M on initial presentation. (See Plate 9.)

## Disease Highlights

**A.** Description of lesion: small 0.5–1.5-cm, round or slightly oval lesions with characteristic overlying silvery scales. (See Figure 24–9.)

**B.** Character of the lesion

    **1.** Lesions tend to occur over the upper trunk and proximal extremities.

    **2.** Face, ears, and scalp may also be involved.

    **3.** The lesions may localize to sites of minor skin trauma, such as scrapes (Koebner phenomenon).

    **4.** Eruption generally persists for 3–4 months and then remits spontaneously.

**C.** Most commonly seen in young adults, frequently preceded by a streptococcal throat infection.

**D.** Affected patients are at increased risk for development of psoriasis vulgaris in the next 3–5 years.

**E.** There is an increased incidence of psoriasis in families.

## Evidence-Based Diagnosis

**A.** The diagnosis is often made based on the clinical presentation.

**B.** Finding of a streptococcal pharyngitis is supportive.

**C.** A skin biopsy of an established lesion may demonstrate classic histologic findings of psoriasis vulgaris.

## Treatment

**A.** Guttate psoriasis is typically a self-limited eruption, although clearance can take weeks to months.

**B.** Remission can be hastened with the use of UV light treatments.

**C.** Antibiotics such as erythromycin and tetracycline can be additionally helpful for flares.

    **1.** There is an infectious trigger in most cases.

    **2.** These antibiotics also function as suppressors of inflammation in the skin.

**D.** Topical corticosteroids can be effective on individual lesions.

**E.** Systemic corticosteroids should be avoided in psoriasis because withdrawal may trigger flares.

## MAKING A DIAGNOSIS

Based on the lesion's morphology, family history, and recent pharyngitis, guttate psoriasis was considered the likely diagnosis. A throat culture was sent. A skin biopsy was considered but not performed.

 Have you crossed a diagnostic threshold for the leading hypothesis, guttate psoriasis? Have you ruled out the active alternatives? Do other tests need to be done to exclude the alternative diagnoses?

## Alternative Diagnosis: Pityriasis Rosea

### Textbook Presentation

Pityriasis rosea commonly presents as a "herald patch" and then progresses to small, oval, scaly plaques over the trunk. The rash is mildly pruritic.

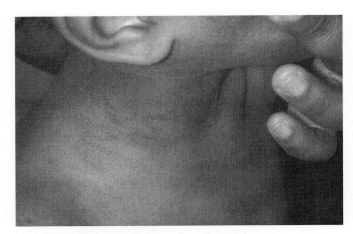

***Figure 24–10.*** Pityriasis rosea. (See Plate 10.)

## Disease Highlights

**A.** Description of lesion: oval or round plaque with scale (Figure 24–10).

**B.** Character of the lesion

    **1.** The primary eruption appears as a single oval or round, pink to brownish plaque with a collarette of scale around the inner margin of the lesion (the herald patch). This herald patch most often occurs on the trunk and is often misdiagnosed as tinea corporis.

    **2.** One to 2 weeks after the appearance of the herald patch, the secondary eruption emerges as generalized smaller but similar oval scaly plaques distributed along skin tension lines in a "fir tree" pattern.

    **3.** Variable degrees of pruritus

    **4.** Spontaneous resolution occurs over 8–12 weeks, often with subsequent postinflammatory hypopigmentation or hyperpigmentation.

**C.** A history of a mild prodrome of malaise, nausea, headache, and low-grade fever may be present.

**D.** Pityriasis rosea is a common worldwide disease without genetic or racial predilection, occurring sporadically throughout the year.

**E.** A viral cause is postulated; evidence suggests but does not confirm a role for human herpesvirus 7.

## Evidence-Based Diagnosis

**A.** The diagnosis is clinical, based on morphology and distribution of the skin lesions.

**B.** Skin biopsy demonstrates many nonspecific findings of a subacute dermatitis but can provide supportive evidence for the diagnosis.

## Treatment

**A.** No specific treatment is indicated or effective; the condition resolves over 8–12 weeks.

**B.** In cases with severe pruritus, symptomatic treatments, such as antihistamines and mild topical corticosteroids, may be beneficial.

**C.** UV B phototherapy has been advocated to decrease the severity, particularly when administered early in the course. This treatment may worsen the postinflammatory dyspigmentation.

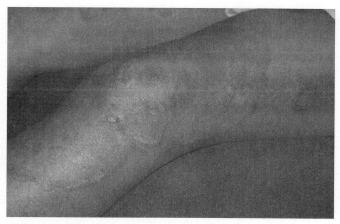

**Figure 24–11.** Tinea corporis. (See Plate 11.)

## Alternative Diagnosis: Tinea Corporis

### Textbook Presentation

Tinea corporis commonly presents as round, pink, plaques with small peripheral papules and a rim of scales. The neck and back are the most common locations (Figure 24–11).

### Disease Highlights

A. Description of the lesion: multiple lesions are possible.

1. Circular lesions with a sharply marginated raised border and central clearing, arising by centrifugal spread of the fungus from the initial site of infection

2. Inflammatory lesions may demonstrate pustules or vesicles, especially around the margin.

3. Overlying scale is common, typically more prominent at the border of the lesion.

4. Solitary lesions may occur, or there may be multiple plaques that remain discrete or become confluent.

B. The degree of associated inflammatory change is variable, depending on the causative species of fungus.

C. The wide variation in clinical presentation depends on the species of fungus, size of the inoculum, body site infected, and immune status of the patient.

### Evidence-Based Diagnosis

A. Identification of the fungus by microscopic examination of scales after application of 5–20% potassium hydroxide

B. Culture of tissue material (such as the scale)

C. Histopathology is rarely necessary to make the diagnosis of a superficial infection, but with the use of fungal stains the cell walls may be visible in fixed sections.

### Treatment

A. Both topical and systemic antifungal agents are effective.

B. Decision of which to use is based on the extent and location of the infection.

C. Hair-bearing sites often require systemic therapy.

## Alternative Diagnosis: Nummular Dermatitis

### Textbook Presentation

Nummular dermatitis generally presents as an extremely pruritic rash of numerous, round, crusted lesions on a patient's legs.

### Disease Highlights

A. Description of lesions: well-demarcated coin-shaped lesions composed of minute vesicles and papules on an erythematous base. The lesions have an overlying crust, frequently with a weeping exudate (Figure 24–12).

B. Nummular dermatitis is an acute eruption of numerous lesions predominantly on the extremities.

C. The lesions are severely pruritic.

D. The eruption runs a remitting and relapsing course.

E. Patients are often atopic.

F. Secondary infection is frequently present.

### Evidence-Based Diagnosis

A. Microscopic examination of a scraping will rule out tinea.

B. Histopathology can assist in the diagnosis by demonstrating the features of an acute dermatitis.

### Treatment

A. If present, secondary infections often require treatment with systemic antibiotics.

B. Antihistamines can help alleviate the pruritus.

C. Skin care, especially bathing practices and appropriate use of emollients, should be stressed.

D. Topical corticosteroids are useful for flares.

## Alternative Diagnosis: Secondary Syphilis

### Textbook Presentation

Secondary syphilis presents as oval macules in sexually active people. The lesions are present diffusely, including on the palms and soles. A history of a transient, painless, genital ulcer in the preceding weeks can often be obtained.

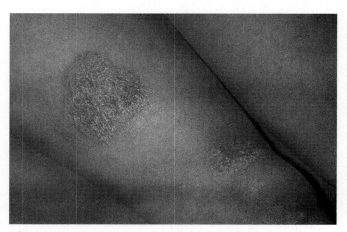

**Figure 24–12.** Nummular dermatitis. (See Plate 12.)

### Disease Highlights

**A.** Description of lesion: papules and plaques distributed over the entire body. They are copper red to hyperpigmented in color.

**B.** Character of the lesion

    **1.** There may be variable lesions at different stages of disease.

        **a.** A fleeting eruption of symmetric, coppery red, round and oval macules may be seen early in the secondary stage, about 8 weeks after the infecting exposure.

        **b.** The later, classic eruption includes involvement of mucosal surfaces and palms and soles.

        **c.** In the latest phases, thick scales may cover the plaques.

    **2.** The rashes of secondary syphilis are nonpruritic.

    **3.** The lesions are generally symmetrically distributed.

### Evidence-Based Diagnosis

**A.** The Venereal Disease Research Laboratories (VDRL) and fluorescent treponemal antibody (FTA) tests are 100% sensitive for secondary syphilis.

**B.** FTA tests have specificities in the high 90% range.

### Treatment

Penicillin is the treatment of choice for secondary syphilis.

## CASE RESOLUTION

The patient's throat culture revealed group A streptococcus. A clinical diagnosis of guttate psoriasis was made. The patient was prescribed a 3-week course of erythromycin as well as topical corticosteroids and topical calcipotriene (a vitamin D derivative). UV B treatments, 3 times weekly, were begun to induce remission of the psoriatic flare. She was counseled on her risk for future development of psoriasis vulgaris.

Guttate psoriasis affects those with a predisposition toward psoriasis. The guttate flares tend to remit quite reliably; however, affected individuals are at increased risk for the development of chronic psoriasis.

## OTHER IMPORTANT CUTANEOUS DISORDERS

## Urticaria

### Textbook Presentation

Urticaria typically presents as an itchy rash with large or small, palpable, red areas over the entire body. The rash is variable, with no one lesion lasting very long. Both the rash and the pruritus respond to antihistamines.

### Disease Highlights

**A.** Description of the lesion: transient pink to red smooth flat-topped papules and plaques that may coalesce into giant lesions. The lesions often leave purple discoloration or central clearing when they fade (Figure 24–13).

**B.** Characteristics of the lesion

    **1.** Individual lesions should resolve within 24 hours while new lesions may continue to develop.

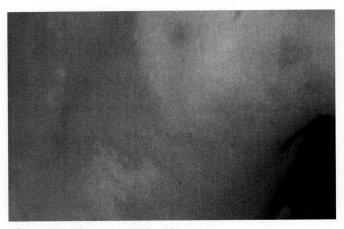

***Figure 24–13.*** Urticaria. (See Plate 13.)

    **2.** The eruption is typically accompanied by itch, but excoriations are rare.

**C.** Mucous membranes, eyelids, hands, and feet may develop deeper subcutaneous swelling manifesting as angioedema.

**D.** Most urticaria is acute, lasting less than 6 weeks.

**E.** Urticaria is a hypersensitivity reaction to numerous insults.

    **1.** Etiologic factors can be remembered with the mnemonic *I-I-I-I-I.*

        **a.** Infection

        **b.** Infestation

        **c.** Ingestion

        **d.** Inhalation

        **e.** Injection

    **2.** Idiopathic should probably be added to this list because the etiologic agent may induce an immunologic cascade that persists in the absence of the inciting agent.

**F.** Chronic urticaria can also be seen in the setting of systemic disease such as collagen vascular disease, malignancy, parasitosis, and chronic infection.

### Evidence-Based Diagnosis

**A.** Clinical findings of typical transient urticaria are diagnostic, and a skin biopsy is rarely indicated.

**B.** The morphologic differential diagnosis often includes the following:

    **1.** Erythema multiforme (because of the targetoid appearance of some urticaria)

    **2.** Insect bite reactions

    **3.** The early phases of bullous pemphigoid

**C.** Urticaria can be distinguished from all of the above disorders because it is the only one with lesions that last less than 24 hours.

**D.** A careful history, including review of medications, recent exposures, and food ingestion, is the most important aspect of the evaluation to determine a cause.

**E.** Laboratory evaluation is sometimes undertaken in cases of chronic urticaria, but studies have shown that relevant results are so rarely found without other symptoms that this approach is discouraged.

## Treatment

**A.** Identification of the inciting agent (medication, supplement, infection) is paramount and should be addressed as the first step in management.

**B.** Antihistamines are the mainstay of therapy. H₁-blockers should be given on a regular dosing schedule until the eruption is suppressed and then tapered gradually to prevent rebound flare.

**C.** Combinations of different H₁-blockers can be effective when a single agent is inadequate.

**D.** Addition of H₂-blockers may be helpful in refractory cases.

## Purpura/Petechiae

### Textbook Presentation

Purpura and petechiae are seen in patients with bleeding diatheses or vascular damage. Petechiae are capillary hemorrhages that present as nonblanching, pinpoint, red spots over dependent body parts, most commonly the lower extremities. Purpura are larger hemorrhages into the skin.

 Purpura are associated with a variety of life-threatening diseases such as vasculitis and sepsis.

### Disease Highlights

**A.** Description of the lesion: petechiae are red, blue or purple, nonblanching, pinpoint spots. Purpura are larger (up to several centimeters) macules, papules, or plaques that may or may not be palpable (Figure 24–14).

**B.** Both purpura and petechiae are, to some degree, nonblanching; (ie, the color cannot be compressed out of the lesion by pressure).

**C.** The shape of these lesions is variable, ranging from stellate to round or oval or targetoid to retiform (netlike).

**D.** The color, texture, and configuration of these lesions will be helpful in constructing a differential diagnosis of the cause.

**E.** The differential diagnosis of purpura/petechiae is vast, and many classification schemes have been proposed. The first step is to differentiate ecchymoses from purpura and petechiae.

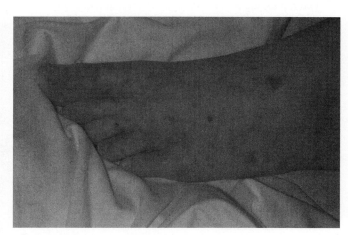

***Figure 24–14.*** Purpura. (See Plate 14.)

**F.** Ecchymoses

   **1.** Ecchymoses are the most common form of hemorrhage in the skin.

   **2.** They are typically induced by trauma and, therefore, are seen on trauma-prone sites such as the dorsal hand, forearm, lateral thigh, and shin.

   **3.** The shape of ecchymoses tends to be geometric (rectangular) or linear because they are induced by an external force.

   **4.** Predisposing factors to ecchymoses include weakening of the dermal structure secondary to age, corticosteroid use, solar damage, and vitamin C deficiency (scurvy), as well as coagulation defects.

**G.** Petechiae are most commonly associated with thrombocytopenia.

 Petechiae are commonly caused by thrombocytopenia.

**H.** Purpura

   **1.** Like petechiae, purpura signify hemorrhage into the skin.

   **2.** The hemorrhage may

     **a.** Be simple extravasation through leaky vessel walls.

     **b.** Be accompanied by inflammation that is damaging vessel walls. (These lesions are often partially blanching because the inflammatory component blanches while the hemorrhagic component does not.)

     **c.** Be the result of occlusion of a vessel leading to ischemic damage to the skin.

   **3.** The degree to which purpuric lesions are palpable is helpful diagnostically.

     **a.** Nonpalpable hemorrhage in the skin is most concerning for thrombocytopenia or abnormal platelet function.

     **b.** Extravasation of blood alone into deep tissue layers can produce a nodule (such as occurs with a hematoma).

     **c.** Edema associated with the vessel injury (such as in cases of inflammatory vasculitis) may cause a palpable lesion.

### Evidence-Based Diagnosis

**A.** An evaluation of clotting (platelet number, function and measures of coagulation) is indicated to determine if purpura and petechiae are symptoms of a coagulopathy or vasculitis.

**B.** A skin biopsy can be helpful in determining

   **1.** The size and location of affected vessels within the dermal and subcutaneous tissues.

   **2.** The degree and character of associated inflammation.

   **3.** The type of vessel damage (leukocytoclastic or granulomatous).

   **4.** The presence and character of any occlusions within vessels (organisms, calcium, fibrin).

**C.** Immunofluorescence studies of histologic specimens can be helpful in identifying antibody and complement deposits on vessels walls.

### Treatment

**A.** Treatment is directed toward management of the underlying cause of the vessel damage.

**B.** Supportive therapy includes local wound care and prevention of secondary infection.

# Skin Cancer

There are innumerable specific forms of skin cancer, deriving from all of the structures of the skin and subcutaneous tissues. In addition, many cancers will metastasize to the skin. The three most common skin cancers are described.

## 1. Basal Cell Carcinoma

### Textbook Presentation

Basal cell carcinoma most commonly presents as a flesh-colored, translucent, or slightly red papule or nodule, classically displaying a rolled border. Most commonly presents on the head or neck of older adults.

### Disease Highlights

A. Description of lesion: the typical lesion is a flesh-colored, translucent, or slightly red papule or nodule, classically displaying a rolled border (Figure 24–15).

   1. Lesions are often friable, bleeding easily and developing crust. Telangiectasias on the surface can be a helpful sign.

   2. Large tumors can be locally destructive.

B. Basal cell carcinoma is the most common malignant tumor in humans.

C. Lesions are typically asymptomatic except for the observation of easy bleeding from a site.

   1. Only rarely is pain associated.

   2. Metastasis from a basal cell carcinoma is rare.

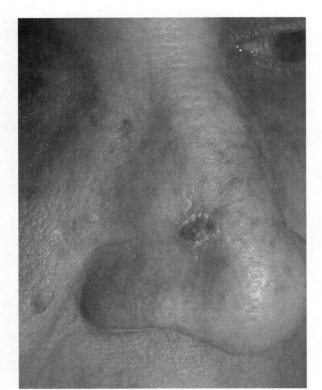

***Figure 24–15.*** Basal cell carcinoma. (See Plate 15.) (Photograph courtesy of Dr. Anne E. Laumann.)

D. Individuals at risk are adults with fair hair and eyes, easy freckling, and propensity for sunburn

   1. Patients with skin of color are less likely to be affected.

   2. Men and women are about equally affected.

   3. Exposure to UV light has long been believed to play a causative role in the development of this tumor, although the exact mechanism is not clear.

   4. Chronic wounds and sites of inflammation as well as immunosuppression can predispose to development of this tumor.

   5. Exposure to arsenic is another risk factor for basal cell carcinoma.

E. The head and neck are the most common sites affected with this tumor.

   1. Only 10–15% of tumors develop on sun-protected skin.

   2. The nose is the most common site, accounting for 20–30% of all cases.

F. Basal cell carcinoma is likely derived from the hair follicle. The name implies a resemblance of the tumor cells to the basal cells of the epidermis, although this is not believed to be their derivation.

G. Patients have up to a 45% risk of developing subsequent basal cell carcinomas in the 5 years after initial diagnosis.

### Evidence-Based Diagnosis

Histologic evaluation of affected tissue is the gold standard for diagnosis.

### Treatment

A. The goal of therapy is to eliminate the tumor and prevent local tissue destruction. Numerous methods are available to accomplish this goal, and selection depends on tumor size, type, and location, patient characteristics, and patient preferences.

B. Five-year recurrence rates vary by treatment modality. The lowest recurrence rate is achieved with Mohs micrographic surgery.

   1. This method involves excision of the visible tumor, followed by microscopic evaluation of frozen tissue sections to visualize tumor margins and repeat local excision until all margins are clear of tumor.

   2. The technique allows for maximal tissue sparing while ensuring complete eradication of tumor.

C. Follow-up of patients for recurrent, or subsequent tumors is critical.

## 2. Squamous Cell Carcinoma

### Textbook Presentation

Squamous cell carcinoma most commonly presents as a firm but somewhat indistinct nodule. It may evolve from actinic keratoses on the sun-exposed skin of middle-aged people.

### Disease Highlights

A. Description of lesion: lesions are firm but somewhat indistinct nodules that may arise from an in situ carcinoma or in normal skin. Tumors may become ulcerated or bleed easily and become crusted (Figure 24–16).

   1. The surface may be smooth, verrucous, or papillomatous, with or without scaling.

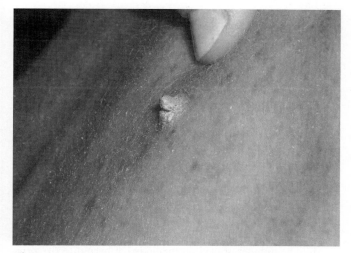

**Figure 24–16.** Squamous cell carcinoma. (See Plate 16.) (Photograph courtesy of Dr. Anne E. Laumann.)

2. Fixation to underlying structures develops as the lesion invades locally.

3. In situ lesions tend to be sharply demarcated erythematous scaling plaques.

B. This tumor most commonly affects fair-skinned individuals with excessive sun exposure.

1. Often evolves from actinic keratoses on sun-exposed skin in these patients.

2. UV radiation is a major risk factor for the development of this tumor.

3. Additional predisposing factors include

   a. Radiation therapy

   b. Chronic scar formation

   c. Chemical carcinogens, such as hydrocarbons

   d. Viral exposures

   e. Thermal exposures

   f. Arsenic

   g. Long-term immunosuppression (such as in renal transplant recipients).

C. Metastasis from squamous cell carcinoma is a significant risk.

1. The incidence of metastasis varies greatly with anatomic location, level of invasion, and cellular differentiation and also depends on the individual tumor precipitants.

2. The incidence of metastasis from squamous cell carcinoma ranges from 1% to 20% in some series and is as high as 42% in others.

3. Cutaneous lesions arising in solar keratosis have the lowest risk for metastasis, and lip lesions have the highest. Mucosal squamous cell carcinomas in general have a higher risk of metastasis.

D. Oral squamous cell carcinoma is predominantly a disease of adult men.

1. Risk factors are alcohol and tobacco use.

2. When detected in the early asymptomatic stage, these cancers are easily curable.

E. Incidence increases with age and varies with geographic location, ethnicity, and behavior patterns.

**Evidence-Based Diagnosis**

A. Histologic evaluation of affected tissue is the gold standard for diagnosis.

B. A high index of suspicion may be necessary to recognize a potential tumor when its appearance or location is unusual. For example, the verrucous form of squamous cell carcinoma can be mistaken for a wart.

**Treatment**

A. The goal of treatment is eradication of the tumor while producing the least disability and dysfunction for the patient.

B. Careful evaluation for the presence of metastatic disease is paramount. This may include lymph node dissection in some instances.

C. Multiple destruction modalities are available and are selected based on size, shape, and location of the tumor as well as patient preferences. These modalities include, but are not limited to

1. Excisional surgery

2. Mohs micrographic surgery

3. Electrosurgery

4. Radiation therapy

5. Local immunotherapy

D. Wide destruction of these tumors usually results in cure as squamous cell carcinomas grow by direct extension. However, residual tumor can invade and extend along peripheral nerves, allowing a deep recurrence on occasion.

E. A large percentage of squamous cell carcinomas could be prevented by avoidance of excessive solar exposure. Routine screening for tumors, especially in high-risk patients, is also imperative.

## 3. Melanoma

### Textbook Presentation

Melanoma presents as a dark brown macule in a middle-aged person. The lesion has pigment variation throughout and irregular borders.

### Disease Highlights

A. Description of lesion: the most common type of melanoma is superficial spreading (Figure 24–17).

1. These tumors may present as a dark brown to black macule or thin plaque, typically with pigment variation throughout and irregular borders.

2. With growth, the surface becomes glossy.

3. The most common location of superficial spreading melanomas is on the upper back in males and the leg in females.

B. These cancers are most commonly diagnosed in the fourth and fifth decades of life.

C. Melanoma may arise in a preexisting melanocytic nevus or de novo.

D. Multiple subtypes exist, including lentigo maligna melanoma, superficial spreading melanoma, nodular melanoma, acral lentiginous melanoma, and amelanotic melanoma among others.

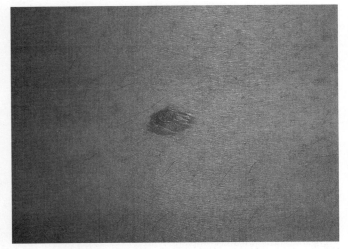

***Figure 24–17.*** Malignant melanoma. (See Plate 17.) (Photograph courtesy of Dr. Anne E. Laumann.)

1. Nodular melanoma is the second most common type of melanoma.

   a. Presents most often on the head, neck, or trunk.

   b. These tumors evolve rapidly over months.

   c. They appear as a blue-black, reddish, purplish, or even a nonpigmented papule or nodule.

2. Acral lentiginous melanoma is the predominant type of melanoma seen in the more pigmented races, such as Africans, Asians, and Indians.

   a. Acral lentiginous melanoma occurs on the palms and soles and beneath the nail plate.

   b. Diagnosis of these lesions is often delayed; therefore, they are often of a more advanced stage at diagnosis.

   c. Affected individuals tend to be older.

3. Lentigo maligna melanoma is a rare type of melanoma found predominantly in the elderly on the sun-exposed portions of the head and neck.

   a. The tumor is usually flat, with irregular borders and a diameter of several centimeters.

   b. Color varies throughout from tan to brown to black and purple and blue.

E. Melanoma is a tumor of melanocytes.

   1. Benign pigmented nevi are composed of altered melanocytes, termed "nevomelanocytes."

   2. Malignant transformation of melanocytes and nevomelanocytes can result in melanoma, arising de novo from normal skin, or from a preexisting nevomelanocytic lesion (nevus).

F. The incidence of cutaneous melanoma is increasing steadily in the United States. In 1935, the lifetime risk of an American developing melanoma was 1 in 1500 individuals, whereas in 2002 the risk was 1 in 68 individuals.

   1. In 2003, it is estimated that melanoma will be diagnosed in 54,200 Americans, and 7600 will die of the disease.

   2. Melanoma will be the fifth most common cancer among males and the seventh most common cancer among females.

G. Epidemiologic studies strongly suggest that sun exposure is a major risk factor for the development of cutaneous melanoma in the light-skinned populations.

   1. Intense intermittent episodes of sun exposure before 18 years of age are thought to engender the highest risk in susceptible populations.

   2. Phenotypic features have been associated with increased risk for cutaneous melanoma: light skin pigmentation, ease of sunburning, blond or red hair, prominent freckling, and blue or green eyes.

H. Familial melanoma accounts for 8–12% of cases. Those with at least 2 first-degree relatives with a history of melanoma are at particularly high risk.

I. Dysplastic nevi (clinically atypical appearing nevi) are thought to be markers of an individual with an increased risk of development of cutaneous melanoma.

   1. The number of nevi on the body has been directly correlated with the magnitude of melanoma risk.

   2. About one-third of melanomas have been associated with an underlying nevus.

J. Recurrences of disease generally occur in a stepwise manner, first locally, then in regional lymph nodes, and lastly as distant metastases.

## Evidence-Based Diagnosis

A. An excisional biopsy is the preferred method for obtaining tissue for diagnosis. This preserves the extent of the primary tumor and all associated histologic features without disrupting the lymphatic architecture.

B. Full-thickness incisional or punch biopsies of lesions too large to excise fully or in anatomically sensitive locations are satisfactory.

C. The histologic diagnosis of melanoma is based on a constellation of features; no single feature is diagnostic. Both cytologic and architectural features are evaluated.

D. The staging system for melanoma focuses on tumor thickness and presence of ulceration as the most important initial prognostic variables in localized disease (stages I and II). Stage III has regional nodal involvement, and stage IV has distant metastases.

## Treatment

A. Management of cutaneous melanoma is guided by stage of disease. Wide excision of tumors is the general rule.

B. Sentinel lymph node mapping may be beneficial diagnostically in more advanced stages, decreasing the complications associated with full lymph node dissections.

C. Adjuvant treatment options for advanced stage disease include interferon alpha-2b, radiation of nodal basins, chemotherapy, and other novel strategies such as tumor vaccines.

D. Follow-up of melanoma patients is critical to detect recurrences as well as new primary tumors and to provide ongoing education.

E. Melanoma prevention strategies focus on education about the risks of UV exposure via sunlight or tanning machines, sun protection guidelines, and the importance of routine self-skin exams.

   1. Early detection is important for improving outcomes.

**2.** Patients should be instructed on the importance of their own skin examination and what constitutes a worrisome mole, easily remembered by the *ABCDE*s of mole evaluation.

**a.** A: asymmetry

**b.** B: borders that are irregular or changing

**c.** C: color that is irregular or changing

**d.** D: diameter > 6 mm (or larger than a pencil eraser)

**e.** E: evolution of the lesion in general

## REFERENCES

Gnann JW Jr, Whitley RJ. Clinical practice. Herpes zoster. N Engl J Med. 2002;347:340–6.

Kotani N, Kushikata T, Hashimoto H et al. Intrathecal methylprednisolone for intractable postherpetic neuralgia. N Engl J Med. 2000;343:1514–9.

Kozel MM, Mekkes JR, Bossuyt PM, Bos JD. The effectiveness of a history-based diagnostic approach in chronic urticaria and angioedema. Arch Dermatol. 1998;134:1575–80.

Lens MB, Dawes M. Global perspectives of contemporary epidemiological trends of cutaneous malignant melanoma. Br J Dermatol. 2004;150:179–85.

Oxman MN, Levin MJ, Johnson GR et al; Shingles Prevention Study Group. A vaccine to prevent herpes zoster and postherpetic neuralgia in older adults. N Engl J Med. 2005;352(22):2271–84.

Roujeau JC, Kelly JP, Naldi L et al. Medication use and the risk of Stevens-Johnson syndrome or toxic epidermal necrolysis. N Engl J Med. 1995;333:1600–7.

Simor AE, Phillips E, McGeer A et al. Randomized controlled trial of chlorhexidine gluconate for washing, intranasal mupirocin, and rifampin and doxycycline versus no treatment for the eradication of methicillin-resistant *Staphylococcus aureus* colonization. Clin Infect Dis. 2007;44(2):178–85.

Viard I, Wehrli P, Bullani R et al. Inhibition of toxic epidermal necrolysis by blockade of CD95 with human intravenous immunoglobulin. Science. 1998;282:490–3.

Whitley RJ, Weiss H, Gnann JW Jr et al. Acyclovir with and without prednisone for the treatment of herpes zoster. Ann Intern Med. 1996;125:376–83.

## Summary Table

| Primary Lesion Morphology | Diagnosis | Clinical Clues | Distribution | Figure |
|---|---|---|---|---|
| Folliculopapular eruptions | Acne | Presents in adolescence<br>Waxing and waning lesions<br>Inflammatory papules, pustules, comedones, and nodulocysts | Face, chest, and back | 24-1 |
| | Rosacea | Present in adults<br>Telangiectasias and persistent centrofacial erythema occasionally with inflammatory red papules and papulopustules | Face | 24-2 |
| Blistering disorders | Herpes zoster | Closely grouped vesicles on an erythematous base<br>Over 2-3 days, the lesions become pustular and then crust over after 7-10 days<br>Pain and paresthesias over involved dermatome may precede the rash | Single, unilateral dermatome | 24-3 |
| | Bullous impetigo | Presents as flaccid, transparent bullae that rupture easily and leave a rim of scale and shallow moist erosion<br>Usually seen in children | Intertriginous areas | 24-4 |
| | Bullous arthropod bites | A cluster of large, tense blisters on exposed skin | Most common on the extremities | 24-6 |
| | Bullous pemphigoid | Seen in elderly patients<br>Sudden onset of 1-2 cm tense blisters and bright, red, urticarial plaques | Begin on the lower extremities and progresses upward | 24-7 |
| | Stevens-Johnson syndrome | Macular rash that subsequently blisters and then rapidly erodes<br>The skin is usually excruciatingly tender | Begins on chest and face and then spreads<br>Palms and soles often involved | 24-8 |
| Papulosquamous eruptions | Psoriasis | Well-demarcated erythematous plaques with silvery, adherent scales | Extensor surfaces, umbilicus, and scalp (Trunk and proximal extremities for guttate psoriasis) | 24-9 |
| | Pityriasis rosea | "Herald patch" progressing to small, oval, scaly plaques in a "fir tree pattern" | Trunk | 24-10 |
| | Tinea corporis | Round, pink, plaques with small peripheral papules and an advancing scaling border | Anywhere | 24-11 |
| | Nummular dermatitis | Extremely pruritic rash of numerous, round, crusted lesions | Legs | 24-12 |
| | Secondary syphilis | Oval macules presenting diffusely, including palms and soles<br>A history of a transient, painless, genital ulcer in the preceding weeks can often be obtained | Rash can be diffuse including palms and soles | |
| Skin cancers | Basal cell carcinoma | Flesh-colored, translucent, or slightly red papule or nodule, classically displaying a rolled border | Head, neck, or other sun-exposed skin | 24-15 |
| | Squamous cell carcinoma | Firm, but somewhat indistinct nodule or plaque | Sun-exposed skin | 24-16 |
| | Melanoma | Dark brown macule with pigment variation and irregular borders | Anywhere | 24-17 |
| Purpura and petechiae | Petechiae | Non-blanching, pinpoint, red spots | Dependent body parts, most commonly the lower extremities | |
| | Purpura | Red, blue or purple macules, papules or plaques, may or may not be palpable, up to several centimeter in diameter | Anywhere | 24-14 |

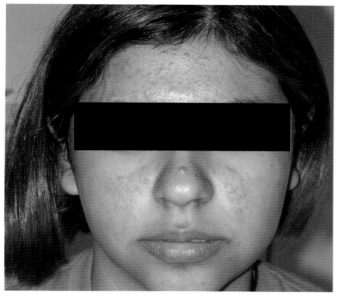

Plate 1. Ms. N. on initial presentation.

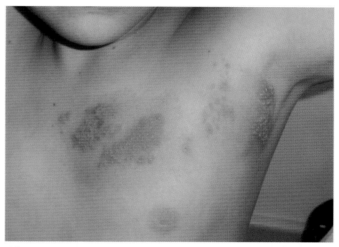

Plate 3. Mr. B. on initial presentation.

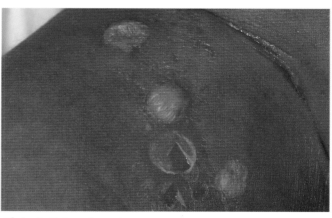

Plate 4. Bullous impetigo.

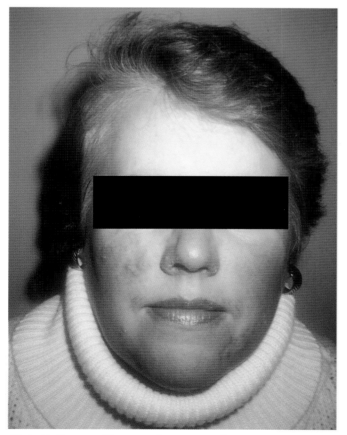

Plate 2. Rosacea (Photograph courtesy of Dr. Anne E. Laumann.)

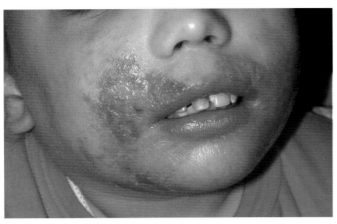

*Plate 5.* Impetigo.

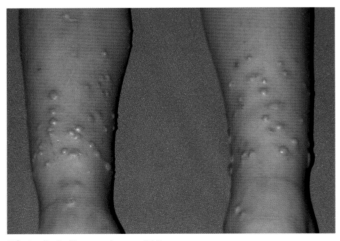

*Plate 6.* Bullous arthropod bites.

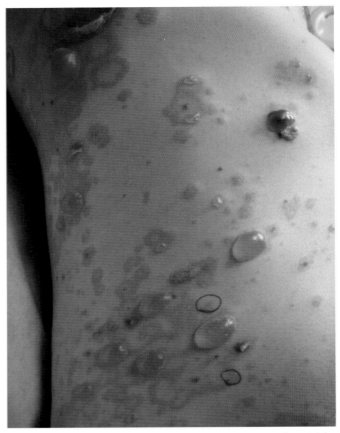

*Plate 7.* Bullous pemphigoid. (Photograph courtesy of Dr. Keith Duffy.)

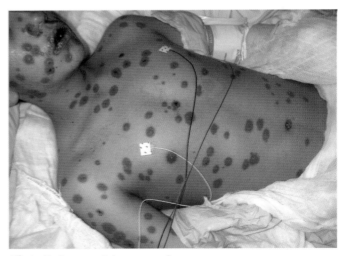

*Plate 8.* Stevens-Johnson syndrome.

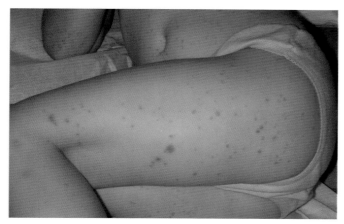

Plate 9. Ms. M on initial presentation.

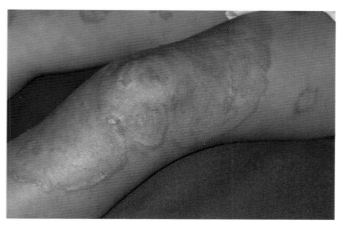

Plate 11. Tinea corporis.

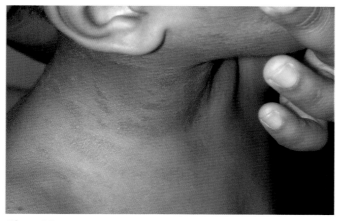

Plate 10. Pityriasis rosea.

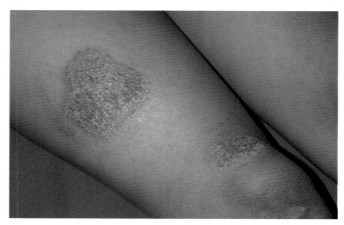

Plate 12. Nummular dermatitis.

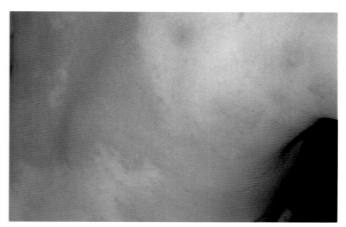

Plate 13. Urticaria.

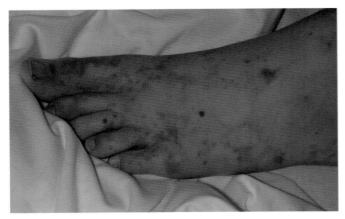

Plate 14. Purpura.

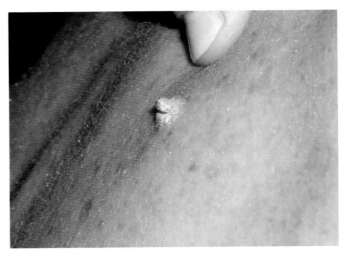

Plate 16. Squamous cell carcinoma. (Photograph courtesy of Dr. Anne E. Laumann.)

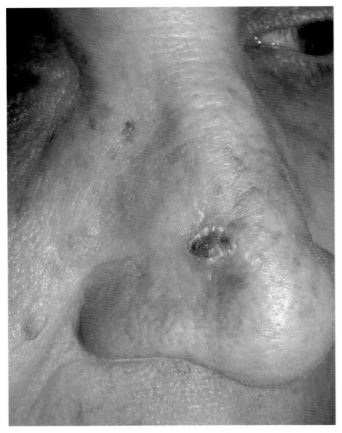

Plate 15. Basal cell carcinoma. (Photograph courtesy of Dr. Anne E. Laumann.)

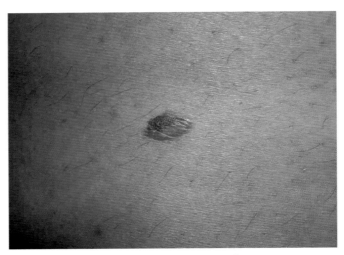

Plate 17. Malignant melanoma. (Photograph courtesy of Dr. Anne E. Laumann.)

# I have a patient with acute renal failure. How do I determine the cause?

## CHIEF COMPLAINT

PATIENT ▽ 1

Mr. T is 77-year-old man with acute renal failure (ARF).

☑ What is the differential diagnosis of ARF? How would you frame the differential?

## CONSTRUCTING A DIFFERENTIAL DIAGNOSIS

ARF is defined as an abrupt decrease in glomerular filtration rate (GFR), with a concomitant increase in serum creatinine, resulting in an inability to maintain fluid and electrolyte balance. It occurs over hours or days and can occur in the presence of previously normal renal function or in patients with chronic kidney disease (CKD). There is no standard definition, and criteria commonly used include an increase in serum creatinine of > 0.5 mg/dL, an increase of more than 20% above baseline, or a decrease in GFR of at least 50%.

The framework for the differential diagnosis is a combination of anatomic and pathophysiologic:

A. Prerenal (due to renal hypoperfusion)
1. Hypovolemia
   a. GI fluid loss
   b. Renal loss
   c. Hemorrhage
   d. Third spacing
   e. Decreased effective circulating volume
      (1) Heart failure (HF)
      (2) Cirrhosis
2. Hypotension
   a. Sepsis
   b. Cardiogenic shock
   c. Anaphylaxis
   d. Anesthesia- and medication-induced
   e. Relative hypotension below patient's autoregulatory level
3. Changes in renal hemodynamics
   a. Nonsteroidal antiinflammatory drugs (NSAIDs)/cyclooxygenase (COX)-2 inhibitors
   b. ACE inhibitors/angiotensin receptor blockers (ARBs)
   c. Renal artery thrombosis or embolism
   d. Abdominal aortic aneurysm

B. Intrarenal
1. Vascular
   a. Vasculitis
   b. Malignant hypertension
   c. Cholesterol emboli
   d. Thrombotic microangiopathies
      (1) Thrombotic thrombocytopenic purpura
      (2) Hemolytic uremic syndrome
      (3) Disseminated intravascular coagulopathy
2. Glomerular
   a. Inflammatory
      (1) Postinfectious glomerulonephritis (GN)
      (2) Cryoglobulinemia
      (3) Henoch-Schönlein purpura
      (4) Systemic lupus erythematosus
      (5) Antineutrophil cytoplasmic antibody associated GN
      (6) Anti-glomerular basement membrane disease
   b. Thrombotic microangiopathies
3. Tubular injury (acute tubular necrosis [ATN])
   a. Ischemic, due to prolonged renal hypoperfusion
   b. Toxin induced
      (1) Medications (such as aminoglycosides)
      (2) Radiocontrast media
      (3) Heavy metals (cisplatinum)
      (4) Intratubular pigments (myoglobin, hemoglobin), crystals (uric acid, oxalate), or proteins (myeloma)
4. Interstitial
   a. Acute interstitial nephritis
   b. Bilateral pyelonephritis
   c. Infiltration (lymphoma, sarcoidosis)

C. Postrenal
1. Mechanical
   a. Ureteral (must be bilateral obstruction to cause ARF)
      (1) Stones
      (2) Tumors
      (3) Hematoma
      (4) Retroperitoneal adenopathy or fibrosis
   b. Bladder neck
      (1) Benign prostatic hyperplasia (BPH) or prostate cancer
      (2) Tumors
      (3) Stones

   **c.** Urethral

   **(1)** Strictures

   **(2)** Tumors

   **(3)** Obstructed indwelling catheters

**2.** Neurogenic bladder

An algorithm outlining the diagnostic approach to acute renal failure appears at the end of the chapter.

## Measuring Kidney Function

**A.** GFR

**1.** Best overall measure of kidney function

**2.** Normal = 130 mL/min/1.73m² in young men (120 mL/min/1.73m² in women)

**3.** Difficult to accurately measure in clinical practice

**B.** Creatinine

**1.** Generation determined by muscle mass and dietary intake

**2.** Level varies with age, sex, race or ethnic group, muscle mass, diet, nutritional status

**3.** The relationship between creatinine and GFR varies inversely and exponentially, so that relatively small changes in serum creatinine may reflect significant decreases in GFR (Figure 25–1).

**C.** Creatinine clearance

**1.** Creatinine is filtered by glomeruli *and* secreted by proximal tubule, so creatinine clearance exceeds GFR.

**2.** Must be calculated with a 24-hour urine collection, which is inconvenient for patients and often incomplete.

**D.** Cystatin C

**1.** Freely filtered by glomerulus

**2.** Less variable than creatinine

**3.** Not yet in widespread use

**E.** Estimating GFR

**1.** Cockcroft-Gault formula (multiply by 0.85 for women):

$$C_{cr} = \frac{[(140 - age) \times weight\ in\ kg]}{72 \times creatinine\ in\ mg/dL}$$

**a.** Systematically overestimates GFR

**b.** Does not adjust for body surface area

**2.** Modification of Diet in Renal Disease Study Equation (MDRD) study equation:

$$GFR = 175 \times (standardized\ creatinine)^{-1.154} \times (age)^{-0.203} \times 0.742\ (if\ female)\ or\ \times 1.212\ (if\ African\ American)$$

**a.** Online calculator available: http://www.kidney.org/professionals/kdoqi/gfr_calculator.cfm

**b.** Most accurate in nonhospitalized patients known to have CKD

**c.** Less accurate in patients without kidney disease; values > 60 mL/min/1.73m² should be reported as "above 60" rather than an exact number

**d.** Overall, more accurate and now more commonly used than Cockcroft-Gault formula or 24-hour urine measurement of creatinine clearance.

Mr. T felt well until last night, when he had a shaking chill followed by a fever and the onset of a cough productive of rusty colored sputum. His fever has persisted, his cough has worsened, and he feels lethargic. His past medical history is notable for well-controlled hypertension and prostate cancer treated with radiation therapy 5 years ago. His current medications are hydrochlorothiazide and lisinopril. He smokes a few cigarettes a day and has

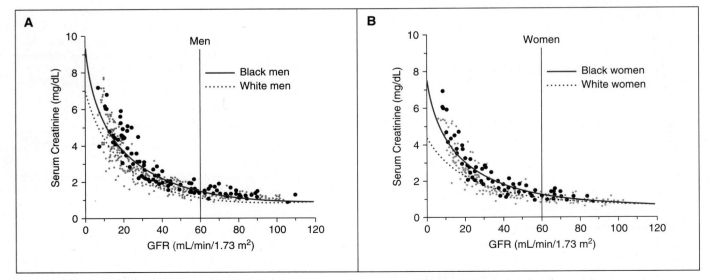

***Figure 25–1.*** Relationship of serum creatinine level to measured GFR. (Reproduced, with permission, from Levey AS, Bosch JP, Lewis JB, Greene T, Rogers N, Roth D. A more accurate method to estimate glomerular filtration rate from serum creatinine: a new prediction equation. Ann Intern Med. 1999;130:461–470.)

1 drink per week. His physical exam shows temperature, 38.6°C; BP, 90/60 mm Hg; pulse, 110 bpm; RR, 24 breaths per minute. His mucous membranes appear dry. Lung exam is notable for decreased breath sounds and crackles at the right lung base.

One month ago, his creatinine was 1.4 mg/dL. Six months ago, his PSA was 1.0. Laboratory test results now include WBC, 16,000/mcL (70% PMNs, 20% bands, 10% lymphocytes); Hgb, 10.2 g/dL; Hct, 32%; MCV, 88 mcm³; Na, 140 mEq/L; K, 5.4 mEq/L; Cl, 100 mEq/L; HCO₃ 19 mEq/L; BUN, 40 mg/dL; creatinine, 3.8 mg/dL; glucose, 102 mg/dL.

 At this point, what is the leading hypothesis, what are the active alternatives, and is there a must not miss diagnosis? Given this differential diagnosis, what tests should be ordered?

## PRIORITIZING THE DIFFERENTIAL DIAGNOSIS

 Although one etiology may be more likely than the others based on the presentation, the initial testing is generally the same for every patient with ARF.

The pivotal point in this patient's presentation is the hypotension, due to hypovolemia, sepsis (presumably pneumococcal based on his classic presentation), or both. Transient hypovolemia or hypotension causes prerenal azotemia, but prolonged hypotension leads to renal ischemia. It is likely he has been hypotensive long enough to have developed renal ischemia and consequent ATN. His history of CKD (baseline creatinine of 1.4 mg/dL), age, and chronic hypertension increase his risk of developing ATN whenever his renal blood flow is reduced. Nevertheless, it is necessary to make sure he does not also have a component of prerenal ARF due to volume depletion. Finally, despite his normal PSA a few months ago, he could have obstruction from BPH or recurrent prostate cancer. Post-streptococcal glomerulonephritis, an intrarenal cause of ARF, is not a consideration since that occurs after group A hemolytic streptococcal infections, not after pneumococcal infections. Table 25–1 lists the differential diagnosis.

 Because hypovolemia and obstruction are such treatable causes of ARF, they are always "must not miss" diagnoses.

The evaluation of ARF always begins with urine electrolytes and a urinalysis.

① Mr. T receives 1 L of normal saline, with no change in his BP. Urine is obtained prior to the fluid bolus and results include urine sodium, 40 mEq/h; urine chloride, 57 mEq/mL; urine creatinine, 45 mg/24 h, and urine urea nitrogen 250 g/24 h; urinalysis showed specific gravity, 1.010; leukocyte esterase, negative; glucose, negative; blood, negative; protein, trace; RBC, 1–2/hpf; WBC, 1–2/hpf; positive granular casts.

**Table 25–1.** Diagnostic hypotheses for Mr. T.

| Diagnostic Hypotheses | Clinical Clues | Important Tests |
|---|---|---|
| **Leading Hypothesis** | | |
| ATN | Hypotension from any cause<br>Exposure to toxins (especially radiocontrast media, aminoglycosides) | $FE_{Na}$<br>Urinalysis |
| **Active Alternative—Must Not Miss** | | |
| Hypovolemia | Orthostatic hypotension<br>Sunken eyes<br>Dry axilla<br>History of vomiting or diarrhea<br>Elderly | BUN/creatinine ratio<br>$FE_{Na}, FE_{urea}$ |
| Obstruction | Incontinence<br>Dribbling<br>Pelvic discomfort | Ultrasound |

 Is the clinical information sufficient to make a diagnosis? If not, what other information do you need?

## Leading Hypothesis: ATN

ATN is not synonymous with ARF; it is 1 cause of ARF.

### Textbook Presentation

The presentation ranges from asymptomatic (with discovery of an increased creatinine on routine laboratory testing) to symptoms of uremia (eg, lethargy, nausea, delirium, seizures, edema, and dyspnea).

### Disease Highlights

A. Etiology

1. Ischemia due to renal hypoperfusion prolonged enough to cause tubular cell damage

   a. Due to autoregulation, patients with normal kidneys and normal renal arteries can maintain normal renal blood flow and GFR with mean arterial pressures as low as 80 mm Hg.

   b. When renal artery pressure decreases, there is a prostaglandin-mediated drop in afferent arteriolar resistance and an angiotensin II–mediated increase in efferent arteriolar resistance; these changes maintain glomerular capillary pressure and GFR.

   c. If renal artery pressure drops below the autoregulatory range, endogenous vasoconstrictors cause an increase

***Table 25–2.*** Factors affecting autoregulation of glomerular pressure and glomerular filtration rate.

| Inability to decrease afferent arteriolar resistance | Inability to increase efferent arteriolar resistance | Vascular obstruction |
|---|---|---|
| Older age<br>Atherosclerosis<br>Chronic hypertension<br>Chronic kidney disease<br>Malignant hypertension<br>NSAIDs/COX-2 inhibitors<br>Sepsis<br>Hypercalcemia<br>Cyclosporine/tacrolimus<br>Renal artery stenosis | ACE inhibitors<br>Angiotensin receptor blockers | Renal artery stenosis |

COX, cyclooxygenase; NSAIDs, nonsteroidal antiinflammatory drugs.

in afferent arteriolar resistance, leading to reduced glomerular capillary pressure and GFR.

   **d.** Despite decreased perfusion, tubules remain intact initially; however, with prolonged ischemia, there is tubular injury and death.

   **e.** Patients with the conditions or exposures listed in Table 25–2, all of which impair autoregulation, are at higher risk for developing ATN.

  **2.** Toxin exposure (radiocontrast media, aminoglycosides, amphotericin B, cisplatin, Hgb, myoglobin, crystals, myeloma proteins)

**B.** Epidemiology and prognosis

  **1.** ATN accounts for 55–60% of ARF in hospitalized patients and for 11% in outpatients.

  **2.** Postoperative ATN and contrast-induced nephropathy (CIN) are the most common causes.

  **3.** Can be oliguric (urinary output < 400 mL/d) or nonoliguric.

  **4.** Mortality in hospitalized patients with ATN is about 37%; in ICU patients, mortality is about 78%.

  **5.** Risk factors for increased mortality include

    **a.** Male sex

    **b.** Advanced age

    **c.** Comorbid illness

    **d.** Malignancy

    **e.** Oliguria

    **f.** Sepsis

    **g.** Mechanical ventilation

    **h.** Multiorgan failure

    **i.** Severity of illness

  **6.** Full renal recovery generally occurs over 1–2 weeks in about 60% of survivors; a "post ATN diuresis," during which urinary output transiently increases, may be seen.

  **7.** Overall, 5–10% of patients with ATN require long-term dialysis; 33% of patients in whom ATN develops in the ICU and who survive require dialysis.

## Evidence-Based Diagnosis

 Urine electrolytes, urinalysis, and serum BUN and creatinine are used to distinguish ATN from prerenal states; ultrasound is used to distinguish ATN from obstruction.

**A.** Urine sodium

  **1.** Hypoperfusion causes increased reabsorption of sodium, water, and urea by the tubules; if prolonged ischemia leads to tubular damage, the tubules can no longer increase reabsorption, leading to urinary sodium loss.

  **2.** Consequently, there should be little sodium in the urine in prerenal ARF, whether measured by the amount of sodium in a spot urine sample, or by the fractional excretion of sodium ($FE_{Na}$).

  **3.**
$$FE_{Na} = \frac{urine\ Na/plasma\ Na}{urine\ creatinine/plasma\ creatinine} \times 100\%$$

$$= \frac{urine\ Na \times plasma\ creatinine}{Plasma\ Na \times urine\ creatinine} \times 100\%$$

  **4.** The test characteristics of urine sodium, $FE_{urea}$, and $FE_{Na}$ are shown in Table 25–3.

  **5.** When are the urine sodium and $FE_{Na}$ misleading?

    **a.** Urine sodium and $FE_{Na}$ will be high if the patient is taking diuretics or has received intravenous saline prior to collection of the urine sample, even if the patient is prerenal.

    **b.** Urine sodium and $FE_{Na}$ can be low in ATN due to rhabdomyolysis, myoglobinuria, hemolysis, sepsis, cirrhosis, HF, and CIN.

 $FE_{Na}$ is a better test than urine sodium for distinguishing prerenal states from ATN.

**B.** Fraction excretion of urea nitrogen ($FE_{urea}$)

  **1.**
$$FE_{urea} = \frac{urine\ urea\ nitrogen/blood\ urea\ nitrogen}{urine\ creatinine/plasma\ creatinine} \times 100\%$$

$$= \frac{urine\ urea\ nitrogen \times plasma\ creatinine}{blood\ urea\ nitrogen \times urine\ creatinine} \times 100\%$$

  **2.** In well-hydrated individuals, the $FE_{urea}$ is 50–65%.

  **3.** In prerenal ARF, the $FE_{urea} < 35\%$; in ATN, it is > 50%.

  **4.** The $FE_{urea}$ is not affected by diuretic use.

  **5.** In patients taking diuretics, the sensitivity of $FE_{urea} < 35\%$ for prerenal ARF is 89%, while the sensitivity of $FE_{Na}$ drops to 48%.

 The $FE_{urea}$ is the best urine index to diagnose prerenal ARF in patients taking diuretics.

**C.** Other urine tests

  **1.** Classically, muddy brown granular casts and renal tubular cells are seen in ATN; the sensitivity and specificity of these findings are unknown.

***Table 25–3.*** Urinary sodium and urea nitrogen test characteristics.

| Test | Classic Pattern | | Test Characteristics of Classic Prerenal Patterns in Patients not Taking Diuretics | | | |
| | Prerenal | ATN | Sensitivity | Specificity | LR+ | LR– |
| --- | --- | --- | --- | --- | --- | --- |
| Urine sodium | < 20 mEq/L | > 20 mEq/L | 90% | 82% | 5 | 0.12 |
| $FE_{Na}$ | < 1% | > 2% | 96% | 95% | 19 | 0.04 |
| $FE_{urea}$ | < 35% | > 50% | 90% | 96% | 22.5 | 0.1 |

ATN, acute tubular necrosis.

2. Specific gravity >1.015 and urine osmolality >400 mOsm/kg are associated with prerenal states.

   a. Osmolality can be falsely low in prerenal states because of impairment of concentrating ability from underlying chronic renal disease, an osmotic diuresis, use of diuretics, or diabetes insipidus.

   b. Sensitivity and specificity of these findings are unknown.

D. BUN/creatinine ratio

   1. Classically, > 20:1 in prerenal states due to reabsorption of urea with sodium

   2. Can also be elevated with GI bleeding, use of corticosteroids, intake of a high-protein diet, or increased catabolism (postoperative or infection)

   3. Can be low with ARF secondary to rhabdomyolysis, or with decreased production due to malnutrition or liver disease

E. Physical exam

   1. See Chapter 26, Syncope, for a discussion of measuring orthostatic vital signs and their usefulness in assessing acute blood loss.

   2. The ability of the physical exam to diagnosis hypovolemia is not well studied. Available data show:

      a. Orthostatic vital signs: pulse increment > 30 bpm and systolic BP decline > 20 mm Hg have moderate specificity (75% for pulse, 81% for BP) but poor sensitivity (43% for pulse, 29% for BP); LR+ and LR– are both ~1.

      b. Sunken eyes (LR+ = 3.4) and dry axilla (LR+ = 2.8) are the best predictors of hypovolemia, but absence of these findings does not rule out hypovolemia.

      c. Dry mucous membranes of mouth is not that helpful in ruling in hypovolemia (LR+ = 2) but has the best LR– (LR– = 0.3).

      d. One study suggests that a combination of findings (eg, confusion, nonfluent speech, dry mucous membranes, dry/furrowed tongue, extremity weakness, and sunken eyes) is highly predictive of hypovolemia.

**Treatment**

A. Normalize intravascular volume.

B. Ensure mean arterial pressure (MAP) is > 70 mm Hg.

   1. MAP = 1/3 systolic BP + 2/3 diastolic BP

   2. Elderly patients may need MAP > 80–90 mm Hg

C. Obtain renal consultation within 48 hours.

D. Avoid CIN

   1. Main risk factors for CIN are estimated GFR <50 mL/min/1.73m², diabetes, hypovolemia

   2. Other risk factors include age over 75, HF, cirrhosis, hypertension, proteinuria, concomitant use of NSAIDs, intra-arterial injection of contrast, and high doses of contrast

   3. Serum creatinine levels peak at 3 days postexposure and usually return to baseline within 10 days.

   4. It is not clear how to best prevent CIN

      a. The lowest dose of contrast possible should be used.

      b. Low osmolar contrast agents may be better.

      c. Hydration with IV 0.9 normal saline may be preventive; the optimal duration of hydration is not clear.

      d. Although N-acetylcysteine and IV sodium bicarbonate are sometimes used, the data demonstrating efficacy are inconsistent.

E. Adjust doses of drugs for renal impairment as necessary.

F. Optimize nutritional support.

G. No evidence to support the use of loop diuretics, such as furosemide, or low-dose dopamine; both may actually be harmful.

H. Indications for acute dialysis

   1. Hyperkalemia

   2. Volume overload

   3. Metabolic acidosis refractory to medical therapy

   4. Uremic pericarditis or encephalopathy

## MAKING A DIAGNOSIS

Mr. T's $FE_{Na}$ is 2.41%, and his $FE_{urea}$ is 53%. He is treated with IV antibiotics and fluids, with normalization of his BP. A repeat creatinine, done several hours later, is again 3.8 mg/dL.

 Have you crossed a diagnostic threshold for the leading hypothesis, ATN? Have you ruled out the active alternatives? Do other tests need to be done to exclude the alternative diagnoses?

The combination of sepsis, a $FE_{urea}$ > 50%, a bland urinalysis, and a lack of exposure to other toxins makes hypotension-induced

ATN the most likely diagnosis. You would not expect his creatinine to improve after just a few hours of normotension, so the repeat creatinine of 3.8 mg/dL is not necessarily alarming. However, it is not possible to rule out obstruction based on the information available so far, so it is necessary to do a renal ultrasound. (ARF due to obstruction will be discussed later in the chapter.)

 Exclude urinary tract obstruction in all patients with ARF.

## CASE RESOLUTION

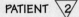

1

The ultrasound shows normal kidneys, with no hydronephrosis. Mr. T's BP remains stable, and at discharge

1 week later, his creatinine is 2.0 mg/dL. He returns to see you 2 weeks later, reporting that his osteoarthritis "flared" after so much time in bed, and he has been using celecoxib for relief. His creatinine is 2.5 mg/dL. You advise him to stop the celecoxib, and a repeat creatinine 2 weeks later is 1.5 mg/dL.

NSAIDs, even selective COX-2 inhibitors, can decrease renal perfusion due to prostaglandin inhibition, leading to a prerenal ARF. Patients with abnormal renal function are at the highest risk for this complication, and such medications should be avoided. Renal function usually returns to baseline after stopping the drug.

## CHIEF COMPLAINT

PATIENT 2

Mr. K is an 80-year-old man brought in by his family with the chief complaint of malaise, anorexia, and confusion for the past 3 days. He is generally healthy and independent, and he had been feeling fine, except for a cold several days ago. Over the last 3 days, his family noticed that he has seemed tired and a little confused. He has been drinking liquids but not eating much. They also report that he has had a couple of episodes of urinary incontinence, something he has never experienced before. His past medical history is notable only for osteoarthritis, for which he takes either acetaminophen or ibuprofen. On physical exam, he is alert and cooperative. His BP is 160/80 mm Hg, pulse is 88 bpm, RR is 16 breaths per minute, and he is afebrile. There is no adenopathy, lungs are clear, and cardiac exam is normal. Abdominal exam shows no masses or tenderness. His prostate is mildly enlarged, without nodules. There is no peripheral edema.

Initial laboratory test results include Na, 138 mEq/L; K 4.8, mEq/L; Cl, 100 mEq/L; $HCO_3$, 20 mEq/L; BUN, 90 mg/dL; creatinine, 7.2 mg/dL.

At this point, what is the leading hypothesis, what are the active alternatives, and is there a must not miss diagnosis? Given this differential diagnosis, what tests should be ordered?

## PRIORITIZING THE DIFFERENTIAL DIAGNOSIS

All 3 etiologies of ARF need to be considered. His age, prostatic enlargement, and urinary incontinence are all pivotal points suggesting urinary tract obstruction. However, he also could have prerenal ARF from either NSAID use or intravascular volume depletion. He has no history suggesting a specific intrarenal cause, so intrarenal causes would be considered only if no postrenal or prerenal cause could be identified. Table 25–4 lists the differential diagnosis.

***Table 25–4.*** Diagnostic hypotheses for Mr. K.

| Diagnostic Hypotheses | Clinical Clues | Important Tests |
|---|---|---|
| **Leading Hypothesis** | | |
| Obstruction | Nocturia<br>Incontinence<br>Dribbling<br>Slow stream<br>Abdominal/pelvic discomfort<br>Palpable bladder | Catheterization<br>Postvoid residual<br>Ultrasound |
| **Active Alternative—Most Common** | | |
| NSAID use | Medication history, including over-the-counter medications | $FE_{Na}$<br>Stopping medication |
| **Active Alternative—Must Not Miss** | | |
| Hypovolemia | Orthostatic hypotension<br>Sunken eyes<br>Dry axilla<br>History of vomiting or diarrhea<br>Elderly | $FE_{Na}$<br>BUN/creatinine ratio<br>Fluid challenge |

Mr. K's urine sodium is 20 mEq/h, with a $FE_{Na}$ of 1%. He is given 500 mL of 0.9% saline intravenously. A couple of hours later, his creatinine is 7.0 mg/dL, and he reports lower abdominal pain. He has had several episodes of dribbling urine since receiving the IV fluids.

Catheterization can be a diagnostic test in ARF.

After he urinates, a Foley catheter is placed and 500 mL of urine quickly fills the bag.

Is the clinical information sufficient to make a diagnosis? If not, what other information do you need?

## Leading Hypothesis: Urinary Tract Obstruction

### Textbook Presentation

Symptoms vary with site, degree, and rapidity of onset of the obstruction, ranging from severe pain with acute obstruction to mild or no pain. Incontinence and dribbling are common.

### Disease Highlights

A. Clinical manifestations

1. Upper ureteral or renal pelvic lesions can cause flank pain; lower obstruction can cause pelvic pain that sometimes radiates to the ipsilateral testicle or labium.

2. Obstruction must be bilateral to cause renal failure; the most common cause is prostatic enlargement.

3. Urinary output

a. Anuria, if obstruction is complete

(1) Anuria is defined as < 100 mL of urine per day.

(2) Also seen in shock, vascular lesions, severe ATN, or severe glomerulonephritis.

b. Output can be normal or increased with partial obstruction.

c. Increased output is due to tubular injury that impairs concentrating ability and sodium reabsorption.

d. Incontinence, dribbling, decreased output, and hematuria may be present.

B. Obstruction accounts for 17% of cases of outpatient ARF, and for 2–5% of cases of inpatient ARF; obstruction is more commonly seen in men than women.

C. Patients can have type 4 renal tubular acidosis with hyperkalemia due to tubular injury.

D. In patients with normal kidneys, unilateral obstruction often is undetected because the unobstructed kidney compensates enough to maintain normal renal function.

E. Prognosis

1. Complete recovery of renal function occurs if total ureteral obstruction is relieved within 7 days; little or no recovery occurs if the total obstruction is present for 12 weeks.

a. Complete or prolonged partial obstruction can lead to tubular atrophy and irreversible loss of renal function.

b. Obstruction is a rare cause of end-stage renal disease.

2. Prognosis of partial obstruction is unpredictable.

### Evidence-Based Diagnosis

A. Urine electrolytes are not very helpful.

B. Postvoid residual is normally < 100 mL; it will be increased only if obstruction is distal to the ureters.

C. Renal ultrasound

1. The best first test to look for obstruction.

2. Has a sensitivity of 80–85% for detecting postrenal ARF, defined as finding dilatation of the collecting system *and* the site of the obstruction.

3. There are 4 settings in which obstruction can occur without dilatation of the complete collecting system.

a. Within the first 1–3 days, due to relative lack of compliance of collecting system

b. When the patient is also volume depleted; sometimes repeating an ultrasound after hydration will demonstrate the dilatation

c. With retroperitoneal fibrosis, which can cause hydronephrosis without ureteral dilatation; the hydronephrosis and fibrosis are better seen on CT scan

d. With obstruction so mild that there is no impairment in renal function

4. Duplex ultrasound can identify unilateral obstruction early by detecting an increased resistive index compared with the other kidney; however, it cannot be used to diagnose bilateral obstruction.

D. CT scan can detect sites of obstruction missed on ultrasound.

E. Intravenous pyelography

1. Used if site of obstruction cannot be seen on ultrasound or CT

2. Especially useful for identifying papillary necrosis or caliceal blunting from previous infection

### Treatment

A. Relieve the obstruction immediately.

1. Modalities

a. Foley catheter for bladder neck obstruction

Remember that indwelling catheters can be obstructed by clots.

b. Suprapubic catheter, if Foley is not possible

c. Percutaneous nephrostomy tubes for ureteral obstruction

2. Consequences

a. Rapid decompression of the bladder can rarely lead to hematuria and even hypotension

b. Will often see a postobstructive diuresis; ie, an initial urinary output of 500–1000 mL/h

  (1) Represents an attempt to excrete fluid retained during the period of obstruction

  (2) Not necessary to replace entire urinary output; doing so will increase the diuresis

  (3) Should treat with normal replacement fluids

  (4) Should monitor electrolytes closely and replace as needed

B. Correct the underlying cause of the obstruction.

## MAKING A DIAGNOSIS

A renal ultrasound shows bilateral ureteral dilatation and hydronephrosis, confirming the diagnosis of urinary tract obstruction. He is admitted to the hospital, and over several days, his creatinine returns to baseline of 1.5 mg/dL. The catheter is removed, and he urinates with his usual mild difficulty starting the stream. Several days after discharge, he arrives in the emergency department, reporting that he cannot urinate at all. As instructed, he has avoided all NSAID use but has been taking pseudoephedrine for cold symptoms.

 Have you crossed a diagnostic threshold for the leading hypothesis, urinary tract obstruction? Have you ruled out the active alternatives? Do other tests need to be done to exclude the alternative diagnoses?

No further tests are necessary to diagnose the cause of his ARF; however, it is important to determine the cause of the urinary tract obstruction, and that of his new, related problem, acute urinary retention.

## Related Diagnoses: Acute Urinary Retention and BPH

### 1. Acute Urinary Retention

Acute urinary retention is most commonly seen in older men with prostatic hypertrophy causing bladder neck obstruction (seen in 10% of men in their 70s and up to 33% of men in their 80s). The risk is increased for older men, for those with moderate to severe lower urinary tract symptoms, for those with a flow rate < 12 mL/sec, and for those with a prostate volume > 30 mL by transrectal ultrasound.

In women, acute urinary retention is usually due to neurogenic bladder, and in younger patients, it is usually due to neurologic disease. Medications that commonly induce urinary retention in susceptible patients include antihistamines, anticholinergics, antispasmodics, tricyclic antidepressants, opioids, and α-adrenergic agonists.

### 2. BPH

#### Textbook Presentation

The classic presentation is urinary frequency, nocturia, reduced stream, and dribbling at the end of urination in an older man.

#### Disease Highlights

A. Defined as microscopic (histologic evidence of cellular proliferation), macroscopic (actual enlargement of the prostate), or clinical (symptoms resulting from macroscopic BPH)

B. Two-thirds of the adult prostate is glandular and one-third is fibromuscular.

  1. Intraprostatic dihydrotestosterone (DHT), synthesized from testosterone by 5-α-reductase type 2, controls glandular growth.

  2. The smooth muscle of the prostate, urethra, and bladder are under $\alpha_1$-adrenergic control.

C. Prostatic enlargement causes symptoms due to compression of the periurethral area and of the bladder; the compression occurs because of the physical enlargement of the prostate and also because of increased muscle tone in the urethra, prostatic fibromuscular tissue, and bladder neck.

D. Symptoms can be categorized as

  1. Storage symptoms (urgency frequency, nocturia, urge incontinence, stress incontinence)

  2. Voiding symptoms (hesitancy, poor flow, straining, dysuria)

  3. Postmicturition symptoms (dribbling, incomplete emptying)

E. Prostate size does not correlate with symptom severity.

  1. Prostate growth is 0.4 mL/year in younger men; 1.2 mL/year in older men.

  2. However, men with prostates > 30 mL, and especially > 40 mL, are more likely to have symptoms.

  3. Can use International Prostate Symptom Score to assess severity of symptoms and assess response to therapy.

    a. There are 7 questions to be answered on a 0 to 5 scale, yielding a potential total of 35 points (Table 25–5).

    b. 0–7 = mild BPH; 8–19 = moderate BPH; 20–35 = severe BPH

#### Evidence-Based Diagnosis

A. Guidelines recommend all patients have a digital rectal exam, urinalysis, and serum creatinine; other testing (urodynamics, imaging) is optional.

B. A prostate specific antigen (PSA) should be checked in those men who would consider treatment for prostate cancer.

C. Urinary flow rates, urodynamic measurements, and amount of postvoid residual do not correlate well with symptoms.

D. Digital rectal exam

  1. Cannot ascertain anterior or posterior extension or feel entire posterior surface.

  2. Therefore, prostate size is underestimated by 25–55% on digital rectal exam, compared with transrectal ultrasound; the underestimation increases the larger the prostate volume.

 The prostate is even bigger than you think it is on digital rectal exam.

#### Treatment

A. α-Blockers (terazosin, doxazosin, alfuzosin, tamsulosin)

  1. Decrease muscle tone in the stroma and prostatic capsule

  2. Provide the most rapid relief of lower urinary tract symptoms

***Table 25–5.*** International Prostate Symptom Score.

| Over the past month, how often ... | Not at All | < 1 Time in 5 | < Than Half the Time | About Half the Time | > Half the Time | Almost Always |
|---|---|---|---|---|---|---|
| have you had a sensation of not emptying your bladder completely after you finished urinating? | 0 | 1 | 2 | 3 | 4 | 5 |
| have you had to urinate again less than 2 hours after you finished urinating? | 0 | 1 | 2 | 3 | 4 | 5 |
| have you found you stopped and started again several times when you urinated? | 0 | 1 | 2 | 3 | 4 | 5 |
| have you found it difficult to postpone urination? | 0 | 1 | 2 | 3 | 4 | 5 |
| have you had a weak urinary stream? | 0 | 1 | 2 | 3 | 4 | 5 |
| have you had to push or strain to begin urination? | 0 | 1 | 2 | 3 | 4 | 5 |
| did you most typically get up to urinate from the time you went to bed at night until the time you got up in the morning? | 0 | 1 | 2 | 3 | 4 | 5 |

Scoring Key: 0-7, mild; 8-19 moderate; 20-35, severe.
Modified, with permission, from Barry MJ et al. The American Urological Association symptoms index for benign prostatic hyperplasia. *J Urol.* 1992;148:1549.

**B.** 5-α-reductase inhibitors (finasteride, dutasteride)

1. Reduce prostate size by blocking conversion of testosterone to DHT.

2. Finasteride has been shown to reduce symptoms when the prostate is > 40 mL.

   **a.** Slow onset of action: weeks to months

   **b.** Might also reduce risk of acute urinary retention and need for surgery.

   **c.** Should check PSA prior to starting finasteride, at 6 months, and at 18 months; it should decrease by about 50%.

**C.** There is some evidence that combination therapy with α-blockers and finasteride may be more effective than α-blockers alone.

**D.** Indications for surgical intervention include moderate to severe symptoms not responsive to medical therapy, acute urinary retention, recurrent infections or hematuria, and azotemia.

## CASE RESOLUTION

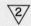

He is catheterized, and 500 mL of urine is obtained. Because the urinary retention was precipitated by the use of an α-adrenergic agent (pseudoephedrine), he is given tamsulosin and the catheter is removed on a trial basis. He is again unable to urinate. He then undergoes transurethral resection of the prostate (TURP) with resolution of his urinary symptoms. His creatinine stays at 1.5 mg/dL throughout these events.

## CHIEF COMPLAINT

PATIENT 3

Mrs. F is a 63-year-old woman with a history of diastolic dysfunction, hypertension, and osteoarthritis. Her usual medications are atenolol, lisinopril, and acetaminophen, and her usual serum creatinine is 1.5 mg/dL. Three weeks ago, she came to see you reporting severe pain, erythema, and swelling of her right first metatarsophalangeal joint.

You diagnosed gout, and prescribed indomethacin 25 mg 3 times daily to use until the gout resolved. She returned for follow-up yesterday, reporting that the gout had resolved in a few days, but that she kept taking the indomethacin because it helped her arthritis so much. Despite your reservations, you agree to refill the prescription because she clearly feels so much better than usual. Today you receive the results of the blood tests you ordered during the visit: Na, 141 mEq/24 h; K, 5.0 mEq/24 h; Cl, 100 mEq/24 h; HCO₃, 20 mEq/L; BUN, 32 mg/dL; creatinine, 2.5 mg/dL.

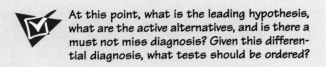

At this point, what is the leading hypothesis, what are the active alternatives, and is there a must not miss diagnosis? Given this differential diagnosis, what tests should be ordered?

## PRIORITIZING THE DIFFERENTIAL DIAGNOSIS

At this point, the differential for her new renal insufficiency is quite broad, but it is logical to focus on the pivotal point in this case, the recent use of indomethacin. Through prostaglandin inhibition, NSAIDs can cause decreased renal blood flow, leading to a prerenal state. NSAIDs are also 1 of the classes of drugs most commonly associated with an intrarenal disease, interstitial nephritis. Although obstruction must always be considered, she is having no urinary symptoms and has no risk factors. Table 25–6 lists the differential diagnosis.

Mrs. F's urine sodium is 35 mEq/h, and the $FE_{Na}$ is 1.5%. Urinalysis shows 1+ protein, 3 RBCs/hpf, 5–10 WBCs/hpf, and no casts.

Is the clinical information sufficient to make a diagnosis? If not, what other information do you need?

## Leading Diagnosis: NSAID-Induced Renal Hypoperfusion

### Textbook Presentation

ARF caused by NSAIDs is usually asymptomatic and is most commonly detected by finding an increased serum creatinine.

### Disease Highlights

A. Can occur with nonselective NSAIDs and COX-2 inhibitors.

B. Seen within 3–7 days of starting therapy.

**Table 25–6.** Diagnostic hypotheses for Mrs. F.

| Diagnostic Hypotheses | Clinical Clues | Important Tests |
|---|---|---|
| **Leading Hypothesis** | | |
| NSAID-induced renal hypoperfusion | Use of NSAIDs History of renal disease HF | $FE_{Na}$ Stopping the medication |
| **Active Alternative** | | |
| Interstitial nephritis | Flank pain Hematuria | Stopping the medication Urine eosinophils Renal biopsy |

C. Renal prostaglandins are not important regulators of blood flow in normal kidneys.

D. As discussed in the first case, prostaglandins are important in the autoregulation of glomerular pressure and GFR.

E. Patients with CKD, hypertension, volume depletion, HF, and cirrhosis already have impaired autoregulation.

F. Prostaglandin inhibition in such patients can lead to significant decreases in renal blood flow, consequent reversible renal ischemia, and ARF.

### Evidence-Based Diagnosis

A. $FE_{Na}$ should be < 1%. (Sensitivity and specificity are unknown.)

B. Should reverse when the drug is stopped.

### Treatment

Stop the exposure.

## MAKING A DIAGNOSIS

You call Mrs. F and tell her to stop taking the indomethacin. One week later, her creatinine is still 2.5 mg/dL. Urine eosinophils are negative.

Have you crossed a diagnostic threshold for the leading hypothesis, NSAID-induced renal hypoperfusion? Have you ruled out the active alternatives? Do other tests need to be done to exclude the alternative diagnoses?

Mrs. F's $FE_{Na}$ is higher than expected for NSAID-induced renal hypoperfusion. She has not used diuretics or received IV fluids, both of which can cause a falsely elevated urine sodium and $FE_{Na}$. In addition, her creatinine has not improved. Therefore, it is unlikely that prostaglandin inhibition is the reason for her renal insufficiency.

## Alternative Diagnosis: Interstitial Nephritis

### Textbook Presentation

Classic symptoms include renal insufficiency, hematuria, pyuria with WBC casts, fever, and eosinophilia. The full syndrome is rarely seen today since it occurs primarily with methicillin-induced acute interstitial nephritis.

### Disease Highlights

A. Interstitial nephritis is found in 2–3% of all renal biopsies, and in up to 15% of patients who had a biopsy done for ARF.

B. Etiology

1. In 1 case series, 10% of cases were caused by infection, 85% of cases were caused by medications, and 4% of cases were idiopathic.

2. Can be caused by many medications, including but not limited to

a. Antibiotics—most commonly ampicillin, ciprofloxacin, penicillin G, rifampin, sulfonamides

**b.** NSAIDs—most commonly fenoprofen, ibuprofen, indomethacin, naproxen, aspirin, phenylbutazone, piroxicam

**c.** COX-2 inhibitors

**d.** Diuretics—most commonly furosemide

**e.** Anticonvulsants—most commonly phenytoin

**f.** Cimetidine, omeprazole, allopurinol

**3.** Can be caused by viral infections (eg, cytomegalovirus, Epstein-Barr virus, herpes simplex virus, HIV, mumps, and others), bacterial infections (staphylococci, streptococci, *Yersinia, Legionella,* and others), other infections such as mycobacteria, toxoplasmosis, syphilis

**4.** Can be seen in vasculitis, systemic lupus erythematosus, and lymphoproliferative disorders

**C.** Clinical manifestations

**1.** Renal manifestations develop within 3 weeks in 80% of patients, with an average delay of 10 days (range 1 day to 18 months; longer delays often seen with NSAIDs).

**2.** Symptoms develop more rapidly if patient is rechallenged with the offending drug.

**3.** Clinical presentation is often incomplete.

**a.** The most suggestive presentation, a combination of renal insufficiency, mild proteinuria, abnormal urinalysis, normal BP, no edema, and flank pain, is seen in < 25% of cases.

**b.** Hematuria (usually microscopic), pyuria, and flank pain are each seen in about 50% of cases.

**c.** Extrarenal symptoms (fever, rash) are seen in < 50% of cases (< 10% of cases of NSAID-induced interstitial nephritis)

**d.** Proteinuria is more prominent in NSAID-induced interstitial nephritis (often nephrotic range with NSAIDs; otherwise, usually < 1 g/d)

**e.** Less than 20% of patients are oliguric.

 The absence of fever, rash, eosinophilia, or eosinophiluria does *not* rule out interstitial nephritis.

**D.** Prognosis

**1.** Most patients improve within 6–8 weeks and return to baseline renal function.

**2.** Predictors of irreversible injury are diffuse infiltrates and frequent granulomas on biopsy, intake of the offending drug for longer than 1 month, delayed response to prednisone, and persistent renal failure after 3 weeks.

## Evidence-Based Diagnosis

**A.** Sensitivity of urine eosinophils is 67% and specificity is 83% (LR+ = 3.9; LR− = 0.39).

**B.** $FE_{Na}$ usually > 1%

**C.** Gallium scan

**1.** Substantial renal uptake in acute interstitial nephritis, but also see uptake in glomerulonephritis, pyelonephritis, and other conditions

**2.** Sensitivity and specificity are not well defined.

**3.** No uptake with ATN, so possibly useful in distinguishing ATN from acute interstitial nephritis

**D.** Renal biopsy is gold standard.

## Treatment

**A.** Stop exposure, if possible.

**B.** Corticosteroids are sometimes used, but there are no prospective randomized clinical trials.

**1.** Consider in patients whose renal function does not improve within 1 week of stopping exposure, after biopsy confirms diagnosis.

**2.** Consider empiric trial in patients who have worsening renal function and suspected acute interstitial nephritis, and who are poor candidates for biopsy.

**3.** NSAID-induced acute interstitial nephritis is less responsive to corticosteroid therapy.

**4.** Should see improvement in 2–3 weeks.

## CASE RESOLUTION

3

*Her urinalysis is consistent with interstitial nephritis, and the lack of urine eosinophils does not rule out the diagnosis. Renal biopsy is performed, which shows inflammatory infiltrates in the interstitium. Her renal function returns to baseline several weeks after the NSAIDs are discontinued. She is cautioned to never use NSAIDs in the future to avoid recurrent interstitial nephritis.*

## REVIEW OF OTHER IMPORTANT DISEASES

### Acute Glomerulonephritis

Acute GN is caused by one of several disease processes, all of which involve immunologically mediated proliferative GN. The classic clinical "nephritic syndrome" consists of the *acute* onset of hematuria (with red cell casts), proteinuria, elevated creatinine, hypertension, and edema. In rapidly progressive GN (RPGN), also called crescentic GN because of the "crescent" shaped changes around the glomerulus, the nephritic syndrome develops *subacutely,* over weeks to months (see Table 25-7).

### Vascular Causes of ARF

Vascular events are serious, but rare, causes of ARF. There are 3 mechanisms of acute vascular compromise: renal artery thrombosis, thromboembolism of the renal arteries, and atheroembolism.

### 1. Renal Artery Thrombosis

**Textbook Presentation**

The classic presentation is severe flank pain, hematuria, nausea, vomiting, fever, and hypertension.

**Disease Highlights**

**A.** Blunt trauma is most common cause.

**B.** Nontraumatic causes include

**1.** Dissecting aortic or renal artery aneurysms

***Table 25–7.*** Causes of acute glomerulonephritis (GN).

| Type | Serologic markers | Diseases | Highlights |
|---|---|---|---|
| Anti-GBM GN | 100% anti-GBM ab +<br>80% ANCA(−)<br>20% ANCA +<br>C3 normal | Anti-GBM disease<br>Goodpasture syndrome<br>(GN plus pulmonary<br>hemorrhage) | Incidence 0.5/million<br>Pulmonary symptoms usually predate GN<br>Diagnosed by renal biopsy<br>Treated with plasmapheresis, corticosteroids,<br>immunosuppressives<br>30% develop ESRD |
| Pauci-immune GN | > 90% ANCA +<br>Anti-GBM (−)<br>C3 normal | Idiopathic crescentic GN<br>Microscopic polyangiitis (GN +<br>systemic vasculitis<br>Wegener (GN + vasculitis of<br>respiratory tract) | 80% of patients with Wegener have renal disease<br>Treated with corticosteroids and cyclophosphamide<br>ESRD develops in 15% |
| Immune Complex GN | C3 low<br>Anti-GBM (−)<br>ANCA (−)<br>ASO high (post strep only) | Idiopathic<br>Postinfectious<br>Lupus nephritis<br>Cryoglobulinemia<br>Bacterial endocarditis | Poststreptococcal GN<br>  Most common postinfectious GN<br>  10-14 days after infection with nephritogenic<br>  strain group A β-hemolytic streptococci<br>  Supportive treatment only; residual renal<br>  impairment rare |

**2.** Vasculitis

**3.** Cocaine abuse

**4.** Antiphospholipid antibody syndrome

### Evidence-Based Diagnosis

**A.** Angiogram is the gold standard.

**B.** Infused CT is often diagnostic.

### Treatment

**A.** Nephrectomy, if renal infarction occurs

**B.** Revascularization or thrombolysis

**C.** Sometimes observation and medical management

## 2. Thromboembolism of the Renal Arteries

### Textbook Presentation

Most patients have flank pain, often with hematuria or anuria.

### Disease Highlights

**A.** Clinical features depend on severity and location of emboli.

**B.** Bilateral emboli or emboli to a solitary kidney more likely to produce ARF and anuria.

**C.** 75% of patients have abdominal or flank pain.

**D.** Variably see nausea, vomiting, hematuria

**E.** Fever and hypertension are common, but fever is often delayed until second or third day.

**F.** Sources of emboli

    **1.** Cardiac: atrial fibrillation, myocardial infarction, rheumatic valvular disease, prosthetic valves, subacute bacterial endocarditis

    **2.** Aortic or renal aneurysms

    **3.** Intra-arterial catheterization

### Evidence-Based Diagnosis

**A.** Diagnosed at onset of symptoms in only 30% of patients

**B.** Usually have leukocytosis, increased lactate dehydrogenase (LDH) and transaminases; the LDH is increased more than the transaminases.

**C.** Alkaline phosphatase elevated in 30–50% of patients.

**D.** Angiography is gold standard for diagnosis; infused CT can be diagnostic.

### Treatment

**A.** Unilateral embolism and normal contralateral kidney: streptokinase and/or angioplasty, followed by anticoagulation; no indication for surgery

**B.** Bilateral emboli, or embolus to solitary kidney: same as above, but try surgical reconstruction if cannot restore blood flow

## 3. Atheroembolism

### Textbook Presentation

The classic presentation is a white man over age 60 with hypertension, smoking, and vascular disease in whom livedo reticularis and acute or subacute renal failure develop after an inciting event.

### Disease Highlights

**A.** Cholesterol crystal embolism from an atherosclerotic aorta

**B.** 3 syndromes: abrupt onset of renal failure after an inciting event (such as angiography), subacute worsening of renal function a few weeks after an event, and chronic renal impairment

C. Risk factors include male sex, age > 60, hypertension, smoking, diabetes, vascular disease

D. Can occur spontaneously or after vascular surgery procedures, angiograms (especially coronary angiograms), and with anticoagulation

E. Incidence probably quite low (< 1–2%) but may be as high as 5-6% in high-risk patients

F. Clinical manifestations (from 5 case series)

1. Skin lesions (livedo reticularis) in 35–90%

2. GI symptoms in 8–30%

3. Eosinophilia in 22–73%

4. CNS involvement in 4–23%

5. Dialysis needed in 28–61%

### Evidence-Based Diagnosis

A. Renal or skin biopsy

B. Can sometimes be diagnosed on fundoscopic exam

### Treatment

A. Best approach beyond supportive therapy unknown

B. Avoid anticoagulation

C. Consider aggressive lipid management

## Chronic Kidney Disease (CKD)

### Textbook Presentation

Patients are often asymptomatic, or may have nonspecific symptoms such as fatigue. Patients with kidney failure can present with fluid overload, uremic symptoms (fatigue, nausea, delirium), or manifestations of electrolyte abnormalities (such as arrhythmias).

### Disease Highlights

A. There are 5 stages of CKD. GFR is estimated using the MDRD equation, and kidney damage is defined as an albumin/creatinine ratio of > 17 mg/g in men or > 25 mg/g in women on 2 separate measurements 3 months apart.

1. Stage 1: Kidney damage with normal or increased GFR (> 90 mL/min/1.73m$^2$)

2. Stage 2: Kidney damage with mild decrease in GFR (60–89 mL/min/1.73m$^2$)

3. Stage 3: Moderate decrease in GFR (30–59 mL/min/1.73m$^2$)

4. Stage 4: Severe decrease in GFR (15–29 mL/min/1.73m$^2$)

5. Stage 5: Kidney failure (GFR < 15 mL/min/1.73m$^2$)

B. Risk factors for CKD

1. Clinical conditions: history of hypertension, diabetes, autoimmune disease, systemic infections, urinary tract infections, urinary stones, urinary tract obstruction, recovery from ARF

2. Sociodemographic factors: older age (> 60 years), racial or ethnic minority, family history of CKD, low birth weight, low income or educational level

3. Exposure to nephrotoxic drugs or chemicals

C. Epidemiology

1. 16.5% of the US population has stage 1, 2, or 3 CKD, about one-third at each stage

2. 0.4% of the US population has stage 4 or 5 CKD

D. Etiologies of CKD

1. Diabetic nephropathy

a. Largest single cause of kidney failure in the United States

b. Found in ~40 of dialysis patients

2. Nondiabetic kidney diseases

a. Glomerular diseases (such as autoimmune, drug induced); prevalence in dialysis patients ~18%

b. Vascular diseases (such as large vessel disease, hypertensive nephrosclerosis); prevalence in dialysis patients ~20%

c. Tubulointerstitial diseases (recurrent urinary tract infection, drug toxicity); prevalence in dialysis patients ~7%

d. Cystic kidney diseases; found in ~5% of dialysis patients

E. Evaluation

1. All patients should have an estimation of GFR (the MDRD equation discussed above is the best estimation); a random urine specimen for albumin-creatinine ratio; a urinalysis including specific gravity, pH, and microscopic examination for RBCs, WBCs, and casts; a renal ultrasound; and serum electrolytes

2. Selected patients will need further evaluation including renal biopsy

F. Complications

1. Volume overload

2. Hyperkalemia

3. Metabolic acidosis

4. Hyperphosphatemia

5. Secondary hyperparathyroidism and renal osteodystrophy

6. Hypertension

7. Anemia

8. Hyperlipidemia

9. Uremic pericarditis

10. Uremic neuropathy

11. Uremic encephalopathy

### Treatment

A. Identify and treat reversible causes of renal dysfunction such as hypovolemia, urinary tract obstruction, administration of nephrotoxic drugs

B. Prevent or slow the progression of disease using ACE inhibitors or ARBs to reduce protein excretion; the addition of other drugs is often necessary to reach the BP treatment goal of < 130/80 mm Hg.

C. Treat the complications listed above (a full discussion is beyond the scope of this chapter).

D. Optimize cardiovascular risk factors.

E. Refer patients with a GFR < 30 mL/min/1.73m$^2$ to a nephrologist for comanagement of complications and discussion of potential need for dialysis.

F. Adjust doses of medications that are excreted by the kidneys.

# REFERENCES

Abuelo JG. Normotensive ischemic acute renal failure. N Engl J Med. 2007;357:797–805.

Barrett BJ, Parfrey PS. Preventing nephropathy induced by contrast medium. N Engl J Med. 2006;354:379–386.

Carvounis CP, Nisar S, Guro-Razuman S. Significance of the fractional excretion of urea in the differential diagnosis of acute renal failure. Kidney Int. 2002;62:2223–29.

Hilton R. Acute renal failure. BMJ. 2006;333:786–90.

Levey AS, Coresh J, Balk E, et al. National Kidney Foundation guideline for chronic kidney disease: evaluation, classification, and stratification. Ann Intern Med. 2003;139:137–47.

Levy A, Samraj GP. Benign prostatic hyperplasia: when to 'watch and wait,' when and how to treat. Cleve Clin J Med. 2007;74(suppl 3):S15–S20.

McGee S, Abernethy WB, Simel DL. Is this patient hypovolemic? JAMA. 1999;281:1022–29.

Singri N, Ahya SN, Levin ML. Acute renal failure. JAMA. 2003;289:747–51.

Stevens LA, Coresh J, Greene T, Levey AS. Assessing kidney function—measured and estimated glomerular filtration rate. N Engl J Med. 2006;354:2473–83.

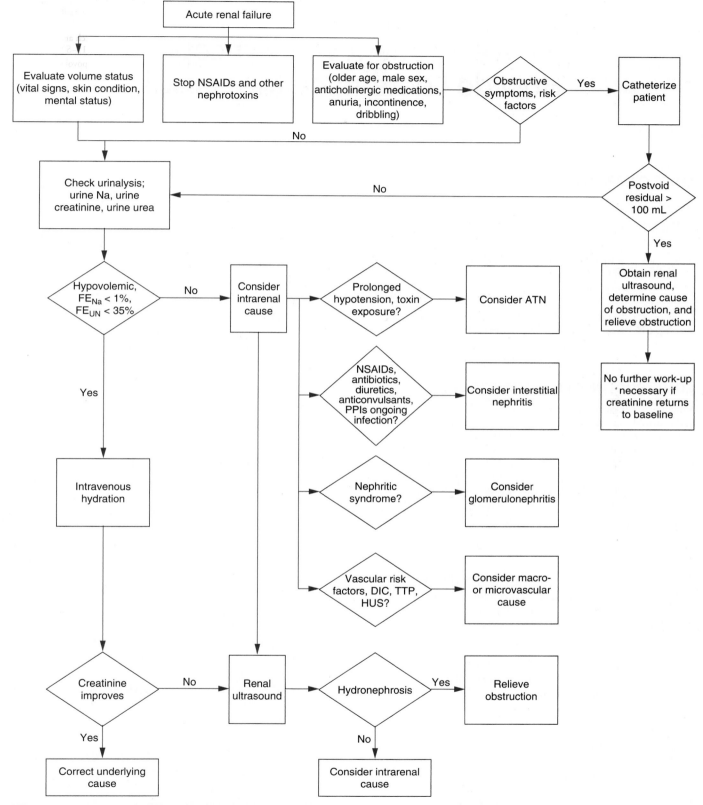

ATN, acute tubular necrosis; DIC, disseminated intravascular coagulation; HUS, hemolytic uremic syndrome;
NSAIDS, nonsteroidal antiinflammatory drugs; PPIs, proton pump inhibitors; TTP, thrombotic thrombocytopenic purpura.

**Diagnostic Approach: Acute Renal Failure**

# I have a patient with syncope. How do I determine the cause?

## CHIEF COMPLAINT

PATIENT 1

Mr. M is a 23-year-old medical student who had an episode of syncope this morning after entering his anatomy lab for the first time. He is quite alarmed (and embarrassed).

**What is the differential diagnosis of syncope? How would you frame the differential?**

## CONSTRUCTING A DIFFERENTIAL DIAGNOSIS

Syncope is the abrupt, transient complete loss of consciousness and postural tone. Syncope may be a warning sign that the patient is at risk for sudden cardiac death; therefore, a careful evaluation is critical to identify and treat patients with potentially life-threatening etiologies of syncope. The differential diagnosis is easily remembered by considering the brain's requirements to maintain consciousness. Derangement of any of these requirements may result in syncope. Consciousness requires the following:

1. Organized cortical electrical activity
2. Glucose
3. Oxygen
4. A functional delivery system to deliver oxygen and glucose.

This in turn requires open vascular conduits and an adequate BP. By far, most causes of syncope result from hypotension. Therefore, it is useful to look at the determinants of BP.

BP = cardiac output (CO) × total peripheral resistance (TPR)

CO = stroke volume (SV) × heart rate (HR)

Simple substitution: BP = SV × HR × TPR

SV = end-diastolic volume (EDV) − end-systolic volume (ESV)

Simple substitution: BP = (EDV − ESV) × HR × TPR

In summary, the differential diagnosis of syncope can be remembered by considering the requirements for consciousness (ie, BP [determined by EDV, ESV, HR, TPR], organized cortical electrical activity, glucose, oxygen, and open vascular conduits).

## Differential Diagnosis of Syncope

A. BP = (EDV − ESV) × HR × TPR
  1. Inadequate EDV (poor filling)
    a. Dehydration
    b. Hemorrhage
    c. Pulmonary embolism (PE)
    d. Cardiac tamponade
  2. Elevated ESV (inadequate emptying)
    a. Aortic stenosis (AS)
    b. Hypertrophic cardiomyopathy
  3. Heart rate disorders
    a. Tachycardias
      (1) Ventricular tachycardia (VT)
      (2) Supraventricular tachycardia associated with accessory pathway (Wolff-Parkinson-White [WPW] syndrome)
    b. Bradycardias
      (1) Neurally mediated syncope (cardio-inhibitory type)
        (a) Neurocardiogenic syncope
        (b) Situational syncope
        (c) Carotid sinus syndrome
      (2) Sinus node disorders
        (a) Sinus bradycardia (< 35 beats per minute)
        (b) Sinus pauses (> 3 seconds or > 2 seconds with symptoms)
      (3) Atrioventricular (AV) block (second- or third-degree)
  4. Decreased TPR (vasodilatation)
    a. Neurocardiogenic syncope (vasodepressor type)
    b. Drugs (α-blockers, vasodilators, nitrates, tricyclic antidepressants, and phenothiazines)
    c. Hypersensitive carotid (vasodepressor type)
    d. Sepsis (usually causes protracted hypotension rather than syncope)
    e. Addison disease (usually causes protracted hypotension rather than syncope)
B. Disorganized electrical activity: Generalized seizures
C. Hypoglycemia
  1. Iatrogenic (eg, insulin and sulfonylureas)
  2. Insulinomas (exceedingly rare)
D. Hypoxemia (usually results in impaired consciousness or coma rather than syncope)
E. Obstructed vascular conduits
  1. Vertebrobasilar insufficiency
  2. Subclavian steal

Mr. M reports that he was in his usual state of health and felt perfectly well prior to entering the anatomy dissection room. Upon viewing the cadaver, he felt queasy and warm. He became diaphoretic and collapsed to the floor. When he regained consciousness, he was not confused. The instructor told him that he was unconscious for only a few seconds.

At this point, what is the leading hypothesis, what are the active alternatives, and is there a must not miss diagnosis? Given this differential diagnosis, what tests should be ordered?

## PRIORITIZING THE DIFFERENTIAL DIAGNOSIS

The evaluation of all syncopal patients must include a thorough history, physical exam, and ECG. A detailed history of the event is critical (including what the patient was doing and feeling). **Pivotal clues** include any findings on history or physical exam that suggest cardiac disease, since patients with syncope and heart disease are at a markedly increased risk for VT and sudden death. Such clues include a history of coronary artery disease (CAD), structural heart disease, heart failure (HF), syncope during exertion, a family history of sudden cardiac death, advanced age, or significant murmurs. Other **pivotal clues** may suggest alternate hypotheses such as neurocardiogenic syncope, seizures, hypoglycemia, PE, or significant valvular disease (see Figures 26–7, 26–8). The physical exam should evaluate vital signs and orthostatic BPs in addition to a thorough cardiac and neurologic exam. Finally, the ECG is scrutinized to look for signs of ischemia, hypertrophy, AV block, bundle-branch block (BBB), or other abnormalities (see below).

Mr. M's history is classic for neurocardiogenic syncope. Neurocardiogenic syncope is often precipitated by a highly emotional event or painful stimulus. Patients may experience nausea, diaphoresis, and then brief syncope with a rapid return to normal consciousness. It is also important to consider other common causes of syncope such as dehydration or medications. "Must not miss" diagnoses include cardiac syncope or seizures. In young patients the most common "must not miss" form of cardiac syncope is hypertrophic cardiomyopathy. Table 26–1 lists the differential diagnosis.

Mr. M reports no diarrhea or vomiting, and he is not taking any medications. He has no known heart disease and exercises vigorously without symptoms. There is no family history of sudden cardiac death. There is no history of confusion following the syncope, tonic-clonic activity, or incontinence. On physical exam, his BP and pulse are normal and do not change with standing. Cardiac exam reveals a regular rate and rhythm without a significant murmur, JVD, or $S_3$ gallop. His ECG is normal.

Is the clinical information sufficient to make a diagnosis? If not what other information do you need?

**Table 26–1.** Diagnostic hypotheses for Mr. M.

| Diagnostic Hypotheses | Clinical Clues | Important Tests |
|---|---|---|
| **Leading Hypothesis** | | |
| Neurocardiogenic syncope (faint) | Preceding pain, anxiety, fear or prolonged standing; rapid normalization of consciousness; absence of heart disease | Tilt table if recurrent |
| **Active Alternatives—Most Common** | | |
| Dehydration | History of vomiting, diarrhea, poor oral intake | Orthostatic measurement of BP and pulse |
| Medications | History of α-blockers, other antihypertensive medication | Orthostatic measurement of BP and pulse |
| **Active Alternatives—Must Not Miss** | | |
| Hypertrophic cardiomyopathy | History of exertional syncope, Family history of sudden death Systolic murmur, which increases on standing | ECG Echocardiogram |
| Seizure | Prolonged period of lethargy, confusion or amnesia following syncope suggesting postictal period Tonic-clonic activity, incontinence, tongue biting | EEG Neuroimaging |

## Leading Hypothesis: Neurocardiogenic (Vasovagal) Syncope

### Textbook Presentation

Neurocardiogenic syncope typically develops in young patients during prolonged standing at times precipitated by pain or anxiety (ie, phlebotomy). Lightheadedness, nausea, and diaphoresis may precede syncope, which is brief.

### Disease Highlights

**A.** Most common cause of syncope (20–33% of cases)

**B.** Pathophysiology (Figure 26–1)

1. Patients are often in a low preload state due to venous pooling (from prolonged standing) or dehydration.

2. Superimposed anxiety, pain or fear triggers a sympathetic surge.

3. Sympathetic surge augments ventricular contraction.

4. Vigorous contraction coupled with low preload results in low ESV, which triggers intracardiac mechanoreceptors.

5. The mechanoreceptors trigger the vagal reflex.

6. Vagal reflex triggers bradycardia, vasodilatation, or both, resulting in hypotension and syncope.

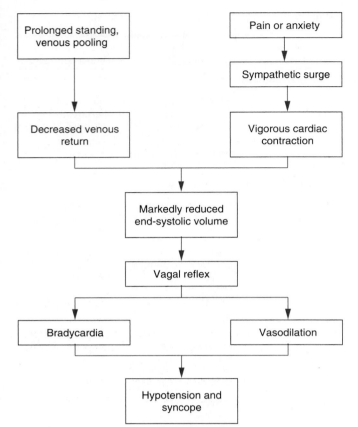

**Figure 26-1.** Pathophysiology of neurocardiogenic syncope.

C. Other forms of neurally mediated syncope include situational syncope and carotid sinus syndrome (see end of chapter).

### Evidence-Based Diagnosis

A. History

1. Provocative circumstances include prolonged standing (37%), hot weather (42%), lack of food (23%), fear (21%), and acute pain (14%).

2. No single finding is very sensitive for neurocardiogenic syncope (14–40%).

3. However, certain findings are fairly specific and increase the likelihood of neurocardiogenic syncope when present.

   a. Feeling warm (LR+ 12)

   b. Prolonged standing (LR+ 9.0)

   c. Abdominal discomfort prior to syncope (LR+ 8)

   d. Occurring during injection/cannulation (LR+ 7)

   e. Dehydration (LR+ 3.7)

   f. Nausea after syncope (LR+ 3.5)

   g. Although neurocardiogenic syncope can occur *after* exercise it is rare *during* exercise. Syncope during exercise should raise the suspicion of *cardiogenic* syncope.

B. Laboratory and radiologic tests

1. Patients with a typical history, a normal physical exam and ECG, and no evidence of heart disease or red flags (Figure 26–7), do not require further testing.

2. Patients with an atypical history (ie, without a clear precipitant) require an echocardiogram, and occasionally tilt-table testing.

3. Tilt-table testing is particularly useful in patients with recurrent events in whom the diagnosis is unclear.

   a. The patient is initially supine for 20–45 minutes.

   b. The table is then tilted to 60–80 degrees and the patient kept upright for 30–45 minutes during which time the pulse and BP are continuously monitored.

   c. Criteria for a positive test include the reproduction of the presyncopal or syncopal symptoms with hypotension, bradycardia, or both.

   d. Sensitivity is 26–80% and specificity is about 90%, but they cannot be precisely determined due to the lack of a gold standard.

      (1) Furthermore, estimates vary depending on tilt-table angle, duration, and medications used.

      (2) A variety of medications can increase sensitivity but decrease specificity (eg, isoproterenol and nitrates).

### Treatment

A. Patients should be reassured, instructed to avoid triggers, and lie down if they notice the premonitory signs of an impending faint.

B. Vasodilators and diuretics should be eliminated or decreased (ie, α-blockers and diuretics).

C. Isometric arm and leg contractions in which the muscles are tensed for 2 minutes significantly raises BP. 94% of clinical events are aborted with this maneuver.

D. Midodrine is an α-agonist that has prevented neurocardiogenic syncope in a few small studies.

E. Orthostatic training programs have been effective in patients with drug refractory recurrent neurocardiogenic syncope.

F. Other therapies have included fludrocortisone and selective serotonin reuptake inhibitors.

G. β-Blockers slow HR and improve ventricular filling. While successful in short-term trials, long-term placebo-controlled trials have not demonstrated a benefit over placebo. The use of β-blockers is therefore controversial.

H. "Rate drop" dual chamber pacemakers (triggered by a sudden drop in HR) may be effective in select patients with recurrent severe neurocardiogenic syncope, when syncope is due to profound bradycardia or asystole. This should only be considered in severe drug refractory cases.

## MAKING A DIAGNOSIS

Mr. M's well-defined precipitant for neurocardiogenic syncope and typical premonitory symptoms combined with the absence of red flags for serious cardiac syncope (such as HF, ischemic heart disease, advanced age, abnormal physical exam or ECG) makes neurocardiogenic syncope the most likely diagnosis. You still wonder if you need to consider hypertrophic cardiomyopathy.

**Have you crossed a diagnostic threshold for the leading hypothesis, neurocardiogenic syncope? Have you ruled out the active alternatives? Do other tests need to be done to exclude the alternative diagnoses?**

# Alternative Diagnosis: Hypertrophic Cardiomyopathy

## Textbook Presentation

Patients with hypertropic cardiomyopathy may be asymptomatic and discovered due to a family history of sudden cardiac death, during the evaluation of an asymptomatic systolic murmur, during pre-participation athletic screening, or when symptoms occur (syncope, heart failure, atrial fibrillation, or cardiac arrest).

## Disease Highlights

A. The most common cause of cardiovascular death among young athletes

B. A large number of different autosomal dominant mutations in genes that encode sarcomere constituents result in myocyte hypertrophy with disarray, increased cardiac fibrosis, and diastolic dysfunction.

C. Affects 1/500 adults in the general population

D. Left ventricular hypertrophy (LVH) is the hallmark of the disease.

   1. LVH may develop in childhood, adolescence, or adult life.

   2. LVH can affect any part of the LV, although often preferentially affects the ventricular septum which can cause outflow tract obstruction.

   3. Outflow tract obstruction increases the risk of progression to heart failure, stroke, and sudden cardiac death. The outflow obstruction can be fixed or dynamic (variable).

   4. The obstruction may generate high velocities, which draw the mitral valve leaflet toward the septum (known as systolic anterior motion of the mitral valve). This further aggravates the outflow obstruction and simultaneously causes mitral regurgitation.

   5. Chamber size affects magnitude of obstruction. Smaller chamber size brings the anterior leaflet of mitral valve closer to the hypertrophied septum and increases obstruction. This occurs when preload decreases (such as with standing), or when afterload decreases or contractility increases.

E. Most patients are asymptomatic or mildly symptomatic.

F. Complications include HF, angina, mitral regurgitation, atrial fibrillation, stroke, syncope, and sudden cardiac death.

   1. HF

      a. More common in patients with outflow obstruction

      b. Develops due to a combination of outflow obstruction and diastolic dysfunction

      c. Dyspnea on exertion is the most common symptom.

      d. Aggravated by concomitant mitral regurgitation when present

   2. Angina

      a. May be typical or atypical in quality

      b. Develops in 25–30% of patients with hypertrophic cardiomyopathy

      c. Ischemia is not primarily due to epicardial CAD, but results from a mismatch of oxygen supply and demand.

      d. Aggravated by massive LVH and abnormal microvasculature

      e. Concomitant CAD may be present

   3. Syncope

      a. Develops in 15–25% of patients with hypertrophic cardiomyopathy

      b. Secondary to a variety of mechanisms, including ventricular arrhythmias, outflow tract obstruction, ischemia and, rarely, conduction blocks

   4. Sudden cardiac death is the most dreaded complication.

      a. Often occurs in previously asymptomatic patients

      b. Secondary to ventricular tachyarrhythmias (which may in turn be triggered by outflow tract obstruction and ischemia)

      c. Annual risk among all patients with hypertrophic cardiomyopathy: 0.6–1%

      d. *Major* risk factors include the following:

         (1) Prior events

            (a) Prior cardiac arrest

            (b) Spontaneous sustained VT

         (2) High risk clinical factors

            (a) Family history of sudden cardiac death in first-degree relative

            (b) Unexplained syncope (particularly if repetitive, exercise-induced, or occurs in children)

            (c) Massive LVH (≥ 30 mm)

            (d) Abnormal BP response to exercise

            (e) Nonsustained VT on Holter monitoring

   5. Atrial fibrillation

      a. Left atrial enlargement may develop secondary to decreased LV compliance or mitral regurgitation and creates a substrate for the development of atrial fibrillation.

      b. Atrial fibrillation decreases LV filling and worsens the outflow tract obstruction.

      c. Amiodarone is often used for these patients.

   6. Stroke usually secondary to concomitant atrial fibrillation and subsequent embolization.

F. Annual evaluation

   1. History and physical exam

   2. Family history

   3. Echocardiography

   4. 48-hour Holter monitoring

   5. Exercise stress testing (to assess BP response to exercise and evaluate ischemia)

## Evidence-Based Diagnosis

A. The classic murmur of hypertrophic cardiomyopathy is a harsh systolic murmur heard at the apex and lower left sternal border.

   1. It is accentuated by maneuvers that decrease chamber size (resulting in an increased obstruction).

   2. The murmur increases as a patient goes from a squatting to a standing position (sensitivity 95%, specificity 84%; LR+ 5.9, LR– 0.06).

   3. Passive leg elevation decreases the murmur (sensitivity 85% specificity 91%; LR+ 9.4, LR– 0.16).

B. ECG findings

   1. Abnormal in 92% of patients (73% in asymptomatic patients without obstruction)

2. Repolarization abnormalities (ST-segment elevation, depression or T-wave inversions) are found in 86% of patients although less common in asymptomatic, nonobstructed patients (58%).

3. LVH present in 81% obstructed patients and 48% nonobstructed patients

4. Other abnormalities include: Prominent Q waves, left atrial enlargement, and left axis deviation.

5. ECG abnormalities may *precede* echocardiographic abnormalities and may increase in frequency with age.

C. Echocardiogram

1. May be normal in affected young children

2. Often first appears abnormal during adolescence

3. LV wall thickening (≥ 15 mm) in the absence of other conditions known to cause LVH (ie, hypertension or aortic stenosis).

   a. LVH can occur in any part of the LV and in an array of distributions but is often asymmetric in distribution.

   b. The classic pattern that has specific consequences is marked septal hypertrophy.

D. DNA analysis for mutant genes is not widely available but is the most definitive method for establishing hypertrophic cardiomyopathy. This is particularly useful when another family member has been affected and the particular mutation is known.

### Treatment

A. Medical therapy

1. Patients should be told to avoid dehydration and strenuous exertion.

2. β-Blockers

   a. Decrease contractility and slow HR, augmenting diastolic filling and thereby decreasing dynamic outflow obstruction

   b. May also decrease ischemia

3. Many drugs are contraindicated and medications should be instituted cautiously.

B. Implantable cardioverter defibrillator (ICD) therapy is recommended by The American College of Cardiology for patients with a history of a prior cardiac arrest, spontaneous sustained VT, or ≥ 1 of the major risk factors listed above.

C. Surgical therapy (septal myomectomy) can decrease the degree of obstruction in severely symptomatic patients (ie, sudden cardiac death, syncope, heart failure) with documented gradients of > 30 mm at rest or 50 mm with exercise.

D. Catheter-based alcohol septal ablation can induce septal infarction and is another option.

1. However, compared with surgical myomectomy, there appears to be an increased risk of subsequent life-threatening arrhythmias, complications, and less reliable symptom relief.

2. Surgical therapy remains the gold standard over alcohol infusion.

E. Family members of affected patients should be screened for the specific mutation (if it is known) or with annual echocardiograms and ECG (from 12 to 18 years of age) if the mutation is not known. After age 18, recommendations call for screening every 5 years.

F. Preparticipation screening of all young competitive athletes has been demonstrated to reduce the incidence of sudden cardiac death by 79% primarily due to a reduction in deaths from cardiomyopathy.

## CASE RESOLUTION

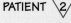

As noted above Mr. M's history and physical exam and normal ECG suggest neurocardiogenic syncope. There is no family history of sudden cardiac death, significant murmur, or ECG abnormality to suggest hypertrophic cardiomyopathy. There is no history of dehydration or offending medications (eg, vasodilators). Tilt-table testing is not indicated in patients with isolated episodes of well-defined neurocardiogenic syncope. Mr. M is reassured, and although embarrassed, he feels much better. After explaining the pathophysiology of his disorder, you initiate standard recommendations for the prevention of further episodes.

## CHIEF COMPLAINT

### PATIENT 2

Mr. C is a 65-year-old man who comes to see you with a chief complaint of syncope. He reports that he was sitting at home watching television when he suddenly lost consciousness without any warning. His wife reports that he was unresponsive for approximately 30 seconds. There was no tonic-clonic activity or incontinence, and the patient was not confused after regaining consciousness.

At this point, what is the leading hypothesis, what are the active alternatives, and is there a must not miss diagnosis? Given this differential diagnosis, what tests should be ordered?

## PRIORITIZING THE DIFFERENTIAL DIAGNOSIS

Mr. C's syncope sudden loss of consciousness without warning or precipitant and his age raise the possibility of some form of cardiac syncope. Active alternatives include orthostatic syncope (secondary to dehydration, hemorrhage, or drugs) and hypoglycemia-induced syncope. Hypoglycemia-induced syncope is usually preceded by either confusion or sympathetic stimulation producing tremulousness, nervousness, or diaphoresis and occurs almost exclusively in diabetic patients taking insulin, sulfonylureas, or thiazolidinediones. "Must not miss" alternatives include PE, which is an uncommon cause of syncope. Neurocardiogenic syncope is unlikely because syncope occurred while Mr. C was sitting and was not preceded by any pain or anxiety. The absence of any post syncopal confusion makes seizure unlikely. Table 26–2 lists the differential diagnosis.

**Table 26–2.** Diagnostic hypotheses for Mr. C.

| Diagnostic Hypotheses | Clinical Clues | Important Tests |
|---|---|---|
| **Leading Hypothesis** | | |
| Cardiac syncope | History of CAD, HF, or valvular heart disease Syncope while supine or with exercise Palpitations S$_3$, JVD, or significant murmur | ECG Echocardiogram Stress test Event monitor EP study |
| **Active Alternatives—Most Common** | | |
| Dehydration or hemorrhage | History of vomiting, diarrhea, poor oral intake History of melena or rectal bleeding Positive fecal occult blood test | Orthostatic measurement of BP and pulse |
| Medications | History of α-blockers, other antihypertensive medication | Orthostatic measurement of BP and pulse |
| Hypoglycemia | Insulin, sulfonylureas, or thiazolidinediones therapy | Glucose measurement at time of event |
| **Active Alternatives—Must Not Miss** | | |
| PE | Risk factors for PE Pleuritic chest pain or dyspnea Loud S$_2$ Unexplained persistent hypotension Right heart strain on ECG (right bundle-branch block, right axis deviation) or right ventricular dilatation on echocardiogram | CT angiogram Ventilation-perfusion scan Leg Dopplers Angiogram |

2

Past medical history reveals that Mr. C has suffered from 2 myocardial infarctions (MI). Subsequently, he has dyspnea upon walking more than 20 yards. Mr. C also has diabetes mellitus. His medications include atenolol, aspirin, atorvastatin, insulin, and lisinopril. On physical exam, his BP is 128/70 mm Hg with a pulse of 72 bpm, which is regular. There is no significant change upon standing. His lung exam is clear, and cardiac exam reveals prominent JVD and a loud S$_3$ gallop. There is no significant murmur. He has 2+ pretibial edema, and his rectal exam reveals guaiac-negative stool. Finally, Mrs. C reports that she took Mr. C's blood glucose when he passed out and that the reading was 120 mg/dL.

☑ **Is the clinical information sufficient to make a diagnosis? If not, what other information do you need?**

Mr. C's history of myocardial infarction (MI) is **a pivotal clue** and dramatically increases the likelihood of some form of cardiac syncope. Furthermore, his history of dyspnea on minimal exertion, jugular venous distention (JVD), and S$_3$ gallop all suggest HF. HF in turn markedly increases the likelihood of VT. His lack of postural BP change argues against orthostatic syncope from dehydration, hemorrhage, or medications. His normal blood glucose at the time of the event effectively rules out hypoglycemia. PE is possible but less likely.

## Leading Hypothesis: Cardiac Syncope

### Textbook Presentation

Cardiac syncope refers to syncope secondary to a disorder arising within the heart. Arrhythmias (either tachyarrhythmias or bradyarrhythmias) are the most common disorders, although occasionally syncope may be secondary to severe valvular heart disease (eg, aortic stenosis). Rare causes of cardiac syncope include aortic dissection, cardiac tamponade, and atrial myxoma. Classically, patients with cardiac syncope are elderly patients with known heart disease (ie, HF or CAD) who experience sudden syncope, which may occur without warning. Patients may have palpitations.

### Disease Highlights

A. The presence of heart disease is the single most important prognostic factor in patients with syncope.

   1. Cardiac syncope is associated with increased mortality. The 1-year mortality rate in patients with cardiac syncope is 18–33%, compared with 6% in patients with syncope of unknown cause.

   2. Subsequent mortality in patients experiencing syncope increases with the severity of heart disease.

      a. Class 1–2 HF, OR 7.7

      b. Class 3–4 HF, OR 13.5

   3. Patients in whom cardiac syncope is suspected should be admitted for evaluation (see Figures 26–7, 26–8).

   4. Among patients with dilated cardiomyopathy, sudden cardiac death (presumably arrhythmogenic) accounts for 30% of the mortality.

B. Although there are a large number of cardiac dysrhythmias, only a relative few produce syncope. Most supraventricular tachyarrhythmias will not cause syncope because the AV node limits the ventricular response rate. The most common arrhythmias associated with syncope include

   1. Tachycardias

      a. VT

      b. Supraventricular tachycardias associated with an accessory pathway (ie, WPW syndrome [see end of chapter]).

   2. Bradycardias: 34% of patients with heart disease have significant bradycardias.

      a. Sinus node dysfunction

         (1) Sinus bradycardia (< 35 bpm)

         (2) Sinus pauses defined as > 3 seconds (or > 2 seconds with symptoms)

      b. AV heart block (second- or third-degree)

      c. Atrial fibrillation with a *slow* ventricular response

***Table 26–3.*** Sensitivity, specificity, and LRs for cardiac syncope.

| Clinical Feature | Sensitivity | Specificity | LR+ | LR– |
|---|---|---|---|---|
| **Patients with suspected or certain heart disease** | | | | |
| Prior history of cardiac disease | 95% | 45% | 2.1 | 0.09 |
| Syncope while supine | 12% | 98% | 6 | 0.90 |
| Syncope with effort | 14% | 96% | 3.5 | 0.90 |
| **Patients without suspected or certain heart disease** | | | | |
| Palpitations | 75% | 87% | 5.8 | 0.29 |

## Evidence-Based Diagnosis

A. History

1. Syncope in patients with suspected or certain heart disease

   a. Preexistent cardiac disease increases the risk of cardiac syncope, and the absence of cardiac disease markedly decreases the risk of cardiac syncope (Table 26–3).

   b. Syncope while supine or during exertion increases the likelihood of cardiac syncope (LR+ 6 and 3.5, respectively). However, since neither of these features is sensitive for cardiac syncope, their absence does not diminish the likelihood of cardiac syncope.

2. Syncope in patients without known or suspected heart disease: Palpitations increased the likelihood of cardiac syncope (LR+ 5.8)

B. Laboratory tests

1. An abnormal ECG increases the OR of cardiac arrhythmias in patients without neurocardiogenic syncope (OR, 23.5 [CI, 7–87]).

2. Certain ECG findings may suggest particular cardiac etiologies.

   a. ECG evidence of prior MI or a long QT interval increases the likelihood of VT.

   b. ECG findings of significant bradycardia, second- or third-degree AV block increase the likelihood of a significant bradycardia.

   c. BBB suggests intermittent AV block.

   d. RV strain (S1Q3T3) or right BBB suggests PE.

   e. Ischemic changes suggest MI.

   f. Delta wave or short PR interval suggests an accessory pathway (eg, WPW syndrome).

3. Echocardiograms

   a. Used to assess LV function

   b. Used to assess valve function (eg, aortic stenosis)

   c. VT is much more common in presence of LV dysfunction.

4. Exercise testing

   a. Particularly useful in patients with exertional syncope

   b. Also obtained in patients with cardiac disease

5. Holter monitoring: External cardiac leads are applied to the patient and a 24- to 48-hour recording of the cardiac rhythm is made.

   a. Diagnostic only if

      (1) Arrhythmia captured *and* patient symptomatic during arrhythmia or

      (2) Rhythm normal during symptoms (excludes an arrhythmia)

   b. Often nondiagnostic due to

      (1) Absence of arrhythmia during study

      (2) Absence of symptoms during arrhythmia

6. External loop recorders

   a. External devices that can be worn for up to 1 month. A continuous recording is made.

   b. If symptoms occur, most recent 2–5 minutes can be frozen in memory and transmitted by telephone.

   c. Relative short duration of monitoring (1 month) still limits sensitivity.

   d. Often used in patients with nondiagnostic Holter monitoring, particularly when symptoms are infrequent. Sensitivity is 14%, compared with long-term *implantable* loop recorder.

7. Implantable loop recorders have been used successfully in some patients with recurrent unexplained syncope. The yield in such patients has been reported at 90%. This may be particularly useful at detecting bradycardias missed by electrophysiologic (EP) studies.

8. EP studies are invasive procedures that use a right heart catheterization. During EP studies, stimuli are delivered to the heart in order to detect bradyarrhythmias and accessory pathways as well as to elicit tachyarrhythmias.

   a. Sensitivity is 90% for VT.

   b. Sensitivity for bradyarrhythmias is low (33%).

   c. Overall diagnostic yield of EP studies

      (1) 36–70% in patients with heart disease

      (2) 22% in patients with abnormal ECGs

      (3) 14% in select patients with normal ECGs without heart disease

   d. Indications for EP studies in patients with unexplained syncope include

      (1) Prior MI

      (2) Structural heart disease

      (3) Impaired LV function

**(4)** Bifascicular block

**(5)** Monitoring suggests sinus node dysfunction or AV block

**e.** Risk of EP studies include cardiac perforation, MI, AV fistulae (< 3%), deep venous thrombosis, and PE.

Mr. C's serum troponin levels are undetectable (thus excluding acute MI). The ECG shows Q waves in leads V1–V4 and II, III and aVF consistent with prior anterior and inferior MI. The PR interval is normal. There is no evidence of sinus bradycardia, sinus pause, or AV block. The QRS width is normal, excluding BBB. An echocardiogram reveals severe LV dysfunction with hypokinesis of the anterior and inferior walls. The ejection fraction is estimated to be 25%. The aortic valve is normal without evidence of aortic stenosis.

Mr. C's ECG and echocardiogram confirm severe LV dysfunction, markedly increasing the likelihood of some form of cardiac syncope. In particular, patients with LV dysfunction are at high risk for VT. There are no ECG findings to suggest bradycardia (ie, heart block, BBB, sinus bradycardia). The leading hypothesis is revised to VT.

## Revised Leading Hypothesis: VT

### Textbook Presentation

Patients with VT may be asymptomatic or have symptoms that range from palpitations to lightheadedness, near syncope, syncope, or sudden cardiac death.

VT occurs most commonly in patients with CAD and HF and should be seriously considered when patients with preexisting CAD or HF present with syncope.

### Disease Highlights

**A.** Etiology and associations

  **1.** Ischemic heart disease

  **a.** Associated with CAD in 80% of cases

  **b.** May be secondary to acute ischemia/MI or prior scar

  **2.** Heart failure

  **3.** Hypertrophic cardiomyopathy

  **4.** Valvular heart disease

  **5.** Drugs (antiarrhythmic, antipsychotic, tricyclic antidepressant and other drugs that prolong the QT interval)

  **6.** Electrolyte disorders (hypokalemia, hypocalcemia, hypomagnesemia)

  **7.** Congenital disorders

  **a.** Congenital heart disease

  **b.** Long QT syndrome

    **(1)** The ECG of affected families demonstrates long refractory periods (long QT intervals)

    **(2)** Affected patients are at risk for sudden cardiac death from a form of VT called torsades de pointes.

    **(3)** Arrhythmias may be precipitated by emotional or physical stress.

    **(4)** Associated with congenital neural deafness

    **(5)** A variety of drugs and electrolyte disturbances may also prolong the QT interval and predispose to VT and sudden cardiac death.

  **c.** Brugada syndrome

    **(1)** Unusual disorder secondary to mutation in the sodium channel gene, which predisposes patients to polymorphic VT and sudden death.

    **(2)** Suggestive baseline ECG abnormalities include a right BBB pattern with ST elevation in the right precordial leads.

**B.** ECG criteria

  **1.** ≥3 consecutive wide complex (QRS ≥ .12 seconds) beats (Figure 26–2)

  **a.** Supraventricular tachycardias can also occasionally manifest wide QRS complexes.

  **b.** ECG criteria that increase the likelihood that the wide complex tachycardia is VT include fusion beats, capture beats, AV dissociation, or a QRS width > .14 seconds.

  **c.** A history of CAD or HF increases the likelihood that the wide complex tachycardia is VT.

  **2.** Sustained VT is defined as VT lasting longer than 30 seconds.

**C.** Evaluation

  **1.** Obtain baseline ECG to look for evidence of ischemia, long QT syndrome

  **2.** Stress testing (and coronary angiography in selected patients) is recommended for patients with exercise-induced syncope or chest pain or an intermediate or greater probability of CAD.

  **3.** Obtain echocardiogram to evaluate LV function and rule out valvular heart disease.

  **4.** EP testing is recommended for selected patients (see above).

**D.** Prognosis

  **1.** VT is a potentially life-threatening arrhythmia.

  **2.** Predictors of mortality in patients with VT include prior cardiac arrest, LV dysfunction, post MI, or inducible VT on EP studies.

### Treatment

**A.** The management of *acute* VT evolves rapidly and is beyond the scope of this text. Please see appropriate ACLS guidelines.

**B.** Prevention of recurrent VT and sudden cardiac death

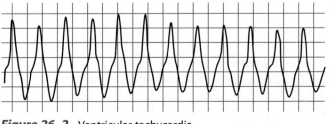

***Figure 26–2.*** Ventricular tachycardia.

   1. Treat underlying conditions
      a. Treat ischemic heart disease (including revascularization if necessary)
      b. Treat HF (ACE inhibitors, β-blockade, and spironolactone have all been shown to decrease mortality)
      c. Optimize electrolytes, including magnesium
   2. Specific therapy for the treatment and prevention of VT includes antiarrhythmic drugs (especially β-blockers and possibly amiodarone), catheter ablation, ICDs, and combinations of the above.
      a. ICDs are implanted devices that monitor the cardiac rhythm and automatically detect and shock patients in VT.
      b. ICDs are used in selected patients at high risk of sudden death including survivors of sudden death and patients in whom syncope was believed to have been caused by VT.
      c. Indications for ICD therapy include
         (1) Patients with syncope and heart disease and documented prior spontaneous VT or inducible VT (during EP testing)
         (2) Patients with syncope and significant LV dysfunction (ejection fraction ≤ 30%) in whom VT cannot be documented or induced but in whom syncope remains unexplained (and presumed due to VT)
         (3) Patients with unexplained syncope and inducible sustained VT or ventricular fibrillation during EP studies.

## MAKING A DIAGNOSIS

The pretest probability of VT is very high. You elect to admit Mr. C for inpatient monitoring. You still wonder if a significant bradyarrhythmia or a PE might be responsible for Mr. C's syncope.

 Have you crossed a diagnostic threshold for the leading hypothesis, VT? Do other tests need to be done to exclude the alternative diagnoses?

## Alternative Diagnosis: Bradycardia from Sick Sinus Syndrome (SSS)

### Textbook Presentation

The presentation of SSS depends on the duration and severity of the bradyarrhythmia. When the bradyarrhythmia is severe and prolonged, patients may experience sudden syncope. With less severe bradycardia, patients may experience weakness, dyspnea on exertion, angina, transient ischemic attacks, or near syncope. Since the bradyarrhythmia may be short lived, patients may recover without intervention.

### Disease Highlights

A. Episodic or persistent failure of sinus node

B. Most common indication for pacemaker placement

C. Often seen in the elderly (mean age 68) due to fibrosis and degeneration of sinus node

D. Underlying CAD is common and contributes to the pathogenesis of SSS in some patients.

E. A variety of medications can depress sinus node function and aggravate SSS, including β-blockers, verapamil, diltiazem, digoxin, clonidine, methyldopa, and other antiarrhythmics

F. Electrical manifestations may include
   1. Sinus bradycardia < 40 bpm
   2. Sinus pauses > 2 seconds
   3. Sinus arrest (with an escape junctional rhythm)
   4. Sinoatrial exit block (inability of the sinus impulse to exit the sinus node)

G. Concomitant AV conduction disturbances are present in over 50% of patients with SSS.

H. Associated with supraventricular *tachy*arrhythmias, in 40–60% of patients, particularly atrial fibrillation (tachy-brady syndrome). Such patients may complain of palpitations. The bradycardia often follows termination of the tachycardia. Tachy-brady syndrome markedly increases the risk of death or nonfatal stroke (2- to 3-fold) compared with SSS alone.

### Evidence-Based Diagnosis

A. Simultaneous symptoms and ECG findings (sinus bradycardia, significant pauses or sinus exit block) establishes the diagnosis.

B. Holter monitoring may be used but is often nondiagnostic due to the intermittent nature of the arrhythmia.

C. External cardiac event monitors allow for a longer period of monitoring and correlation with symptoms.

D. Carotid sinus massage (CSM) may cause prolonged pauses in patients with SSS (> 3 seconds).

E. Internal loop recorders have also been used.

F. Pharmacologic studies
   1. Adenosine slows sinus node activity.
   2. Small studies suggest patients with SSS have delayed sinus node recovery following adenosine administration.
   3. The diagnostic accuracy is similar to EP studies.

G. EP studies
   1. Useful in patients with severe symptoms when simultaneous rhythm abnormalities and symptoms are unavailable.
   2. Sinus node recovery time (SNRT) and sinoatrial conduction time (SACT) can be measured. Abnormal responses are 70% sensitive, 90% specific. Normal results do not rule out SSS.

### Treatment

A. Discontinue any medications that may adversely affect sinus function (see above). (If β-blockers or other drugs cannot be discontinued, patients may require pacemaker.)

B. Pacemakers
   1. Indications
      a. Documented **symptomatic** sinus node dysfunction
      b. Chronotropic incompetence: In this condition, the sinus rate does not increase appropriately with physical activity, leading to a relative bradycardia and symptoms.
      c. Pacemakers are used in certain situations when SSS is suspected but cannot be confirmed.
         (1) Patients with HR < 40 bpm and prior symptoms
         (2) EP study shows long SNRT in patients with prior unexplained syncope.

**2.** Atrial pacing is associated with a lower incidence of complications (eg, HF, atrial fibrillation, embolization, and possibly mortality) than isolated ventricular pacing.

**C.** Anticoagulation is indicated for certain patients with SSS.

**1.** Patients with concurrent tachy-brady syndrome and atrial fibrillation (persistent or intermittent)

**2.** Patients with a ventricular pacemaker (rather than an atrial pacemaker)

**3.** For the remaining patients, the risk of embolization is low (1.2–1.4%/y) and the benefits of anticoagulation must be weighed against the risks.

## Alternative Diagnosis: Bradycardia due to AV Heart Block

### Textbook Presentation

Depending on the duration and severity of the heart block, patients with AV block may be asymptomatic or complain of syncope, near syncope, palpitations, angina or transient ischemic attacks.

### Disease Highlights

**A.** Secondary to conduction abnormalities in the AV node, bundle of His, or bundle branches.

**B.** Classification (Table 26–4)

**1.** In first-degree AV block *all* of the sinus impulses (P waves) are conducted (but the PR interval is prolonged), whereas in third-degree AV block, *none* of the P waves are conducted (Figure 26–3).

**2.** In second-degree block, *some* of the impulses are conducted.

**C.** In second- or third-degree AV block, the ventricular rate slows and may depend on lower intrinsic pacemakers residing within the ventricle. The bradycardia can result in dyspnea, angina, hypotension, syncope, or death.

**D.** AV nodal disease should also be suspected in patients with atrial fibrillation who have a slow ventricular response and are not on drugs that slow AV conduction (eg, digoxin, β-blockers, verapamil, or diltiazem).

**E.** Etiology

**1.** Fibrosis of the conduction system

**2.** Ischemic heart disease

**3.** Drugs (eg, β-blockers, verapamil, diltiazem, digoxin, amiodarone)

 The combination of verapamil and β-blockers should always be avoided. There is a high incidence of subsequent AV block and HF.

**4.** Hyperkalemia

**5.** Valvular heart disease (due to extension of calcification into the conduction system)

**6.** Increased vagal tone

**7.** Miscellaneous other causes (Lyme disease, sarcoidosis, etc)

### Treatment

**A.** Withdraw drugs that impair AV conduction.

**B.** Treat ischemia.

**C.** Correct electrolyte abnormalities.

**D.** Atropine can be useful in emergent situations.

**E.** Pacemakers

**1.** Precise indications are complex.

**2.** In general, pacing is recommended for patients with third-degree AV block or Mobitz II second-degree AV block.

**3.** Pacing is not usually indicated in asymptomatic first-degree AV block or Mobitz I second-degree AV block.

## Alternative Diagnosis: Pulmonary Embolism

### Textbook Presentation

PE is an unusual cause of syncope (about 1%) and is covered extensively in Chapter 14, Dyspnea. This discussion will focus on

**Table 26–4.** Classification of heart block.

| Atrial Ventricular Type | Conduction | ECG Findings | Clinical Findings | Treatment |
|---|---|---|---|---|
| First degree | 1:1 | PR interval > 0.2 seconds<br>QRS width usually within normal limits | None | None |
| Second degree Mobitz I | Intermittent | Progressive lengthening of PR interval until P wave is not conducted and QRS absent. Next PR interval shorter than PR prior to dropped beat<br>QRS width usually within normal limits | Associated with inferior MI. Rarely progresses to third-degree AV block | Observation or atropine |
| Second degree Mobitz II | Intermittent | Intermittent non-conduction of P waves. More severe infranodal damage, QRS may be widened, BBB may be seen | Associated with anterior MI. Often progresses to third-degree AV block | Pacemaker |
| Third-degree | ∅ | P waves not conducted. Complete AV disassociation. Ventricular rate depends on escape pacemakers | Associated with CAD, drugs, degeneration, abnormal electrolytes, bradycardia, hypotension | Pacemaker |

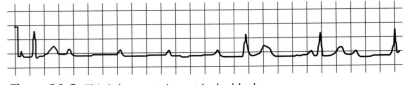

**Figure 26–3.** Third-degree atrioventricular block.

patients who experience syncope due to PE. Between 9% and 14% of patients with PE experience syncope. Syncope in PE is usually secondary to massive embolization involving more than 50% of the pulmonary vascular bed. This massive embolization increases the likelihood of findings consistent with more extensive PE including hypotension (ranging from 14% to 76% in various studies), cardiac arrest (24%), and ECG evidence of cor pulmonale (S1Q3T3 or new complete or incomplete right BBB in 60%.) Despite this, the subset of patients with PE and syncope who survive to arrive at the hospital have often stabilized due to clot fragmentation and may be hemodynamically stable and relatively asymptomatic. Dyspnea has been reported in 50–90% of patients, hypoxia (PaO$_2$ < 60 mm Hg) in 91%. PE should be considered as a cause of syncope in patients with dyspnea, hypoxia, a history of risk factors for PE, pleuritic chest pain or physical exam findings of unexplained hypotension, tachycardia, JVD, a loud S$_2$ or a right-sided S$_3$ gallop. Suggestive ECG findings include a S1Q3T3 pattern, right axis deviation, or right BBB. Echocardiographic findings suggestive of PE include right atrial or right ventricular enlargement. An unexplained pulmonary infiltrate may be a sign of infarction from pulmonary embolus.

## CASE RESOLUTION

After 24 hours, Mr. C is feeling well. He is anxious to go home. The telemetry reveals normal sinus rhythm without evidence of intermittent AV block or VT. Stress testing is performed and shows evidence of prior MI but no acute ischemia.

The sensitivity of telemetry is inadequate to exclude life-threatening arrhythmias such as VT. Furthermore, none of the alternative diagnoses are suggested by the history, physical exams, or laboratory test results (such as AS, hypoglycemia, dehydration, orthostatic hypotension, PE, SSS, or AV heart block). After careful discussion with Mr. C, you order an EP study.

The EP study demonstrates inducible sustained VT, placing the patient at high risk for spontaneous lethal ventricular arrhythmias. An ICD is placed. At follow-up 12 months later, Mr. C is doing well and has no subsequent syncopal events. His ICD has delivered 5 shocks.

## CHIEF COMPLAINT

PATIENT 3

Mrs. S is a 60-year-old woman who arrives at the emergency department via ambulance after an episode of syncope. The patient reports that she was eating dinner, and the next thing she knew she was in the emergency department. Mr. S reports that he found his wife lying on the floor next to the dining room table when he came home. At that time, Mrs. S was conscious but lethargic. The food and plate were scattered on the floor. There was no evidence of incontinence. On physical exam, her vital signs are normal. HEENT exam reveals a contusion over the right eye and bruising along the right half of her tongue. Cardiac and pulmonary exams are normal. Abdominal exam is unremarkable. Stool is guaiac negative. Neurologic exam is nonfocal.

 At this point, what is the leading hypothesis, what are the active alternatives, and is there a must not miss diagnosis? Given this differential diagnosis, what tests should be ordered?

## PRIORITIZING THE DIFFERENTIAL DIAGNOSIS

The remarkable feature of Mrs. S's history is the prolonged period of lethargy and confusion that persisted until she reached the emergency department. This **pivotal clue** is highly suggestive of a postictal period following a seizure. Furthermore, the patient's bruised tongue is a diagnostic **fingerprint** that markedly increases the likelihood of a seizure. Another consideration is hypoglycemia, which can also cause a prolonged period of lethargy or confusion. This contrasts with patients suffering from cardiac or neurocardiogenic syncope who tend to regain consciousness almost immediately and do not usually suffer from prolonged confusion, lethargy, or memory loss. Therefore, despite the absence of witnessed tonic-clonic activity, the prolonged period of confusion, amnesia and bruised tongue are highly suggestive of seizures. Table 26–5 lists the differential diagnosis.

Patients with syncope should be asked, "What was the next thing you remember?" Patients who do not remember the ambulance ride or suffer a period of amnesia **following the event** (> 5 minutes) should be evaluated for seizures.

**Table 26–5.** Diagnostic hypotheses for Mrs. S.

| Diagnostic Hypotheses | Clinical Clues | Important Tests |
|---|---|---|
| **Leading Hypothesis** | | |
| Seizure | Prolonged period of lethargy, confusion, amnesia suggesting postictal period<br>Tonic-clonic activity<br>Incontinence<br>Prior stroke, CNS tumor, or neurologic disease<br>Abnormal neurologic exam | EEG<br>Contrast-enhanced CT or MRI scan |
| **Active Alternatives—Most Common** | | |
| Hypoglycemia | Diabetes mellitus treated with either insulin, thiazolidinediones, or sulfonylureas | Glucose measurement at time of event |

③

The patient reports no prior history of epilepsy, CNS tumor, or stroke. She has no history of cerebrovascular disease or head trauma. She has no history of diabetes and is not taking any medications. She does not remember any antecedent event. She has no cardiac history and walks 2 miles every day without dyspnea or chest pain. She reports no history of melena or hematochezia.

Is the clinical information sufficient to make a diagnosis? If not, what other information do you need?

## Leading Hypothesis: Seizures

### Textbook Presentation

Generalized seizures classically present with tonic-clonic activity, loss of postural tone, incontinence, and a prolonged postictal period of lethargy. The purpose of this review is to focus on features that help distinguish seizures from syncope.

### Disease Highlights

A. 3% of US population suffers a seizure in their lifetime

B. Seizures are the cause of syncope in 1–7% of patients.

C. Etiology of seizure and prevalence in patients over age 60

   1. Idiopathic, 35%

   2. Ischemic, 49%

   3. CNS tumor, 11%

      a. Primary CNS tumor, 35%

      b. Metastatic, 59%

   4. CNS trauma, 3%

   5. CNS infection, 2%

   6. Metabolic disturbances

      a. Hypoglycemia and hyperglycemia (marked)

      b. Hypoxia

      c. Hyponatremia

      d. Hypocalcemia

      e. Uremia

   7. Medications (Numerous medications have been implicated. Some commonly used medications that rarely cause seizures include cyclosporine, fentanyl, meperidine, lidocaine, phenothiazines, quinolones, theophylline, tricyclic antidepressants, and bupropion)

   8. Illicit drugs (ie, methylenedioxymethamphetamine [MDMA; Ecstasy], cocaine)

   9. Withdrawal states (ie, alcohol, baclofen, benzodiazepines, and opioids)

### Evidence-Based Diagnosis

A. Postictal confusion is the most sensitive clinical feature (Table 26–6). The absence of a postictal period makes seizures an unlikely cause of syncope. (sensitivity 94%, LR– 0.09).

FP

B. Tongue laceration, head turning, and unusual posturing are the most specific clinical features and substantially increase the likelihood of seizure (specificity 97%, LR+ 12–15).

C. Certain symptoms are unusual in patients with seizures and reduce the likelihood of seizure.

   1. Diaphoresis preceding spell, LR 0.17

   2. Chest pain preceding spell, LR 0.15

   3. Palpitations, LR 0.12

   4. Dyspnea prior to spell, LR 0.08

   5. CAD, LR 0.08

   6. Syncope with prolonged standing, LR 0.05

**Table 26–6.** Sensitivity, specificity, and LRs for seizures.

| Clinical Feature | Sensitivity (%) | Specificity (%) | LR+ | LR– |
|---|---|---|---|---|
| Cut tongue | 45 | 97 | 15 | 0.57 |
| Head turning | 43 | 97 | 14 | 0.59 |
| Unusual posturing | 35 | 97 | 12 | 0.67 |
| Bedwetting | 24 | 96 | 6.4 | 0.79 |
| Limb jerking noted by others | 69 | 88 | 5.8 | 0.35 |
| Prodromal trembling | 29 | 94 | 4.8 | 0.76 |
| Prodromal preoccupation | 8 | 98 | 4.0 | 0.94 |
| Prodromal hallucinations | 8 | 98 | 4.0 | 0.94 |
| Postictal confusion | 94 | 69 | 3.0 | 0.09 |

***Table 26–7.*** A point score to distinguish seizures from syncope.[1]

| Criteria | Points |
| --- | --- |
| Waking with cut tongue | 2 |
| Abnormal behavior (eg, limb jerking, prodromal trembling, preoccupation, hallucinations) | 1 |
| Lost consciousness with emotional stress | 1 |
| Postictal confusion | 1 |
| Head turning to 1 side | 1 |
| Prodromal deja vu | 1 |
| Any presyncope | −2 |
| Lost consciousness with prolonged standing | −2 |
| Diaphoresis before a spell | −2 |

[1]Point scores of ≥ 1 suggest seizures.

D. Convulsive syncope
   1. Limb jerking is not entirely specific for seizures.
   2. 15–90% of patients with syncope not related to seizures experience limb jerking, a phenomenon referred to as **convulsive syncope**. Limb jerking due to syncope is associated with myoclonic jerks, which should be distinguished from tonic-clonic activity.
      a. Myoclonic jerks tend to be arrhythmic and asymmetric, whereas the opposite is true of tonic-clonic activity.
      b. Myoclonic jerks tend to be briefer than tonic-clonic activity (average of 6.6 seconds).
      c. Myoclonic jerks never precede collapse, whereas tonic-clonic activity may precede collapse.
   3. Finally, unlike generalized seizures, which are usually associated with a significant postictal period, convulsive syncope is not associated with a significant postictal period (< 1 minute).
   4. Patients who appear to have refractory "seizure disorders" and nonspecific abnormalities on EEG should undergo tilt-table testing to rule out neurocardiogenic syncope with myoclonic jerks.
E. A point score to distinguish seizures from syncope has been developed (Table 26–7). Point scores of ≥ 1 suggest seizures (sensitivity, 94%; specificity, 94%; LR+, 16; LR−, 0.06).
F. Evaluation
   1. EEG
      a. Sensitivity (between episodes) of the spike and wave pattern is 35–50% (increased with sleep deprivation)
      b. Specificity 98%
      c. Indicated in the evaluation of patients with possible seizures
   2. Neuroimaging
      a. 37% of adults with new-onset seizures have structural lesions (eg, tumors, strokes)

   b. 15% of adults with new-onset seizures and nonfocal neurologic exams have structural lesions on neuroimaging.
   c. Indicated in all adults with new-onset seizures.
   d. In acute cases, a noncontrast CT is often performed to rule out an intracranial bleed. Follow-up MRI is recommended due to its increased sensitivity for both tumor and stroke.
3. Sodium, calcium, glucose, BUN, and creatinine
4. Oxygen saturation
5. Lumbar puncture
   a. A lumbar puncture should be considered if CNS infection is suspected (ie, patient is immunocompromised or has fever, meningismus, headache, or persistent confusion).
   b. Elevated intracranial pressure should be excluded (usually with neuroimaging) prior to a lumbar puncture in order to prevent lumbar puncture–induced herniation.
   c. Platelet count, prothrombin time (PT), and partial thromboplastin time (PTT) should be checked prior to lumbar puncture. (Thrombocytopenia and coagulopathies increase the risk of bleeding at the lumbar puncture site and subsequent spinal cord compression secondary to hemorrhage.)
6. Toxicology screen should be ordered if illicit drug use is suspected.
7. Prolactin measurement: American Academy of Neurology concluded that serum prolactin levels cannot be used to distinguish seizures from syncope.

## Treatment

Anticonvulsant therapy is complex and evolves rapidly (see neurology texts).

## MAKING A DIAGNOSIS

The patient's EEG revealed intermittent right temporal spike and wave pattern.

The patient's history of a postictal period and tongue biting are highly suggestive of seizures, which was confirmed on the EEG. Since structural lesions and ischemia are common in adults with new-onset seizures, neuroimaging is required.

## CASE RESOLUTION

An MRI scan revealed a solitary right temporal lobe mass. Subsequent biopsy demonstrated a glioblastoma multiforme. The patient underwent surgical resection and was treated with anticonvulsant therapy. She died approximately 6 months later.

## CHIEF COMPLAINT

PATIENT 4

Mrs. P is a 39-year-old woman who arrives at the emergency department via ambulance with abdominal pain and syncope. She was in her usual state of health until the morning of admission when increasing left lower quadrant abdominal pain developed. The pain increased in intensity and became quite severe. Upon standing, she lost consciousness and collapsed to the floor. She recovered quickly and was helped to a chair by her husband. When she stood several minutes later, she briefly lost consciousness again. The patient reports that her abdominal pain is much better. Her vital signs are BP, 105/60 mm Hg; pulse, 85 bpm; temperature, 37.0°C; and RR, 18 breaths per minute. Her cardiac and pulmonary exams are normal, and abdominal exam reveals mild left lower quadrant tenderness. Her ECG is normal and her Hct is normal at 36.0%.

At this point, what is the leading hypothesis, what are the active alternatives, and is there a must not miss diagnosis? Given this differential diagnosis, what tests should be ordered?

## PRIORITIZING THE DIFFERENTIAL DIAGNOSIS

Several features of Mrs. P's syncope are noteworthy. First, her syncope occurred in association with abdominal pain raising the possibility of neurocardiogenic syncope. Second, she had 2 episodes of syncope upon standing. This **pivotal clue** raises the possibility of orthostatic syncope from either dehydration, hemorrhage or medications. PE is another possibility. Reviewing the remaining differential diagnoses at the beginning of the chapter, her young age, absence of preexistent cardiovascular disease, and normal ECG argue against cardiac syncope. Aortic stenosis is unlikely in patients without a significant systolic murmur. Her rapid restoration of consciousness argues against a seizure. Table 26–8 lists the differential diagnosis.

4

Further history reveals that Mrs. P is not taking any medications and did not have any chest pain or dyspnea. She has no risk factors for PE (eg, oral birth control pills, prolonged immobilization, recent surgery or postpartum period, cancer, or known hypercoagulable state). Your initial assessment is neurocardiogenic syncope secondary to transient abdominal pain.

As discussed in the first case presentation, neurocardiogenic syncope is often precipitated by pain, is brief, and is followed by a rapid restoration of consciousness. Many of Mrs. P's features are consistent with this diagnosis. However, both episodes of syncope occurred immediately after standing providing a clue that her syncope was in fact orthostatic. In addition, although her abdominal pain is improved, it is still unexplained. You elect to check her BP and pulse for orthostatic change.

***Table 26–8.*** Diagnostic hypotheses for Mrs. P.

| Diagnostic Hypotheses | Clinical Clues | Important Tests |
|---|---|---|
| **Leading Hypothesis** | | |
| Neurocardiogenic syncope (faint) | Preceding pain, anxiety, fear or prolonged standing Rapid normalization of consciousness Absence of heart disease | Tilt table if recurrent |
| **Active Alternatives—Most Common** | | |
| Syncope due to orthostatic hypotension | History of vomiting, diarrhea, decreased oral intake, melena, bright red blood per rectum or other blood loss | Orthostatic measurement of BP and pulse |
| Medications | History of α-blockers, other antihypertensive medication | Orthostatic measurement of BP and pulse |
| **Active Alternatives—Must Not Miss** | | |
| PE | Risk factors for PE Pleuritic chest pain or dyspnea Loud $S_2$ Unexplained persistent hypotension Right heart strain on ECG (right bundle-branch block, right axis deviation) or right ventricular dilatation on echocardiogram | CT angiogram Ventilation-perfusion scan Leg Dopplers Angiogram |

4

Mrs. P's BP while supine was 105/60 mm Hg with a pulse of 85 bpm, which changed when sitting to BP of 95/50 mm Hg with a pulse of 90 bpm. Upon standing her BP fell to 60/0, her pulse was 140 bpm, and she lost consciousness. She was quickly laid down and again rapidly regained consciousness.

The patient's volume status is always assessed based on the clinical, **not laboratory** exam. Orthostatic measurement of BP and pulse are critical. Life-threatening hypovolemia may be overlooked if the BP and pulse are not measured while the patient is standing.

Mrs. P's profound drop in BP upon standing, reflex tachycardia, and recurrent syncope is a key **pivotal clue** and clearly indicate that she is syncopal due to orthostatic hypotension. This is not consistent with neurocardiogenic syncope. You revise the leading hypothesis to syncope due to orthostatic hypotension.

Is the clinical information sufficient to make a diagnosis? If not, what other information do you need?

# Leading Hypothesis: Orthostatic Hypotension

## Textbook Presentation

The distinguishing feature of orthostatic hypotension is the occurrence of syncope or symptoms (near syncope, visual blurring) when arising. Patients often have obvious sources of fluid or blood loss. Common causes include vomiting, diarrhea, inadequate fluid intake, or GI bleeding (presenting as hematemesis, melena, or bright red blood per rectum). Occasionally, orthostatic hypotension may develop secondary to massive but occult internal bleeding (rupture of abdominal aortic aneurysm, splenic rupture, retroperitoneal hemorrhage, or ruptured ectopic pregnancy). Finally, orthostatic hypotension may occur without volume loss, particularly in the elderly.

## Disease Highlights

A. Accounts for 20–30% of patients with syncope

B. Definition

  1. > 20 mm Hg decrease in systolic BP within 3 minutes of standing

  2. > 10 mm Hg decrease in diastolic BP within 3 minutes of standing

  3. Or > 30 bpm increase in pulse within 3 minutes of standing

C. Etiology

  1. Dehydration

    a. Decreased oral intake

    b. GI losses (vomiting, diarrhea)

    c. Urinary losses

      (1) Uncontrolled diabetes mellitus

      (2) Salt losing nephropathy

      (3) Adrenal insufficiency

    d. Over-dialysis

  2. Hemorrhage

    a. GI

    b. Ruptured abdominal aortic aneurysm

    c. Ruptured spleen

    d. Ruptured ectopic pregnancy

  3. Medications

    a. α-Blockers

    b. Diuretics

    c. Vasodilators (ie, nitrates, calcium channel blockers)

    d. Tricyclic antidepressants

    e. Phenothiazines

    f. Alcohol and opioids

  4. Prolonged bed rest

  5. Autonomic insufficiency (characterized by a fall in BP upon standing *without* a concomitant increase in pulse)

    a. Diabetes mellitus

    b. Other neurologic disorders (ie, Parkinson disease, multiple sclerosis, and numerous others)

  6. Elderly (20–30% of patients > 65-years-old have orthostatic hypotension although most are asymptomatic.)

  7. Postprandial hypotension, particularly common in the elderly

  8. Hot environments (hot tubs, baths, saunas)

**Table 26–9.** Accuracy of physical exam for large blood loss (630–1150 mL).

| Clinical Finding | Sensitivity | Specificity | LR+ | LR– |
|---|---|---|---|---|
| Postural increase in pulse > 30 bpm | 97% | 98% | 48.0 | 0.03 |
| Supine HR > 100 bpm | 12% | 96% | 3.0 | 0.9 |
| Supine hypotension < 95 mm Hg | 33% | 97% | 11.0 | 0.7 |

Modified, with permission, from McGee S, Abernethy WB 3rd, Simel DL. Is this patient hypovolemic? JAMA. 1999;281:1022–9.

## Evidence-Based Diagnosis

Several studies assessed the impact of phlebotomy on volunteers. Phlebotomy removed a moderate (450–630 mL) to large (630–1150 mL) volume of blood.

A. An increase in pulse of > 30 bpm with standing is both highly sensitive for large volume blood loss (97%) and highly specific (98%, LR+ 48) (Table 26–9). The sensitivity falls dramatically if the patient sits instead of stands (39–78%).

B. Simple supine measurements of BP and pulse were not sensitive for even large blood loss (sensitivity 12–33%).

C. Any abnormal finding on orthostatic maneuvers strongly suggested volume loss (specificity 94–98%; LR+, 3.0–48).

D. The sensitivity of orthostatic measurements is greatest if the supine and standing BPs are compared. If the supine BP is not measured, 67% of orthostatic patients may not be identified.

E. Patients should stand for 1 minute before the measurement of the upright BP.

F. No measure was very sensitive for moderate blood loss (0–27%).

G. Profound blood loss may occasionally paradoxically produce bradycardia. (The reduction in ESV may trigger the neurocardiogenic reflex.)

H. The admission Hct does not accurately reflect the severity of acute hemorrhage. A fall in Hct may take 24–72 hours.

## Treatment

A. Acute blood loss: Blood transfusion is appropriate in the orthostatic patient with acute blood loss.

B. Acute plasma loss (diarrhea, vomiting, or decreased oral intake)

  1. Patients able to tolerate oral intake: oral rehydration

  2. Patients unable to tolerate oral intake: IV hydration

    a. Normal saline is preferred.

    b. Usually 500 mL to 1 L boluses are given over 1 hour.

    c. Smaller boluses may be given to fragile patients (eg, those with a history of renal failure or HF).

    d. Repeat orthostatic BP measurements are made following each bolus as well as a lung and cardiac exam to ensure the patient has not received excessive fluid.

    e. Bolus therapy should be continued until orthostatic hypotension resolves.

C. Chronic orthostatic hypotension

  1. Hydration (water, soup, or sports drinks)

  2. Discontinue offending agents (diuretics, α-blockers, nitrates, tricyclic antidepressants, phenothiazines)

3. Patients are advised to arise slowly (sitting on the side of the bed, prior to standing), avoid large meals and excessive heat, and use waist high support hose.

4. Fludrocortisone is initial drug of choice. Monitor patients for hypokalemia and hypertension.

5. α-Agonists (ie, midodrine) have also been used successfully. Side effects include urinary retention, hypertension, and worsening HF.

6. Caffeine can be useful.

7. Erythropoietin is helpful in anemic patients.

## MAKING A DIAGNOSIS

Mrs. P reports that she has not suffered from any diarrhea or vomiting and has taken in normal amounts of fluid. She denies any hematemesis, melena, or bright red blood per rectum.

It is important to remember that Mrs. P presented with syncope *and* abdominal pain. Although the pain has improved, it has not resolved; it may provide an important clue to the underlying etiology. Given the profound orthostatic hypotension and the lack of external blood or volume loss, internal bleeding must be considered as a source of her abdominal pain and syncope. In the differential diagnosis you consider ruptured spleen, ruptured abdominal aortic aneurysm, and ruptured ectopic pregnancy. The lack of trauma argues against splenic rupture and the patient's age and gender are atypical for abdominal aortic aneurysm. You wonder if in fact she has suffered from a ruptured ectopic pregnancy.

It is important to remember the patient's chief complaint because it usually holds the most important clues to the diagnosis.

## CASE RESOLUTION

Mrs. P reports that she missed her last menstrual period. An abdominal ultrasound is performed and reveals 750 mL of fluid (presumed to be blood) in the pelvis. A urine pregnancy test is positive.

Although the final diagnosis of ectopic pregnancy was not considered initially, a careful clinical exam confirmed orthostatic syncope. Once that pivotal clue was discovered, the differential diagnosis could be narrowed and the underlying cause determined. It is instructive to note that her initial Hct was normal because the remaining intravascular blood had not yet been diluted by any oral or IV fluids.

Initial Hct measurements will not accurately reflect the magnitude of blood loss in a patient with recent hemorrhage.

Mrs. P had 2 large bore IVs placed and was typed and crossed for RBC transfusions. CBC, PT, PTT, and platelet counts were measured and a 1 L bolus of normal saline was given while waiting for the packed RBCs. After volume and blood resuscitation, she underwent surgical exploration and removal of her ruptured fallopian tube.

## REVIEW OF OTHER IMPORTANT DISEASES

### Aortic Stenosis

#### Textbook Presentation

Aortic stenosis is usually diagnosed incidentally during routine exam rather than due to symptoms. Typically, aortic stenosis produces a loud crescendo-decrescendo systolic murmur at the right second intercostal space, which may radiate to the neck and apex. When aortic stenosis becomes very severe, patients may have any of the 3 cardinal symptoms: HF (dyspnea), syncope, or angina.

#### Disease Highlights

A. Thickening and calcification of valve leaflets results in **progressive** obstruction to blood flow.

B. LVH develops to compensate for the obstruction.

C. Pathophysiology of symptoms is shown in Figure 26–4.

D. Prevalence 3% in patients ≥ 75-years-old

E. Etiology
   1. Degeneration of a previously normal valve
   2. Congenital bicuspid valve
      a. 1–2% of population is born with congenital bicuspid valve.
      b. Severe aortic stenosis develops in 66% of patients and at an earlier age than in patients with tricuspid valves.
      c. Aortic root structure is usually abnormal and often associated with progressive dilation of the aortic root that may require repair to prevent rupture or dissection.
   3. Rheumatic heart disease

F. Severe aortic stenosis is characterized by valve area < 1 cm or mean aortic valve gradient > 40 mm Hg.

G. Prognosis: Mortality increases markedly when symptoms develop (HF, angina, or syncope). The most common symptoms are decreased exercise tolerance and dyspnea on exertion. The mortality for symptomatic patients not undergoing valve replacement follows:
   1. Aortic stenosis and angina: 50% 5-year mortality
   2. Aortic stenosis and syncope: 50% 3-year mortality
   3. Aortic stenosis and dyspnea: 50% 2-year mortality

H. Other late manifestations: Atrial fibrillation (which is poorly tolerated) and an increased bleeding tendency secondary to disruption of large von Willebrand multimers by the abnormal aortic valve.

#### Evidence-Based Diagnosis

A. History and physical exam: Most studies demonstrate only a fair kappa between examiners.
   1. Findings that help **rule in** aortic stenosis

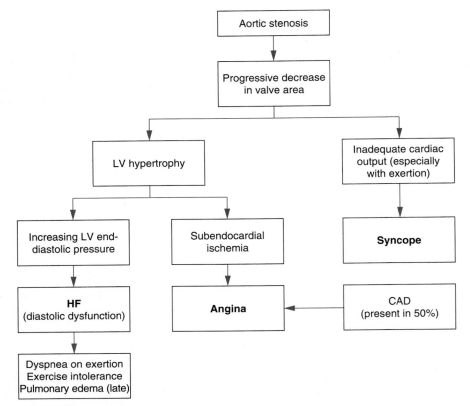

CAD, coronary artery disease; HF, heart failure, LV, left ventricular.

**Figure 26–4.** Pathophysiology of symptoms in aortic stenosis.

   **a.** Effort syncope in patients with a systolic murmur (LR+ 1.3–∞, LR– 0.76)

   **b.** Slow carotid upstroke (sensitivity, 15–42%; specificity, 95–100%; LR+ 9.2–∞)

   **c.** Murmur radiating to right carotid (sensitivity, 71–73%; specificity, 90%; LR+ 7.5)

   **2.** Findings that help **rule out** aortic stenosis

   **a.** Absence of any murmur (LR– 0.0)

   **b.** Absence of murmur below right clavicular head (LR– 0.1)

   **3.** Murmurs may be less intense in patients with superimposed HF.

B. Doppler echocardiogram

   **1.** The initial test of choice to assess for aortic stenosis

   **2.** Aortic stenosis is graded as mild if the valve area is > 1.5 cm², moderate if the valve area is 1–1.5 cm², and severe if the valve area < 1.0 cm².

   **3.** Recommended for patients with a systolic murmur ≥ grade III/VI

   **4.** Also recommended to monitor progression in patients with known aortic stenosis (annually for severe aortic stenosis, every 1–2 years for moderate aortic stenosis, and every 3–5 years for mild aortic stenosis).

Treatment

A. Mechanical correction

   **1. Symptomatic** patients should be treated with valve replacement, not medical therapy. Subsequent survival approaches the age-matched normal population.

   **2.** Definite indications for valve replacement

   **a.** Severe aortic stenosis in **symptomatic** patients

   **b.** Severe aortic stenosis in **asymptomatic** patients undergoing coronary artery bypass grafting (CABG) or other valve surgery.

   **c.** Severe aortic stenosis in asymptomatic patients with ejection fraction < 50%.

   **3.** Possible indication: Moderate aortic stenosis in asymptomatic patients undergoing CABG or other valve surgery

   **4.** Standard preoperative evaluation includes angiography in many patients to determine whether the patient needs concomitant CABG. This includes patients with symptoms of CAD or CAD risk factors (including men ≥ 35, postmenopausal women, or premenopausal women ≥ 35 with CAD risk factors).

   **5.** Mechanical and bioprosthetic valves have been used.

   **a.** Mechanical valves have greater durability and a significantly lower rate of failure and need for replacement. They are associated with a lower all-cause mortality than bioprosthetic valves.

   **b.** Mechanical valves are associated with an increased risk of thromboembolism and infection. Patients with mechanical valves require lifelong anticoagulation therapy. In addition to warfarin, aspirin is recommended at 75–100 mg/day.

   **c.** Bioprosthetic valves are reserved for patients who have a contraindication to warfarin therapy or are believed to be noncompliant. They may also be used in patients over 65 (whose life expectancy makes replacement unlikely).

    **d.** Another alternative is the Ross procedure in which the pulmonary valve is removed and used as the aortic valve. The pulmonary artery is reconstructed to create the pulmonary valve. The survival of these grafts is good and patients do not require anticoagulation therapy. In-hospital surgical mortality may be higher with this procedure.

   **6.** Balloon valvotomy is a poor option. It provides only temporary relief (6–12 months) and does not improve survival. Complications occur in 10–20%. It is reserved for palliation in patients with other serious (or lethal) comorbidities. An exception to this is the young adult with non-calcific aortic stenosis in whom balloon valvotomy is a viable option.

**B.** Vigorous exercise should be discouraged in patients with moderate to severe aortic stenosis.

## Situational Syncope

This is a variant of neurocardiogenic syncope, in which syncope occurs during or immediately after micturition, defecation, swallowing, or coughing.

## Carotid Sinus Syndrome

### Textbook Presentation

Carotid sinus syndrome is another variant of neurally mediated syncope. In affected individuals pressure applied to the carotid (eg, head turning, buttoning collar, shaving or cervical motion) produces bradycardia and/or hypotension with syncope or near syncope.

### Disease Highlights

**A.** 47% of patients report symptoms precipitated by head movement of looking upward.

**B.** More common in the elderly in whom it may account for 15% of recurrent syncopal events.

**C.** 15–56% of affected patients experience retrograde amnesia and complain of falls but deny syncope.

**D.** One study documented carotid hypersensitivity in 46% of patients presenting with non-accidental falls (compared with 11% in patients with accidental falls).

### Evidence-Based Diagnosis

**A.** CSM is applied for 5–10 seconds during continuous ECG and BP monitoring. CSM needs to be performed on each side separated in time by ≥ 1 minute. (The inhibitory response is unilateral in 81% of patients.)

**B.** Criteria for a positive response include reproduction of symptoms (ie, syncope) and ≥ 3-second pause or ( 50 mm Hg drop in BP.

**C.** CSM is significantly more sensitive when performed in the upright position on the tilt table than when the patient is supine.

**D.** Carotid hypersensitivity is not specific for carotid sinus syndrome.

   **1.** 12–35% of asymptomatic elderly patients experience carotid hypersensitivity during CSM (specificity, 65-88%).

   **2.** The specificity of CSM is higher when symptoms occur in addition to hemodynamic findings.

   **3.** Other diagnoses still need to be considered in elderly patients with syncope who demonstrate carotid hypersensitivity during CSM.

**E.** CSM is contraindicated in patients with carotid bruits, recent cerebrovascular accident or transient ischemic attack, MI (within 6 months), or severe dysrhythmias.

**F.** CSM has been complicated by transient and permanent neurologic symptoms in 0.3% and 0.05% of patients, respectively.

### Treatment

Pacemakers are clearly indicated in patients with cardioinhibitory carotid sinus syndrome in whom they have been demonstrated to reduce the incidence of subsequent syncope and falls.

## Wolff-Parkinson-White (WPW) Syndrome

### Textbook Presentation

WPW syndrome may be asymptomatic or present with palpitations, near syncope, syncope, or sudden death. In asymptomatic cases, the diagnosis may only be made after typical findings are discovered on an ECG performed for some other reason.

### Disease Highlights

**A.** A congenital disorder in which an accessory bundle directly connects the atria and ventricular muscle bypassing the AV node.

**B.** A variety of life-threatening arrhythmias may develop that cause syncope or sudden cardiac death. These include

   **1.** Antidromic tachycardia in which an impulse spreads down the accessory pathway and then back up the His-Purkinje system in a retrograde fashion. This reentrant loop can result in rapid tachycardias, hypotension, syncope and sudden death.

   **2.** The reentrant loop may run in the opposite direction (orthodromic tachycardia, Figure 26–5).

   **3.** Finally, atrial fibrillation or flutter can develop. In patients with atrial fibrillation or flutter, the accessory pathway facilitates rapid conduction of the atrial tachycardia into the ventricles allowing rapid ventricular depolarization and putting patients at risk for syncope or sudden death.

### Evidence-Based Diagnosis

**A.** Baseline ECG abnormalities during normal sinus rhythm may reveal a combination of a short PR interval and a delta wave.

   **1.** Short PR interval

      **a.** In healthy persons, the normal PR interval is produced by a built-in delay at the AV node (designed to allow atrial emptying prior to ventricular systole.)

      **b.** In WPW syndrome, the accessory pathway bypasses the AV node and initiates ventricular depolarization without such a delay; this results in a shortened PR interval in 75% of patients (Figure 26–6).

   **2.** Delta wave

      **a.** In most patients with WPW syndrome, the accessory pathway inserts directly into ventricular muscle (rather than into the specialized His-Purkinje system).

      **b.** Ventricular depolarization spreads slowly from cell to cell through gap junctions, rather than rapidly through the specialized rapid His-Purkinje conduction system.

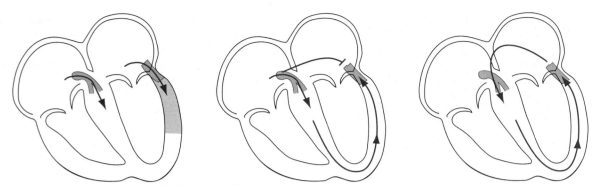

***Figure 26–5.*** Orthodromic tachycardia in patients with the Wolff-Parkinson-White syndrome. (Reproduced, with permission, from McPhee SJ: Pathophysiology of Disease, fifth edition. McGraw-Hill, 2006.)

**c.** This results in slow ventricular depolarization and the slow initial upstroke of the QRS complex known as the delta wave (Figure 26-6).

**d.** Finally, as this ventricular depolarization progresses, the AV node is also processing the supraventricular impulse. Eventually, the impulse passes through the AV node, activates the His-Purkinje system and causes rapid depolarization. This results in a narrow *terminal* portion of the QRS complex.

**B.** EP studies can provide detailed information about the presence, location, and conduction characteristics of the bypass tracts.

### Treatment

Therapy includes calcium channel blockers, β-blockers, digoxin, and radiofrequency catheter ablation of the bypass tract.

## Cerebrovascular Disease & Syncope

Although physicians commonly consider carotid artery obstruction in the differential diagnosis of patients with syncope, unilateral obstruction of the carotid will not result in syncope. Therefore, evaluation of the anterior circulation is not indicated in the patient with syncope. On the other hand, impairment of the posterior circulation may cause syncope due to interruption of blood flow to the reticular activating system. This may occur in the subclavian steal syndrome, vertebrobasilar insufficiency, and basilar artery occlusion. These disorders should be considered whenever patients have syncope and other symptoms referable to the brainstem (ie, diplopia, vertigo, ataxia, weakness). Finally, patients in whom subarachnoid hemorrhage develops can present with syncope. Such patients inevitably also complain of severe headache or confusion. Evaluation includes emergent noncontrast head CT scan.

## REFERENCES

Alboni P, Brignole M, Menozzi C et al. Diagnostic value of history in patients with syncope with or without heart disease. J Am Coll Cardiol. 2001;37(7):1921–8.

American College of Cardiology/American Heart Association Task Force on Practice Guidelines; Society of Cardiovascular Anesthesiologists; Society for Cardiovascular Angiography and Interventions; Society of Thoracic Surgeons, Bonow RO, Carabello BA, Kanu C et al. ACC/AHA 2006 guidelines for the management of patients with valvular heart disease: a report of the American College of Cardiology/American Heart Association Task Force on Practice Guidelines (writing committee to revise the 1998 Guidelines for the Management of Patients With Valvular Heart Disease): developed in collaboration with the Society of Cardiovascular Anesthesiologists: endorsed by the Society for Cardiovascular Angiography and Interventions and the Society of Thoracic Surgeons. Circulation. 2006;114(5):e84–231.

Bell WR, Simon TL, DeMets DL. The clinical features of submassive and massive pulmonary emboli. Am J Med. 1977;62(3):355–60.

Calvo-Romero JM, Perez-Miranda M, Bureo-Dacal P. Syncope in acute pulmonary embolism. Eur J Emerg Med. 2004;11(4):208–9.

Castelli R, Tarsia P, Tantardini C, Pantaleo G, Guariglia A, Porro F. Syncope in patients with pulmonary embolism: comparison between patients with syncope as the presenting symptom of pulmonary embolism and patients with pulmonary embolism without syncope. Vasc Med. 2003;8(4):257–61.

Colman N, Nahm K, van Dijk JG, Reitsma JB, Wieling W, Kaufmann H. Diagnostic value of history taking in reflex syncope. Clin Auton Res. 2004;14 Suppl 1:37–44.

Elliott PM MW. Clinical manifestations of hypertrophic cardiomyopathy. In: UpToDate; 2006.

Epstein AE, DiMarco JP, Ellenbogen KA et al. ACC/AHA/HRS 2008 Guidelines for Device-Based Therapy of Cardiac Rhythm Abnormalities: a report of the American College of Cardiology/American Heart Association Task Force on Practice Guidelines (Writing Committee to Revise the ACC/AHA/NASPE 2002 Guideline Update for Implantation of Cardiac Pacemakers and Antiarrhythmia Devices): developed in collaboration with the American Association for Thoracic Surgery and Society of Thoracic Surgeons. Circulation. 2008;117(21):e350–408.

Etchells E, Bell C, Robb K. Does this patient have an abnormal systolic murmur? JAMA. 1997;277(7):564–71.

Etchells E, Glenns V, Shadowitz S, Bell C, Siu S. A bedside clinical prediction rule for detecting moderate or severe aortic stenosis. J Gen Intern Med. 1998;13(10):699–704.

European Heart Rhythm Association; Heart Rhythm Society, Zipes DP, Camm AJ, Borggrefe M et al; American College of Cardiology; American Heart Association Task Force; European Society of Cardiology Committee for Practice Guidelines. ACC/AHA/ESC 2006 guidelines for management of patients with ventricular arrhythmias and the prevention of sudden cardiac death: a report of the American College of Cardiology/American Heart Association Task Force and the European Society of Cardiology Committee for Practice Guidelines (Writing Committee to Develop Guidelines for Management of Patients With Ventricular Arrhythmias and the Prevention of Sudden Cardiac Death). J Am Coll Cardiol. 2006;48(5):e247–346.

Grubb BP. Clinical practice. Neurocardiogenic syncope. N Engl J Med. 2005;352(10):1004–10.

Lembo NJ, Dell'Italia LJ, Crawford MH, O'Rourke RA. Bedside diagnosis of systolic murmurs. N Engl J Med. 1988;318(24):1572–8.

Maron BJ, McKenna WJ, Danielson GK et al; American College of Cardiology/European Society of Cardiology clinical expert consensus document on hypertrophic cardiomyopathy. A report of the American College of Cardiology Foundation Task Force on Clinical Expert Consensus Documents and the European Society of Cardiology Committee for Practice Guidelines. J Am Coll Cardiol. 2003;42(9):1687–713.

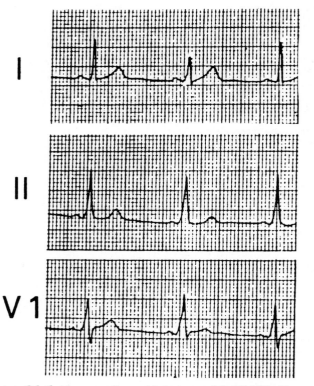

***Figure 26–6.*** Electrocardiographic features of the Wolff-Parkinson
White-syndrome. (Reproduced, with permission, from Fuster V:
Hurst's The Heart, 12th edition. McGraw-Hill, 2008.)

McGee S, Abernethy WB 3rd, Simel DL. The rational clinical examination. Is this patient hypovolemic? JAMA. 1999;281(11):1022–9.

McKeon A, Vaughan C, Delanty N. Seizure versus syncope. Lancet Neurol. 2006;5(2):171–80.

Nishimura RA, Holmes DR Jr. Clinical practice. Hypertrophic obstructive cardiomyopathy. N Engl J Med. 2004;350(13):1320–7.

Sheldon R, Rose S, Connolly S, Ritchie D, Koshman ML, Frenneaux M. Diagnostic criteria for vasovagal syncope based on a quantitative history. Eur Heart J. 2006;27(3):344–50.

Sheldon R, Rose S, Ritchie D et al. Historical criteria that distinguish syncope from seizures. J Am Coll Cardiol. 2002;40(1):142–8.

Strickberger SA, Benson DW, Biaggioni I et al. AHA/ACCF Scientific Statement on the evaluation of syncope: from the American Heart Association Councils on Clinical Cardiology, Cardiovascular Nursing, Cardiovascular Disease in the Young, and Stroke, and the Quality of Care and Outcomes Research Interdisciplinary Working Group; and the American College of Cardiology Foundation: in collaboration with the Heart Rhythm Society: endorsed by the American Autonomic Society. Circulation. 2006;113(2):316–27.

Warren J. The Effect of Venesection and the Pooling of Blood in the Extremities on the Atrial Pressure and Cardiac Output in Normal Subjects with Observations on Acute Circulatory Collapse in Three Instances. 1944.

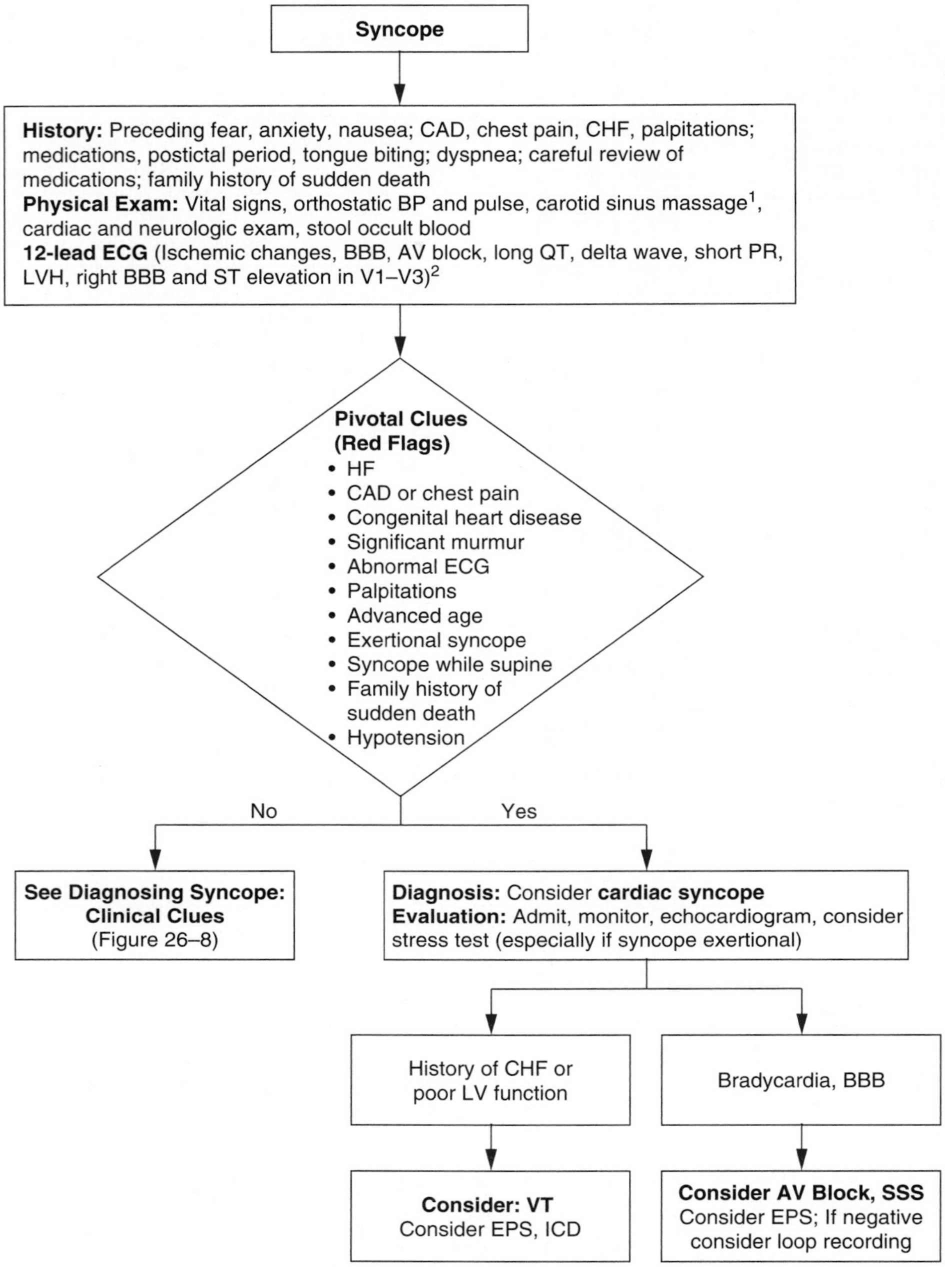
Syncope
History: Preceding fear, anxiety, nausea; CAD, chest pain, CHF, palpitations; medications, postictal period, tongue biting; dyspnea; careful review of medications; family history of sudden death
Physical Exam: Vital signs, orthostatic BP and pulse, carotid sinus massage[1], cardiac and neurologic exam, stool occult blood
12-lead ECG (Ischemic changes, BBB, AV block, long QT, delta wave, short PR, LVH, right BBB and ST elevation in V1–V3)[2]
Pivotal Clues (Red Flags)
• HF
• CAD or chest pain
• Congenital heart disease
• Significant murmur
• Abnormal ECG
• Palpitations
• Advanced age
• Exertional syncope
• Syncope while supine
• Family history of sudden death
• Hypotension
No
Yes
See Diagnosing Syncope: Clinical Clues (Figure 26–8)
Diagnosis: Consider cardiac syncope
Evaluation: Admit, monitor, echocardiogram, consider stress test (especially if syncope exertional)
History of CHF or poor LV function
Bradycardia, BBB
Consider: VT
Consider EPS, ICD
Consider AV Block, SSS
Consider EPS; If negative consider loop recording

[1]Carotid sinus massage is contraindicated in patients with carotid bruits, recent TIA, CVA, MI, or dysrhythmias
[2]Ischemic changes suggest CAD and possible VT. Sinus bradycardia may suggest SSS. BBB suggests possible intermittent AV block. Right BBB suggests possible PE. Long QT interval suggests long QT syndrome and possible VT. A delta wave and short PR interval suggests WPW syndrome. LVH may suggest hypertrophic cardiomyopathy. A right BBB pattern with ST elevation in V1–V3 suggests Brugada syndrome and VT. Low voltage in limb leads suggests pericardial effusion.

AV, atrioventricular block; BBB, bundle-branch block; CAD, coronary artery disease; HF, heart failure; CVA, cerebrovascular accident; EPS, electrophysiologic study; ICD, implantable cardiac defibrillator; LV, left ventricular; LVH, left ventricular hypertrophy; MI, myocardial infarction; PE, pulmonary embolism; SSS, sick sinus syndrome; TIA, transient ischemic attack; VT, ventricular tachycardia; WPW, Wolff-Parkinson-White.

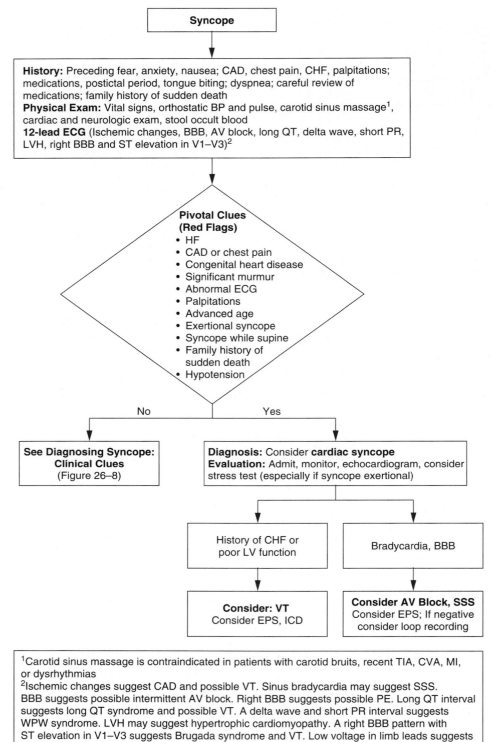

***Figure 26–7.*** Diagnostic approach to syncope.

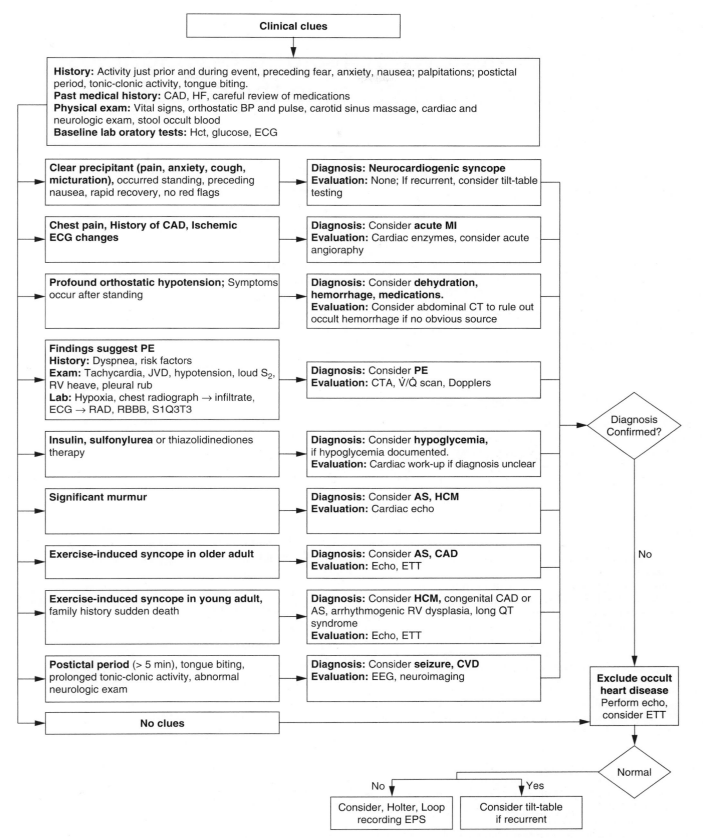

**Figure 26–8.** Diagnosing syncope: clinical clues.

AS, aortic stenosis; CAD, coronary artery disease; CTA, CT angiogram; CVD, cerebrovascular disease; ECG, electrocardiogram; EEG, electroencephalogram; EPS, electrophysiologic study; ETT, exercise tolerance test; HCM, hypertrophic cardiomyopathy; HF, heart failure; JVD, jugular venous distention; MI, myocardial infarction; PE, pulmonary embolism; RAD, right axis deviation; RBBB, right bundle-branch block; RV, right ventricular; V̇/Q̇, ventilation-perfusion.

# 27

# I have a patient with involuntary weight loss. How do I determine the cause?

## CHIEF COMPLAINT

PATIENT ▽ 1

Mrs. M is an 85-year-old woman who comes to the office complaining of weight loss. She is quite concerned that she has something dreadful.

☑ **What is the differential diagnosis of involuntary weight loss? How would you frame the differential?**

## CONSTRUCTING A DIFFERENTIAL DIAGNOSIS

Significant involuntary weight loss (IWL) is defined as > 5% loss of usual body weight in the last 6–12 months. Significant IWL can be a harbinger of serious underlying disease. One study documented significantly increase mortality in men with IWL compared with men whose weight was stable or increased (36% vs ≈15%). There are a large number of diseases that can cause IWL, which are best organized by system (see below). The 4 most common causes of IWL are cancer (GI, lung, and lymphoma), ≈25%; nonmalignant GI diseases, 17%; depression and alcoholism, 14%; and unknown, 22%. Endocrine disorders account for 7% of IWL. Although cancer is the most common cause, it is not the cause in most patients.

Three **pivotal points** are worth remembering when evaluating the patient with IWL. First, the weight loss should be documented, because 25–50% of patients who complain of IWL, have not in fact lost weight. Elderly adults often lose muscle mass and simply look like they lost weight. Weight loss should be documented by comparing prior weights or if these are unavailable by finding a significant decrease in a patient's clothing size.

 Clinicians should verify the weight loss or document significant changes in the patient's clothing or belt size.

Second, inquire about symptoms of diarrhea or malabsorption. Symptoms of diarrhea, or large difficult to flush, malodorous stools suggests small bowel or pancreatic disease and directs the diagnostic search.

Third, obtain a truly comprehensive history (including a psychosocial history) and perform a detailed head to toe physical exam and a baseline laboratory evaluation to search for any subtle diagnostic clues that may help focus the evaluation (Figure 27–1).

## Differential Diagnosis of Involuntary Weight Loss

A. Cardiovascular
1. Heart failure (severe)
2. Subacute bacterial endocarditis (SBE)

B. Endocrine
1. Adrenal insufficiency
2. Diabetes mellitus
3. Hyperthyroidism

C. GI (organized from mouth to rectum)
1. Poor dentition (50% of patients edentulous by age 65)
2. Anosmia
3. Esophageal disorders
   a. Esophageal stricture or web
   b. Dysmotility
   c. Esophageal cancer
4. Gastric disorders
   a. Peptic ulcer disease (PUD)
   b. Gastric cancer
   c. Gastroparesis
   d. Gastric outlet obstruction
5. Small bowel diseases
   a. Mesenteric ischemia
   b. Crohn disease
   c. Celiac sprue
   d. Bacterial overgrowth syndromes
   e. Lactose intolerance
6. Pancreatic disease
   a. Acute pancreatitis
   b. Chronic pancreatitis
   c. Pancreatic insufficiency
   d. Pancreatic cancer
7. Hepatic disease
   a. Hepatitis
   b. Cholelithiasis
   c. Cirrhosis
   d. Hepatocellular carcinoma
8. Colonic diseases
   a. Chronic constipation
   b. Colon cancer

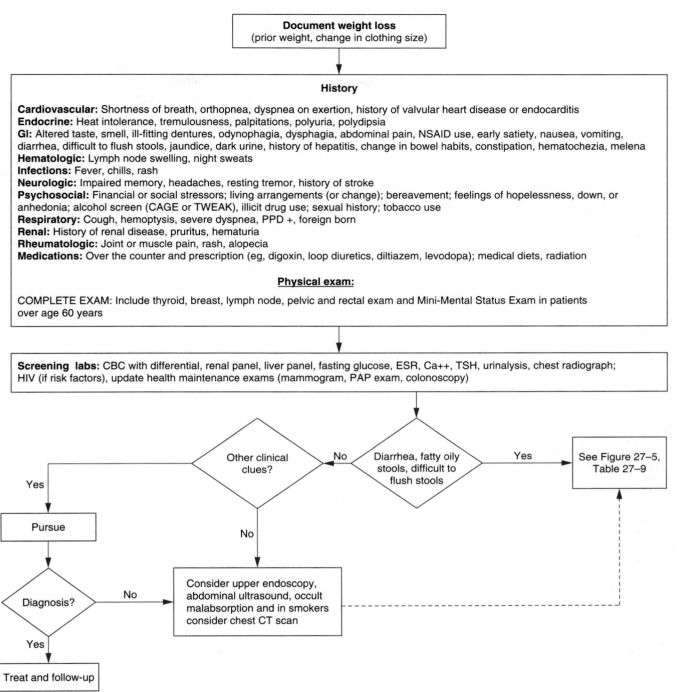

ESR, erythrocyte sedimentation rate; NSAID, nonsteroidal antiinflammatory drug.

***Figure 27–1.*** Diagnostic approach: involuntary weight loss.

**9.** Chronic GI infectious
   **a.** *Giardia lamblia*
   **b.** *Clostridium difficile*
   **c.** *Entamoeba histolytica*

**D.** Hematologic/oncologic
   **1.** Lung cancer
   **2.** Pancreatic cancer
   **3.** GI cancers

4. Lymphoma

5. Miscellaneous others

E. Infectious: HIV infection or complications

F. Neurologic

1. Dementia

2. Stroke

3. Parkinson disease

G. Psychiatric

1. Depression

2. Anxiety

3. Bipolar

4. Schizophrenia

H. Psychosocial

1. Poverty (15% of patients over age 65 live below the poverty line)

2. Isolation

3. Immobility or inadequate transportation

4. Alcoholism

I. Renal/metabolic

1. Uremia

2. Hypercalcemia

J. Respiratory

1. Chronic obstructive pulmonary disease (severe)

2. Tuberculosis

K. Rheumatologic

1. Polymyalgia rheumatica

2. Temporal arteritis

3. Rheumatoid arthritis

4. Systemic lupus erythematosus

L. Miscellaneous

1. Drugs (eg, digoxin, loop diuretics, diltiazem, levodopa)

2. Medical diets

3. Radiation

4. Chronic pain

Mrs. M reports that she has lost weight over the last 6 months. She denies any diarrhea, loose, or difficult to flush stools. She reports that her appetite is poor and she feels fatigued.

☑ At this point, what is the leading hypothesis, what are the active alternatives, and is there a must not miss diagnosis? Given this differential diagnosis, what tests should be ordered?

## PRIORITIZING THE DIFFERENTIAL DIAGNOSIS

The patient's history is typical of many patients complaining of weight loss. Patients report an unspecified amount of weight loss, associated with anorexia. The first pivotal step in the evaluation is to verify that weight loss did in fact occur.

▽ Mrs. M does not remember her prior weight but reports that her clothes are much too loose. Indeed, she has gone out to buy clothes 2 sizes smaller.

Mrs. M's change in clothing size suggests true and significant weight loss. The second pivotal step in evaluating patients with documented weight loss determines whether the patient has symptoms suggestive of diarrhea or malabsorption. Since the history does not suggest diarrhea or malabsorption, the third pivotal step in the evaluation of these patients is a comprehensive, system-based approach utilizing a thorough history and physical exam as well as basic laboratory exams (CBC, urinalysis, renal panel, calcium, liver panel, fecal occult blood test (FOBT), erythrocyte sedimentation rate (ESR), TSH, and chest radiograph). The myriad of diseases associated with IWL make it vital to search for clues before beginning a more expensive and indiscriminate investigation. In the absence of specific clues, focus first on cancer (the most common cause of IWL and the leading hypothesis) and then on other common causes, including nonmalignant GI disease, psychosocial disease, and hyperthyroidism (active alternatives). SBE, HIV, temporal arteritis, and tuberculosis are "must not miss" alternatives.

Finally, malabsorption should be reconsidered if the evaluation is negative, since patients with malabsorption may not have diarrhea or foul stools. Table 27–1 lists the differential diagnosis.

**Table 27–1.** Diagnostic hypotheses for Mrs. M. (*Continued*)

| Diagnostic Hypotheses | Clinical Clues | Important Tests |
|---|---|---|
| **Leading Hypothesis** | | |
| Cancer | | |
|   Stomach | Early satiety | EGD or upper GI |
|   Colon | Change in stools Hematochezia Positive FOBT, iron deficient anemia | Colonoscopy |
|   Lung | Cough, hemoptysis Tobacco use | Chest radiograph, chest CT scan |
|   Pancreas | Abdominal pain Jaundice, dark urine (bilirubinuria) | Abdominal ultrasound or CT scan |
| **Active Alternatives—Most Common** | | |
| Nonmalignant GI disease | | |
|   Dental | New ill-fitting dentures | |
|   Esophageal disease | Dysphagia | EGD or upper GI |
|   PUD | Epigastric pain, early satiety, nausea, melena, NSAID use | EGD *H pylori* breath test or stool antigen |

(*Continued*)

**Table 27–1.** Diagnostic hypotheses for Mrs. M. (*Continued*)

| Diagnostic Hypotheses | Clinical Clues | Important Tests |
|---|---|---|
| **Active Alternatives—Most Common** | | |
| Chronic pancreatitis | Epigastric pain, History of alcohol use or acute pancreatitis | Calcification on plain abdominal films or CT scan, lipase, fecal fat stain |
| Hepatitis | Alcohol use, injection drug use, jaundice | AST, ALT, bilirubin |
| IBD | Diarrhea, hematochezia, anemia, + FOBT, family history of IBD | Colonoscopy |
| Psychosocial Depression | History of loss, personal or family history of depression, postpartum state, > 6 somatic symptoms, overestimation of weight loss | Complaints of feeling down or anhedonia |
| Alcoholism | Quantity of alcohol use Family or work-related problems Family history of alcoholism Elevated AST and MCV Resistant hypertension | Alcohol screen |
| Hyperthyroidism | Increased sweating Nervousness Goiter Tachycardia Atrial fibrillation Lid lag or retraction Fine tremor Hyperactive reflexes Exophthalmos Frightened stare | TSH |
| **Active Alternatives—Must Not Miss** | | |
| HIV | Fevers, lymphadenopathy, recurrent pneumonias History of high-risk sexual contacts, sexually transmitted disease, or injection drug use | HIV |
| Subacute bacterial endocarditis | History of valvular heart disease, fevers, murmur | Blood cultures ESR, TEE |
| Temporal arteritis | Proximal muscle soreness Headache Visual loss Temporal artery tenderness Jaw claudication | ESR Temporal artery biopsy |
| Tuberculosis | Fever, cough, hemoptysis, foreign born, exposure | PPD, γ interferon Chest radiograph |

Mrs. M reports no early satiety, nausea, or vomiting. She reports that she never smoked cigarettes, has no unusual cough, and has not experienced any episodes of hemoptysis. She has had no change in her bowel habits or blood in her stool. She has had dentures for many years without change. She has not experienced dysphagia, odynophagia, abdominal pain, jaundice, change in the color of her urine, and has no history of hepatitis. She has not noticed any tremulousness, heat intolerance, or swelling over her thyroid. She denies having any headaches, fevers, or history of known valvular heart disease or injection drug use.

On physical exam, Mrs. M looks quite cachectic. She appears apathetic (Figure 27–2). Her vital signs are normal. HEENT exam reveals no oral lesions or adenopathy. Lungs are clear to percussion and auscultation. Cardiac exam reveals a regular rate and rhythm, with a grade I-II flow systolic murmur along the left sternal border. Her abdomen is scaphoid, without hepatosplenomegaly or mass. Rectal exam reveals guaiac-negative stool. Neurologic exam is normal, including a Mini-Mental State Exam.

> **Is the clinical information sufficient to make a diagnosis? If not what other information do you need?**

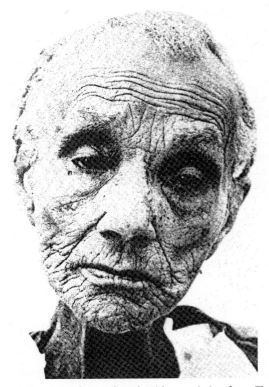

**Figure 27–2.** Mrs. M. (Reproduced, with permission from Thomas FB et al. Ann Intern Med. 1970;72:679–685.)

Mrs. M's history and physical exam do not clearly point to a specific disease process. There are no clues to suggest a GI disorder or a particular systemic disease. Given her cachectic appearance, your primary concern is that she has an underlying malignancy. Her apparent apathy also raises the possibility of depression. Hyperthyroidism seems unlikely given her sluggish demeanor.

## Leading Hypothesis: Cancer Cachexia

### Textbook Presentation

Patients with cancer cachexia often have advanced disease. They suffer from anorexia, fatigue, and other symptoms specific to their particular malignancy. The cancer may have been diagnosed before the weight loss or the weight loss may lead to the diagnosis.

### Disease Highlights

A. Cancer diagnoses account for ≈ 25% of cases of unexplained weight loss.

B. The most common malignancies associated with weight loss are GI, lung, and lymphoma.

C. Weight loss is 1 of the most common presenting symptoms in patients with lung cancer (comparable to cough). It is more frequent than dyspnea, hemoptysis, or chest pain.

D. IWL is common in cancer patients. At the time of diagnosis, 24% of patients with cancer have lost weight.

E. Patients with IWL due to cancer have a higher 2-year mortality than patients with IWL due to unknown causes (62% vs 18%).

F. Weight loss increases the risk of immobility, deconditioning, and adversely affects immunity. The risk of pulmonary embolism, decubitus ulcers, and pneumonia are increased.

### Evidence-Based Diagnosis

A. Several studies have evaluated a battery of history, physical exam, and initial laboratory studies to aid in the detection of cancer in patients with IWL.

B. Laboratory studies usually included a CBC, chemical survey (including glucose, calcium, BUN, creatinine, and liver function tests), HIV when appropriate, ESR, TSH, urinalysis, and chest radiograph. Several of these studies also incorporated abdominal ultrasound.

C. Further work-up was dictated by abnormalities detected in the initial battery. (For instance, GI evaluation with endoscopy and colonoscopy would be initiated in patients with GI complaints or iron deficiency anemia; hepatobiliary and pancreatic imaging would be done in those with abdominal pain or abnormal liver function tests, etc).

1. Cancer was detected in 28% of patients in these studies.

2. The battery was 93% sensitive for the detection of cancer in patients with IWL.

3. Occult cancer was diagnosed in only 2.6% of patients with a negative battery and evaluation.

### Treatment

A. Nutritional support

1. In many patients, artificial nutritional support is not effective.

2. Certain subgroups of patients may benefit from nutritional support.

   a. Head and neck cancer (after radiation therapy)

   b. Bowel obstruction

   c. Surgery patients (particularly upper GI tract cancer)

   d. Patients receiving high-dose chemotherapy

   e. Enteral support is appropriate if the bowel is functional and always preferred if feasible

B. Treat underlying malignancy

C. Medroxyprogesterone and megestrol

1. Decreases nausea and anorexia and increases weight gain

2. May increase the risk of thromboembolic events.

3. Other side effects include hyperglycemia, endometrial bleeding, edema, hypertension, and adrenal suppression and insufficiency.

D. Corticosteroids

1. Decrease anorexia and nausea

2. Increase appetite, quality of life, and feeling of well-being

3. Because of the side effects, corticosteroids are often reserved for patients with terminal disease.

E. A variety of other medications have been tried with limited to no success.

1. Prokinetic drugs (metoclopramide) can decrease anorexia and nausea but did not increase appetite or caloric intake.

2. The cannabinoid dronabinol was less effective than progestins.

3. Other agents under study include gherlin, melatonin, ATP infusions, and oxandrolone.

## MAKING A DIAGNOSIS

Clearly, a diagnosis is not yet apparent on history or physical exam. The data suggest that when the cause of IWL is malignant, there are usually clues on history, physical exam, or on laboratory testing. You elect to check a CBC, liver panel, renal panel, urinalysis, chest radiograph, and screening mammogram. Finally, you elect to schedule Mrs. M for a colonoscopy, since she has never undergone colon cancer screening.

Surprisingly, Mrs. M's laboratory evaluation is strikingly normal. Her CBC is normal without evidence of iron deficiency anemia (which could have suggested gastric or colon cancer). The chest radiograph is also normal, making lung cancer unlikely, particularly in a patient who never smoked. ALT (SGPT), AST (SGOT), alkaline phosphatase, and bilirubin are normal (an elevation can suggest hepatic metastasis or obstruction due to pancreatic cancer), and her renal panel is normal. There was no hematuria on urinalysis (which could suggest renal cell carcinoma or bladder cancer). Her mammogram and colonoscopy were normal.

**Have you crossed a diagnostic threshold for the leading hypothesis, cancer cachexia? Have you ruled out the active alternatives? Do other tests need to be done to exclude the alternative diagnoses?**

## Alternative Diagnosis: Depression

### Textbook Presentation

Depression may follow a recognizable loss or occur without a clear precipitant. Classically, patients complain of profound sadness, lack of interest in activities (anhedonia), sleep and appetite disturbances, impaired concentration, and other symptoms. Patients may lose or gain weight. Patients may experience suicidal or homicidal thoughts.

## Disease Highlights

**A.** Point prevalence of major depressive disorder (MDD) is 5.4–8.9%. Lifetime prevalence 16.2%. Minor depression is twice as common.

**B.** Depression is the second most common condition seen in primary care practices and the fourth leading cause of disability.

**C.** Recurrences are common. Many patients require lifelong therapy.

**D.** Risk factors for major depression
   1. Prior episode of depression
   2. Postpartum period
   3. Comorbid medical illness
   4. Older age (including concomitant neurologic disease)
   5. Chronic pain
   6. Absence of social support
   7. Female sex (2–3 times more common than in males)
   8. Family history (first-degree relative)
   9. Stressful life events
   10. Substance abuse

**E.** Associated anxiety: 50% of patients have anxiety symptoms
   1. 10–20% of patients with MDD have evidence of panic disorder and 30–40% have evidence of generalized anxiety disorder.
   2. Patients with anxiety and MDD are at higher risk for suicide.

**F.** Minor depression
   1. 10–18% progress to major depression within 1 year.
   2. 20% have moderate to severe disability.

## Evidence-Based Diagnosis

**A.** Criteria for MDD requires 5 of the following (1 of which is depressed mood or anhedonia) for at least 2 weeks:
   1. Depressed mood
   2. Anhedonia
   3. Significant appetite or weight change
   4. Sleep disturbance
   5. Psychomotor agitation or retardation
   6. Fatigue
   7. Feelings of worthlessness
   8. Impaired concentration
   9. Suicidal ideation

**B.** Minor depression requires 2–4 of the above symptoms, including anhedonia or depressed mood for > 2 weeks.

**C.** Depression is often missed on routine evaluation. In patients in whom depression was subsequently diagnosed, only 8.8% were found to be depressed during routine interview.

**D.** Screening tools increase identification of patients with depression by 2- to 3-fold (an absolute increase of 10–47%) and are recommended by the US Preventive Services Task Force.

**E.** 2 screening questions perform well (a positive response to either question is considered positive).

1. "Over the past 2 weeks, have you felt down, depressed, or hopeless?"

2. "Over the past 2 weeks, have you felt little interest or pleasure in doing things?"

3. Sensitivity, 96%; specificity, 57%; LR+, 2.2; LR–, 0.07)

4. Patients with a positive response to either question should undergo a full evaluation.

**F.** Clinical clues that might suggest a patient is depressed include
   1. Recent stress or loss
   2. Chronic medical illness, chronic pain syndromes
   3. > 6 physical symptoms
   4. Higher patient ratings of symptom severity
   5. Lower patient rating of overall health
   6. Physician perception of encounter as difficult
   7. Substance abuse (23% have MDD)
   8. Overestimation of weight loss
      **a.** In patients who overestimated their weight loss (by more than .5 kg), cancer was unlikely (6%) and no organic cause was found in 73%.
      **b.** In patients who underestimated their weight loss (by more than 1 kg), cancer was diagnosed in 52%.
   9. The patient appears more functionally restricted than explained by their medical illness.
   10. The language used to describe their condition is extreme (terrible, unbearable, etc).
   11. Sleep disturbances

**G.** Even in patients with depression, care must be taken before ascribing weight loss solely to depression. Many medical illnesses that cause weight loss are also associated with depression (eg, 20–45% of patients with cancer are depressed, and 40% of patients with Parkinson disease are depressed).

 The diagnosis of depression does not exclude other serious illnesses causing IWL. Patients should be monitored to ensure weight gain following treatment of their depression.

## Treatment

**A.** Work-up should include a full psychosocial history, including degree of functional impairment, history of domestic violence, and a drug history to look for agents that can worsen or precipitate depression (alcohol, interferon, L-dopa, glucocorticoids, oral contraceptives, propranolol, cocaine).

**B.** Patients should be screened for a history of manic symptoms that suggest bipolar illness (periods of reduced need for sleep, impulsivity, euphoric mood, racing thoughts, increased sexual activity, and grandiosity).

**C.** Screening tests (ie, TSH, basic metabolic panel, liver function tests, CBC) are recommended to rule out medical conditions (eg, hypothyroidism) that can simulate or cause depression.

**D.** Assess suicide risk: Ideation, intent, or plan
   1. Have you been having thoughts of dying?
   2. Do you have a plan?
   3. Does patient have the means (eg, weapons) to succeed?
   4. Other risk factors include
      **a.** Older men
      **b.** Psychotic symptoms

    **c.** Alcohol or illicit substance abuse

    **d.** History of prior attempts

    **e.** Family history of suicide or recent exposure to suicide

  **5.** Risk factors for suicide attempts in blacks included young age (OR 9.4), less than high school education (OR 3.6), mood disorder (OR 3.8), anxiety disorder (OR 6.0), and substance abuse (OR 4.5).

  **6.** Emergent psychiatric evaluation should be performed in patients with risk factors for suicide, who appear intoxicated, who cannot contract for safety, or have poor social support.

**E.** Pharmacotherapy

  **1.** Based on a number of symptoms *and* functional impairment

  **2.** *Not* influenced by whether or not there is well-defined precipitant (ie, stress). Therapy should be strongly considered in grieving patients with persistent symptoms of MDD for more than 2 months after a loss.

  **3.** Multiple classes of medications are effective; selective serotonin reuptake inhibitors (SSRIs), serotonin and norepinephrine reuptake inhibitors (SNRIs), tricyclic antidepressants (TCAs), and monoamine oxidase inhibitors (MAOIs).

  **4.** SSRIs are often used as first-line agents due to low frequency of adverse effects and safety in overdose. SSRIs and SNRIs may cause sexual dysfunction. Venlafaxine (an SNRI) can be lethal in overdose.

  **5.** Mirtazapine may be useful in patients with weight loss and insomnia and bupropion may be useful in patients with daytime lethargy and fatigue.

  **6.** TCAs frequently cause troubling anticholinergic side effects, significant weight gain (> 20 lbs) and are dangerous in overdose so are used less often. High-dose TCAs may increase the risk of sudden cardiac death.

  **7.** MAOIs interact with a variety of tyramine-containing foods and medications and may precipitate a hypertensive crisis. These are typically prescribed only by psychiatrists.

  **8.** Patients with a prior history of manic symptoms should be referred for psychiatric evaluation prior to the institution of antidepressant therapy. Antidepressant therapy can trigger mania.

  **9.** Treat for 6–9 months *after* clinical recovery.

  **10.** Patients with multiple recurrences (≥ 2–3) may require lifetime therapy.

**F.** Psychotherapy

  **1.** Equally effective as pharmacotherapy in patients with mild to moderate depression. Options include cognitive behavioral therapy, problem solving therapy, and interpersonal psychotherapy.

  **2.** Less effective than pharmacotherapy in patients with severe depression. Combined psychotherapy and pharmacotherapy may be the best option.

**G.** Exercise programs may be helpful in older adults with mild to moderate depression.

**H.** Electroconvulsive therapy (ECT) is an alternative therapy for patients with severe, refractory depression, particularly those with psychotic or suicidal features.

**I.** Indications for referral include psychotic features, substance abuse, panic disorder, agitated depression, severe depression, bipolar features, suicidality, relapsing depression, dysthymia.

---

Mrs. M reports no unusual stresses or losses. She has been widowed for 15 years and feels that she has come to terms with her husband's death. She lives with her daughter and regularly sees family members and remains actively involved in her church. She denies feeling down, depressed or hopeless in the last month and denies loss of interest or pleasure in doing things.

Mrs. M's answers to the screening questions make depression highly unlikely (LR– 0.07). Although her appearance seems antithetical to hyperthyroidism, you wonder if that possibility should be pursued.

## Alternative Diagnosis: Hyperthyroidism

### Textbook Presentation

Classically, patients with hyperthyroidism present with a myriad of symptoms and signs obvious to the experienced observer. Symptoms include palpitations, heat intolerance, increased sweating, insomnia, tremulousness, diarrhea, and *weight loss.* Signs of hyperthyroidism include sinus tachycardia, systolic hypertension, frightened stare, an enlarged goiter, a fine resting tremor, and exophthalmos (only if hyperthyroidism is secondary to Graves disease). Exophthalmos may be unilateral or bilateral. Other manifestations may include hyperpigmentation, irregular menses, pruritus, and thinning of hair. Complications include osteoporosis, tracheal obstruction (from the goiter), tachyarrhythmias (particularly atrial fibrillation), high output heart failure, anemia, and proximal muscle weakness.

### Disease Highlights

**A.** Prevalence, 0.3%.

**B.** Hyperthyroidism is actually an endocrine syndrome caused by several distinct pathophysiologic entities (Table 27–2).

### Evidence-Based Diagnosis

**A.** History and physical exam

  **1.** Certain findings of hyperthyroidism are quite specific (ie, lid lag and lid retraction) and help rule in the diagnosis (specificity, 99%; LR+, 17–32).

  **2.** Clinical findings are not highly sensitive. Therefore, absent clinical findings do not allow hyperthyroidism to be ruled out.

    **a.** Goiter is present in 70–93% of cases.

    **b.** HR > 90 bpm is present in 80% of cases.

    **c.** Lid lag is present in 19% of cases.

    **d.** Ophthalmopathy is present in 25–50% of patients with Graves disease.

    **e.** Hyperreflexia is variable depending on the age of the patient (see below).

**B.** Elderly patients

  **1.** Prevalence of hyperthyroidism in elderly is 2–3%.

  **2.** Hyperthyroidism often presents atypically in elderly patients. Expected adrenergic findings are often absent, whereas atrial fibrillation, depression, and weight loss are more common, resulting in the phenomenon referred to as *apathetic hyperthyroidism of elderly.*

***Table 27–2.*** Distinguishing features of several hyperthyroid states.

| Disease | Pathogenesis/Important features | TSH | T4, FTI or T3 | Thyroid Scan and Other Tests |
|---|---|---|---|---|
| Graves disease | Autoimmune production of thyroid-stimulating antibody binds and stimulates TSH receptor Exophthalmos unique to Graves | ↓ | ↑ | Homogenously increased uptake Elevated TSI |
| Toxic multinodular goiter | Most common form in elderly | ↓ | ↑ | Patchy increased uptake |
| Painful subacute thyroiditis | Viral or immune inflammatory attack on thyroid resulting in neck pain, tenderness, fever and release of hormone | ↓ | ↑ | Decreased uptake Elevated ESR |
| Toxic adenoma | Autonomously functioning benign thyroid nodule | ↓ | ↑ | Hot nodule, uptake in rest of gland is suppressed |
| Iodine or amiodarone | Amiodarone[1] may cause the release of T4 and T3 | ↓ | ↑ | Usually decreased uptake |
| TSH-producing pituitary adenoma | Autonomously functioning benign *pituitary* adenoma May cause bitemporal hemianopsia Galactorrhea develops in 33% of women | ↑ | ↑ | Diffusely increased uptake |
| Factitious or iatrogenic | Self or physician induced | ↓ | ↑ | Decreased uptake T4/FTI more elevated than T3 Thyroglobulin concentration low |

[1]Amiodarone causes *hypothyroidism* in 20% of patients by impairing conversion of T4 to T3.
ESR, erythrocyte sedimentation rate; FTI, free thyroxine index; TSI, thyroid-stimulating immunoglobin.

Table 27–3 compares the findings in young and older patients with hyperthyroidism.

 Consider hyperthyroidism in elderly patients with weight loss (OR 8.7), tachycardia (OR 11.2), atrial fibrillation, or apathy (OR 14.8). Hyperthyroidism was not even considered in 54% of admitted patients in whom hyperthyroidism was subsequently diagnosed.

***Table 27–3.*** Sensitivity of findings in patients with hyperthyroidism.

| Signs and Symptoms | Patients Aged 70 Years or Older | Patients Aged 50 Years or Younger |
|---|---|---|
| Sinus tachycardia | 41% | 94% |
| Atrial fibrillation | 35–54% | 2% |
| Fatigue | 56% | 84% |
| Anorexia | 32–50% | 4% |
| Weight loss | 50–85% | 51–73% |
| Goiter | 50% | 94% |
| Ophthalmopathy | 6% | 46% |
| Tremor | 44–71% | 84–96% |
| Nervousness | 31% | 84% |
| Hyperactive reflexes | 28% | 96% |
| Increased sweating | 24–66% | 92–95% |
| Heat intolerance | 15% | 92% |

C. Laboratory tests

1. TSH is the test of choice (in the absence of pituitary disease) (sensitivity > 99%, specificity > 99%, LR+ > 99, LR− < .01).

   a. Low TSH indicates hyperthyroidism.

   b. Normal TSH indicates euthyroidism.

   c. High TSH indicates hypothyroidism.

2. Exception occurs when the pituitary itself is diseased (rare).

   a. Pituitary adenomas can produce TSH causing hyperthyroidism with increased TSH and FTI.

   b. Pituitary destruction (eg, sarcoidosis) results in hypothyroidism with decreased TSH and FTI.

3. T4 measurements

   a. Thyroid hormone exists in the serum bound to thyroid-binding globulin (TBG) and free

   b. Free T4 (FT4) is active and more accurately reflects thyroid activity than the total T4.

   c. The FTI estimates the FT4.

   d. Many conditions alter the TBG and total T4. However, they do not affect the FT4 level (or FTI), and patients remain euthyroid. (For example, pregnancy raises the TBG and total T4; however, the FT4 and FTI are normal and the patient is euthyroid.)

4. Occasionally, patients with hyperthyroidism have isolated elevations in T3, or T3 thyrotoxicosis. In such patients, the TSH is still suppressed.

5. An approach to thyroid function tests is shown in Figure 27–3.

6. Established hyperthyroidism

   a. Certain features can help distinguish the *etiology* of hyperthyroidism, including thyroid-stimulating immunoglobulin and radioactive iodine uptake scan (see Table 27–2).

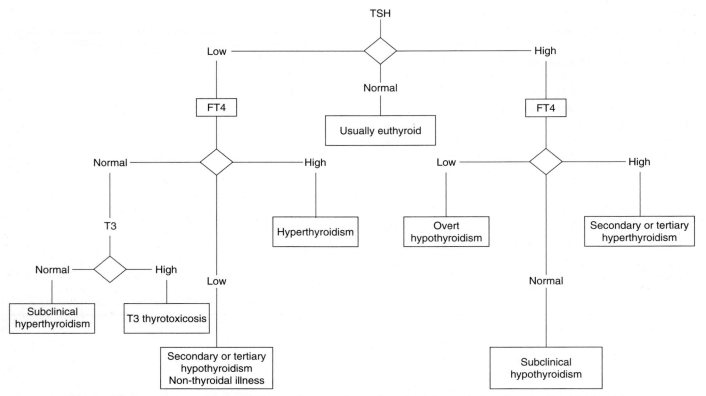

***Figure 27–3.*** Diagnosis of thyroid function disorders. (Reproduced, with permission, from Muller AF. Thyroid function disorders. Neth J Med. 2008;66(3):134–42.)

**b.** Doppler flow can be useful in patients unable to undergo the radioactive uptake scan. Increased flow correlates with increased uptake.

**c.** Women of child-bearing years should have a pregnancy test performed prior to iodine scanning or instituting therapy.

**d.** Imaging with ultrasound or occasionally CT scan or MRI can be useful in patients with large goiters, particularly if there is a suggestion of airway obstruction.

**Treatment**

**A.** β-Blockers can be used to decrease the sympathetic stimulation and the tremor, palpitations, and sweating.

**B.** Definitive treatment of hyperthyroidism depends on underlying etiology.

  **1.** Graves disease

    **a.** Antithyroid drugs (methimazole and propylthiouracil)

      **(1)** May cause agranulocytosis (0.1–0.3%)

      **(2)** ≈ 40% of patients relapse

    **b.** Radioactive iodine

      **(1)** Used successfully for over 60 years.

      **(2)** ≈ 21% relapse rate

      **(3)** Patients usually require subsequent lifelong thyroid hormone replacement because the radioactive iodine induces hypothyroidism.

    **c.** Surgery is occasionally used, particularly if the goiter is troublesome.

  **2.** Toxic multinodular goiter

    **a.** Elderly: Consider radioactive iodine; monitor for hypothyroidism.

    **b.** Large goiter: Consider surgery.

  **3.** Subacute thyroiditis

    **a.** Aspirin or nonsteroidal antiinflammatory drugs (NSAIDs) decrease thyroid inflammation.

    **b.** β-Blockers decrease symptoms of hyperthyroidism until inflammation subsides.

    **c.** Prednisone and ipodate can be used in severe cases.

## CASE RESOLUTION

A TSH on Mrs. M is completely suppressed (< 0.1 mcU/mL). The T4 is elevated at 20 mcg/dL (nl 5–11.6) and the FTI is 22 (nl 6–10.5). You diagnose hyperthyroidism. A thyroid scan reveals heterogeneous uptake consistent with a toxic multinodular goiter.

 Check the TSH on every patient evaluated for weight loss.

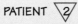

Due to her advanced age, you elect to have her treated with radioactive iodine. Six months later she returns; she is taking replacement levothyroxine for the radioactive iodine–induced hypothyroidism. Laboratory exam reveals that she is euthyroid. She complains that her clothes are now too tight.

## CHIEF COMPLAINT

PATIENT

Mr. O is a 55-year-old man who complains of weight loss. He reports that he has tried for years to lose weight (unsuccessfully) but that recently he has lost more and more weight without effort. He was initially pleased but recently has become concerned. He reports that altogether he has lost 30 pounds in the last 6 months (from 200 lbs to 170 lbs).

At this point, what is the leading hypothesis, what are the active alternatives, and is there a must not miss diagnosis? Given this differential diagnosis, what tests should be ordered?

## PRIORITIZING THE DIFFERENTIAL DIAGNOSIS

As noted above the first pivotal step in the evaluation of IWL is to verify the weight loss. Mr. O clearly suffered from verifiable significant IWL. The second pivotal step in the evaluation of patients with *documented* weight loss is to determine whether or not the patient is having symptoms that suggest diarrhea or malabsorption.

Mr. O reports no diarrhea, large foul-smelling stools, or difficult to flush stools. He reports that he previously moved his bowels once a day but lately only once every other day. He attributes this to his decreased appetite.

Since Mr. O's weight loss is not clearly secondary to malabsorption or diarrhea, the focus turns to the third pivotal step, which takes a system-based approach and utilizes a comprehensive history, physical exam, and basic laboratory studies to look for clues.

Mr. O notes that he has a decreased appetite and feels full quickly after starting to eat. He has not noticed any melena or hematochezia or any jaundice. He has never been a tobacco smoker. He denies night sweats or swollen lymph nodes. He denies any dysphagia or odynophagia but does admit to NSAID use. He reports that he takes 600 mg of ibuprofen 2–3 times a day for his arthritis. He denies any abdominal pain. He reports that he has not felt down, depressed, or hopeless during the past month nor has he been bothered by a lack of interest in activities. He drinks 2 beers about once a month. Finally, he denies symptoms associated with a variety of systemic diseases including fevers, muscle aches, or headaches.

Physical exam reveals a thin but otherwise healthy appearing middle-aged man. Vital signs are normal. The remainder of his exam is completely normal.

Laboratory tests, including CBC, differential, hepatic panel, renal panel, urinalysis, ESR, and TSH, are normal. A chest radiograph is normal without mass or adenopathy.

The cause of Mr. O's weight loss is not obvious. However, his early satiety and NSAID use are clues that he might have PUD or gastric cancer. You consider PUD your leading hypothesis. Gastric cancer is an alternative hypothesis, and colon cancer is a must not miss hypothesis given his change in bowel habits. Table 27–4 lists the differential diagnosis.

All medications (prescription and over the counter) should be carefully scrutinized in patients complaining of IWL. Some medications cause anorexia directly, others through various organ toxicities.

**Table 27–4.** Diagnostic hypotheses for Mr. O.

| Diagnostic Hypotheses | Clinical Clues | Important Tests |
| --- | --- | --- |
| **Leading Hypothesis** | | |
| PUD | Epigastric pain, early satiety, nausea, melena, NSAID use | EGD *H pylori* breath test or stool antigen |
| **Active Alternatives—Most Common** | | |
| Stomach cancer | Early satiety | EGD or upper GI |
| **Active Alternatives—Must Not Miss** | | |
| Colon cancer | Change in stools Hematochezia Positive FOBT, iron deficient anemia | Colonoscopy |

Colon cancer causing subtotal obstruction may present a change in bowel habits, either constipation *or* diarrhea.

Is the clinical information sufficient to make a diagnosis? If not what other information do you need?

## Leading Hypothesis: PUD

### Textbook Presentation

The pain of PUD is classically described as a dull or hunger-like pain in the epigastrium that is either exacerbated or improved by food intake. The pain is often worse on waking and may radiate to the back. Symptomatic periods often last for several weeks. Nausea and early satiety may be seen.

### Disease Highlights

**A.** 250,000 cases per year in the United States

**B.** Etiology: Most ulcers are secondary to NSAID use, *Helicobacter pylori* infection or both.

  **1.** *H pylori* infection

    **a.** Asymptomatic in 70% of patients

    **b.** Peptic ulcer develops in 15% of infected patients.

    **c.** May cause duodenal or gastric ulcers. Gastric ulcers are also associated with diffuse gastritis, and rarely, gastric cancer.

  **2.** NSAIDs

    **a.** 25% of all adverse drug reactions involve NSAIDs

    **b.** 16,500 deaths/year from NSAID-associated GI bleeding

    **c.** Gastric ulcers 5 times more common than duodenal ulcers.

    **d.** Ulcers are visible on esophagogastroduodenoscopy (EGD) in 20% of NSAID users, dyspepsia occurs in 10%, hospitalizations in 0.5%, and deaths in 0.15%.

    **e.** Ulcers are most likely in the first 1–3 months of NSAID use.

    **f.** Factors that increase the risk of NSAID-associated ulcers or their complications include concurrent warfarin use (10×), high-dose NSAIDs (10×), age > 60 (4–6×), concurrent glucocorticoid use (4–5×), *H pylori* infection (3.3×), and nonselective NSAIDs.

    **g.** NSAIDS may be nonselective, inhibiting both cyclooxygenase (COX)-1 and COX-2, or selective, inhibiting only COX-2.

      **(1)** Selective COX-2 inhibitors have less GI toxicity.

      **(2)** However, several selective COX-2 inhibitors *increase* the risk of adverse cardiovascular outcomes (ie, myocardial infarction) and several have been withdrawn from the market. Celecoxib is still available.

      **(3)** Alternate strategies to decrease the risk of NSAID-related PUD include concurrent use of proton pump inhibitors (PPIs) with nonselective NSAIDS (see below).

  **3.** Zollinger-Ellison syndrome is a rare cause of PUD.

**C.** Complications: Bleeding can vary from massive hemorrhage (with hematemesis and melena or hematochezia) to occult GI blood loss and iron deficiency anemia (see Chapter 17, GI Bleeding).

### Evidence-Based Diagnosis

**A.** History and physical exam

  **1.** Pain is not a good predictor of PUD.

    **a.** Ulcers are often asymptomatic.

      **(1)** 60% of NSAID-associated ulcers are asymptomatic.

      **(2)** 25% of non-NSAID ulcers are asymptomatic.

    **b.** Pain often reflects nonulcer dyspepsia rather than PUD.

      **(1)** Less than one-third of patients with epigastric discomfort have PUD.

      **(2)** Among patients undergoing endoscopy, patients with nonulcer dyspepsia have more severe and more numerous symptoms than patients with PUD.

    **c.** Surprisingly, several clinical predictors are not good at discriminating ulcer from nonulcer dyspepsia including

      **(1)** Response to antisecretory therapy

      **(2)** Epigastric tenderness

      **(3)** The quality of the pain

  **2.** Best predictors of PUD are a history of NSAID use and *H pylori* infection (Table 27–5).

  **3.** First sign of ulcer may be life-threatening complication (hemorrhage or perforation): > 50% of patients with serious to life-threatening complication had no prior symptom.

  **4.** IWL may be a sign of a benign gastric ulcer.

    **a.** 31–55% of patients with benign gastric ulcer noted weight loss.

    **b.** ~50% lost 10–20 lbs; 21% lost > 20 lb

    **c.** PUD is found more often in patients undergoing EGD for weight loss than for dyspepsia.

A significant number of patients with NSAID-induced ulcers do not experience pain. Anemia, GI bleeding, early satiety, or weight loss can be the only symptom of PUD.

**B.** Laboratory studies

  **1.** *H pylori* testing

    **a.** Eradication markedly decreases recurrence from 60–100% to < 10%. All patients with documented PUD, whether or not they are taking NSAIDs, should be tested for *H pylori*.

    **b.** Patients with a prior history of PUD who have not previously been treated for *H pylori* should also be tested.

**Table 27–5.** Prevalence of PUD in patients with dyspepsia.

| Age | Neither H pylori nor NSAIDs | Current NSAID use | H pylori infection |
|---|---|---|---|
| 40 years | 1% | 5% | 20% |
| 75 years | 3% | 20% | 30% |

NSAID, nonsteroidal antiinflammatory drug; PUD, peptic ulcer disease.

**Table 27–6.** Test characteristics for detecting *Helicobacter pylori* infection.

| Test | Sensitivity (%) | Specificity (%) | LR+ | LR− |
|---|---|---|---|---|
| **Invasive tests** | | | | |
| Rapid urease test | 67 | 93 | 9.8 | 0.35 |
| Histology | 70 | 90 | 7 | 0.33 |
| Culture | 45 | 98 | 22.5 | 0.56 |
| **Noninvasive tests** | | | | |
| Urea breath test | 93 | 92 | 11.6 | 0.08 |
| Stool antigen | 87 | 70 | 2.9 | 0.2 |
| Serology | 88 | 69 | 2.8 | 0.2 |

c. Testing for *H pylori* is also recommended for patients with dyspepsia. Eradication of *H pylori* is recommended in symptomatic patients. (EGD is only recommended for those with "alarm" symptoms (see below) or those who do not respond to therapy.)

d. Options for diagnosing *H pylori* infection include invasive and noninvasive testing (Table 27–6).

   (1) Urea breath tests and *H pylori* stool antigen are preferred in patients not undergoing EGD.

   (2) Rapid urease test and histology are preferred in patients undergoing EGD.

   (3) Serology does not distinguish active from prior infection.

   (4) Active bleeding from PUD decreases the sensitivity of rapid urease tests. Patients with bleeding and negative rapid urease tests and negative histology should undergo urea breath tests several weeks after completing PPI therapy.

e. Stool antigen, breath test, or the rapid urease can also assess eradication.

f. PPI therapy for even 1 day markedly decreases the sensitivity of histology, rapid urease test, stool antigen test, and urea breath test. Serology is not affected but cannot distinguish active from prior infection.

2. Ulcer diagnosis

a. EGD is more sensitive than upper GI series (92% vs 54%) and is useful to rule out other serious pathology.

b. Indications for EGD (Figure 27–4)

   (1) Bleeding

   (2) Anemia

   (3) Weight loss

   (4) Early satiety

   (5) Dysphagia

   (6) Recurrent vomiting

   (7) Prior esophagogastric malignancy or family history of GI cancer

   (8) Patients who do not respond to initial therapy

   (9) Age > 55 years

**Treatment**

A. The 3 components of therapy for PUD include eradication of *H pylori*, if present; discontinuation of NSAIDs, if possible; and use of proton pump inhibitors. In addition, gastric ulcers warrant biopsy to rule out adenocarcinoma.

B. Regardless of the cause of the ulcer, and the presence or absence of bleeding, PPIs dramatically suppress acid secretion and are the mainstay of therapy. For patients infected with *H pylori*, PPIs are given during the course of antibiotics therapy and longer for larger ulcers (> 1- 2 cm) or patients with complications.

C. *H pylori* eradication

   1. Regimens require multiple simultaneous medications using a PPI and usually 2 or 3 distinct antibiotics. Recent evidence suggests the sequential use of antibiotics increases the eradication rate. (Amoxicillin with a PPI followed by clarithromycin, 5-nitroimidazole and a PPI.)

   2. Increased incidence of *H pylori* resistance has led to the recommendation for posttreatment testing to confirm eradication. Appropriate tests would include the stool antigen or urea breath tests 4–6 weeks after completing therapy.

D. NSAID-associated ulcers

   1. Prevention: Consensus guidelines suggest prophylactic PPIs for patients who are at high risk for PUD on NSAID therapy. Patients who should receive prophylactic therapy include those receiving

      a. Dual antiplatelet therapy ie, aspirin (any dose) with any NSAID (nonselective, COX-2 selective or over the counter) or clopidogrel

      b. Antiplatelet *and* anticoagulant therapy

      c. Antiplatelet therapy with a history of PUD

      d. Antiplatelet therapy with ≥ 1 of the following risk factors: aged over 60 years, corticosteroid use, dyspepsia, or GERD symptoms.

   2. Documented ulcers

      a. Test for *H pylori* infection and eradicate if present.

      b. Strategies for patients who require continuation of NSAIDS (even low-dose aspirin) should include:

         (1) Continue PPI therapy for duration of NSAID (even after *H pylori* eradication). (H$_2$-receptor blockers are ineffective.)

         (2) Minimize dose and duration of NSAIDs

         (3) Avoid certain high-risk nonselective NSAIDS, such as ketorolac, piroxicam, indomethacin, diclofenac, and naproxen, all of which increase the relative risk of PUD.

## MAKING A DIAGNOSIS

Despite the absence of pain, Mr. O's history of NSAID use, the early satiety, and weight loss convinces you to order an EGD.

2

The EGD reveals 2 gastric ulcers 1.5 cm in size. Pathology reveals organisms consistent with *H pylori*.

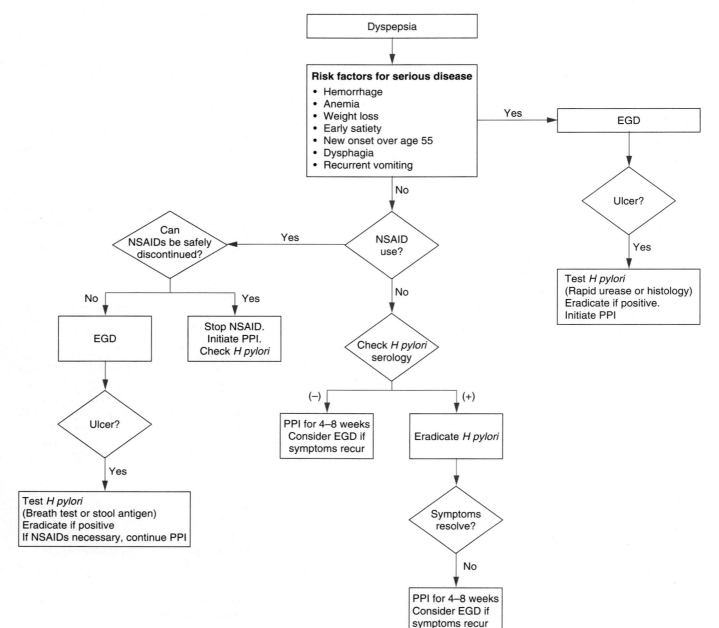

EGD, esophago gastro duodenoscopy; NSAID, nonsteroidal antiinflammatory drug; PPI, proton pump inhibitor.

***Figure 27–4.*** Indications for EGD.

Have you crossed a diagnostic threshold for the leading hypothesis, gastric ulcer? Have you ruled out the active alternatives? Do other tests need to be done to exclude the alternative diagnoses?

You conclude that the likely cause of Mr. O's weight loss is gastric ulcer. You elect to initiate therapy without further testing.

Altogether, malignant and nonmalignant GI diseases are the cause of IWL in 28% of patients. The yield of EGD in patients with IWL is 12–44%.

EGD should be considered in the evaluation of patients with unexplained weight loss.

## CASE RESOLUTION

Mr. O received eradication therapy, a PPI, and stopped the ibuprofen. Three months later, his appetite is excellent. He is advised to use acetaminophen for his arthritis pain and to perform nonimpact physical activities.

## CHIEF COMPLAINT

PATIENT 3

Mr. A. is a 62-year-old man who complains of recent weight loss. He reports that he has lost 15 pounds over the last 6–9 months, and that his clothes no longer fit. He denies diarrhea but admits to abdominal bloating and having several large stools a day that are difficult to flush. He reports that his appetite is not what it used to be but attributes that to his recent separation from his wife. He confides that they have not gotten along for years. She seemed to blame everything on his drinking, but he assures you that alcohol was definitely not a problem. Further, he reports that he is glad she is out of his life.

 At this point, what is the leading hypothesis, what are the active alternatives, and is there a must not miss diagnosis? Given this differential diagnosis, what tests should be ordered?

## PRIORITIZING THE DIFFERENTIAL DIAGNOSIS

The first step in IWL is to verify Mr. A's weight loss. This is clearly established by his history and a review of his medical records. The second and third steps look for signs of malabsorption and clues from the history and physical exam. Mr. A's social history raises several possibilities. First, you suspect that his drinking is a problem and might be contributing to his weight loss. Alternatively, he may be more depressed than he acknowledges or simply adjusting to lifestyle changes precipitated by his separation. Finally, although he denies frank diarrhea, his large frequent stools raise the possibility of some form of malabsorption. Table 27–7 lists the differential diagnosis.

3

On further questioning, Mr. A reports that he drinks 2 or so alcoholic beverages a night. He proudly states that he has never missed work due to a hangover and never drinks before noon. When you ask him how much alcohol he uses in each drink and whether anyone else has commented on his drinking, he gets defensive and reminds you he is here because he is losing weight.

 Is the clinical information sufficient to make a diagnosis? If not, what other information do you need?

Mr. A's defensiveness increases your suspicion of alcoholism. You wonder how much alcohol consumption is normal and how to screen him more thoroughly for alcoholism.

***Table 27–7.*** Diagnostic hypotheses for Mr. A.

| Diagnostic Hypotheses | Clinical Clues | Important Tests |
|---|---|---|
| **Leading Hypothesis** | | |
| Alcoholism | Quantity of alcohol use Family or work-related problems Injury Family history of alcoholism Resistant hypertension | Alcohol screen Elevated AST or MCV |
| **Active Alternatives—Most Common** | | |
| Depression | History of loss, personal or family history of depression, postpartum state > 6 somatic symptoms | Admission of feeling down or anhedonia |
| Chronic pancreatitis | Epigastric pain History of alcohol use or acute pancreatitis Diarrhea or large difficult to flush stools | Calcifications on radiograph and CT scan, ERCP |
| Crohn disease | Diarrhea Chronic abdominal pain Family history of IBD Jewish descent Vitamin $B_{12}$ deficiency Uveitis, erythema nodosum Sclerosing cholangitis Hematochezia, anemia, rectal abscess, aphthous ulcers Polymicrobial urinary tract infection | Colonoscopy Capsule endoscopy pANCA and ASCA antibodies Fecal lactoferrin or calprotectin |
| Ulcerative colitis | Bloody diarrhea Family history of IBD Jewish descent Uveitis, erythema nodosum Sclerosing cholangitis | Colonoscopy |
| Bacterial overgrowth | Diarrhea Prior bowel surgery, stricture, blind loop Chronic pancreatitis Small bowel diverticula | Quantitative jejunal aspirates D-xylose breath test |
| Celiac disease | Diarrhea Family history Iron deficiency anemia Neurologic disorders (ataxia, headaches) Dermatitis herpetiformis | IgA endomysial Ab IgA-tGT Ab |
| Chronic infection (eg, *Clostridium difficile, Giardia lamblia, Entamoeba histolytica*) | Diarrhea Recent antibiotic use Hospitalization, long-term facility Fresh water intake Travel | Stool *C difficile* toxin Stool *Giardia* antigen Stool O & P |

# Leading Hypothesis: Alcoholism

## Textbook Presentation

Alcohol intake varies from low risk use to risky use, problem drinking, abuse, and finally alcohol dependence. Patients with alcoholism present along a continuum, from the functioning executive to the homeless alcoholic. Psychosocial complications include job loss, marital difficulties, loss of driving license, and violent behavior. Medical complications may include injury, pancreatitis, gastritis, cirrhosis, vitamin deficiency, cardiomyopathy, hypertension, malnutrition, weight loss, and death. Weight loss may be multifactorial secondary to decreased caloric intake during intoxication or due to alcohol-related illnesses (gastritis, pancreatitis, cirrhosis). Alcoholism is difficult to recognize early, when intervention may prevent progression.

## Disease Highlights

A. Alcohol is involved in 40% of all traffic fatalities and 20–37% of emergency department trauma and responsible for 85,000 deaths per year in the United States. Other causes of alcohol-related deaths include drownings, suicides, cirrhosis, and an increased risk of several cancers (esophageal, pharyngeal, laryngeal, and hepatocellular cancer).

B. Women are more likely to deny alcohol-related problems and to have associated eating disorders, depression, and panic disorders.

C. 37% of adults with alcohol abuse or dependence have concomitant mood or personality disorders.

D. Categories and definitions of patterns of alcohol use (1 drink is defined as 12 g of alcohol or 1.5 oz of liquor, 5 oz of wine, or 12 oz of beer)

   1. Risky use: Prevalence 4–29%

      a. Men: > 14 drinks/wk or > 4 drinks per occasion

      b. Women: > 7 drinks/wk or > 3 drinks per occasion

      c. Persons > 65 years: > 7 drinks/wk or 3 drinks per occasion

   2. Hazardous drinking: At risk for consequences from alcohol

   3. Alcohol abuse: ≥ 1 of the following events in 1 year:

      a. Recurrent use resulting in failure to fulfill major role or obligations

      b. Recurrent use in physically hazardous situations

      c. Recurrent alcohol-related legal problems (eg, driving while intoxicated)

      d. Continued use despite social or interpersonal problems caused by or exacerbated by alcohol

   4. Alcohol dependence: Prevalence 2–9%. Defined as ≥ 3 of the following events in 1 year:

      a. Tolerance (increased amounts to achieve effect)

      b. Withdrawal

      c. Alcohol is often taken in larger amounts or over a longer period than was intended.

      d. Persistent desire or unsuccessful efforts to cut down or control alcohol use.

      e. A great deal of time spent obtaining, using, or recovering from alcohol

      f. Important social, occupational, or recreational activities are given up or reduced because of alcohol use.

      g. Continued use despite knowledge of a physical or psychological problem caused by or exacerbated by alcohol

## Evidence-Based Diagnosis

A. The US Preventive Services Task Force recommends screening all adults. A variety of clinical clues can suggest alcohol misuse including:

   1. Injury

   2. Resistant hypertension

   3. Family, work, or legal problems

   4. Violence

   5. Depression

   6. Substance abuse

   7. Chronic pain

   8. Abnormal liver enzymes

   9. Macrocytosis

   10. Anemia

   11. Thrombocytopenia

   12. Family history of alcoholism

B. Recommendations suggest asking patients about the quantity of alcohol they ingest as well as the administration of a validated screening questionnaire.

   1. Self-reporting of alcohol ingestion may be inaccurate, particularly in patients who have recently ingested alcohol (sensitivity 20–47%).

   2. A variety of validated screening questionnaires exist including the CAGE, AUDIT, AUDIT-C, and TWEAK questionnaires.

      a. The CAGE questionnaire is easy to remember and frequently used but insensitive for heavy alcohol use.

      b. AUDIT (Alcohol Use Disorder Identification Test) is the best validated tool and available online, but it is lengthy.

      c. The TWEAK questionnaire is the optimal screening tool in women and the short Michigan Alcohol Screening Test-Geriatric version is an accurate tool in older adults.

      d. The accuracy of these screening tools and biochemical abnormalities is shown in Table 27–8.

C. The National Institutes of Health, and National Institute on Alcohol Abuse and Alcoholism recommend screening patients by asking if in the last year they have consumed 5 or more drinks in 1 day (4 or more drinks in women).

   1. Alternatively, the AUDIT score can be used.

   2. Patients with a positive response to the single question screen or men with an AUDIT score of ≥ 8 (≥ 4 for women or men over age 60) should complete a screening intervention.

   3. The pocket guide to this intervention can be found at http://pubs.niaaa.nih.gov/publications/Practitioner/pocketguide/pocket_guide.htm

D. Laboratory abnormalities (Table 27–8)

   1. A variety of laboratory abnormalities may be seen in patients with heavy alcohol use, including an elevated GGT (gamma glutamyl transpeptidase), MCV (mean corpuscular volume), or CDT (carbohydrate deficient transferrin).

   2. Elevated levels may increase the suspicion of alcoholism but are insensitive and should not be used to rule out the diagnosis.

   3. The sensitivity increases in patients with alcohol dependency in whom the diagnosis is increasingly obvious.

***Table 27–8.*** Accuracy of detecting unhealthy drinking using questionnaires and laboratory tests.

| | Sensitivity (%) | Specificity (%) | LR+[1] | LR– |
|---|---|---|---|---|
| **Questionnaires** | | | | |
| CAGE | 53–69 | 81–95 | 5.1 | 0.44 |
| AUDIT | 51–97 | 78–96 | 5.3 | 0.3 |
| AUDIT-C | 86 | 72 | 3.1 | 0.19 |
| (women) | 84 | 85 | 5.6 | 0.19 |
| TWEAK | 79–87 | 83–87 | 5.5 | 0.2 |
| (women) | | | | |
| **Laboratory tests** | | | | |
| Increased GGT | 65 | 80 | 3.3 | 0.44 |
| CDT | 26–60 | 80–92 | 3.1 | 0.66 |
| % CDT | 36–66 | 87–96% | 5.1–8.8 | 0.39–0.66 |
| Macrocytosis | 24 | 96 | 6 | 0.79 |

[1]LRs are calculated using average values for sensitivity and specificity.

## Treatment

**A.** Components of effective interventions for hazardous drinkers include:

1. Feedback on clinical assessment
2. Comparison to drinking norms
3. Discussion of the adverse effects of alcohol
4. Statement of the recommended drinking limits
5. Prescription to "Cut down on your drinking"
6. Patient educational material (www.niaaa.nih.gov)
7. Drinking diary
8. Follow-up office sessions and phone contact

**B.** Physician feedback, discussion, and prescription to cut down have been demonstrated to reduce drinking (OR 1.95), binge drinking, hospitalizations, total costs, and mortality.

**C.** Patients at moderate to high risk of alcohol withdrawal, a potentially fatal condition, should be hospitalized in a detoxification unit (see Chapter 10, Delirium & Dementia). Other patients who may benefit from inpatient treatment include those with concomitant psychiatric disorders (especially suicidal ideation) and unstable home environments.

**D.** Relapse prevention: Several options

1. Alcoholics Anonymous (AA), a 12-step program
2. Motivational enhancement therapy
3. Therapy to develop cognitive behavioral coping skills.
4. Naltrexone, acamprosate, and disulfiram have reduced drinking in patients with alcohol dependence. Pharmacotherapy is most effective when combined with behavioral support. Detailed documents that outline clinician support and include patient education materials are available.
   a. Naltrexone is an opioid antagonist that blunts the pleasurable effects of alcohol.
      (1) It can be taken orally or given monthly as a depot injection.

      (2) Naltrexone should be avoided in patients using opioids and those with acute hepatitis or liver failure.
   b. Acamprosate should not be given to patients who are actively drinking. It is contraindicated in patients with severe renal impairment (CrCl < 30 mL/min).
   c. Disulfiram acts as an alcohol deterrent by making patients sick who consume alcohol while taking disulfiram.
      (1) It is contraindicated in patients who are actively drinking, patients with coronary artery disease, and those taking metronidazole.
      (2) Disulfiram can cause hepatic toxicity; liver function tests should be monitored.
5. Treatment of depression, if present.

## MAKING A DIAGNOSIS

Mr. A's history of "2 or so" drinks per night suggest at-risk drinking. Furthermore, his marital separation, while possibly multifactorial, raises the real possibility of alcohol abuse. You ask Mr. A the screening question if he has had 5 or more drinks on any day in the last year.

Mr. A reports that he probably drinks that much at least once a month when he is "partying."

Mr. A's intake raises your concern further. You elect to administer the CAGE questionnaire.

Mr. A reports that he tried to **cut** down while he was married. Since his separation, he no longer feels that restraint. He admits to feeling **annoyed** with other family members who have suggested he cut down. (He is certain that his wife turned them against him.) He denies feeling **guilty** about his drinking and has never taken an **eye** opener. Mr. A reports that he has always been able to "hold his liquor" and that 6 drinks in an evening is not uncommon if he is having fun **(tolerance)**. He acknowledges that occasionally he hears funny stories about himself from these parties that he cannot recollect **(amnesia)**.

Mr. A reluctantly reports that he received 2 tickets for driving while intoxicated within the past year. He feels mildly guilty about this but assures you he knows better than to make that mistake again. He reiterates that he has never missed work due to his drinking but did miss several family events because he was "partying."

Mr. A has 2 positive responses to the CAGE questionnaire and his history of driving while intoxicated and missed family engagements defines his pattern as alcohol abuse. He meets 2 criteria (but not the necessary 3 criteria) for alcohol dependence (tolerance and missed engagements). You elect to check a CBC and a liver panel. The CBC shows macrocytosis and the liver panel shows a mildly elevated AST and ALT. The elevation in AST is more marked than the elevation in ALT, a pattern commonly seen in alcoholic hepatitis.

Clearly, Mr. A suffers from alcohol abuse. This may be the sole cause or a contributing cause of his IWL. You elect to initiate a treatment plan and reevaluate him once he is abstinent.

## CASE RESOLUTION

You have a frank discussion of the issues with Mr. A. You acknowledge that his marital difficulties are complex, but

that many features of his alcohol use suggest dependence and abuse. The missed family gatherings, alcoholic blackouts, tolerance, tickets for driving while intoxicated, and abnormal blood test results all suggest this is a serious medical problem. Mr. A confides that he is frightened to go "cold turkey." He feels shaky and agitated whenever he stops drinking. You suggest admission to a detoxification unit. Mr. A listens carefully and agrees to be admitted.

## FOLLOW-UP OF MR. A

Two months later, Mr. A returns to your office. His mood is clearly better. He proudly reports that he is "on the wagon" and feeling better. He attends AA meetings 5–7 nights per week. However, he remains concerned about his weight. He reports that his appetite is better and he is eating well but has not regained any weight.

At this point, what is the leading hypothesis, what are the active alternatives, and is there a must not miss diagnosis? Given this differential diagnosis, what tests should be ordered?

Mr. A's response to your intervention is rewarding. It is surprising that his weight is not improving particularly in light of his improved appetite. During his previous visit, he mentioned difficult to flush, large stools and you wonder if part of his weight loss is secondary to malabsorption. You revisit the common causes of malabsorption and diarrhea (Table 27–9 and Figure 27–5).

**Table 27–9.** Differential diagnosis of diarrhea organized by mechanism.

**Most common causes:** IBS, lactose intolerance, chronic infections, IBD, celiac disease

**Osmotic diarrhea:**
- Diagnostic clue: increased osmolar gap
- Lactose intolerance
- Mg++ laxatives, antacids

**Fatty diarrhea:**
- Diagnostic clue: Stool fecal fat
- Celiac disease
- Crohn disease
- Short bowel syndrome
- Bacterial overgrowth
- Pancreatic insufficiency

**Inflammatory diarrhea:**
- Diagnostic clue: Fecal calprotectin, fecal lactoferrin
- Inflammatory bowel disease
- Infectious
- Ischemic colitis
- Radiation colitis
- Neoplasia

**Secretory diarrhea:**
- Diagnostic clue: no osmolar gap
- Laxative abuse (nonosmotic laxative)
- Bacterial toxin
- Inflammatory bowel disease
- Collagenous colitis
- Ileal bile salt malabsorption
- Microscopic colitis
- Motility disorders: diabetic neuropathy, hyperthyroidism, IBS
- Neuroendocrine: Mastocytosis, carcinoid syndrome, VIPoma
- Neoplasia: Colon cancer, lymphoma, villous adenoma

Infections include invasive bacteria, C difficile, TB, HSV, CMV, amebiasis, giardiasis
Osmolar gap ≡ Measured fecal osmolarity − calculated fecal osmolarity NI < 50 osm/L. Calculated fecal osmolarity = 2 × (fecal Na+ + fecal K+)
IBD, inflammatory bowel disease; IBS, irritable bowel syndrome

## PRIORITIZING THE DIFFERENTIAL DIAGNOSIS

Mr. A denies ever being diagnosed with acute pancreatitis. He does remember multiple episodes of abdominal pain over the years following a night of binging. He did not seek medical care but remained at home drinking only clear fluids for several days until the pain subsided. He denies any history of bowel surgery, family history of inflammatory bowel disease (IBD), hematochezia, recent antibiotic use, or travel.

Mr. A's history of alcohol abuse and recurrent pain leads you to suspect that he may have chronic pancreatitis. This becomes the leading hypothesis.

Is the clinical information sufficient to make a diagnosis? If not, what other information do you need?

## Leading Hypothesis: Chronic Pancreatitis

### Textbook Presentation

Patients typically seek medical attention for long-standing postprandial abdominal pain. Frequent, loose, malodorous bowel movements are common, and weight loss occurs. Patients may note that several flushes are required to clear the toilet. A prior history of alcoholism and acute pancreatitis are clues to the diagnosis.

### Disease Highlights

A. Usually secondary to recurrent acute pancreatitis, primarily from alcohol abuse (70% of adult cases). Less common causes in adults include cystic fibrosis, hereditary pancreatitis, ductal obstruction (ie, stones, tumor), autoimmune disease, hypercalcemia, and hypertriglyceridemia.

B. Progressive destruction results in both exocrine and endocrine insufficiency.

C. Manifestations include

  1. Chronic, disabling, mid-epigastric postprandial pain is very common (80–100% of patients) and a major cause of morbidity. The pain may radiate to the back and be relieved by sitting forward.

  2. Weight loss secondary to anorexia and steatorrhea

  3. Steatorrhea

    a. Defined as fat malabsorption ≥ 14 g/d (nl ≤ 7 g/d fecal fat on 75–100 g fat diet. Patients with primarily watery diarrhea may excrete up to 13 g/d of fecal fat.)

    b. Manifestations include difficult to flush oily stools and weight loss. Elderly patients may not have diarrhea.

    c. Floating stools not specific for steatorrhea (bacterial gas may also result in floating stools)

    d. Diarrhea may develop secondary to bacterial overgrowth, which develops in 40% of patients with chronic pancreatitis.

  4. Diabetes develops in over 40% of patients due to the concomitant destruction of islet cells.

    a. Ketoacidosis is rare.

    b. Hypoglycemia is common due to loss of glucagon-producing pancreatic alpha cells.

  5. Complications include pseudocysts, obstruction of the common bile duct or duodenum and pancreatic ascites. Splenic vein thrombosis may also develop, leading to gastric varices.

  6. Pancreatic cancer develops in 4% of patients.

### Evidence-Based Diagnosis

A. One study reported IWL and diarrhea in 68%, and bloating in 30%. Diabetes was found in 28%.

B. Amylase and lipase are often normal or slightly elevated.

C. Abdominal radiographs may reveal pancreatic calcifications. Sensitivity is only 30%.

D. Routine abdominal ultrasound is 60–70% sensitive and 80–90% specific.

E. CT scan is test of choice. It may demonstrate ductal calcification (74–90% sensitive, 85% specific) and can demonstrate pancreatic pseudocysts or tumor.

F. Endoscopic retrograde cholangiopancreatography (ERCP) is invasive and typically reserved for patients in whom it might be therapeutic (ie, stenting) (sensitivity, 75–95%; specificity ≈ 90%).

G. Endoscopic ultrasound (EUS) is 97% sensitive and 60% specific.

H. Magnetic resonance cholangiopancreatography (MRCP) is being evaluated for the diagnosis of chronic pancreatitis.

I. ERCP, EUS, and MRCP are less sensitive in patients with mild disease (55–72%).

J. Secretin stimulation test can document pancreatic exocrine insufficiency. This test is highly accurate but invasive and rarely performed.

K. Tests for steatorrhea

  1. Stool Sudan III stain (qualitative) is 90% sensitive for fecal fat ≥ 10 g/d.

  2. Acid steatocrit (performed on spot stool specimen) is 100% sensitive and 95% specific.

  3. Can also be confirmed by low levels of fecal fat elastase (sensitivity and specificity 93%).

### Treatment

A. Abstinence from drinking is vital (but not universally effective at halting progression).

B. Pain management

  1. Exclude other causes of increasing or persistent pain

  2. NSAIDS, TCAs, and opioids are often used. Opioid dependence is a common problem.

  3. Pancreatic enzymes can decrease pain and improve nutritional status.

    a. Give with meals and low fat diets (< 20 g/d).

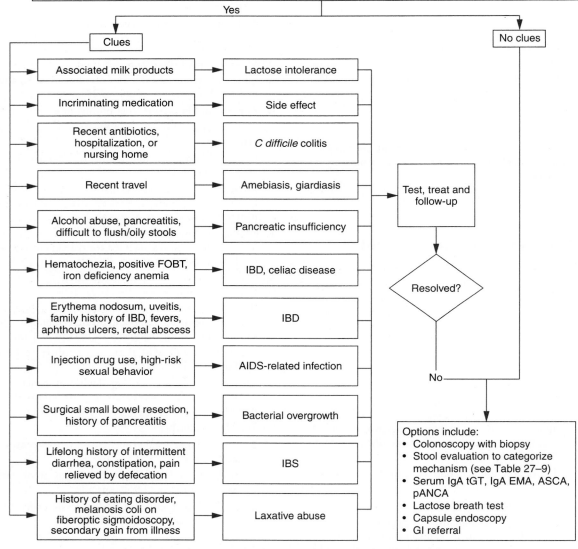

**History**

Dietary history: Association with milk products, sorbitol-containing mints or gums, caffeine, ruffage
Medication history: Including over-the-counter medications, antacids, recent antibiotics, metformin
Social history: Recent travel, alcohol use, risk factors for HIV
Family history: Jewish descent, family history of IBD or celiac disease
Clinical clues: Weight loss, stool appearance (bloody, oily), history of pancreatitis, alcohol use,
    manifestations of IBD (hematochezia, erythema nodosum, uveitis, aphthous ulcers, rectal abscess, fever);
Past medical history: Prior small bowel or gastric resection, cholecystectomy, radiation

**Physical exam**: Include comprehensive exam, weight, thyroid and abdominal exam, FOBT. Pallor, edema,
easy bruisability

**Laboratory studies**: CBC with differential, stool cultures, O & P (or stool *Giardia* antigen), stool *C difficile* toxin,
TSH, LFTs, BMP, serum albumin, cholesterol, HIV if appropriate

Yes

Clues         No clues

| Associated milk products | → | Lactose intolerance |
| Incriminating medication | → | Side effect |
| Recent antibiotics, hospitalization, or nursing home | → | *C difficile* colitis |
| Recent travel | → | Amebiasis, giardiasis |
| Alcohol abuse, pancreatitis, difficult to flush/oily stools | → | Pancreatic insufficiency |
| Hematochezia, positive FOBT, iron deficiency anemia | → | IBD, celiac disease |
| Erythema nodosum, uveitis, family history of IBD, fevers, aphthous ulcers, rectal abscess | → | IBD |
| Injection drug use, high-risk sexual behavior | → | AIDS-related infection |
| Surgical small bowel resection, history of pancreatitis | → | Bacterial overgrowth |
| Lifelong history of intermittent diarrhea, constipation, pain relieved by defecation | → | IBS |
| History of eating disorder, melanosis coli on fiberoptic sigmoidoscopy, secondary gain from illness | → | Laxative abuse |

Test, treat and follow-up

Resolved?

No

Options include:
• Colonoscopy with biopsy
• Stool evaluation to categorize mechanism (see Table 27–9)
• Serum IgA tGT, IgA EMA, ASCA, pANCA
• Lactose breath test
• Capsule endoscopy
• GI referral

BMP, basic metabolic panel; FOBT, fecal occult blood test; IBD, inflammatory bowel disease;
IBS, irritable bowel syndrome; LFTs, liver function tests; O & P, ova and parasite.

***Figure 27–5.*** Diagnostic approach: malabsorption and diarrhea.

**b.** Nonenteric coated enzymes may provide superior pain relief.

**c.** Coadministration of PPIs is recommended to prevent the inactivation of the enzymes.

**C.** Diabetes should be treated, with care to avoid hypoglycemia. Metformin should be avoided due to concomitant alcoholism.

**D.** ERCP, stenting, and surgery are useful in selected patients to relieve obstruction and pain.

**E.** Pseudocysts require surgical or endoscopic drainage.

## MAKING A DIAGNOSIS

A CT scan of the abdomen reveals multiple areas of pancreatic calcifications consistent with chronic pancreatitis. A Sudan stain for fecal fat is positive consistent with fat malabsorption.

 Have you crossed a diagnostic threshold for the leading hypothesis, chronic pancreatitis? Have you ruled out the active alternatives? Do other tests need to be done to exclude the alternative diagnoses?

## Alternative Diagnosis: Bacterial Overgrowth

### Textbook Presentation

Classically, patients have previously undergone GI surgery that resulted in some type of surgical blind loop that allows for bacterial multiplication. Patients may experience long-standing diarrhea, bloating, and weight loss.

### Disease Highlights

**A.** Mechanism of diarrhea is multifactorial.

1. Bacteria digest carbohydrates producing gas and osmotically active byproducts promoting an osmotic diarrhea

2. Bacteria and their fatty acid byproducts injure mucosa and contribute to diarrhea.

3. Mucosal injury can create lactase deficiency.

4. Bacterial deconjugation of bile salts interferes with fat absorption and the absorption of fat-soluble vitamins.

**B.** Etiologies

1. Stasis

   **a.** Strictures (surgical, Crohn disease, radiation enteritis)

   **b.** Anatomic abnormalities (surgical blind loops or diverticula)

   **c.** Dysmotility (diabetic autonomic neuropathy, scleroderma)

   **d.** Chronic pancreatitis (obstruction or opioid therapy can promote stasis).

2. Abnormal small to large intestine connections (ie, fistula or resection of ileocecal valve (allows retrograde colonization from heavily colonized colon into ileum)

3. Achlorhydria (ie, PPI therapy or autoimmune)

4. Miscellaneous (cirrhosis up to 60% of patients, end-stage renal disease)

**C.** Bacteria may utilize $B_{12}$, leading to $B_{12}$ deficiency.

**D.** Unusual complications include tetany (due to hypocalcemia) and night blindness due to vitamin A deficiency.

### Evidence-Based Diagnosis

**A.** Healthy older patients may also have bacterial overgrowth without any symptoms, making diagnosis difficult.

**B.** Gold standard is quantitative jejunal aspirates demonstrating $> 10^5$ bacteria.

**C.** A variety of tests detect bacterial byproducts in exhaled breath as an aid to diagnosis. Since bacteria normally reside in the colon, but only in low levels in the small intestine, early peaks in the concentration of these byproducts suggests small intestinal bacterial overgrowth. False-positives and false-negatives occur when other conditions increase or decrease bowel transit time, respectively.

1. D xylose breath test is usually abnormal secondary to bacterial digestion of xylose-releasing radiolabeled C14.

   **a.** Sensitivity 30–95%, specificity 89–100%.

   **b.** Avoid in fertile women.

   **c.** Antibiotics can interfere with the breath tests.

2. Hydrogen breath tests measure bacterial hydrogen production (measured in the patients breath) after patients ingest sugar.

   **a.** Their accuracy is similar to the xylose tests and avoids radioactivity.

   **b.** Some bacteria produce methane, and this measurement may increase accuracy.

**D.** Consider bacterial overgrowth if upper GI series demonstrates hypomotility, obstruction, or diverticula.

**E.** Weight loss may occur without diarrhea.

**F.** Therapeutic trials of antibiotics may be necessary.

### Treatment

**A.** Eliminate drugs that reduce intestinal motility or reduce gastric acidity.

**B.** A variety of oral antibiotics have been used for 7–10 days. Rotating course of antibiotics has been used in some patients. Rifaximin is a nonabsorbable antibiotic that has been useful.

**C.** Correct calcium, vitamin A, D, K and $B_{12}$ deficiency.

**D.** Minimizing carbohydrates, especially lactose, can be helpful.

## Alternative Diagnosis: IBD

IBD (Crohn disease and ulcerative colitis) are complex diseases. Genetic factors and commensal bacterial factors play a role. They are found most commonly in patients of Jewish descent and among patients with a family history of IBD. Crohn disease is a transmural process that may affect the entire GI tract whereas ulcerative colitis is a mucosal disease limited to the colon. Manifestations may be intestinal or extraintestinal (uveitis, erythema nodosum, large joint peripheral arthritis, ankylosing spondylitis, sclerosing cholangitis, secondary amyloidosis, and venous thromboembolism). Chronic colitis increases the risk of colon cancer in proportional to the amount of the colon involved and the duration of disease.

# 1. Crohn Disease

## Textbook Presentation

Common complaints include chronic abdominal pain, diarrhea, fever, weight loss, enterocutaneous fistulas, and acute abdominal pain, (which can mimic acute appendicitis).

## Disease Highlights

A. Transmural inflammation leads to fistula formation, strictures, and obstruction. Complications of fistulas include abscess formation, peritonitis, enterocutaneous fistulas (most commonly perianal), and enterovesicular fistulas (resulting in polymicrobial urinary tract infection).

B. Manifestations

1. Can involve any part of GI tract with normal "skip areas" between involved areas

   a. 80% of patients have small bowel involvement (most often in terminal ileum)

   b. 50% of patients have ileocolitis

   c. 20% of patients have isolated colitis

2. Nonspecific symptoms may precede diagnosis by many years.

3. Diarrhea may occur due to

   a. Small bowel disease impairing absorption

   b. Ileal disease, may decrease ileal bile absorption allowing bile salts into the colon which, in turn, causes irritation and diarrhea. Alternatively, when bile salt malabsorption is severe, it leads to bile salt deficiency and steatorrhea.

   c. Bacterial overgrowth secondary to strictures

4. Abdominal pain, weight loss, and fever

5. $B_{12}$ deficiency (secondary to ileal disease)

6. Calcium oxalate renal stones

   a. Normal oxalate absorption is limited by intraluminal intestinal binding of oxalate to calcium.

   b. Intraluminal fat is increased in malabsorption and binds intraluminal calcium decreasing calcium's availability to oxalate.

   c. This leads to increased oxalate absorption.

   d. Increased oxalate absorption causes hyperoxaluria and predisposes patients to kidney stones.

7. Osteoporosis due to vitamin D deficiency, calcium malabsorption, and corticosteroid therapy.

8. Gross bleeding is less frequent than in ulcerative colitis

9. Aphthous ulcers

## Evidence-Based Diagnosis

A. Colonoscopy with ileoscopy is often useful with biopsy.

B. Noninvasive markers

1. Serum markers (ASCA and pANCA) and stool markers (calprotectin and lactoferrin) can *suggest* IBD (Table 27–10).

2. Negative ASCA and pANCA do not rule out IBD.

3. Other inflammatory intestinal diseases can result in positive ASCA studies and fecal markers. ASCA is positive in 38% of patients with celiac disease and 67% of patients with intestinal tuberculosis.

4. C-reactive protein is insensitive for IBD (64%).

C. Diagnostic imaging

1. A variety of imaging techniques are available to image the small bowel when colonoscopy/ileoscopy fails to establish the diagnosis, including

   a. Small bowel follow through

   b. Enteroclysis

   c. CT enterography (CTE)

   d. MR enterography (MRE)

   e. Small bowel ultrasound

   f. Capsule endoscopy (CE)

2. Recent reviews and meta-analysis suggest CE has a greater diagnostic yield than

   a. Small bowel barium studies (43% vs 13%)

   b. Colonoscopy/ileoscopy (33% vs 26%)

   c. CTE (70% vs 21%)

   d. MRE (72% vs 50%)

3. CE was also superior to push enteroscopy.

4. There are two major limitations to capsule enteroscopy.

   a. First, CE is not completely specific. Small mucosal breaks can be caused by NSAIDs and be seen in normal patients.

   b. Second, the capsule can get stuck in strictures necessitating surgical removal. The risk of this in patients undergoing CE for the diagnosis of Crohn disease is ≈ 3% and may be minimized by avoiding CE in patients with known or suspected strictures.

5. A new capsule that disintegrates within the GI tract may markedly decrease this risk (Patency capsule). Some authorities recommend a small bowel study prior to CE to rule out a stricture.

***Table 27–10.*** Test characteristics of markers for the diagnosis of IBD.

| Test | Comments | Sensitivity (%) | Specificity (%) | LR+ | LR– |
|------|----------|-----------------|-----------------|-----|-----|
| Either ASCA or pANCA + | Suggests IBD | 62.6 | 92.6 | 8.5 | 0.4 |
| ASCA+/pANCA– | Suggests Crohn disease | 54.6 | 92.8 | 7.6 | 0.49 |
| ASCA–/pANCA+ | Suggests ulcerative colitis | 51.3 | 94.3 | 9 | 0.5 |
| Stool calprotectin | Suggests IBD | 90 | 80 | 4.5 | 0.13 |
| Stool lactoferrin | Suggests IBD | 87 | 96 | 21.8 | 0.14 |

IBD, inflammatory bowel disease.

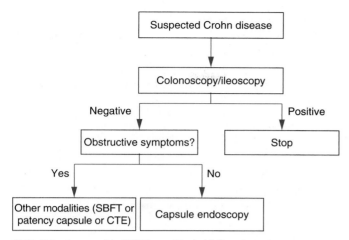

Suspected Crohn disease

↓

Colonoscopy/ileoscopy

Negative ↙ ↘ Positive

Obstructive symptoms? | Stop

Yes ↙ ↘ No

Other modalities (SBFT or patency capsule or CTE) | Capsule endoscopy

CTE, CT enterography; SBFT, small bowel follow through.

***Figure 27–6.*** Imaging approach: Crohn disease. (Reproduced, with permission, from Kornbluth A, Colombel JF, Leighton JA, Loftus E; ICCE. ICCE consensus for inflammatory bowel disease. Endoscopy. 2005;37(10):1051–4.)

6. One approach to imaging in Crohn disease is presented in Figure 27–6.

D. Active infection with the following organisms should be excluded in patients presenting with diarrhea: *Salmonella, Shigella, Campylobacter, Yersinia, Escherichia coli 0157:H7, Yersinia, Giardia, C difficile,* and *E histolytica.*

## Treatment

A. Primary therapy often uses 5-aminosalicylic acid (5-ASA), often with antibiotics.

B. Options for nonresponders or patients with severe disease include corticosteroids, 6 mercaptopurine (6MP), methotrexate, and tumor necrosis factor (TNF) antagonists.

C. Adjunctive therapy

1. Treat lactose intolerance if present

2. Antibiotics, CT-guided drainage of abscesses

3. Total parenteral nutrition (TPN) and multivitamins

   a. Necessary if patient is unable to maintain adequate nutrition.

   b. May also produce remission in refractory cases.

4. Bile acid resins for patients with watery diarrhea and ileal disease

5. Monitor for colon cancer if colonic involvement.

6. Surgery

   a. May be required for the management of massive hemorrhage, fulminant colitis, abscesses, peritonitis, obstruction, or disease refractory to medical therapy.

   b. High rate of recurrence following surgery (10–15%/y clinical recurrence, 80% endoscopic recurrence).

   c. 5-ASA, metronidazole, and 6MP have been demonstrated to reduce postoperative recurrences.

## 2. Ulcerative Colitis

### Textbook Presentation

Typically, bloody diarrhea and fecal urgency are the presenting symptoms.

### Disease Highlights

A. Primarily mucosal disease. (Occasionally, severe inflammation may extend deeper, involving muscular layers resulting in dysmotility and toxic megacolon.)

B. Strictly limited to colon

C. Starts at rectum and proceeds proximally in a *continuous fashion;* may be limited to rectum or involve rectosigmoid or entire colon. Rectal sparing suggests another disease (ie, Crohn disease).

D. Decreased risk among smokers (opposite of Crohn disease)

E. Anemia, fever, and increasing diarrhea are seen with more extensive disease.

F. Complications

1. Massive hemorrhage (rare)

2. Toxic megacolon

3. Stricture

4. Colon cancer

   a. The cancer risk is increased except in patients with just proctitis or very distal colitis.

   b. Increased risk begins 7–8 years after onset of disease.

### Evidence-Based Diagnosis

A. Sigmoidoscopy or colonoscopy demonstrates loss of vascular markings, erythema, friability, and exudates in a continuous fashion extending from the rectum proximally.

B. Biopsy specimen reveals crypt abscesses, branching crypts, and glandular atrophy.

C. Serologic and stool studies can suggest IBD (see Crohn disease) but are less helpful in ulcerative colitis since colonoscopy can rule in or rule out ulcerative colitis.

D. Exclude acute infectious processes (*Salmonella, Shigella, Campylobacter, E coli 0157:H7, C difficile, E histolytica*).

E. NSAIDs may cause colitis and their use should also be excluded.

### Treatment

A. For distal disease, options include oral 5–ASA preparations or topical preparations of 5-ASA or corticosteroids (suppositories, enemas, or foams).

1. Enemas can be used for disease that extends to 30–40 cm from the rectum.

2. Oral preparations are necessary for more proximal disease.

B. Oral or systemic corticosteroids can be added for more severe disease or nonresponders.

C. 5-ASA preparations (but not topical corticosteroids) are effective at maintaining remission.

D. Cyclosporine, 6MP, and infliximab have been effective in some patients with severe, corticosteroid refractory disease.

E. Antibiotics may be useful in select ill patients, particularly those with toxic megacolon or peritonitis.

**F.** Surgery (colectomy) is curative. Indications include:

1. Patients with high-grade dysplasia, carcinoma in situ or cancer on surveillance colonoscopy. Low-grade dysplasia should also prompt consideration for colectomy.

2. Other severe complications including massive hemorrhage, perforation, and toxic megacolon.

3. Intractable disease

**G.** Adjuvant therapy

1. Persistent diarrhea
   a. Test for lactose intolerance
   b. Avoid fresh fruits, vegetables, and caffeine

2. Surveillance colonoscopy for colon cancer for ulcerative colitis and Crohn disease begins 8 years after diagnosis and then every 1–2 years.

3. Supplemental iron

4. Fish oils and nicotine (transdermal) have been demonstrated to induce remission in some patients.

5. TPN if patients are unable to maintain adequate nutrition

6. Antidiarrheals may *increase* the increased risk of toxic megacolon.

7. Screen patients who have been taking corticosteroids for > 3 months for osteoporosis.

## CASE RESOLUTION

Mr. A's history and CT scan point strongly toward chronic pancreatitis. It would be reasonable to exclude chronic infection (*C difficile*, *Giardia*, and *E histolytica*) with a single stool for ova and parasites and stool for *C difficile* toxin. IBD is possible but unlikely. Since bacterial overgrowth can complicate chronic pancreatitis, an empiric trial of antibiotics could be given if therapy for chronic pancreatitis is unsuccessful.

Mr. A is given pancreatic enzymes. He reports that his diarrhea and bloating are greatly improved. Six months later he is back to his baseline weight.

## REVIEW OF OTHER IMPORTANT DISEASES

### Celiac Disease

**Textbook Presentation**

Classically, chronic diarrhea, steatorrhea, and weight loss are present. Iron and vitamin deficiencies may be seen.

**Disease Highlights**

**A.** Prevalence ≈ 1% in Northern Europeans; affects women 2–3 times more often than men.

**B.** Secondary to immune reaction to gliadin, a component of the wheat protein gluten. Antibodies develop to gliadin, transglutaminase (tTG), and endomysin (EMA).

**C.** Celiac disease is only seen in patients who carry either the HLA DQ2 or HLA DQ8 alleles.

**D.** Immune reaction results in villous atrophy and malabsorption.

**E.** Clinical manifestations

1. Usually presents between ages 10 and 40 years, although may be recognized in patients aged 60–80 years

2. Symptoms precipitated by exposure to wheat protein (gluten) and resolve within weeks to months on gluten-free diet.

3. Diarrhea and weight loss are seen in 68% of patients. Patients may also have unexplained iron deficiency anemia, osteoporosis, or abnormal liver function tests; however, they could be asymptomatic.

4. Vitamin deficiencies may cause ataxia and headaches.

5. Osteopenia and osteoporosis may develop due to vitamin D deficiency and subsequent secondary hyperparathyroidism.

6. Strongly associated with dermatitis herpetiformis, which develops secondary to antibodies against epidermal transglutaminase.

7. Far more common in patients with Down syndrome

8. Increase risk of other autoimmune disorders including thyroiditis and type 1 diabetes mellitus

9. Patients with celiac disease are at increased risk for intestinal adenocarcinoma and enteropathy-associated T cell lymphoma.

**Evidence-Based Diagnosis**

**A.** Diagnostic options include duodenal biopsy (the gold standard), serology, and clinical response to gluten-free diet.

**B.** Small bowel biopsy is the gold standard and useful but invasive. Strategies can help determine when biopsies are necessary (see below).

**C.** Serologic testing is highly accurate but not perfect.

1. Endomysial antibody (IgA EMA)
   a. 81–97% sensitive, 99% specific
   b. LR+ ≈ 100, LR− 0.03–0.19

2. Tissue glutaminase antibody (IgA tGT)
   a. 81–95% sensitive, 91–99% specific
   b. LR+ 10.1–90, LR+ 0.05–0.19

3. There are several causes of false-negative serologies including
   a. IgA deficiency: IgG tGT antibodies can be tested when the suspicion is high and IgA levels are low or absent.
   b. Gluten-free diets: IgA levels fall (and may become negative) in patients on gluten-free diet. (Increasing titers in celiac patients suggest dietary noncompliance.)
   c. One paper suggested EMA was less sensitive (50–60%) in patients over age 35 years who smoke.

**D.** HLA typing

1. Virtually all patients with celiac disease express HLA-DQ2 or HLA-DQ8 heterodimers.
   a. 100% sensitive but only 57–75% specific
   b. LR+ 2.3, LR− 0

2. Celiac disease can be virtually ruled out in patients who are negative for HLA-DQ2 or HAL-DQ8.

3. May be useful in patients in patients who instituted a gluten-free diet before evaluation in whom IgA-tGT and IgA EMA antibody levels may be low due to decreased disease activity. If the patient expressed neither HLA DQ haplotype, celiac disease could be excluded.

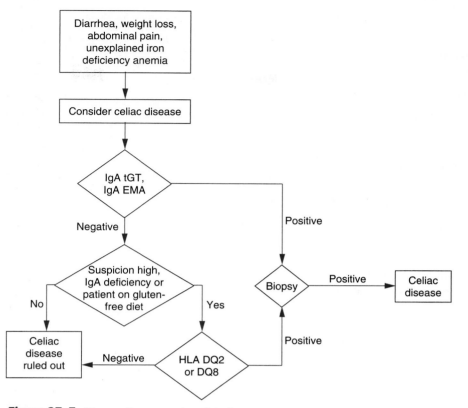

***Figure 27–7.*** Diagnostic approach: celiac disease.

**E.** Surprisingly, due to the low prevalence of celiac disease, positive EMA and tGT serologies do not confirm the diagnosis, despite the high specificity.

    **1.** The PPV ranges from 29% to 76% and biopsy is necessary to confirm the diagnosis.

    **2.** On the other hand, negative EMA and tGT serologies make the diagnosis very unlikely (NPV ≈ 99%) and essentially rule out the disease.

    **3.** If concern remains despite a negative result, HLA typing could help completely exclude the disease.

    **4.** One approach is shown in Figure 27–7.

## Treatment

**A.** Gluten-free diet (no wheat, rye, and barley)

**B.** Oats that are uncontaminated with gluten are usually tolerated in patients with celiac disease.

**C.** Lactose avoidance may be necessary due to concomitant lactase deficiency.

**D.** Correct iron, folic acid, vitamin $B_{12}$, and vitamin D deficiencies.

**E.** Pneumococcal vaccine is recommended by some experts.

**F.** Corticosteroids or other immunosuppressives have rarely been necessary in patients with refractory celiac sprue.

**G.** Osteoporosis screening is recommended.

## REFERENCES

Bergstrom JP, Helander A. Clinical characteristics of carbohydrate-deficient transferrin (% disialotransferrin) measured by HPLC: sensitivity, specificity, gender effects, and relationship with other alcohol biomarkers. Alcohol Alcohol. 2008;43(4):436–41.

Bhatt DL, Scheiman J, Abraham NS. ACCF/ACG/AHA 2008 Expert Consensus Document on Reducing the Gastrointestinal Risks of Antiplatelet Therapy and NSAID Use. Circulation. 2008;118.

Bilbao-Garay J, Barba R, Losa-Garcia JE et al. Assessing clinical probability of organic disease in patients with involuntary weight loss: a simple score. Eur J Intern Med. 2002;13:240–5.

Bradley KA, Boyd-Wickizer J, Powell SH, Burman ML. Alcohol screening questionnaires in women: a critical review. JAMA. 1998;280(2):166–71.

Brent GA. Clinical practice. Graves' disease. N Engl J Med. 2008;358(24):2594–605.

Callery MP, Freedman SD. A 21-year-old man with chronic pancreatitis. JAMA. 2008;299(13):1588–94.

Gisbert JP, Abraira V. Accuracy of *Helicobacter pylori* diagnostic tests in patients with bleeding peptic ulcer: a systematic review and meta-analysis. Am J Gastroenterol. 2006;101(4):848–63.

Gisbert JP, de la Morena F, Abraira V. Accuracy of monoclonal stool antigen test for the diagnosis of *H. pylori* infection: a systematic review and meta-analysis. Am J Gastroenterol. 2006;101(8):1921–30.

Hadithi M, von Blomberg BM, Crusius JB et al. Accuracy of serologic tests and HLA-DQ typing for diagnosing celiac disease. Ann Intern Med. 2007;147(5): 294–302.

Hernandez JL, Riancho JA, Matorras P, Gonzalez-Macias J. Clinical evaluation for cancer in patients with involuntary weight loss without specific symptoms. Am J Med. 2003;114(8):631–7.

Hopper AD, Cross SS, Hurlstone DP et al. Pre-endoscopy serological testing for coeliac disease: evaluation of a clinical decision tool. BMJ. 2007;334(7596):729.

Metalidis C, Knockaert DC, Bobbaers H, Vanderschueren S. Involuntary weight loss. Does a negative baseline evaluation provide adequate reassurance? Eur J Intern Med. 2008;19(5):345–9.

Nakao H, Konishi H, Mitsufuji S et al. Comparison of clinical features and patient background in functional dyspepsia and peptic ulcer. Dig Dis Sci. 2007;52(9):2152–8.

Pignone MP, Gaynes BN, Rushton JL et al. Screening for depression in adults: a summary of the evidence for the U.S. Preventive Services Task Force. Ann Intern Med. 2002;136(10):765–76.

Reese GE, Constantinides VA, Simillis C et al. Diagnostic precision of anti-Saccharomyces cerevisiae antibodies and perinuclear antineutrophil cytoplasmic antibodies in inflammatory bowel disease. Am J Gastroenterol. 2006; 101(10):2410–22.

Saitz R. Clinical practice. Unhealthy alcohol use. N Engl J Med. 2005;352(6): 596–607.

Schoepfer AM, Trummler M, Seeholzer P, Seibold-Schmid B, Seibold F. Discriminating IBD from IBS: comparison of the test performance of fecal markers, blood leukocytes, CRP, and IBD antibodies. Inflamm Bowel Dis. 2008; 14(1):32–9.

Talley NJ, American Gastroenterological A. American Gastroenterological Association medical position statement: evaluation of dyspepsia. Gastroenterology. 2005;129(5):1753–5.

Triester SL, Leighton JA, Leontiadis GI et al. A meta-analysis of the yield of capsule endoscopy compared to other diagnostic modalities in patients with non-stricturing small bowel Crohn's disease. Am J Gastroenterol. 2006;101(5): 954–64.

US Preventive Services Task Force. Screening and behavioral counseling interventions in primary care to reduce alcohol misuse: recommendation statement. Ann Intern Med. 2004;140(7):554–6.

# I have a patient with wheezing or stridor. How do I determine the cause?

## CHIEF COMPLAINT

PATIENT 1

Mr. C is a 32-year-old man with occasional wheezing.

> What is the differential diagnosis of wheezing? How would you frame the differential?

## CONSTRUCTING A DIFFERENTIAL DIAGNOSIS

Wheezing and stridor are symptoms of airflow obstruction. These sounds are caused by the vibration of the walls of pathologically narrow airways. **Wheezing** is a musical sound produced primarily during expiration by airways of any size. **Stridor** is a single pitch, inspiratory sound that is produced by large airways with severe narrowing.

> Stridor is often a sign of impending airway obstruction and should be considered an emergency.

The differential diagnosis for airway obstruction is large. It is best remembered by an anatomic approach. Stridor may be caused by severe obstruction of any proximal airway (see A through D in the differential diagnosis outline below). A more clinical approach to the differential appears in the algorithm at the end of the chapter.

A. Nasopharynx and oropharynx
  1. Tonsillar hypertrophy
  2. Pharyngitis
  3. Peritonsillar abscess
  4. Retropharyngeal abscess
B. Laryngopharynx and larynx
  1. Epiglottitis
  2. Paradoxical vocal cord movement (PVCM)
  3. Anaphylaxis and laryngeal edema
  4. Postnasal drip
  5. Benign and malignant tumors of the larynx and upper airway
  6. Vocal cord paralysis
C. Trachea
  1. Tracheal stenosis
  2. Tracheomalacia
  3. Goiter

D. Proximal airways
  1. Foreign-body aspiration
  2. Bronchitis
E. Distal airways
  1. Asthma
  2. Chronic obstructive pulmonary disease (COPD)
  3. Pulmonary edema
  4. Pulmonary embolism
  5. Bronchiectasis
  6. Bronchiolitis

1

Mr. C has been having symptoms for 1–2 years. His symptoms have always been so mild that he has never sought care. Over the last month, he has been more symptomatic with wheezing, chest tightness, and shortness of breath. His symptoms are worse with exercise and worse at night. He notes that he often goes days without symptoms.

> At this point, what is the leading hypothesis, what are the active alternatives, and is there a must not miss diagnosis? Given this differential diagnosis, what tests should be ordered?

## PRIORITIZING THE DIFFERENTIAL DIAGNOSIS

The presence of wheezing, chest tightness, and shortness of breath are pivotal clues that place asthma at the top of the differential diagnosis. Although asthma is by far the most likely diagnosis, other diseases that could account for recurrent symptoms of airway obstruction should be considered. Allergic rhinitis can cause cough and wheezing but it would be very unusual for it to cause shortness of breath. Vocal cord dysfunction, such as PVCM, is frequently confused with asthma. COPD can also cause intermittent pulmonary symptoms. Table 28–1 lists the differential diagnosis.

1

On further history, Mr. C reports that he had asthma as a child and was treated for years with theophylline. He was without symptoms until he moved 2 years ago.

***Table 28–1.*** Diagnostic hypotheses for Mr. C.

| Diagnostic Hypotheses | Clinical Clues | Important Tests |
|---|---|---|
| **Leading Hypothesis** | | |
| Asthma | Episodic and reversible airflow obstruction | Peak flow PFTs Methacholine challenge Response to treatment |
| **Active Alternative** | | |
| Allergic rhinitis | Rhinitis with seasonal variation | Response to treatment |
| Vocal cord dysfunction | Voice pathology accompanies airflow obstruction | Abnormal vocal cord movement visualized |
| **Active Alternative—Must Not Miss** | | |
| COPD | Presence of smoking history | PFTs |

He reports that his symptoms are worst when he has a cold, when he jogs, and when he is around dogs or cats. His most common symptoms are chest tightness and dyspnea. Only when his symptoms are at their worst does he hear wheezing. He has never smoked cigarettes.

On physical exam he appears well. His vital signs are BP, 120/76 mm Hg; RR, 14 breaths per minute; pulse, 72 bpm; temperature, 36.9°C. His lung exam is normal without wheezes or prolonged expiratory phase. His peak flow is 550 L/min (87% of predicted).

 **Is the clinical information sufficient to make a diagnosis? If not, what other information do you need?**

## Leading Hypothesis: Asthma

### Textbook Presentation

Asthma commonly presents as recurrent episodes of dyspnea, often with chest tightness, cough, and wheezing. Patients usually report stereotypical triggers (eg, allergens, cold weather, exercise) and rapid response to β-agonist inhalers. Asthma is so common that most patients have diagnosed themselves prior to presentation.

### Disease Highlights

**A.** Definition: The NIH/NHLBI definition of asthma is "A chronic inflammatory disease of the airways in which many cells and cellular elements play a role." "In susceptible individuals, this inflammation causes recurrent episodes of wheezing, breathlessness, chest tightness, and cough, particularly at night and/or in the early morning. These episodes are usually associated with widespread but variable airflow limitation that is often reversible either spontaneously or with treatment."

**B.** Clinical manifestations

**1.** Asthma is recurrent and intermittent. Patients will have periods with no or only mild symptoms unless severe disease develops when patients have persistent symptoms.

**2.** Asthma usually presents during childhood but presentation as an adult is not uncommon.

**3.** People with asthma have fluctuation of airway function.

   **a.** Airway function is most commonly measured by peak expiratory flow (PEF).

   **b.** Values are generally lowest in the morning and highest at mid-day.

   **c.** PEF will vary by more than 20% in asthmatic patients over the course of the day.

**4.** Identifying exacerbating factors and timing of symptoms is important. It aids in the diagnosis of asthma (exacerbating factors are stereotypical) and in treatment (if the factors are reversible).

   **a.** Asthma frequently worsens at night (probably related to decreased mucociliary clearance, airway cooling, and low levels of endogenous catecholamines).

   **b.** Asthma frequently worsens with exercise (probably related to airway cooling and drying).

   **c.** Viral infections are a common cause of asthma exacerbations.

   **d.** Occupational agents may cause or exacerbate asthma by a number of mechanisms:

      **(1)** Corrosive agents (ammonia)

      **(2)** Pharmacologic agents (organophosphates)

      **(3)** Reflex bronchoconstriction (ozone)

      **(4)** IgE-mediated (latex)

 Asthma should be in the differential diagnosis of any patient with intermittent respiratory symptoms.

**C.** Classification: The present classification scheme for asthma helps focus attention on the severity of the asthma and dovetails nicely with treatment considerations (Table 28–2). It should be noted, however, that by necessity this scheme simplifies asthma phenotypes and many patients do not fit well into a single category.

**D.** Exacerbations or "flares"

**1.** Asthma exacerbations are periods of increased disease activity identified by increased airflow obstruction (and therefore increased symptoms) and increased medication use.

**2.** Exacerbations may or may not be caused by an identifiable trigger.

**3.** Management of an exacerbation depends on an accurate assessment of the cause of the exacerbation and the risk to the patient.

## EVIDENCE-BASED DIAGNOSIS

**A.** There is no 1 specific test to diagnose asthma; the diagnosis is a clinical one, based on multiple findings in the history, physical, and a few simple tests.

**B.** Asthma is easily recognized when it presents with intermittent wheezing; in fact the diagnosis is often made by the patient.

**Table 28–2.** Classification of asthma severity.

| Classification | Symptoms | Lung Function |
|---|---|---|
| Mild intermittent | Symptoms less than twice a week<br>Asymptomatic between exacerbations and brief exacerbations<br>Nighttime symptoms < twice monthly | PEF > 80% of predicted |
| Mild persistent | Symptoms between once a day and twice a week<br>Asymptomatic between exacerbations but exacerbations may limit activity<br>Nighttime symptoms > twice monthly | PEF > 80% of predicted |
| Moderate persistent | Daily symptoms<br>Exacerbations limit activity<br>Nighttime symptoms > weekly. | PEF 60-80% of predicted |
| Severe persistent | Continual symptoms<br>Symptoms chronically limit physical activity<br>Frequent nighttime symptoms | PEF < 60% of predicted |

PEF, peak expiratory flow.

**Table 28–3.** Test characteristics of symptoms for the diagnosis of asthma.

| Criteria | Sensitivity | Specificity | LR+ | LR− |
|---|---|---|---|---|
| Wheezing | 74.7% | 87.3% | 5.77 | 0.29 |
| Dyspnea at rest | 47.1% | 94.9% | 9.23 | 0.56 |
| Wheezing without URI symptoms | 59.8% | 93.6% | 9.34 | 0.43 |
| Nocturnal dyspnea | 46.2% | 96% | 11.55 | 0.56 |
| Wheezing and exertional dyspnea | 54.2% | 95.7% | 12.60 | 0.48 |
| Wheezing and dyspnea | 65.2% | 95.1% | 13.30 | 0.37 |
| Wheezing and nocturnal chest tightness | 40.9% | 97.5% | 16.44 | 0.61 |
| Wheezing and nocturnal dyspnea | 37.5% | 98.6% | 26.79 | 0.61 |
| Wheezing and dyspnea at rest | 38.4% | 98.7% | 29.54 | 0.62 |

URI, upper respiratory infection.
Adapted from Sistek D et al. Clinical diagnosis of current asthma: predictive value of respiratory symptoms in the SAPALDIA study. Swiss Study on Air Pollution and Lung Diseases in Adults. Eur Respir J. 2001;17:214–219.

C. Diagnosing asthma is challenging when it presents in atypical ways. Asthma should be high in the differential diagnosis when a patient has any of the following intermittent symptoms:

1. Wheezing
2. Dyspnea
3. Cough
4. Chest tightness

D. The key points in establishing the diagnosis of asthma are:

1. Episodic symptoms of airflow obstruction
2. Reversibility of the airflow obstruction
3. Exclusion of other likely diseases

E. There are not great data on the test characteristics of various symptoms of asthma.

1. One large study interviewed nearly 10,000 healthy, community dwelling people regarding pulmonary symptoms in the preceding 12 months.

   a. 225 of these people had asthma, defined as reporting that they had asthma and that a medical professional had confirmed the diagnosis.

   b. The test characteristics of the most predictive historical features are shown in Table 28–3.

   c. It is important to note that these test characteristics were derived in a healthy population. Specificities would be lower in a population containing patients with other cardiopulmonary diseases.

2. In another study, which used a methacholine challenge test to diagnose asthma, 90% specificity was achieved for

making the diagnosis of asthma with the question, "Do you cough during or after exercise?"

F. Other clues that make the diagnosis more likely are outlined in the NIH/NHLBI guidelines:

1. Diurnal variability in PEF (> 20% variability between best and worst)
2. Symptoms occur or worsen in the presence of:

   a. Exercise
   b. Viral infections
   c. Animals with fur or feathers
   d. House dust mites
   e. Mold
   f. Smoke
   g. Pollen
   h. Weather changes
   i. Laughing or hard crying
   j. Airborne chemicals or dust

3. Symptoms occur or worsen at night.

G. There is some evidence that persons with asthma describe their dyspnea differently from people with other cardiorespiratory disease. They are more likely to refer to symptoms of chest tightness or constriction.

H. Pulmonary function tests (PFTs)

1. PFTs are recommended for patients with suspected asthma both as a diagnostic test and to provide objective data to be used in the assessment of management.

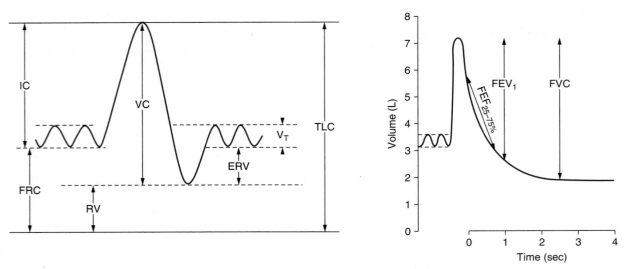

***Figure 28–1.*** Pulmonary function tests. ERV, expiratory reserve volume; FEF 25–75%, forced expiratory flow measured during exhalation of 25–75% of the FVC; $FEV_1$, forced expiratory volume in 1 second; FRC, functional reserve capacity; FVC, forced vital capacity; IC, inspiratory capacity; RV, residual volume; TLC, total lung capacity; VC, vital capacity; $V_T$, tidal volume.

**2.** PFTs should be done in all patients other than those with mild disease and no diagnostic uncertainty.

**3.** Figure 28–1 show a schematic diagram of many of the lung volumes, capacities, and flows measured in PFTs.

**4.** The following all support the diagnosis of asthma:

  **a.** Decreased $FEV_1$, the volume of air exhaled in the first second during a forced expiratory maneuver.

  **b.** Decreased $FEV_1$/forced vital capacity (FVC) ratio

  **c.** Reversibility (defined as at least a 200 mL increase in $FEV_1$ and > 12% improvement with bronchodilators)

**I.** Other tests

  **1.** Chest radiography is useful mainly in excluding other diseases.

  **2.** Methacholine challenge

    **a.** Can be very helpful in diagnosing asthma in patients who have a suspicious history but normal PFTs

    **b.** A decrease in $FEV_1$ of < 20% has a 95% negative predictive value.

## Treatment

**A.** The goals of asthma therapy are to

  **1.** Prevent chronic symptoms such as nighttime wakening

  **2.** Maintain normal pulmonary function (assessed by PEF and spirometry)

  **3.** Maintain normal levels of physical activity. It can be challenging to achieve this goal. Many patients become accustomed to being limited by their breathing and thus may not report that their breathing limits their activity.

  **4.** Prevent exacerbations

**B.** One of the first steps in treating asthma is to treat exacerbating factors. These factors, some of which are listed below, are treated with pharmacologic and nonpharmacologic interventions.

  **1.** Tobacco use and secondhand smoke

  **2.** Air pollution (ozone, $SO_2$, $NO_2$)

  **3.** Gastroesophageal reflux disease (GERD)

  **4.** Common allergens

  **5.** Dander, dust, mold, insects

**C.** Medical therapy for asthma itself is aimed at treating the factors that cause the disease and its symptoms. The drugs are summarized in Table 28–4.

**D.** A usual course of therapy follows:

  **1.** Short-acting $\beta_2$-agonists are used as needed for mild intermittent asthma and exercise-induced asthma.

  **2.** In patients with mild persistent asthma (or once a patient is using short-acting $\beta_2$-agonists more than twice weekly) inhaled corticosteroids are added. The dose of inhaled corticosteroids is escalated for control of symptoms.

  **3.** Long-acting $\beta_2$-agonists are considered for control of nocturnal symptoms and for maintenance after short-acting $\beta_2$-agonists and inhaled corticosteroids are used.

  **4.** Because of data showing an increase in complications from asthma in patients using long-acting $\beta_2$-agonists alone, these drugs should be reserved for patients already using inhaled corticosteroids.

  **5.** Leukotriene antagonists and theophylline can also be used for maintenance after short-acting $\beta_2$-agonists and inhaled corticosteroids are used.

  **6.** Systemic corticosteroids are reserved for the treatment of exacerbations and refractory cases.

 At each visit, review a patient's medications and carefully review symptoms. Focus on any limitations of activity related to asthma.

**Table 28–4.** Pharmacotherapy of asthma.

| Medication | Purpose | Common Adverse Effects |
|---|---|---|
| Short-acting β₂-agonists | Immediate relief of symptoms | Tachycardia, jitteriness |
| Inhaled corticosteroids | Mainstay of long-term therapy | Thrush, dysphonia, potentially osteopenia at high doses |
| Long-acting β₂-agonists | Long-term therapy when inhaled corticosteroids have not adequately controlled symptoms Useful for nocturnal symptoms | Tachycardia, jitteriness |
| Leukotriene antagonists | Long-term therapy when inhaled corticosteroids have not improved symptoms | No significant adverse effects |
| Systemic corticosteroids | Immediate therapy for exacerbations or long-term therapy in patients with refractory asthma | Traditional corticosteroid side effects (weight gain, hyperglycemia, bone loss) |
| Theophylline | Similar to long-acting β₂-agonists but used less frequently | Dose-related tachycardia, nausea, jitteriness |

E. Refractory cases

1. Most cases of asthma can be well controlled. There are a number of considerations if asthma is refractory to treatment.

2. Is the patient compliant? This includes poor inhaler technique (which is very common) and poor understanding of the use of maintenance and as-needed medications.

3. Are there unaccounted for or untreated precipitants? (Consider GERD, sinusitis, and allergies.)

4. Is the diagnosis correct? (Consider other causes of chronic intermittent airway obstruction such as those listed in the algorithm at the end of this chapter.)

5. Are there rare diseases present that can cause or worsen asthma? (Consider Churg-Strauss disease, allergic bronchopulmonary aspergillosis.)

F. Exacerbations

1. History

   a. Duration of exacerbation

   (1) Exacerbations that are very recent (hours) and mild may improve with β-agonists alone while more established and more severe exacerbations require corticosteroids.

   (2) Because early treatment leads to better outcomes, it is important that patients monitor their own disease

and know how to initiate appropriate treatment and contact their physician when necessary.

   b. Precipitants

   (1) Consider if there is a clear precipitant of the exacerbation that needs to be treated or removed (eg, sinusitis, allergen exposure).

   (2) Consider if there is an exacerbating factor that hospital admission might avoid (eg, house painting, recent insect extermination).

   c. Severity of disease. The following patients are at risk for asthma-related death. Hospital admission is nearly always indicated for patients with an exacerbation and 1 of these factors:

   (1) History of sudden severe exacerbations

   (2) Prior admission to an ICU

   (3) Recent emergency department visits or hospitalizations

   (4) Use of more than 2 canisters of β-agonist in the past month

   (5) Current use or recent discontinuation of systemic corticosteroids

   (6) Difficulty perceiving airflow obstruction

   (7) Comorbid medical or psychiatric disease

2. Physical exam

   a. The lung exam is generally a poor marker of the severity of disease.

   b. Lack of wheezing can either reflect improved or worsening airflow.

Patients whose decreased wheezing is accompanied by worsening distress or decreased mental status probably have worsening airflow obstruction. Conversely, a patient whose decreased wheezing is accompanied by lessened respiratory distress likely has improved airflow obstruction.

3. Other tests

   a. Chest radiograph is only helpful for identifying the uncommon concomitant infection or complication (eg, pneumothorax).

   b. Spirometry is most helpful in determining severity of exacerbation.

   (1) A moderate exacerbation will have an FEV₁ or PEF 50–80% of predicted and moderate symptoms.

   (2) A severe exacerbation will have an FEV₁ or PEF 50–80% of predicted with severe symptoms, physical findings, or concerning history.

Spirometry and the history of the patient's prior exacerbations are the most important pieces of information for making admission decisions.

   c. Arterial blood gases are useful in patients whose peak flows are not improving with treatment. ABGs during severe exacerbations should reveal a respiratory alkalosis. A respiratory acidosis (or even a normal PCO₂ during a severe exacerbation) is very worrisome as it suggests severe airway narrowing.

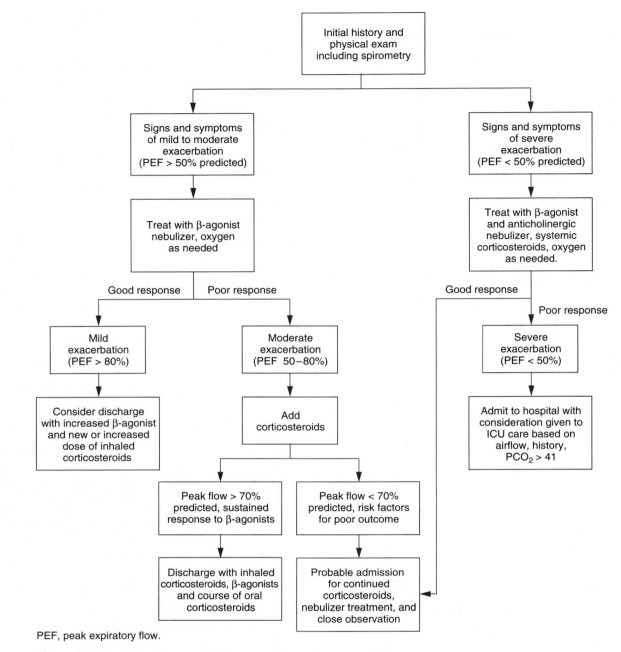

PEF, peak expiratory flow.

***Figure 28–2.*** Initial evaluation and treatment of an asthma exacerbation.

4. Treatment of exacerbations

   a. Figure 28–2 is adapted from the NIH/NHLBI Guidelines for the Diagnosis and Management of Asthma and is a guide to the management of asthma exacerbations.

   b. Recognize that the differentiation of mild, moderate and severe exacerbations is based not only on spirometry but on history and physical as well.

## MAKING A DIAGNOSIS

Mr. C's clinical history is consistent with asthma. He has intermittent symptoms of wheezing, dyspnea, and chest tightness. Multiple points in his history raise the probability of asthma as the diagnosis. These include the childhood history of asthma and the exacerbating factors. His normal peak flow does not exclude the diagnosis because he is presently symptomatic. At this point, a diagnostic and therapeutic trial of asthma medication would be reasonable.

Mr. C was given an albuterol inhaler. He was told to use 2 puffs as needed as well as about 30 minutes before exercise or expected animal exposure. On follow-up 6 weeks later, Mr. C reported improvement in his symptoms. He was able to exercise without difficulty as long as he was using his inhalers and could spend short amounts of time around friends' pets. He suffered one upper respiratory tract infection during the last 6 weeks. He found his symptoms worse during this time. On average, he was using his inhaler about 4 times daily with good relief of symptoms.

 Have you crossed a diagnostic threshold for the leading hypothesis, asthma? Have you ruled out the active alternatives? Do other tests need to be done to exclude the alternative diagnoses?

Because asthma is very common and the initial treatment is benign, the treatment threshold is low. A therapeutic and diagnostic trial of medication is nearly always appropriate.

## CASE RESOLUTION

The patient's history and response to therapy confirms the diagnosis of asthma. The patient has no nasal symptoms that would suggest allergic rhinitis. COPD is unlikely without a smoking history. Vocal cord dysfunction will be discussed below and is also unlikely. Heart failure (HF) is unlikely given the patient's age, the absence of a history of heart disease, and his response to bronchodilators.

Given the frequency of his use of albuterol, the patient was given low-dose inhaled corticosteroids. His symptoms subsequently improved with only rare need for albuterol. The following year, Mr. C's symptoms worsened after a move into a new house. His asthma was eventually controlled with higher doses of inhaled corticosteroids. He was able to wean these medications after he had carpets in his house replaced with hardwood floors.

## CHIEF COMPLAINT

PATIENT

Mrs. P is a 62-year-old woman who arrives at the emergency department with shortness of breath and wheezing. She says that the symptoms have been present for 3 days. The symptoms are present both at rest and with exertion and have not improved with an albuterol inhaler.

She reports that she has had these symptoms intermittently for 6 years. When the symptoms occur, they generally last for hours to a few days. She had been diagnosed with asthma and took long- and short-acting β-agonists and inhaled and systemic corticosteroids, before coming off all medications 1 year ago. She stopped her medications herself out of frustration with side effects and perceived lack of efficacy. She decided instead to treat herself with yoga and meditation. She reports no episodes since this decision.

Presently she denies cough, chest pain, fever, or rhinitis. She does report hoarseness that occurs when her breathing is bad.

Past medical history is remarkable only for depression and hypertension. Her only medication is enalapril. She has no known drug allergies. She does not smoke cigarettes.

At this point, what is the leading hypothesis, what are the active alternatives, and is there a must not miss diagnosis? Given this differential diagnosis, what tests should be ordered?

## PRIORITIZING THE DIFFERENTIAL DIAGNOSIS

As discussed above, asthma is very common and should be considered in anyone with intermittent pulmonary symptoms. There are some pivotal points in Mrs. P's history that argue against asthma. Her symptoms did not improve with a β-agonist and it seems that she came off an aggressive asthma regimen without ill effects. The patient also describes hoarseness associated with her symptoms; this would be atypical for asthma in which hoarseness only occurs if there is associated GERD, postnasal drip, or thrush caused by inhaled corticosteroids. PVCM is a syndrome of episodic adduction of the vocal cords producing wheezing and stridor. The lack of response to bronchodilators and associated hoarseness are clues to this diagnosis. GERD is a very common diagnosis (see Chapter 8, Chest Pain). It can cause and worsen asthma and can cause hoarseness via irritation of the vocal cords. Angioedema occurs when vascular permeability increases leading to swelling of subcutaneous tissues. Airway compromise can occur. It is usually associated with other signs such as facial swelling, tongue swelling, or hives. Table 28–5 lists the differential diagnosis.

On further history, she reports that her present symptoms are moderate for her.

On physical exam, the patient is in some respiratory distress. Her voice is hoarse and "squeaky." Her vital signs are temperature, 37.1°C; pulse, 110 bpm; BP, 140/90 mm Hg; RR, 32 breaths per minute. There is a harsh wheeze heard throughout the lungs that is loudest in the anterior neck. The remainder of the physical exam was normal.

PEF is 300 L/min, 70% of predicted.

***Table 28-5.*** Diagnostic hypotheses for Mrs. P.

| Hypotheses Diagnostic | Clinical Clues | Important Tests |
|---|---|---|
| **Leading Hypothesis** | | |
| Paradoxical vocal cord movement | Episodic airflow obstruction associated with stridor | Laryngoscopy demonstrating abnormal vocal cord movement |
| **Active Alternative—Most Common** | | |
| Asthma | Episodic and reversible airflow obstruction | Peak flow PFTs Methacholine challenge Response to treatment |
| **Active Alternative** | | |
| Gastroesophageal reflux disease | May cause or worsen asthma and cause voice pathology | Identification of esophageal and laryngeal abnormalities on endoscopy |
| **Active Alternative—Must Not Miss** | | |
| Angioedema | Often associated with hives and causative exposure | Clinical presentation with or without risk factors |

 Is the clinical information sufficient to make a diagnosis? If not, what other information do you need?

## Leading Hypothesis: PVCM

### Textbook Presentation

PVCM typically presents as episodic attacks of respiratory distress accompanied by wheezing or stridor or both. The respiratory distress is often accompanied by voice pathology and a lack of response to traditional asthma therapy.

### Disease Highlights

A. PVCM has gone by many names including vocal cord dysfunction, episodic laryngeal dyskinesia, Munchausen stridor, psychogenic stridor, and factitious asthma.

B. Most commonly occurs in younger patients (< 35 years) but can be seen in any age.

C. Female predominance

D. The symptoms are not produced consciously.

E. During asymptomatic disease, there are no abnormalities of lung function:

1. Spirometry is normal.
2. There is none of the increased variability in airway function seen with asthma.
3. Bronchoprovocation tests are normal.

### Evidence-Based Diagnosis

A. Given the prevalence of asthma and the similarity of the presentation, asthma needs to be excluded in any patient with PVCM. This is especially true as the 2 disorders may coexist.

B. Clues to the differentiation of the diseases are:

1. The lack of exacerbating factors (eg, exercise, allergens) and diurnal variation seen with asthma.
2. The lack of response to asthma medications.
3. The occasional disappearance of symptoms during sleep.
4. The striking voice pathology during attacks.
5. The preponderance of auscultatory findings in the neck.
6. A flattened inspiratory limb on flow-volume loops suggesting variable extrathoracic airway obstruction.

C. The definitive diagnosis is made on laryngoscopy.

1. There is adduction of the vocal cords often leaving only a diamond-shaped opening between the cords during flares.
2. There is generally normal vocal cord function between flares.

### Treatment

A. There are no controlled trials of treatments for PVCM.

B. Speech therapy, concentrating on laryngeal relaxation seems to be the most effective therapy.

C. Psychiatric intervention is suggested for patients with psychiatric illness.

D. Acute attacks may be quite hard to manage.

1. Helium/oxygen mixtures have been suggested to obtain better flow through the narrowed larynx though there is no evidence to support its utility.
2. Instructing the patient to lay his tongue on the floor of the mouth and breathe through pursed lips may also help.

## MAKING A DIAGNOSIS

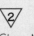 Given Mrs. P's history and physical findings, PVCM was suspected, but the history of asthma and the severity of the dyspnea were concerning. An albuterol nebulizer was started and an otolaryngologist was called to evaluate the patient.

 Have you crossed a diagnostic threshold for the leading hypothesis, PVCM? Have you ruled out the active alternatives? Do other tests need to be done to exclude the alternative diagnoses?

The diagnosis of PVCM is certainly likely given the patient's history and physical exam findings. Asthma still needs to be ruled out with spirometry and, if necessary, bronchoprovocation. The other important diagnosis to consider is angioedema.

Asthma is significantly more prevalent than PVCM. Any patient in whom the diagnosis of PVCM is considered should have asthma ruled out.

## Alternative Diagnosis: Angioedema

### Textbook Presentation

The presentation of angioedema is usually an acute swelling of soft tissue, especially the face, lips, tongue, larynx, or foreskin. Patients nearly always have a history of angioedema or a risk factor for it.

### Disease Highlights

**A.** The onset of angioedema is usually rapid, over minutes to hours.

**B.** Angioedema may be caused by:

  **1.** ACE inhibitors

  **2.** Allergic reactions

  **3.** Hereditary and acquired forms of C1-inhibitor deficiency

**C.** The presentation can range from mild, only sensed by the patient; to disfiguring, obvious to the casual observer; to life-threatening laryngeal involvement.

**D.** The diverse causes of angioedema produce symptoms by different mechanisms, have different presentations, and different treatments.

  **1.** Histamine-related angioedema

    **a.** Almost always accompanied by pruritus and urticaria (hives).

    **b.** Usually related to an allergic exposure such as an insect bite or a food.

    **c.** Urticaria can also be chronic, caused by allergy, drug effect, autoimmune phenomena, or malignancy.

  **2.** Nonhistamine-related angioedema (caused by elevated levels of bradykinin)

    **a.** Most commonly the result of ACE inhibitor therapy

    **b.** Deficiency of C1-inhibitor also causes elevated bradykinin levels as well as elevated C2b levels, another cause of angioedema.

### Evidence-Based Diagnosis

**A.** A diagnosis of angioedema is clinical, based on the recognition of angioedema and associated symptoms.

**B.** Angioedema most commonly presents as swelling of the lips, tongue, or both.

**C.** Figure 28–3 presents a useful algorithm for considering the differential diagnosis and treatment of angioedema.

### Treatment

**A.** The most critical aspect of the management of angioedema is airway stabilization.

**B.** All patients receive $H_1$- and $H_2$-blockers as well as corticosteroids.

**C.** Patients with airway compromise or any intraoral swelling should also receive epinephrine.

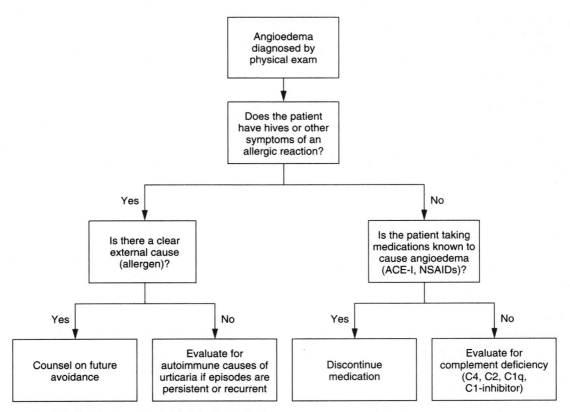

ACE-I, angiotensin-converting enzyme inhibitors; NSAIDs, nonsteroidal antiinflammatory drugs.

***Figure 28–3.*** Differential diagnosis and treatment of angioedema.

**D.** Patients need to be closely monitored because intubation is sometimes necessary.

**E.** Patients with C1-inhibitor deficiency can be treated with androgens, which increase the production of C1-inhibitor, or C1-inhibitor concentrate.

## CASE RESOLUTION

A helium oxygen mixture was given to the patient briefly before laryngoscopy was performed. The findings on

laryngoscopy were consistent with PVCM. The patient was counseled in the emergency department on ways to improve her airflow and symptoms subsided over the next hour. The patient spent 2 days in the hospital, experiencing only 1 mild episode of dyspnea during the period of observation.

The findings on laryngoscopy are diagnostic of PVCM. Except for ACE inhibitor therapy, there is little evidence or history supporting angioedema; the patient has no facial swelling, and there are no consistent findings on laryngoscopy.

## CHIEF COMPLAINT

PATIENT ▽3

Mr. S is a 50-year-old man who arrives at the emergency department with sore throat, fever, and wheezing. He reports being well until 2 days ago when his sore throat started. Over the next 2 days, the sore throat became progressively more severe and he lost his voice. On the morning of admission, a fever of 38.0°C and wheezing developed. He was also unable to eat because of the pain. He has never had similar symptoms before.

At this point, what is the leading hypothesis, what are the active alternatives, and is there a must not miss diagnosis? Given this differential diagnosis, what tests should be ordered?

### PRIORITIZING THE DIFFERENTIAL DIAGNOSIS

The pivotal points in Mr. S' presentation are the acuity of the illness and the fever. Both of these points make an infectious etiology likely. Because the symptoms are not recurrent, asthma, the most common cause of airway obstruction, is unlikely. Acute infectious causes need to be considered first. These include common conditions, such as pharyngitis, and rare but serious causes, such as epiglottitis and retropharyngeal abscess. Angioedema is a possibility, but the infectious symptoms (fever and pain) and the lack of visible swelling make this less likely. Aspiration of a foreign body could cause either a pneumonia or infection of the soft tissues of the neck resulting in fever. Table 28–6 lists the differential diagnosis.

▽3

On physical exam, Mr. S is in obvious distress. He is uncomfortable, is sitting upright, and speaks in a muffled voice. His vitals signs are temperature, 38.3°C; pulse, 110 bpm; BP, 128/88 mm Hg; RR, 18 breaths per minute. Examination of the oropharynx is notable only for mild tonsillar edema without exudates. There is diffuse cervical lymphadenopathy and significant tenderness over the anterior neck. The neck is supple. Lungs are clear, but there is stridor transmitted from the neck.

**Table 28–6.** Diagnostic hypotheses for Mr. S.

| Diagnostic Hypotheses | Clinical Clues | Important Tests |
|---|---|---|
| **Leading Hypothesis** | | |
| Pharyngitis | Sore throat often with fever, exudates and lymphadenopathy | Clinical exam Throat culture |
| **Active Alternative—Must Not Miss** | | |
| Epiglottitis | Sore throat with muffled voice, stridor, and anterior neck tenderness | Direct visualization with laryngoscopy |
| Retropharyngeal abscess | Similar to epiglottitis with more prominent neck symptoms (stiff, painful) | Lateral neck radiograph or CT scan of the neck |
| **Other Alternative** | | |
| Foreign body aspiration | Usually history of acute-onset pain or airway obstruction | Documentation of foreign body directly or radiographically |

Is the clinical information sufficient to make a diagnosis? If not, what other information do you need?

The patient's physical exam makes pharyngitis a less likely cause of his symptoms. His pharynx is patent, and there is more distal stridor.

### Leading Hypothesis: Epiglottitis

#### Textbook Presentation

Fever and sore throat are usually the presenting symptoms. There can be evidence of varying degrees of airway obstruction including wheezing, stridor, and drooling. The disease has become significantly less common in children since the use of the *Haemophilus influenzae B* vaccine.

## Disease Highlights

**A.** Epiglottitis is an infectious disease, classically caused by *H influenzae,* that causes swelling of the epiglottis and supraglottic structures.

**B.** Can rapidly cause airway compromise so the diagnosis is always considered an airway emergency.

**C.** Classic presentation is a patient with sore throat, muffled "hot potato" voice, drooling, and stridor.

**D.** *H influenzae* is cultured in only a small percentage of adult patients; respiratory viruses are the likely cause of most cases of epiglottitis.

**E.** Epiglottitis is a difficult diagnosis because initial presentation is often identical to pharyngitis.

## Evidence-Based Diagnosis

**A.** The gold standard for diagnosis is visual identification of swelling of the epiglottis.

  **1.** Otolaryngology consultation is thus mandatory in any patient with a high suspicion for the disease.

  **2.** Visualization can be achieved with direct or indirect laryngoscopy.

  **3.** In patients with signs of severe disease (eg, muffled voice, drooling, and stridor), an experienced physician should perform direct laryngoscopy and be prepared to intubate the patient or perform a tracheostomy (if airway control cannot be obtained).

**B.** The classic symptoms of muffled voice, drooling, and stridor are seen very rarely and signify imminent airway obstruction.

  **1.** Sitting erect and stridor are independent predictors of subsequent airway intervention (RRs of 4.8 and 6.2, respectively).

  **2.** In 1 study of patients with epiglottitis, the test characteristics of sitting erect at presentation and stridor were as follows:

    **a.** Sitting erect at presentation: Sensitivity, 47%; specificity, 90%; LR+, 4.7; LR−. 0.59.

    **b.** Stridor: Sensitivity, 42%; specificity, 94%; LR+, 7; LR−, 0.61.

**C.** Common symptoms and signs of patients with epiglottitis are shown in Table 28–7.

**D.** Lateral neck films, a commonly used diagnostic tool, have a sensitivity of about 90%. The classic finding is the "thumb sign" of a swollen epiglottis.

A normal lateral neck film does not rule out epiglottitis. Laryngoscopy should be performed in a patient with a high clinical suspicion of epiglottitis, even if the neck film is normal.

## Treatment

**A.** Airway control

  **1.** All patients should be admitted to the ICU for close monitoring.

  **2.** Patients with signs or symptoms of airway obstruction should be intubated electively.

**Table 28–7.** Prevalence of the signs and symptoms of epiglottitis.

| Symptoms and Signs | Frequency |
| --- | --- |
| Sore throat | 95% |
| Odynophagia | 94% |
| Muffled voice | 54% |
| Pharyngitis | 44% |
| Fever | 42% |
| Cervical adenopathy | 41% |
| Dyspnea | 37% |
| Drooling | 30% |
| Sitting erect | 16% |
| Stridor | 12% |

  **3.** Elective intubation is preferred because intubation in a patient with epiglottitis can be very difficult.

  **4.** Some advocate prophylactic intubation of all patients.

Epiglottitis is an airway emergency. Patients need to be monitored extremely closely and not left alone until the airway is stable. Otolaryngology consultation is mandatory.

**B.** Antibiotics

  **1.** Necessary to cover *H influenzae.*

  **2.** Second- or third-generation cephalosporins are usually recommended.

## MAKING A DIAGNOSIS

Mr. S's history is very concerning. His upright posture, voice changes, and stridor are not only indicative of epiglottitis but also of imminent airway closure. None of these findings would be seen with pharyngitis. Foreign-body aspiration does not fit the history. Retropharyngeal abscess remains a possibility.

Given the concern for epiglottitis, lateral neck films were obtained, and an otolaryngologist was called to examine the patient's upper airway.

Have you crossed a diagnostic threshold for the leading hypothesis, epiglottitis? Have you ruled out the active alternatives? Do other tests need to be done to exclude the alternative diagnoses?

## Alternative Diagnosis: Retropharyngeal Abscess

### Textbook Presentation

Retropharyngeal abscess can be seen in either children or adults. Patients usually have symptoms similar to those seen in epiglottitis but commonly have a history of a recent upper respiratory infection or trauma from recently ingested materials (bones), or procedures (pulmonary or GI endoscopy).

### Disease Highlights

**A.** Symptoms that suggest retropharyngeal abscess rather than epiglottitis are:

    **1.** Patients with retropharyngeal abscesses often will sense a lump in their throat.

    **2.** Patients are often most comfortable supine with neck extended (very different from epiglottitis).

### Evidence-Based Diagnosis

**A.** The diagnosis of retropharyngeal abscess is made when a thickening of the retropharyngeal tissues is seen on lateral neck radiographs.

**B.** Radiographs are probably not 100% sensitive, so when radiographs are normal and clinical suspicion is high, CT scanning should be done to verify the diagnosis.

### Treatment

**A.** Retropharyngeal abscesses are usually polymicrobial.

**B.** Treatment is both medical and surgical.

    **1.** Surgical drainage should be accomplished as soon as possible.

    **2.** Many antibiotics have been suggested. Coverage of gram-positive organisms and anaerobes make clindamycin a common choice.

## CASE RESOLUTION

The patient's lateral neck radiograph showed probable acute epiglottitis with a thumb sign. An otolaryngologist visualized the epiglottis and, given the patient's symptoms and severity of the visualized airway obstruction, placed an endotracheal tube. Mr. S was admitted to the ICU and treated with a second-generation cephalosporin. Cultures of the blood and epiglottis were negative.

The patient's infection was diagnosed on the lateral neck radiographs. Intubation was necessary because the patient had signs and symptoms of airway obstruction and the actual obstruction was visualized on laryngoscopy.

---

## CHIEF COMPLAINT

PATIENT 4

Mrs. A is 52-year-old woman who comes to your office with shortness of breath and wheezing. She reports that her symptoms have been present for about 2 years. She reports almost constant, mild dyspnea that is worst with exercise or when she has a cold. Only rarely does she feel "nearly normal." She also complains of a mild cough productive of clear sputum. She does not feel that her cough is much of a problem as it is significantly better since she stopped smoking 2 years ago.

At this point, what is the leading hypothesis, and what are the active alternatives? What other tests should be ordered?

## PRIORITIZING THE DIFFERENTIAL DIAGNOSIS

The pivotal points in this case are the patient's chronic dyspnea wheezing, and smoking history. COPD and asthma should be high in the differential diagnosis. HF is also a possibility. The patient's smoking history is a risk factor for coronary disease, the most common cause of HF, and she suffers from nearly constant dyspnea that is worse with exertion. As noted in Chapter 14, Dyspnea, HF frequently complicates COPD or is misdiagnosed as the pulmonary disease. Bronchiectasis could cause symptoms of dyspnea, cough, and sputum production, but the patient's sputum production seems to be a minor symptom, unlike what is usually seen in bronchiectasis. Tuberculosis (TB) should probably be considered in the differential, since it can cause chronic cough and dyspnea. Given the chronic nature of the symptoms, if TB were the cause, we would expect to hear about weight loss and other constitutional signs. Table 28–8 lists the differential diagnosis.

Mrs. A reports a 60 pack-year history of smoking. She stopped 2 years ago, after smoking 2 packs a day for 30 years, when her chronic cough began to worry her. She reports that she still coughs but only rarely brings up sputum.

She has not experienced fever, chills, weight loss, or peripheral edema. She does say that when her breathing is bad it is worse when lying down. She has never had symptoms consistent with paroxysmal nocturnal dyspnea.

Orthopnea is a very nonspecific symptom. It is found in many types of cardiopulmonary disease.

Is the clinical information sufficient to make a diagnosis? If not, what other information do you need?

**Table 28–8.** Diagnostic hypotheses for Mrs. A.

| Diagnostic Hypotheses | Clinical Clues | Important Tests |
|---|---|---|
| **Leading Hypothesis** | | |
| COPD | Chronic irreversible airway obstruction with a smoking history | Spirometry and sometimes imaging |
| **Active Alternative—Most Common** | | |
| Asthma | Episodic and reversible airflow obstruction | Peak flow PFTs Methacholine challenge Response to treatment |
| **Active Alternative—Must Not Miss** | | |
| HF | Presence of risk factors and consistent physical exam findings | Echocardiography |
| **Other Alternative** | | |
| Bronchiectasis | Chronic, heavy, purulent sputum production | CT scan of the chest |

## Leading Hypothesis: COPD

### Textbook Presentation

Presenting symptoms of COPD include progressive dyspnea, decreased exercise tolerance, cough, and sputum production. The onset is usually slow and progressive with occasional acute exacerbations. A long smoking history is present in almost all patients with COPD who live in industrialized countries.

### Disease Highlights

A. COPD is defined in the WHO/NHLBI Global Strategy for the Diagnosis, Management, and Prevention of Chronic Obstructive Pulmonary Disease as a "disease state characterized by airflow limitation that is not fully reversible. The airflow limitation is usually both progressive and associated with an abnormal inflammatory response of the lungs to noxious particles or gases."

B. COPD should be considered in any patient with a smoking history who has pulmonary complaints. These complaints can be:

   1. Mild (smokers' cough or lingering colds)

   2. Moderate (chronic cough, sputum production, and dyspnea)

   3. Severe (activity-limiting dyspnea with life-threatening exacerbations)

C. COPD can also be seen in patients without a smoking history but with significant exposure to secondhand smoke, occupational dust and chemicals and, especially in less developed countries, indoor air pollution from cooking stoves.

D. Because of the wide variation in disease course, it is impossible to give an average amount of exposure necessary to cause disease.

   1. Pulmonary symptoms usually develop after about 10 years of exposure.

   2. Airflow obstruction may develop later.

E. Diagnosis of early, minimally symptomatic COPD is important because it may allow for more appropriate treatment of mild symptoms (cough) and may provide extra incentive for smoking cessation.

F. Emphysema and chronic bronchitis are currently being used less as descriptors of types of COPD.

   1. Emphysema is a pathologic term not accurately correlating with its general clinical usage.

   2. Chronic bronchitis is the presence of mucus production for most days of the month, 3 months of a year, for 2 successive years. This symptom does not relate to the airflow obstruction that causes the morbidity in COPD.

   3. Due to the overlap and lack of specificity of these 2 terms, COPD should be used as the diagnostic term.

G. Two staging systems provide a way of categorizing patients by symptoms and prognosis.

   1. The WHO/NHLBI outlines stages of COPD (Table 28–9) that are useful for both diagnosis and management of patients. They are based mainly on spirometry and are thus very easy to use.

   2. Other indices, such as the BODE index, take into account other patient features, such as body mass index, degree of dyspnea, and exercise tolerance, and are very useful prognostically.

### Evidence-Based Diagnosis

A. The diagnosis of COPD is based on history, physical exam, and ancillary tests (primarily PFTs).

B. Important aspects of the history are:

   1. Smoker's cough

   2. Lingering colds

**Table 28–9.** WHO/NHLBI stages of COPD.

| Stage | Spirometry | Symptoms |
|---|---|---|
| 0 At Risk | Normal | Chronic cough and sputum production |
| 1 Mild COPD | $FEV_1/FVC < 70\%$ $FEV_1 > 80\%$ | Chronic cough and sputum production often without dyspnea |
| 2A Moderate COPD | $FEV_1 = 50–80\%$ | Chronic dyspnea possibly with intermittent exacerbations |
| 2B Moderate COPD | $FEV_1 = 30–50\%$ | Chronic dyspnea probably with intermittent exacerbations |
| 3 Severe COPD | $FEV_1 < 30\%$ | Also may be diagnosed with $PaO_2 < 60$ mm Hg, $PaCO_2 > 50$ mm Hg or cor pulmonale |

COPD, chronic obstructive pulmonary disease; $FEV_1/FVC$, forced expiratory volume in 1 second/forced vital capacity.
Pauwels RA, Buist AS, Calverley PM, Hurd SS. Global strategy for the diagnosis, management, and prevention of chronic obstructive pulmonary disease. NHLBI/WHO Global Initiative for Chronic Obstructive Pulmonary Disease (GOLD) Workshop Summary. Am J Respir Crit Care Med. 2001. 163: 1256–1276.

  **3.** Chronic cough

  **4.** Sputum production

  **5.** Dyspnea

  **6.** Decreased exercise tolerance

**C.** Physical exam

  **1.** The physical exam is useful mainly in patients with more advanced disease.

  **2.** No findings are sensitive enough to exclude a diagnosis of COPD.

 **3.** The test characteristics for some of the physical exam findings are listed in Table 28–10.

 The absence of wheezing does not rule out, or even significantly decrease the likelihood of, COPD.

**D.** Spirometry

  **1.** Because the results of spirometry are part of the information required to make a diagnosis of COPD, test characteristics cannot be calculated.

  **2.** For the diagnosis of COPD, the most important spirometric values are postbronchodilator, since COPD is defined by irreversible airway obstruction.

  **3.** Typically PFTs in COPD reveal:

    **a.** Increased total lung capacity secondary to decreased elastic recoil

    **b.** Increased functional residual capacity and residual volume secondary to air trapping

    **c.** Decreased $FEV_1$ and FVC due to airflow obstruction

    **d.** Decreased DLCO secondary to destruction of the oxygen/Hgb interface.

**E.** Other tests

  **1.** Spirometry with bronchodilator response is recommended to rule out asthma. Patients with completely reversible airflow obstruction likely have asthma.

  **2.** Chest radiograph is generally not useful in diagnosing COPD.

**Table 28–10.** Test characteristics for physical exam findings in COPD.

| Criteria | Sensitivity | Specificity | LR+ | LR– |
|---|---|---|---|---|
| Subxiphoid cardiac impulse | 4–27% | 97–99% | ≈ 8 | ≈ 1 |
| Absent cardiac dull LLSB | 15% | 99% | 15 | ≈ 1 |
| Diaphragmatic excursion < 2 cm | 13% | 98% | 6.5 | ≈ 1 |
| Early inspiratory crackles | 25–77% | 97–98% | 8–38.5 | ≈ 1 |
| Any unforced wheeze | 13–56% | 86–99% | 1–56 | ≈ 1 |

COPD, chronic obstructive pulmonary disease; LLSB, left lower sternal border.
Modified from McGee SR. Evidence-based physical diagnosis. Philadelphia, PA: Saunders, 2001:382. With permission from Elsevier.

**a.** Some findings are suggestive

  **(1)** Upper lobe bullous disease (uncommon but nearly diagnostic)

  **(2)** Flattened diaphragm on the lateral chest radiograph

  **(3)** Large retrosternal air space

  **(4)** Hyperlucency of the lungs

  **(5)** Diminished distal vascular markings

**b.** Chest radiography is always recommended to rule out other causes of symptoms.

**3.** ABG measurement is recommended in patients with $FEV_1$ < 40% predicted or with right-sided heart failure.

**4.** Testing for $\alpha_1$-antitrypsin deficiency (a rare cause of COPD) is recommended in patients:

  **a.** In whom COPD develops before age 45 years

  **b.** Who do not have a smoking history or suspicious exposure

In general, any patient with a smoking history who complains of chronic cough, sputum production, or dyspnea should be considered to have COPD if no other diagnosis can be made. Additional testing can help establish the diagnosis and assess severity.

## Treatment

**A.** Management of stable disease

  **1.** Nonpharmacologic and preventive therapy

    **a.** Smoking cessation or removal of other inhaled toxic agents

    **b.** Exercise programs if allowable from a cardiovascular standpoint

    **c.** Vaccination against influenza and pneumococcal pneumonia

  **2.** Pharmacologic

    **a.** Anticholinergic inhalers ipratropium or tiotropium

      **(1)** Mainstay of therapy

      **(2)** Initial therapy for symptomatic patients

      **(3)** Also recommended for patients with $FEV_1$ < 50% of predicted regardless of symptoms

      **(4)** Recent data suggest that these medications increase the risk of cardiovascular events.

    **b.** β-Agonists

      **(1)** Short-acting medications are useful if the patient's response to anticholinergic inhalers is insufficient.

        **(a)** Can be used as-needed or on a scheduled basis

        **(b)** Combinations with anticholinergic inhalers are useful

      **(2)** Long-acting medications are especially useful for treatment of nocturnal symptoms.

    **c.** Theophylline

      **(1)** May be used in patients with inadequate response to long-acting β-agonists and anticholinergic inhalers

      **(2)** Narrow therapeutic window limits usefulness

    **d.** Inhaled corticosteroids

      **(1)** Use remains somewhat controversial

      **(2)** There is some evidence that inhaled corticosteroids decrease symptoms and reduce the frequency of exacerbations.

**(3)** They do not seem to effect the rate of decline in pulmonary function and may increase rates of pneumonia.

**e.** Home oxygen is recommended for persons with chronic hypoxia or cor pulmonale.

**B.** Management of exacerbations

**1.** Evaluation

**a.** Patients who are likely to have the worst outcomes have low baseline $FEV_1$, $PaO_2$, pH, and high $PCO_2$. Discharge of such patients from an emergency department should be done with great care.

**b.** Exacerbating factors

**(1)** Factors that likely led to the COPD exacerbation should be sought and addressed during treatment.

**(2)** Historical evidence of infection or exposure (air pollution, ozone) should be sought.

**(3)** All patients should have a chest radiograph to look for pneumonia.

**(4)** As discussed in Chapter 14, Dyspnea, if a cause of the exacerbation is not found, consideration should be given to pulmonary embolism.

**c.** Unlike in the assessment of asthma exacerbations, spirometry is of little value in making admission decisions.

**2.** Therapy

**a.** Anticholinergic inhalers should be given to all patients with addition of β-agonists if necessary.

**b.** Systemic corticosteroids are effective when given for up to 2 weeks. There is no evidence that inhaled corticosteroids are effective.

**3.** Antibiotics are effective for more severe exacerbations. It is unclear which the most effective antibiotic is.

**4.** Oxygen therapy is beneficial.

**a.** Oxygen does carry a risk of hypercapnia and respiratory failure.

**b.** The development of respiratory failure is somewhat predictable.

**c.** The following equation identifies patients who are at high risk for $CO_2$ retention and for requiring mechanical ventilation: $pH = 7.66 - 0.00919 \times PaO_2$. If the calculated pH is greater than the patients true pH, he is at high risk for being intubated. Sensitivity is $\approx 80\%$.

 If a patient with a COPD exacerbation requires oxygen, it should be provided and not withheld for fear of causing $CO_2$ retention. If respiratory failure does ensue, it is caused by COPD and not by the physician who administered the oxygen.

**5.** Noninvasive positive pressure ventilation (eg, bilevel positive airway pressure) decreases rates of intubation, length of stay, and in-hospital mortality in patients with severe exacerbation.

**6.** Mucolytics, theophylline, and chest physiotherapy have no role in the treatment of COPD exacerbations.

## MAKING A DIAGNOSIS

 On the physical exam, Mrs. A appears well. Her vital signs are normal. The only findings on lung exam are decreased breath sounds and a prolonged expiratory phase. Her chest radiograph is normal. Some of the results of her PFTs are shown in Table 28–11.

Have you crossed a diagnostic threshold for the leading hypothesis, COPD? Have you ruled out the active alternatives? Do other tests need to be done to exclude the alternative diagnoses?

The patient's history and physical exam is certainly consistent with the diagnosis of COPD. She has a smoking history, persistent cough, and dyspnea. Her physical exam reveals findings of decreased breath sounds. The chest radiograph does not argue for another diagnosis.

Her PFTs are also supportive of the diagnosis. Most importantly, there is an irreversible decrease in airflow. The severity of disease is surprising given the patient's mild symptoms. The low DLCO (carbon monoxide diffusing capacity), suggests loss of a portion of the Hgb/air interface.

Asthma and HF, the alternative diagnoses, are very unlikely. The irreversibility of the airway disease excludes asthma as a potential cause. The lack of purulent sputum excludes bronchiectasis. HF remains a much less likely possibility not supported by the PFTs.

**Table 28–11.** Pulmonary function test results for Mrs. A.

| Test | Prebronchodilator | | Postbronchodilator | |
|---|---|---|---|---|
| | Result | % of Predicted | Result | % Change |
| Total lung capacity (L) | 6.92 | 128 | | |
| Forced vital capacity (L) | 3.03 | 91 | 2.90 | –4.0 |
| $FEV_1$ (L) | 1.03 | 43 | 1.00 | –4.0 |
| $FEV_1/FVC$ (%) | 34 | NA | 34 | 0 |
| DLCO (mL/min/mm Hg) | | 50 | | |

DLCO, carbon monoxide diffusing capacity of the lungs; $FEV_1/FVC$, forced expiratory volume in 1 second/forced vital capacity.

## Alternative Diagnosis: Bronchiectasis

### Textbook Presentation

Dyspnea and chronic, purulent sputum production are usually present in patients with bronchiectasis. There is usually a history of a chronic infection that has led to airway destruction.

### Disease Highlights

**A.** Chronic sputum production is the hallmark of the clinical presentation of bronchiectasis.

**B.** The disease is caused by the combination of an airway infection and an inability to clear this infection because of impaired immunity or anatomic abnormality (congenital or acquired). Bronchiectasis can be the result of common (viral infection) or rare (Kartagener syndrome) diseases.

  **1.** Pertussis and TB were the classic causes of bronchiectasis.

  **2.** Some of the common causes now are:

    **a.** Postviral, often with lymphadenopathy causing airway obstruction

    **b.** *Aspergillus fumigatus,* mainly in association with allergic bronchopulmonary aspergillosis

    **c.** *Mycobacterium avium* complex infection, usually causing middle lobe disease

    **d.** Cystic fibrosis

    **e.** HIV

**C.** The most common bacteria isolated from the sputum of people with bronchiectasis are *H influenzae, Pseudomonas aeruginosa,* and *Streptococcus pneumoniae.*

**D.** Complications of the disease include hemoptysis and rarely amyloidosis, given the chronic levels of inflammation.

### Evidence-Based Diagnosis

**A.** The diagnosis of bronchiectasis depends on recognizing the clinical symptoms (chronic sputum production) and demonstrating airway destruction, usually by high-resolution CT scanning.

**B.** Symptoms and their prevalence

  **1.** Dyspnea and wheezing, 75%

  **2.** Pleuritic chest pain, 50%

**C.** Signs and their prevalence

  **1.** Crackles, 70%

  **2.** Wheezing, 34%

**D.** Differentiation of bronchiectasis from COPD can sometimes be difficult because both may present with cough, sputum production, dyspnea, and airflow limitation. Important points in the differentiation are as follows:

  **1.** Sputum production is heavy and chronic in bronchiectasis, while it is only truly purulent in COPD during exacerbations.

  **2.** There is usually a smoking history associated with COPD.

  **3.** Spirometry is not helpful since bronchiectasis can cause both airflow limitation and airway hyperreactivity.

  **4.** Imaging (CT scan) will show diagnostic airway changes in bronchiectasis. In COPD, imaging may or may not demonstrate parenchymal destruction.

### Treatment

**A.** Antibiotics are used both to treat flares of disease and to suppress chronic infection.

**B.** Pulmonary hygiene

  **1.** Chest physiotherapy

  **2.** There may be a role for bronchodilators, mucolytics, and antiinflammatory medication.

**C.** Surgery is mainly used to treat airway obstruction, to remove destroyed and chronically infected lung tissue, and to treat life-threatening hemoptysis.

## CASE RESOLUTION

Given the minor role that sputum production plays in Mrs. A's disease, the diagnosis of COPD is nearly definite.

> 4
>
> Mrs. A is given a tiotropium inhaler, and she reports mild improvement in her symptoms. A month later, a long-acting β-agonist inhaler was added. This regimen produced better control of her symptoms. Four months later, she arrives at the emergency department with acute worsening of her symptoms at the time of an upper respiratory tract infection. She is admitted with an exacerbation of COPD.

## REFERENCES

Aaron SD, Vandemheen KL, Fergusson D et al. Tiotropium in combination with placebo, salmeterol, or fluticasone-salmeterol for treatment of chronic obstructive pulmonary disease: a randomized trial. Ann Intern Med. 2007;146(8):545–55.

Bach PB, Brown C, Gelfand SE, McCrory DC. Management of acute exacerbations of chronic obstructive pulmonary disease: a summary and appraisal of published evidence. Ann Intern Med. 2001;134:600–20.

Barker AF. Bronchiectasis. N Engl J Med. 2002;346:1383–93.

Bingham CO. An Overview of Angioedema. UpToDate, accessed 4/2008.

Bone RC, Pierce AK, Johnson RL Jr. Controlled oxygen administration in acute respiratory failure in chronic obstructive pulmonary disease: a reappraisal. Am J Med. 1978;65:896–902.

Calverley PM, Anderson JA, Celli B et al. Salmeterol and fluticasone propionate and survival in chronic obstructive pulmonary disease. N Engl J Med. 2007;356(8):775–89.

Christopher KL, Wood RP 2nd, Eckert RC, Blager FB, Raney RA, Souhrada JF. Vocal-cord dysfunction presenting as asthma. N Engl J Med. 1983;308:1566–70.

Corren J, Newman KB. Vocal cord dysfunction mimicking bronchial asthma. Postgrad Med. 1992;92:153–6.

Mahler DA, Harver A, Lentine T, Scott JA, Beck K, Schwartzstein RM. Descriptors of breathlessness in cardiorespiratory diseases. Am J Respir Crit Care Med. 1996;154:1357–63.

NIH/NHLBI. Guidelines for the Diagnosis and Management of Asthma. Bethesda, 1997:146.

Turcotte H, Langdeau JB, Bowie DM, Boulet LP. Are questionnaires on respiratory symptoms reliable predictors of airway hyperresponsiveness in athletes and sedentary subjects? J Asthma. 2003;40:71–80.

WHO/NHLBI. Global strategy for the diagnosis, management, and prevention of chronic obstructive pulmonary disease. 2001.

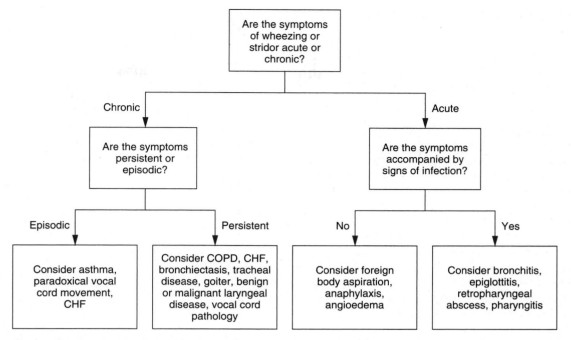

CHF, congestive heart failure; COPD, chronic obstructive pulmonary disease.

**Diagnostic Approach: Wheezing and Stridor**

# Index

Page numbers followed by italic *f* or *t* denote figures or tables, respectively.